WELLNESS

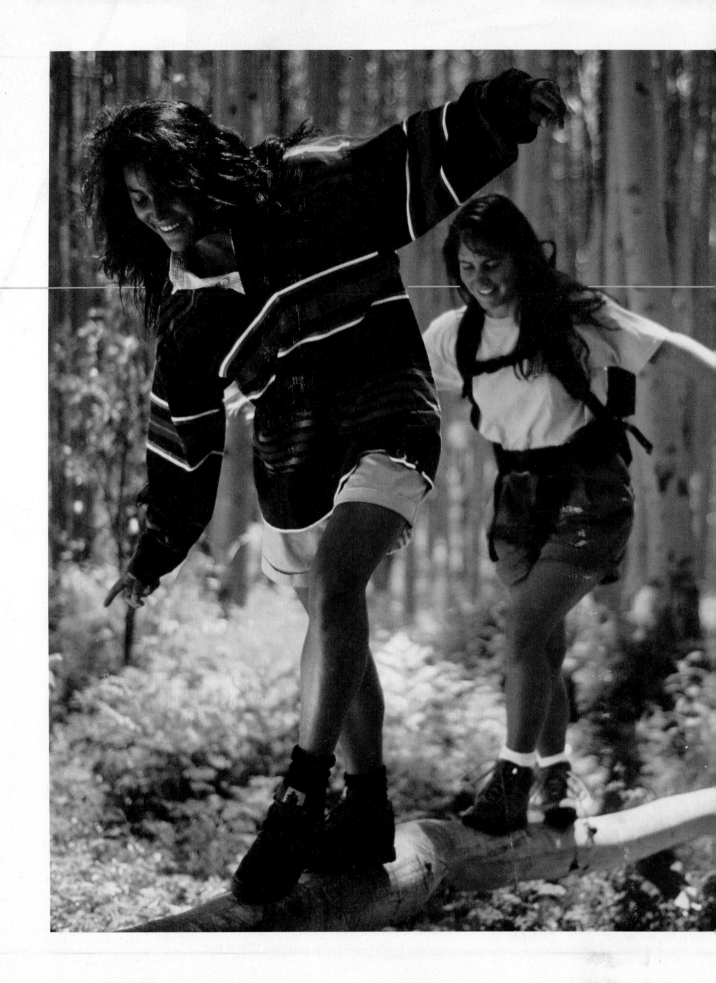

WELLNESS

GUIDELINES FOR A HEALTHY LIFESTYLE

THIRD EDITION

WERNER W.K. HOEGER
BOISE STATE UNIVERSITY

LORI W. TURNER
UNIVERSITY OF ARKANSAS

BRENT Q. HAFEN
BRIGHAM YOUNG UNIVERSITY

WADSWORTH

THOMSON LEARNING™

Australia • Canada • Mexico • Singapore
Spain • United Kingdom • United States

WADSWORTH

THOMSON LEARNING™

Publisher: Peter Marshall
Associate Editor: April Lemons
Assistant Editor: John Boyd
Editorial Assistant: Andrea Kesterke
Marketing Manager: Joanne Terhaar
Marketing Assistant: Justine Ferguson
Advertising Project Manager: Brian Chaffee
Project Manager: Sandra Craig

Print/Media Buyer: Tandra Jorgensen
Permissions Editor: Joohee Lee
Production and Composition: Ash Street Typecrafters, Inc.
Text and Cover Designer: Norman Baugher
Photo Researcher: Myrna Engler
Copy Editor: Carol Lombardi
Cover Images: Hikers: © Tony Stone Images; man spiking volleyball: © Tim
    Pannell/CORBIS; oranges: ©Joseph Sohm/ChromoSohm Inc./CORBIS
Printer: Transcontinental Printing

Printed in Canada

4   5   6   7   05

For permission to use material from this text, contact us by
Web: http://www.thomsonrights.com
Fax: 1-800-730-2215
Phone: 1-800-730-2214

Library of Congress Cataloging-in-Publication Data
Hoeger, Werner W. K.
    Wellness: guidelines for a healthy lifestyle / Werner W. K. Hoeger, Lori Turner, Brent Q. Hafen.—3rd ed.
        p. cm.
    Includes index.
    ISBN 0-534-58923-5
    1. Health. 2. Physical fitness. I. Turner, Lori Waite. II. Hafen, Brent Q.
        III. Title.

RA776 H6816 2001
613—dc21   2001024871

Wadsworth/Thomson Learning
10 Davis Drive
Belmont, CA 94002-3098
USA

For more information about our products, contact us:
Thomson Learning Academic Resource Center
1-800-423-0563
http://www.wadsworth.com

International Headquarters
Thomson Learning
International Division
290 Harbor Drive, 2nd Floor
Stamford, CT 06902-7477
USA

UK/Europe/Middle East/South Africa
Thomson Learning
Berkshire House
168-173 High Holborn
London WC1V 7AA
United Kingdom

Asia
Thomson Learning
60 Albert Street, #15-01
Albert Complex
Singapore 189969

Canada
Nelson Thomson Learning
1120 Birchmount Road
Toronto, Ontario M1K 5G4
Canada

*This book
is dedicated to Brent;
a mentor, colleague, and
friend; with my most
sincere wishes for the
best of health and
continued happiness
throughout life.*

WERNER

BRIEF CONTENTS

CONTENTS

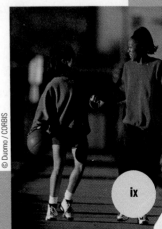
© Duomo / CORBIS

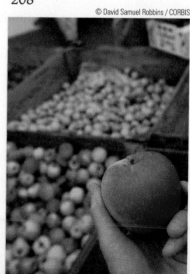

© David Samuel Robbins / CORBIS

C
O
N
T
E
N
T
S

© Ariel Skelly / CORBIS Stockmarket

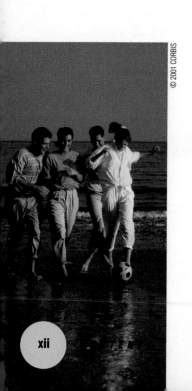

© 2001 CORBIS

PREFACE

THE RESPONSIBILITY FOR enhancing health and wellness and developing a healthy lifestyle rests primarily with the individual. According to research literature, improving happiness, quality of life, and longevity is a matter of personal choice. The purpose of *Wellness: Guidelines for a Healthy Lifestyle* book is not only to increase readers' understanding about health and wellness but also to help assess their own personal attitudes and behavior and, where necessary, to make appropriate changes. This book places a strong emphasis on fitness, because the scientific evidence has shown clearly that one of the most effective ways to enhance wellness and longevity is to increase one's level of physical activity and fitness. Self-responsibility is emphasized throughout the book, with the realization that enhancing wellness requires personal decision making and realistic goal setting, with positive and optimistic follow through.

Contemporary knowledge and ethical considerations suggest a broad approach to health behavior, involving the physical, social, emotional, mental, environmental, occupational, and spiritual natures and consequences. Our book explains, with support from the scientific literature, how each dimension contributes to wellness. In the pages that follow, you will learn what the research literature has to say about traditional wellness-related topics, as well as what we know about how emotions impact health and wellness. What is written here will help you appreciate what we know about the mind/body connection and the tremendous healing power of your mind.

CHANGES TO THE THIRD EDITION

- Chapter 1. The concept of healthy life expectancy, National Health Objectives for the year 2010, and occupational wellness as one of the essential dimensions of wellness have been added to this chapter.

- Chapter 2. This chapter now includes a section on perfectionism, traits of emotionally healthy people including a new table, warning signs of impending suicide and specific suggestions about how to help someone who is suffering from depression and contemplating suicide.

- Chapter 3. A new figure that conveys stressors common to college students, a revised discussion of the stress response and a new figure regarding the stress response ending in recovery or exhaustion are included in this chapter.

- Chapter 4. The contents of this chapter now include descriptions of 4 types of social support (instrumental, emotional, informational, and appraisal), an expanded section regarding ways to enhance your social support network, a new discussion regarding functional, healthy families with a table that describes traits of a healthy family.

- Chapter 5. Contents regarding health benefits of prayer and religious attendance and spirituality were updated citing several scientifically strong studies, the discussion on locus of control was expanded and focuses on health locus of control, a new section regarding contentment has been added, the concept of spiritual health has been expanded including a new table listing traits of spiritual health.

- Chapter 6. Information on world-wide health care costs and health care costs savings in the United States through wellness programs have been added to Chapter 6. A new equation to estimate maximal oxygen uptake (VO_{2max}) according to the 1.0-mile walk test now replaces the one previously used. The new equation was selected because research showed that the previous equation overestimated VO_{2max} in a college-aged population.

Chapter 7. The guidelines for exercise prescription have been updated to incorporate recent changes made by the American College of Sports Medicine (ACSM) in their position stand paper on *The Recommended Quantity and Quality of Exercise for Developing and Maintaining Cardiorespiratory and Muscular Fitness, and Flexibility in Healthy Adults*. The chapter also includes new sections with the ACSM guidelines on exercise and diabetes, specific exercise guidelines for strength-training workouts, the Transtheoretical Model of change (explains the stages of change as people attempt to modify behaviors), and an enhanced section on the prevention and treatment of low-back pain.

Chapter 8. Rewritten by a registered dietitian, this chapter has been revised extensively. Several new sections, tables, and figures have been added. Overnutrition and undernutrition were defined, a new section on food choices was added, a new figure that describes foods and the energy yielding nutrients in them with photos, a new figure with photos of vegetarian protein sources, a new figure on fats and calories with photos of foods with fat, then the same food with fat removed, information regarding sugar and honey, new information regarding sugar substitutes, a new section on the new dietary recommendations or dietary reference intakes (DRIs) and three tables of the new DRIs, a new table regarding strategies for selecting nutritious foods.

Chapter 9. Information on body composition compartments, a body mass index (BMI) table, and an introduction to the air displacement body composition technique were added to this chapter.

Chapter 10. This chapter now provides statistical updates on mortality rates based on body mass index and the ever-growing obesity epidemic in the United States. A new section on "The Diet Craze" that discusses myths and detrimental effects of popular diets on the market today has been added. The glycemic index, effects of high-intensity versus low-intensity exercise in weight loss, and additional tips on behavioral strategies for weight loss were also added to the chapter.

Chapter 11. Extensive revisions were made to the cardiovascular wellness chapter to incorporate advances in this area; including information on strokes, diabetes, homocysteine, treatment of elevated blood lipids, effects of soy foods on cardiovascular risk, and revised blood pressure classification guidelines. The chapter also includes the most recent statistical updates on cardiovascular diseases from the American Heart Association.

Chapter 12. All cancer statistics were updated in this chapter. The general guidelines for cancer prevention have been revised along with risk factors, prevention, and warning signals for many of the specific cancer sites. Risk factors and risk score interpretation were also been added for endometrial cancer in Assessment 12-1.

Chapter 13. This chapter now includes a discussion of physiological versus psychological addiction and two new figures that illustrate the differences, expanded information regarding why people consume alcohol including the influence of advertising, and to help with socialization, more discussion about better ways to develop social skills, expanded discussion of clustering of poor health behaviors such as alcohol abuse, tobacco use, other drug use, and other risk behaviors, the risk-taking personality, a new figure describing the fates of two drinkers (one can drink moderately with no problems, another drinker becomes an alcoholic), expanded discussion about blackouts and the hangover, a new table with a description of a typical 12-step program, strategies for refusing a drink successfully, and a new table with drug-free highs.

Chapter 14 has updated information related to statistics of new cases of STDs, signs and symptoms, and prevention. A new photo that shows genital warts on the female has been added.

ANCILLARIES

Instructor's Manual with Test Bank. The Instructor's Manual with Test Bank helps instructors plan and coordinate their lectures by offering detailed outlines of each chapter with specific transparency and PowerPoint references. Instructor's Activities are included for each chapter. These activities offer instructors ideas for incorporating the material into classroom activities and discussions. A set of Key Point Transparencies is provided. A full test bank containing approximately 30 questions per chapter is also provided.

Transparencies. Approximately 80 color transparency acetates of graphs, tables, and illustrations from the text can be used to enhance lectures. The transparencies will also be available on the Web and on a CD-ROM. Also provided is a set of Key Point Transparencies—text-only transparencies that list important terms from each chapter.

Profile Plus 2002. This interactive CD-ROM includes study guides, quizzes, lecture outlines, and digital video clips. The CD allows students to generate personalized fitness and wellness programs, conduct self-assessments, analyze their diets, and keep an exercise log.

Diet Analysis Plus 5.0 CD-ROM. This interactive nutrition learning tool allows students to create personal profiles and determine the nutritional value of their diet. The program calculates nutrition intakes, goal percentages, and actual percentages of nutrients, vitamins, and minerals, customized according to the student's profile. The information is displayed in colorful, easy-to-read graphs, charts, and spreadsheets.

ExamView ®—Computerized Testing. Create, deliver, and customize tests and study guides (both print and online) in minutes with this easy-to-use assessment and tutorial system. ExamView offers both a Quick Test Wizard and an Online Test Wizard that guide you step-by-step through the process of creating tests, while its unique "WYSIWYG" capability allows you to see the test you are creating on the screen exactly as it will print or display online.

Multimedia Manager for Health, Fitness, and Wellness: A Microsoft PowerPoint® Link Tool. More than 70 PowerPoint® slides. This Link Tool also includes images and PowerPoint slides from other Wadsworth Health, Fitness, and Wellness texts, and digital videos.

CNN Today: Fitness and Wellness Video. Launch your lectures with riveting footage from CNN, the world's leading 24-hour global news television network. The CNN Today: Fitness and Wellness Video allows you to integrate the news gathering and programming power of CNN into the classroom to show students the relevance of course topics to

their everyday lives. Organized by topics introduced in the text, the clips are presented in short 2–5 minute segments, and a new video is available each year.

Relaxation Video. Explores techniques to decrease vulnerability to stress, enhance sports performance, and manage time more effectively.

Wadsworth Video Library for Fitness, Wellness, and Personal Health. A comprehensive library of videos is available to adopters of this textbook. Topics include weight control and fitness, AIDS, sexual communication, peer pressure, compulsive and addictive behaviors and the relationship between alcohol and violence. Contact your local Wadsworth/Thomson Learning representative for a detailed list of video options.

Personal Daily Log. This log contains an exercise pyramid, ethnic foods pyramid, tips for achieving test success, a body composition record form, body mass index chart, cardiorespiratory exercise record forms, strength training record forms, and much more.

Wellness Worksheets. Forty detachable self-assessments and a complete wellness inventory are included.

Trigger Video Series. Exclusive to Wadsworth/Thomson Learning! This video is designed to promote classroom discussion on a variety of important topics related to physical fitness and stress. Each 60-minute video contains five 8–10 minute clips, followed by questions for answer or discussion and material appropriate to the chapters in this text.

InfoTrac® College Edition. This extensive online library gives professors and students access to the latest news and research articles online—updated daily and spanning four years! Conveniently accessible from students' own computers or the campus library, InfoTrac College Edition opens the door to the full text of articles from hundreds of scholarly and popular journals and publications.

The Wadsworth Health & Wellness Resource Center Web Site:

http://health.wadsworth.com

When you adopt *Wellness: Guidelines for a Healthy Lifestyle*, you and your students will have access to a rich array of teaching and learning resources you won't find anywhere else. This outstanding site features both student and instructor resources for this text, including self-quizzes, Web links, suggested online readings, and discussion forums for students—as well as downloadable supplementary resources, PowerPoint® presentations, and more for instructors.

- **Thomson Learning WebTutor™.** Available on WebCT or Blackboard! This content-rich, Web-based teaching and learning tool is rich with study and mastery tools, communication tools, and course content. WebTutor is filled with pre-loaded content and is ready to use as soon as you and your students log on. At the same time, you can customize the content in any way you choose, from uploading images and other resources, to adding Web links, to creating your own practice materials.

ACKNOWLEDGMENTS

We would like to thank the reviewers for their valuable comments and contributions to the Third Edition.

Stephanie Agosta, Ohio University, Lancaster
Kenneth Cameron, United States Military Academy
Richard Fopeano, Rowan University
Lisa Hicks, University of Indianapolis
Ressa Welch, Elon College

We would like to thank the following graduate students from the University of Arkansas for serving as reviewers for selected chapters: Michael Anders, Daniel Bercher, Jeanne Bleeker, Kimberly Bodey, Mary Hawkins, Rebecca Ludwig, Joel Rush, Donald Simpson, Mary Wyandt, and Martha Pickett. Special thanks is also given to Jeanne Bleeker for her valuable research assistance.

1 INTRODUCTION TO WELLNESS

OBJECTIVES

- Identify five of the leading health problems in the United States.
- Identify the characteristics of wellness.
- Identify and describe the dimensions of wellness.
- Identify six risk factors that compromise wellness.
- List the three main goals of the Year 2010 National Health Objectives.
- Discuss at least four things you can do as part of a personalized approach to health and wellness.

1

THE SILVERED BULB of a thermometer is poked under a tongue, and the mercury inches its way along a measured scale. The cold metal of the stethoscope probes for a faintly distinguishable rhythm. A drop of crimson blood is smeared beneath the powerful gaze of a microscope. Using medical tools such as these, we can distinguish between health and disease. Or is it that easy? In reality, health and wellness are not easy to define. Clutching at an elusive definition, the World Health Organization earmarks health as "a state of complete physical, mental, and social well-being, and not merely the absence of disease or infirmity." The key word in that definition is possibly "well-being," and true health may actually be a condition in which we are able to avoid illness, even if we are predisposed to it.

At the beginning of the 20th century, the most common health problems in the United States were infectious diseases such as influenza, diphtheria, polio, and tuberculosis. Scientific advances enabled us to wipe out many of those diseases or, at the least, to reduce dramatically the deaths they caused. Those same scientific advances, however, also heralded an age of convenience characterized by a sedentary lifestyle, more alcohol consumption, and a diet permeated by fats and sugars. The result was America's new health problem, **chronic diseases**, such as heart disease, cancer, diabetes, emphysema, and cirrhosis of the liver.

The focus at the turn of the 20th century was treatment. Researchers confronted with infectious diseases searched for a cure and often met with success. Our focus at the beginning of the 21st century, however, must be on prevention. The health problems that face the population are, in large measure, the result of lifestyle decisions. Emphatic statements released year after year by the U.S. Surgeon General's Office point out that the leading causes of premature death and illness in the United States could be prevented through positive lifestyle habits. The solution to those health problems, then, is largely within our control.

Until recently the American health care system has not addressed prevention. It has been, instead, a sickness-care system. Over $1.035 trillion—more than a fourteenth of the gross national product—is spent on the nation's health care, encompassing hospitals, doctors, health maintenance organizations, pharmaceuticals, and other related companies.

According to the World Health Organization (WHO) figures, the United States spends more per capita ($3,724 per year) on health care than any other country in the world (see Figure 1.1), yet, overall, the health care system ranks only 37th in the world. People in Japan, who spend one-half of what the United States does per person on health care, outlive us by an average of 5 years.

One of the fundamental reasons for this country's low overall ranking is the overemphasis on state-of-the-art cures instead of prevention programs. The United States is the best place in the world to treat someone once they are sick, but the system does a poor job of keeping people healthy in the first place. The U.S. system also fails to provide good health care for all: Forty-four million residents do not have health insurance.

Further, Americans have a higher age-adjusted mortality rate than most industrialized nations. The current U.S. **life expectancy** averages 77 years (73 for men and 80 for women). For the first time, however, in the year 2000, the World Health Organization also calculated **healthy life expectancy** (HLE) estimates for 191 nations. The U.S. ranked 24th in this report with a HLE of 70 years. Japan was first with a HLE of 74.5 years (see Figure 1.2).

The U.S. ranking was a major surprise, given its status as a developed country with one of the best

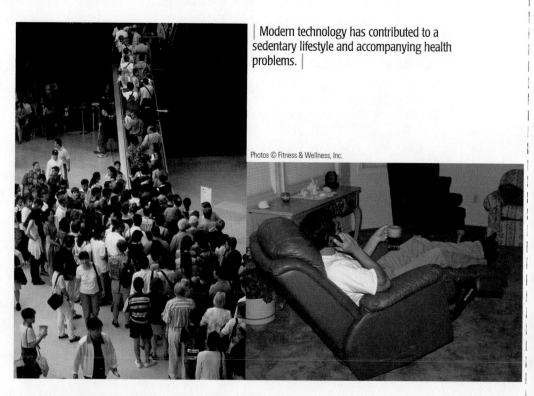

| Modern technology has contributed to a sedentary lifestyle and accompanying health problems. |

Photos © Fitness & Wellness, Inc.

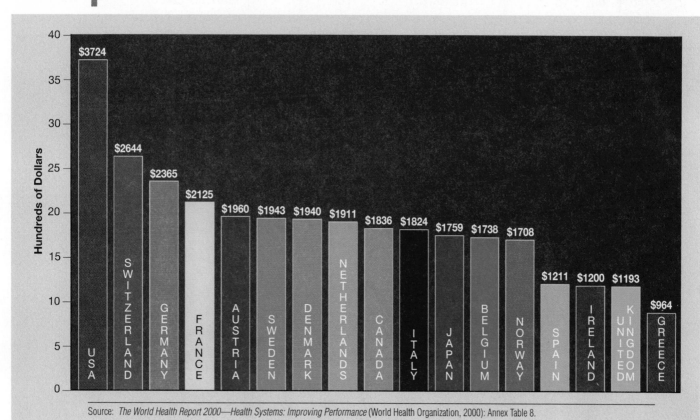

Source: *The World Health Report 2000—Health Systems: Improving Performance* (World Health Organization, 2000): Annex Table 8.

medical care systems in the world. The rating indicates that Americans die earlier and spend more time disabled than people in most other advanced countries. The World Health Organization points to several factors that may account for this unexpected finding:

1. The extremely poor health of some groups such as Native Americans, rural African Americans, and the inner-city poor. Their health status is more characteristic of poor developing nations rather than a rich industrialized country.
2. The HIV epidemic, which causes more deaths and disability than in other developed nations.
3. The high incidence of tobacco use.
4. A high incidence of coronary heart disease.
5. Fairly high levels of violence, notably homicides, as compared with other developed countries.

Further, of 20 countries that researchers at Northwestern University Medical School in Chicago studied, the typical American diet was highest of all in the percentage of fat. Only a few nations ranked higher in the amount of artery-clogging cholesterol consumed. The typical American diet also is the lowest in dietary fiber. As a result, the United States is one of the fattest nations in

the world. Approximately two-thirds of middle-aged U.S. men are overweight, compared with only 3 percent of the middle-aged men in Japan.

As if that isn't enough, the United States has the highest rate of heart disease of all developed nations. The country also has some of the highest rates in the world of cancer of the colon, rectum, breast, and lung.

Considering how much the nation spends on medical care, it should outshine the world in health and wellness, but it doesn't, because it has failed to make prevention a top priority. Critical to a focus on prevention, say health care experts, is a change in attitude by patients and health care providers alike. Patients have to stop demanding medication for every ailment and hospitalization or surgery for every illness. In turn, physicians have to be more conservative in their approach to disease. According to Joseph A. Califano, former Secretary of

Chronic diseases Illnesses that linger over time and may get progressively worse.

Life expectancy Number of years a person is expected to live based on the person's birth year.

Healthy life expectancy (HLE) Number of years a person is expected to live in good health. This number is obtained by subtracting ill-health years from the overall life expectancy.

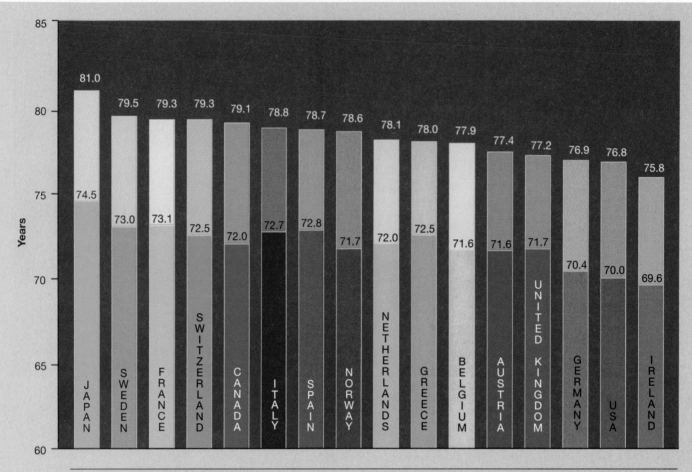

Source: World Health Organization, http://www.who.int/inf-pr-2000/en/pr2000-life.html. Retrieved June 4, 2000.

Health, Education and Welfare, America's doctors need to be "more skeptical in resorting to surgery and less promiscuous in dispensing pills."

> You, the individual, can do more for your health and well-being than any doctor, any hospital, any drug, any exotic medical device.
>
> —Joseph A. Califano (former Secretary of Health, Education, and Welfare)

The problem, in essence, lies with us, not with the medical establishment. Of all the people who die in the United States every year, only about 10 percent die because of inadequate health care, and approximately 20 percent die because of environmental or biological factors. The rest die as the direct result of an unhealthy lifestyle (see Figure 1.3).

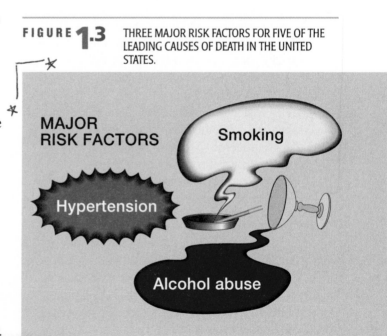

MAJOR RISK FACTORS

Smoking

Hypertension

Alcohol abuse

LEADING HEALTH PROBLEMS IN THE UNITED STATES

According to the U.S. Surgeon General, about 83 percent of all deaths before age 65 in the United States could have been prevented. Almost half of all deaths among people of all ages is attributable to lifestyle factors. An additional 16 percent is caused by environmental factors. More than half of all disease is what researchers call "self-controlled"; that is, we can influence it through lifestyle changes and other preventive methods.

At the beginning of this century, almost one-third of all deaths in the United States resulted from tuberculosis, influenza, and pneumonia. Millions died of influenza in a 1918 epidemic. Fewer than 5 percent died from cancer, and only about 10 percent died of cardiovascular disease. Today, virtually no one dies of tuberculosis. Less than 5 percent die from influenza and pneumonia. Nearly 64 percent of all deaths in the United States are caused by cardiovascular disease and cancer[1] (see Figure 1.4). Close to 80 percent of those deaths could have been prevented by making lifestyle changes—things as basic as eating a diet lower in fat, getting regular exercise, and quitting smoking.

John Crawley

| Health and wellness include physical, mental, emotional, social, environmental, occupational, and spiritual dimensions. |

FIGURE 1.4 LEADING CAUSES OF DEATH IN THE UNITED STATES, 1900 AND 1997.

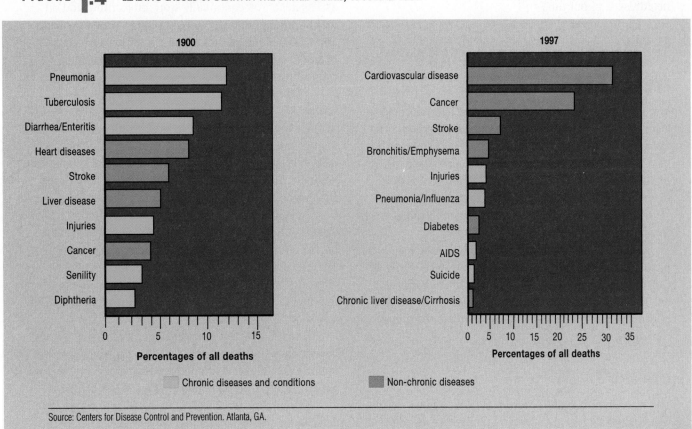

Source: Centers for Disease Control and Prevention. Atlanta, GA.

The other top two causes of death—bronchitis/emphysema, called chronic obstructive pulmonary disease (COPD), and injuries—also are largely preventable. Most COPD cases are caused by cigarette smoking. Many fatal accidents are the result of alcohol abuse, drug abuse, or failure to use seatbelts. And, though our modern-day "epidemic," AIDS, cannot be cured, it can be prevented by lifestyle choices.

According to the American Council on Science and Health, four of the five leading causes of death are related directly to cigarette smoking. Smoking is responsible for an estimated 30 percent of all cancer deaths, 30 percent of all heart disease fatalities, and 83 percent of all deaths from chronic bronchitis and emphysema. It also is an "unquantifiable risk factor" for cerebrovascular disease.

The council has also stated that infant and fetal mortality can be reduced substantially by reducing cigarette smoking. Smoking is responsible for higher rates of spontaneous abortion and stillbirth and accounts for up to 14 percent of all premature births in the United States.

The official position of the World Health Organization on smoking is clear: "The control of cigarette smoking could do more to improve health and prolong life in developed countries than any other single action in the whole field of preventive medicine."[2] And, according to former U.S. Surgeon General C. Everett Koop, cigarette smoking is the number-one preventable cause of death and disease in the United States and the most important health issue of our time.[3]

WHAT ARE HEALTH AND WELLNESS?

More than five decades ago, health care education pioneer Jesse Williams proclaimed that health is a condition that allows one to do the most constructive work, render the best possible service to the world, and experience the highest possible enjoyment of life. "Health as freedom from disease is a standard of mediocrity," he wrote. "Health as a quality of life is a standard of inspiration and increasing achievements."[4]

Williams was ahead of his time. Most Americans have taken decades to catch on to his vision. A series of Gallup polls finally hinted at his much broader scope of health and wellness. In increasing numbers, Americans now are defining health as the energy to do the things we care about.

| Health |

The word **health** is derived from the Old English "hal," which means whole. Researchers on the cutting edge

consider health to be a continuum, a perpetual but ever-changing balance of the various dimensions that make us whole.

Everything with which you interact—the place you live, the air you breathe, the food you eat, the job you have, the people you associate with—affects your position on the health continuum. The same series of Gallup polls shows that Americans are beginning to understand the influence of these interactive factors. When ranking their health priorities, their top concern was staying free of disease, but the third highest was living in an environment with clean air and water.

| Wellness |

Wellness combines seven dimensions of well-being into a quality way of living. It is the ability to live life to the fullest, to have a zest for life, to maximize personal potential in a variety of ways. Illness and health are opposite states, but you can be ill and still enjoy wellness if you have a purpose in life, a deep appreciation for living, a sense of joy.

People who are bound by the strictures of traditionally defined physical health wait until some disease has crept up on them, then consult a professional to evaluate their condition and prescribe treatment. Simply put, they turn over their physical health to someone else. Wellness, on the other hand, places responsibility on the individual. Wellness becomes a matter of self-evaluation and self-assessment. You continually work on learning and on making changes that will enhance your state of wellness. You take the reins. Rather than delegating your physical health to someone else, you make a deep personal commitment to wellness.

Whereas physical health is a fairly simple concept, wellness is multifaceted and involves much more than simple physical condition. Physical health is not available to everyone. On the other hand, everyone can enjoy wellness—despite physical limitations, disease, and handicap. Wellness fully integrates its seven dimensions (see the Dimensions of Wellness, page 7) in a complex interaction that leads to a quality life. It is not something that is "achieved" once and stays with you thereafter; it is a horizon that we move toward throughout life. We move along a continuum, and the important factor is the direction in which we are moving. Finally, wellness affects not only the individual but also can encompass the family and society as a whole.

If we are to accept a definition of wellness that goes beyond mere freedom from disease, we also must accept a notion that calls for a dramatic change in the way we deal with health. For centuries our emphasis has been on identifying bacteria, classifying viruses, and waging a determined war on devastating diseases. We have

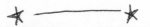

FIGURE 1.5   THE DIMENSIONS OF WELLNESS.

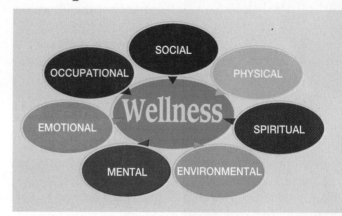

| PHYSICAL | **Physical wellness** is the kind most commonly associated with being healthy. A person who is physically well eats a well-balanced diet, gets plenty of physical activity and exercise, maintains proper weight, gets enough sleep, avoids risky sexual behavior, tries to limit exposure to environmental contaminants, and restricts intake of harmful substances such as alcohol, tobacco, caffeine, and drugs. Physical wellness is characterized by good cardiorespiratory endurance, muscular strength and flexibility, proper body composition, and the ability to carry out daily tasks.

To remain well requires that you take steps to protect your physical health: regularly do self-exams and get thorough physical examinations, including appropriate screening tests, from a physician. It also involves taking effective measures if you do become sick, such as seeking medical care and using medications conservatively.

Physical wellness entails confidence and optimism about one's ability to take care of health problems. These conditions need not prevent one from enjoying life. Physical wellness brings with it a remarkable resistance to disease. The right combination of nutrition, exercise, and sleep renders healthy people capable of resisting the common colds and influenza that wipe out others.

People who enjoy physical wellness are intelligent about their health. When they do develop an unusual or irritating symptom, they do what is necessary to relieve it. If symptoms persist, they check with a doctor.

Irrespective of whether healthy individuals are muscular, they usually are physically powerful. Exercise attunes their muscles and

concentrated on treatment. If we are to redefine health to reflect a condition of wellness, however, we also must redefine the ultimate goal of our health efforts: to prevent disease. Inherent in that challenge is the recognition that behavior plays a key role in the development of disease and also in our ability to resist disease and maintain optimum health.

Embodied in the definition of wellness and behavioral health is a philosophy calling for consideration of the whole person, not a fractionalization into separate parts. We need to consider ourselves as we interact in our environment, not as separate complaints or body parts in a sterile laboratory or in the unnatural environs of a physician's examining room. It stresses a conscious and active commitment by the individual, who understands that optimum health is *not* something that just happens. Most significantly, it calls for concentration on the factors that precede illness instead of concern solely with the anatomy of disease once it strikes.

| The Dimensions of Wellness |

Writing in *The History and Future of Wellness*, author Donald Ardell points out that living by the principles of wellness is considered a richer way to be alive.[5] Optimum wellness balances seven basic dimensions: physical, mental, emotional, social, environmental, occupational, and spiritual. These are depicted in Figure 1.5.

Health A state of complete well-being and not just the absence of disease or infirmity.

Wellness Full integration of physical, mental, emotional, social, environmental, occupational, and spiritual well-being into a quality life.

Physical wellness Flexibility, endurance, strength, and optimism about your ability to take care of health problems.

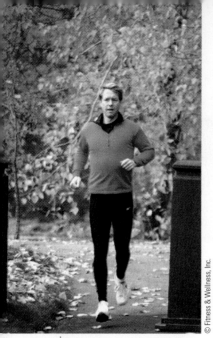

A person who is physically well gets regular exercise.

endows them with a high level of physical coordination and self-confidence. Instead of shying away from physical challenge, they accept it with enthusiasm, confident they can make their body work for them. Reaction time is good, strength is obvious, and endurance is high.

People characterized by physical wellness have an active lifestyle. They like to be outdoors. They enjoy a fast-paced bicycle ride along a roadside choked with apple blossoms or a vigorous game of touch football on a crisp autumn afternoon. They have the energy they need to do the things they enjoy, as well as the energy they need to complete demanding tasks at work, breeze through final exams without feeling exhausted, or clear out all the debris from last year's vegetable garden.

People who are physically well respect and like their own body. They have a natural grace and ease. You can see their health in the way they move. Beauty in the traditional sense of the word has little to do with it. People with physical wellness make the most of their body, and they delight in it.

| MENTAL | Just as the physical dimension of wellness embodies much more than the mere absence of disease, so, too, **mental wellness** is characterized by signs of wellness. Pioneers in the field of psychoneuroimmunology are proving scientifically what philosophers such as Homer, Plato, and Aristotle speculated more than 5,000 years ago: The mind has a striking influence on the body (and, therefore, on health and wellness).

Education shouldn't stop with commencement exercises. A sound mental dimension of wellness involves unbridled curiosity and ongoing learning. This dimension of wellness implies that you can apply the things you have learned (whether at home or on the job), that you create opportunities to learn more, and that you engage your mind in lively interaction with the world around you.

People who are mentally well can think clearly, are quick to pick up new concepts, and catch on rapidly to new ideas. Instead of being intimidated by facts and figures with which they are unfamiliar, they embrace the chance to learn something new. Their confidence and enthusiasm enable them to approach any learning situation with eagerness that leads to success.

Mental wellness breeds creativity. In contrast to people who seem burdened with the task of getting a job done, mentally well people are able to approach the same task in a new way. They don't seem restricted by what they always have done before. They are willing to tackle the chore from a different angle, one that lets them exercise creativity and initiative.

Logic is a basic attribute of mental wellness. People who are confronted suddenly with an unfamiliar situation tend to experience mild panic. Mental wellness brings with it common sense and logic that enable those who are mentally well to reason their way through.

A genuine sense of curiosity leads mentally well people into a world that is always new and challenging. Whereas others accept what life has to offer with quiet resolve, mentally well people grasp each aspect of life with a desire to understand. They are the people who know why the surface of a lake is so blue, how a newspaper is printed, how a robin can tell that spring has arrived. They know the answers because they ask the questions. Some people pass a flowering hedge and notice that it is beautiful. Healthier people want to know why the blooms are pink, what kind of hedge it is, how they can grow one like it.

Along with alertness and brightness, mental wellness brings with it stimulation and capability. Mentally well people have a good memory and use it to their greatest advantage. They are skilled in their chosen area of expertise, and they are open to new ideas and suggestions. They relish the chance to improve themselves and to learn something new.

Mental wellness brings with it vision and promise. More than anything else, mentally well people are open-minded and accepting of others. Instead of being

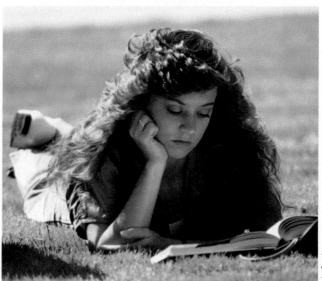

Mental wellness involves curiosity and ongoing learning.

threatened by those who are different from themselves, they show respect and curiosity without feeling they have to conform. They are faithful to their own ideas and philosophies and allow others the same privilege. Their self-confidence guarantees that they can take their place in the world without giving up part of themselves and without requiring others to do the same.

EMOTIONAL Emotions involve both the mind and the body, and, as a result, they can bridge the gap between the two. Emotions are a contributing factor in a number of diseases, such as rheumatoid arthritis, bronchial asthma, peptic ulcer, ulcerative colitis, hypertension, and dermatitis.

What constitutes **emotional wellness**? Foremost is probably the ability to understand your own feelings, to accept your limitations, and to achieve emotional stability. It also involves being comfortable with your emotions. Understanding and accepting your own feelings helps you understand and accept the emotions of others, which leads to the ability to maintain intimate relationships with other people. Emotional wellness also implies the ability to express emotions appropriately, adjust to change, cope with stress in a healthy way, and enjoy life despite its occasional disappointments and frustrations.

The hallmark of emotional wellness is a deep and abiding happiness—not a happiness that depends on some frail set of circumstances but, rather, a happiness that stems from a powerful inner contentment. Instead of being dependent on a certain income or status in life, the happiness that signals real wellness is an emotional anchor that gives meaning and joy to life.

In the Declaration of Independence, Thomas Jefferson promised three things to all Americans: the rights to life, liberty, and the pursuit of happiness. He did not promise happiness itself, because he knew that the government could not deliver it. Happiness is not a fleeting emotion tied to a single event, but a long-term state of mind that permeates the various facets of life and influences our outlook. We can experience true happiness and temporary unhappiness at the same time. Happiness may seem to vanish temporarily, giving way to bursts of depression or disappointment, but it returns. As Harry Emerson Fosdick stated:

> One who expects to completely escape low moods is asking the impossible. Like the weather, life is essentially variable, and a healthy person believes in the validity of his high hours even when he is having a low one.[6]

No one has ever come up with a simple recipe for producing happiness, but researchers agree that certain ingredients seem universal among those who have the kind of true, abiding happiness characteristic of emotional

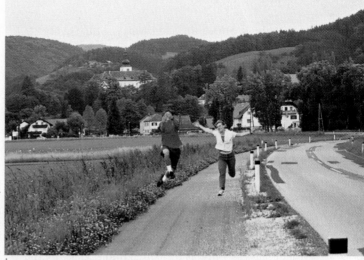

Emotionally well people enjoy friends, play, and leisure time; and they laugh often.

wellness. Those who are happy usually are part of a family. They are partners, parents, or children. They love others, and they feel loved themselves. Healthy, happy people enjoy friends, work hard at something fulfilling, get plenty of exercise, and enjoy play and leisure time. They know how to laugh, and they laugh often. They give of themselves freely to others and seem to have found deep meaning to life.

> Happiness is a long-term state of mind that permeates the various facets of life and influences our outlook.

An attitude of true happiness signals freedom from the tension and depression that many people endure. Emotional wellness is obviously subject to the same kinds of depression and unhappiness that plague all of us once in a while, but the difference lies in the ability to bounce back. Well people take minor setbacks in stride and have the notable ability to enjoy life despite it all. When something unhappy happens, they put it behind them. They don't waste energy or time recounting the situation, wondering how they could have changed it, or dwelling on the past.

The spirit of optimism basic to healthy, happy individuals enables them to focus their energy on the present. They recognize that the past can hold powerful lessons, but they do not let it control the here and now.

In addition to avoiding the pitfalls of the past, they avoid the temptation to pin all their hopes and dreams on the future. They are goal-oriented

Mental wellness A state in which your mind is engaged in lively interaction with the world around you.

Emotional wellness The ability to understand your own feelings, accept your limitations, and achieve emotional stability.

and ambitious, and at the same time are able to enjoy themselves today. They aren't waiting until they graduate from college, until they get married, until they pay off their home, or until they are the president of a company. Instead, they are happy today in the circumstances they are in. They may aspire to graduate with honors, marry their sweetheart, pay off the mortgage, or gain the top spot at the firm, but they are happy regardless. They know that happiness is not the product of a particular thing, but instead is a condition.

Part and parcel of happiness is acceptance of self. Healthy people value themselves as having something to contribute and being worthwhile. Healthy people enjoy a sense of success—not as measured traditionally by the world but as measured against their own standards. They know what is important to them, and they are confident they can achieve it. They are in touch with self to the point that they have a clear definition of their own needs.

Emotional wellness brings with it a certain stability, an ability to look both success and failure squarely in the face and to keep moving along a predetermined course. When success is evident, the emotionally well person radiates the expected joy and confidence. When failure seems evident, the emotionally well person responds by making the best of circumstances and moving beyond the failure. Wellness enables us to learn from failure, identify ways to avoid it in the future, and then go on with the business at hand.

Emotional wellness also embodies the ability to get in touch with your own feelings. Because healthy people have a good self-image, they do not worry about showing their feelings or sharing them with others. They are not concerned with what others think of them. They do not feel the need to prove themselves to others, nor do they feel they have to force others to accept their point of view. They quietly, peacefully accept themselves and are able to move freely beyond that to accept others.

Sensitive, yet independent, emotionally well people accept themselves to an extent that they are extremely insightful about themselves and others. Emotional wellness brings with it a necessary frame of mind that allows involvement with other people. A truly healthy person is one who enjoys others and who is not threatened by what other people might do or say.

Emotional wellness also brings with it a maturity that allows the individual to forgive others. Emotionally well people accept responsibility for their own happiness instead of blaming others when they are unhappy. They are free from anger and resentment because they recognize that anger is almost always destructive. By accepting responsibility for their own emotional well-being, they free themselves to achieve it.

More than dictating happiness and optimism, emotions play a profound part in physical health and avoiding disease. Biobehavioralist Norman Cousins maintained that what you think, what you believe, and how you react to experiences can impair or aid the workings of the body's immune system.

Studies of terminally ill cancer patients reveal that those who survive have one characteristic in common: their utter refusal to give up hope. Cousins said:

> Nothing is more wondrous about the fifteen billion neurons in the human brain than their ability to convert thoughts, hopes, ideas, and attitudes into chemical substances. Every emotion, negative or positive, makes its registrations on the body's systems. . . . The most important thing I have learned about the power of belief is that an individual patient's attitude toward serious illness can be as important as medical help. It would be a serious mistake to bypass or minimize the need for scientific treatment, but that treatment will be far more

A good sense of humor is an important part of wellness.

TEN QUALITIES OF WELLNESS

1. Deeply committed to a cause outside oneself.
2. Physically able to do whatever one wants with intensity and great energy; seldom sick.
3. Caring and loving; a person others can lean on in a crisis.
4. In tune with the spiritual, having a clear sense of purpose and direction.
5. Intellectually sharp, able to handle information, possessing an ever-curious mind and a good sense of humor.
6. Well organized and able to accomplish plenty of work.
7. Able to live in and enjoy the present rather than focusing on the past or looking toward the future.
8. Comfortable with experiencing the full range of human emotions.
9. Accepting of one's limitations, handicaps, and mistakes.
10. Able and willing to take charge of one's life, to practice positive self-care, and to be assertive when necessary.

effective if people put their creative hopes, their faith, and their confidence fully to work in behalf of their recovery.[7]

Harvard-trained surgeon Bernie Siegel, who has spent his medical career working with cancer victims, remarked:

> I can say from my own experience that patients who have given up, who have come to me feeling defeated and desperate, feeling that nothing can possibly help them, have often made their own predictions come true. The fighter-type patients who are willing to try anything that has a chance to help them, who have real faith in their survival, always do better.[8]

| SOCIAL | **Social wellness**, with its accompanying self-image, endows us with the ease and confidence to be outgoing, friendly, and affectionate toward others. Social wellness involves not only a concern for the individual, but also an interest in humanity and the environment as a whole.

One of the hallmarks of social wellness is the ability to relate to others, to reach out to other people, both within the family unit and outside it. Healthy people are honest and loyal. Their own balance and sense of self allow them to extend respect and tolerance to others. They are confident of themselves and don't feel threatened by opening up to others.

People who are socially healthy are able to develop and maintain intimacy but are not promiscuous. They

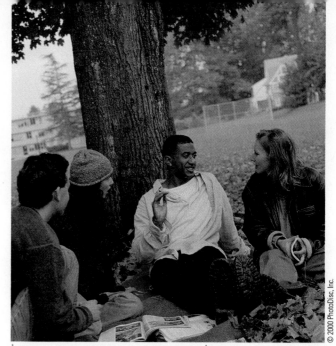

Group activities enhance social wellness.

organize themselves in family groups and are loyal and faithful to family members. They are trustworthy and loyal to those outside the family unit and have the ability to make and keep friends. They treat others with fairness and respect.

Social wellness goes hand in hand with social graces. Socially healthy people are affectionate, polite, and helpful toward others; can handle conflict without exploding; and are true to their ideals and beliefs while allowing others to be true to theirs. They do not interpret a difference of opinion as the basis for destruction. Instead, they are tolerant, respectful, and secure. They can say "no" when they should and are sensitive in responding to others' needs without sacrificing their own.

Socially well people love themselves. This is not a vain, self-centered kind of love that causes them to develop an overinflated image of themselves. Instead, it is the kind of love that enables individuals to feel secure enough, confident enough, and good enough about them-selves to reach out to others. Before you can love others, you must be able to love yourself.

The socially well person relishes touch, especially hugging, as a vital, irreplaceable means of communicating caring and concern for others. Long-term research by experts in a variety of disciplines has confirmed that touch is critical to well-being. San Diego psychologist James Hardison wrote:

> It is through touching that we are able to fulfill a large share of our human needs and, in doing so, to attain happiness. By touching someone, we can

Social wellness The ability to relate well to others, both within and outside the family unit.

BENEFITS OF WELLNESS

Wellness provides benefits not only to the physical body but to the "soul" as well. Achieving a high level of wellness helps you

- Delay the aging process.
- Reduce your risk of chronic illness.
- Be self-confident.
- Boost your muscle strength, endurance, and flexibility.
- Identify and meet your needs.
- Function better.
- Increase your energy.
- Do better at school, on the job, and in everyday living.
- Maintain optimism and hope.
- Get good nutrition.
- Look better.
- Stay stimulated intellectually.
- Bounce back faster after illness or injury.
- Raise your level of cardiovascular health.
- Look at problems as challenges, not stumbling blocks.

affirm our friendship or approval, communicate important messages, promote health, and bring about love.[9]

Unfortunately, Hardison continues, too many people put up barriers to the language of touch, equating touching "with either sex or violence. Consequently many people avoid the simple acts of touching—pats on the back, heartfelt handshakes, cordial hugs—that affirm goodwill."

Socially well people—whether at home, in the classroom, or at work—develop a spirit of teamwork with those around them. They do not view others with suspicion, jealousy, or contempt. They find no satisfaction in the thought of outdoing, putting down, or getting ahead of others. They find great joy in cooperation, mutual support, and working together to accomplish something of lasting value for all.

> Socially well people develop a spirit of teamwork.

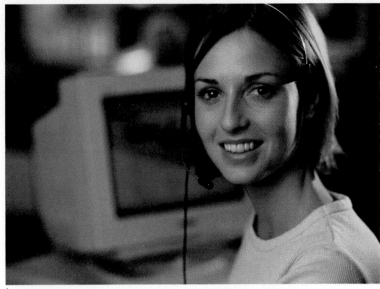

Occupational wellness occurs when a job provides important personal rewards.

OCCUPATIONAL Some models also include a sixth dimension of wellness: **occupational wellness**. Occupational wellness is not tied to high salary, prestigious position, or extravagant working conditions. Any job can bring occupational wellness if it provides rewards that are important to the individual. Salary might be the most important factor to one person, whereas another might place a much greater value on creativity.

People with occupational wellness face demands on the job, and they also have some say over demands that are placed on them. Any job has routine demands, but occupational wellness means that they are mixed with new, unpredictable challenges that keep a job exciting. Occupationally well people are able to maximize their skills, and they have the opportunity to broaden existing skills or gain new ones. There is opportunity for advancement and recognition for achievement.

Occupational wellness also brings some sense of control. People are given the chance to participate in long-term planning and are able to determine some corporate policies, including policies on discipline. People with occupational wellness control the machines they work with, not the other way around. There is ready access to feedback from both customers and management.

Occupational wellness encourages collaboration among co-workers, fostering a sense of teamwork and support. There is good interaction. When problems arise, democratic procedures are used to solve them; those with a grievance have an accepted and effective way to solve it.

A workplace free from physical stressors promotes occupational wellness. Among the many things in the workplace that can cause stress are noise, poor temperature control, crowding, poor arrangement of space, lack of privacy, and problems with lighting (lights are too bright, too dim, too glaring, or flickering). Occupational wellness also implies freedom from safety hazards on the job, such as dangerous machinery, toxic chemicals, air pollution, or the threat of nuclear accidents.

People with occupational wellness consistently work toward a satisfying balance between the time and energy spent at work and the time and energy spent in family and leisure activities. At a healthy job, people share responsibilities so everyone has time (and energy) left for activities away from work.

ENVIRONMENTAL The quality of today's environment has a direct effect on personal wellness. To enjoy health, we require clean air, pure water, quality food, adequate shelter, satisfactory work conditions, personal safety, and healthy relationships.

Health is negatively affected when we live in a polluted, toxic, unkind, and unsafe environment. To enjoy **environmental wellness**, it is our personal responsibility to educate and protect ourselves against environmental hazards. We must also do all that we can to protect the environment so that we, our children, and future generations can also enjoy a safe and clean environment.

SPIRITUAL **Spiritual wellness**—comprising the ethics, values, and morals that guide us—gives meaning and direction to life. Every human being needs the sense

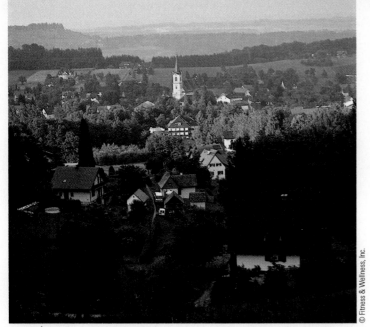

Spiritual wellness includes enjoying the wonder and beauty of nature.

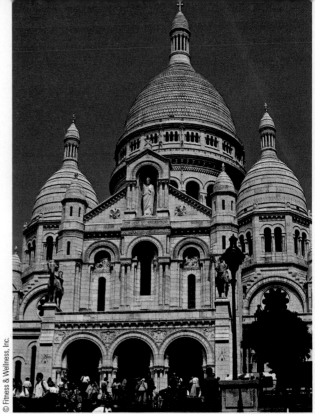

Spiritual wellness recognizes a power higher than oneself.

that life is meaningful, that life has purpose and direction, and that some power (nature, science, religion, or some higher power) brings all of humanity together. In essence, spiritual wellness entails a search for greater value in life.

Spiritual wellness embodies commitment to a worthwhile purpose, faith, and peace, and an undaunted comfort with life and its outcome. It is characterized by faith and optimism, by a hope that sustains us through whatever life has to offer. It entails developing the inner self and identifying a purpose to life. Optimum spiritual wellness occurs when you are able to discover, articulate, and act on that purpose.

Spiritually well people have the unique ability to see beyond the isolated event, to envision the whole picture. A spiritually well person sets realistic goals and goes about reaching them with hope, enthusiasm, and determination. Those goals are never the end result. They are part of the whole, cogs in the larger machine of life. Spiritually healthy people are enthused about what lies ahead, not merely content with what they have accomplished in the past.

That's not to say that spiritually well people never experience disappointment. Spiritually healthy people, however, are able to bridge the gap from one success to another, able to develop the fortitude necessary to keep going. Spiritually healthy individuals don't dwell on discouragement. They mobilize their inner resources to reach the next pinnacle. Instead of envisioning disappointments or setbacks as craggy stone walls, spiritually well people see them as smooth stepping stones, inviting them to keep going, inviting them to make their way, carefully but securely, to the other side.

BEHAVIORAL HEALTH

Behavioral health brings with it solutions that seem simple in comparison to the array of scientific tests, the complex chemical formulas, the powerful lens of the microscope, and the elaborate assortment of available treatments. Researchers have found that the following simple lifestyle habits can add significantly to longevity:

1. Eat a well-rounded diet low in fats and cholesterol and high in dietary fiber and make sure you eat a good breakfast every day.
2. Maintain recommended weight.
3. Get at least 30 minutes of **moderate-intensity physical activity** most days of the week.
4. Get a good night's sleep.
5. Lower your stress levels and surround yourself with a supportive network of friends and family.

Occupational wellness The ability to perform one's job skillfully and effectively under conditions that provide personal and team satisfaction and adequately reward each individual.

Environmental wellness The capability to live in a clean and safe environment that is not detrimental to health.

Spiritual wellness The sense that life is meaningful, that life has purpose, and that some power brings all humanity together; the ethics, values, and morals that guide us and give meaning and direction to life.

Behavioral health The role of lifestyle in health.

Moderate intensity physical activity Activity that uses 150 calories of energy per day, or 1,000 calories per week.

6. Implement personal safety measures—things as simple as wearing seatbelts, observing speed limits, and locking house doors.
7. Stay informed about the environment and avoid potential contaminants whenever you can.
8. Take any medication your doctor prescribes and follow directions precisely.
9. Limit your intake of alcohol.
10. If you smoke, quit.

WELLNESS CHALLENGES OF THE 21ST CENTURY

With the landmark 1979 publication of Healthy People, the U.S. Surgeon General's report on health promotion and disease prevention, the government embarked on a plan to establish broad national goals intended to promote wellness among all Americans. Those goals were converted into specific health objectives a year later, with a precise list of measurable goals we had hoped to attain by the year 1990.

Americans were successful at some; we failed at others. After assessing what had been achieved and what still had to be done, the U.S. Public Health Service conducted hearings across the nation with health professionals from a variety of settings. The result were the Year 2000 National Health Objectives, a set of goals aimed at taking Americans into the 21st century with a higher level of health and wellness. Again, we met a few of the goals but came up short in many others.

Thus, a new set of more realistic goals have been written with the intent to help improve the health of all Americans as we start the first decade of the new millennium. Two unique goals of the new 2010 objectives are that they emphasize increased quality and years of healthy life and they seek to eliminate health disparities among all groups of people (see Figure 1.6).

The objectives address three important points:

1. Personal responsibility. Individuals need to become ever more health-conscious. Responsible and informed behaviors are the key to good health.
2. Health benefits for all people. Lower socioeconomic conditions and poor health are often interrelated. Extending the benefits of good health to all people is crucial to the health of the nation.
3. Health promotion and disease prevention. A shift from treatment to preventive techniques will drastically cut health care costs and help all Americans achieve a better quality of life.

Development of the 2010 Health Objectives involved more than 10,000 people representing 300 national

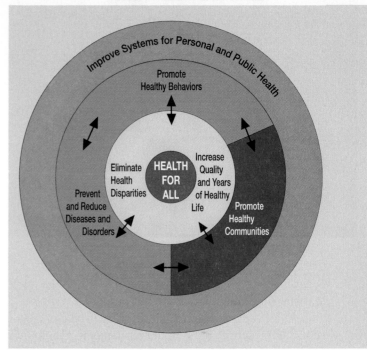

FIGURE 1.6 NATIONAL HEALTH OBJECTIVES 2010: HEALTHY PEOPLE IN HEALTHY COMMUNITIES.

organizations, including the Institute of Medicine of the National Academy of Sciences, all 50 state health departments, and the federal Office of Disease Prevention and Health Promotion. A summary of key 2010 objectives is provided in Figure 1.7. Living the wellness guidelines provided in this book not only will enhance the quality of your life but also will allow you to be an active participant in achieving the Healthy People 2010 Objectives.

Additionally, a major report on the influence of regular physical activity on health was released by the U.S. Surgeon General in 1996. The report states that regular moderate physical activity provides substantial benefits in health and well-being for the vast majority of Americans who are not physically active. This report has become a call to nation-wide action.

According to the Surgeon General, improving health through physical activity is a serious public health challenge that we must meet at once. More than 60 percent of adults do not achieve the recommended amount of physical activity, and 25 percent are not

> The nation's top health goals as we begin the new millennium are: exercise, increased consumption of fruits and vegetables, smoking cessation, and the practice of safe sex.
>
> —David Satcher, U.S. Surgeon General

FIGURE 1.7 SELECTED HEALTH OBJECTIVES FOR THE YEAR 2010.

1. Increase quality and years of healthy life.
2. Eliminate health disparities.
3. Improve the health, fitness, and quality of life of all Americans through the adoption and maintenance of regular, daily physical activity.
4. Promote health and reduce chronic disease risk, disease progression, debilitation, and premature death associated with dietary factors and nutritional status among all people in the United States.
5. Reduce disease, disability, and death related to tobacco use and exposure to secondhand smoke.
6. Increase the quality, availability, and effectiveness of educational and community-based programs designed to prevent disease and improve the health and quality of the American people.
7. Promote health for all people through a healthy environment.
8. Reduce the incidence and severity of injuries from unintentional causes, as well as violence and abuse.
9. Promote worker health and safety through prevention.
10. Improve access to comprehensive, high quality health care.
11. Ensure that every pregnancy in the United States is intended.
12. Improve maternal and pregnancy outcomes and reduce rates of disability in infants.
13. Improve the quality of health-related decisions through effective communication.
14. Decrease the incidence of functional limitations due to arthritis, osteoporosis, and chronic back conditions.
15. Decrease cancer incidence, morbidity, and mortality.
16. Promote health and prevent secondary conditions among persons with disabilities.
17. Enhance the cardiovascular health and quality of life of all Americans through prevention and control of risk factors, and promotion of healthy lifestyle behaviors.
18. Prevent HIV transmission and associated morbidity and mortality.
19. Improve the mental health of all Americans.
20. Raise the public's awareness of the signs and symptoms of lung disease.
21. Increase awareness of healthy sexual relationships and prevent all forms of sexually transmitted diseases.
22. Reduce the incidence of substance abuse by all people, especially children.

physically active at all. Benefits of leading a moderately active lifestyle include a significant reduction in the risk of developing or dying from heart disease, diabetes, colon cancer, and high blood pressure. Regular physical activity also helps to maintain a high quality of life into old age. Additional information on the Surgeon General's report is given in Chapter 6.

Experts who were instrumental in formulating the national objectives and the report on physical activity and health point to the commitment of the government toward achieving wellness goals. They also invite the commitment and involvement of each American in accepting responsibility for their own health and wellness.

A PERSONALIZED APPROACH TO HEALTH AND WELLNESS

Vital to achieving health and wellness is your willingness to take personal responsibility for your behaviors and choices. We know enough about disease and premature death to formulate a set of goals that applies to the nation as a whole. How you achieve those goals, however, requires a personal decision. It entails careful, intelligent planning. How you apply the principles you'll learn in this book has to be highly personalized. What will work for someone else won't necessarily work for you.

As you study the information in this book on achieving wellness, the following personalized approach may be helpful:

- If you're smoking now, determine how you are going to stop. Find out what community resources are available to help you. If you need to, talk to your doctor. Outline a specific course of action that will work for you.
- If you have a drinking problem or a drug dependency, find out specifically where you can get help. Make an appointment. Follow through. Start by figuring out why you started using drugs or alcohol to begin with. Your personal motives have a lot to do with your ability to kick the habit.
- If you have a weight problem, get help. With guidance from your doctor or another health care professional, outline specifically how you are going to change your eating and exercise habits so you can lose weight safely and permanently.
- Increase your level of physical activity. Before you do, however, take a critical look at your situation and determine whether you need a doctor's okay. If you do, schedule an appointment for a thorough physical examination, discuss your objectives with your physician, and get the go-ahead for a safe, effective fitness program. Then design a program that works for you, based on your situation and preferences. If you hate running, try bicycling or swimming instead.

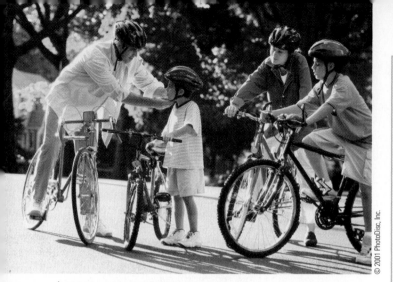

© 2001 PhotoDisc, Inc.

| Objectives for enhancing health and wellness are aimed at protection, promotion, and prevention. |

If you can't afford the fees at the racquetball court, challenge a group of friends to an equally demanding but less expensive competition a couple of times a week.

- Pinpoint your individual sources of stress. You can probably eliminate some of them. You can respond to others differently. If you have a particularly difficult class, for example, get on top of things by scheduling an extra hour every day to study that subject or talk to the professor about getting individualized help from a teaching assistant. Stress has a major impact on disease. A wellness plan demands that you handle stress with determination and commitment.

At the end of this chapter you will find a Health Assessment and a Wellness and Longevity Potential Test. These two assessments will help you determine how well you are living your life and can help you identify areas where you can make improvements. Keep in mind that at the center of wellness is self-responsibility. No one else can make you eat better, exercise more regularly, stop smoking, use alcohol in moderation, or cope with stress. Accepting the challenge to achieve wellness implies that you are willing to make lifelong lifestyle changes. Wellness doesn't happen in a day. It involves an ongoing process of healthy choices throughout the rest of your life.

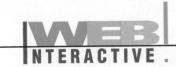

INTERACTIVE.

WEB ACTIVITIES

■ **Healthy People 2010** Healthy People is a national health promotion and disease prevention initiative that lists a series of goals for improving health of all Americans by the year 2010.
http://www.health.gov/healthypeople

■ **Mayo Clinic Online** This comprehensive consumer site, sponsored by the renowned Mayo Clinic, features the following: current health topics, diseases and conditions "A to Z," condition centers (comprehensive resources for cancer, heart disease, and other medical conditions), healthy living centers (practical advice about nutrition, fitness, women's health, men's health, family life, and other topics), "Take Charge of Your Health" (personal health scorecard, healthy lifestyle planners, disease self-management, and health decision guides), drug information, and first-aid and self-care guides.
http://www.mayohealth.org

■ **Your Personalized Health Portrait** Take this confidential health questionnaire to determine your personal lifestyle score, featuring a list of health habits to change, in order of importance. You will also receive a list of screening tests and immunizations to ask your doctor about.
http://www.thriveonline.com/cgi-bin/hmi/healthportrait.cgi

■ **Select Your Health Quiz** Test your general health and medical knowledge; select the "Conventional," "Advanced," and/or "Extreme" Health Quiz.
http://www.mededge.com/quizbb.htm

■ **Self-Care Flow Charts** This excellent, patient-friendly site, sponsored by the *American Family Physician* journal, features a comprehensive list of symptoms and flowcharts to help you seek out the most appropriate type of medical care at the most appropriate time (based on urgency). Some of the symptoms listed include abdominal pain (acute and chronic), chest pain, headaches, fever in adults and children, cold and flu, cough, diarrhea, sore throat, eye problems, foot problems, tooth problems, and lots more.
http://familydoctor.org/flowcharts

InfoTrac
You can find additional readings related to wellness via InfoTrac College Edition, an on-line library of more than 900 journals and publications. Follow the instructions for accessing InfoTrac that came packaged with your textbook, then search for articles using a key word search.

Suggested Reading Rosemarie Sweeney and Verna L. Rose, "'Healthy People 2010' Initiative to Guide Prevention Agenda for the Next Ten Years," *American Family Physician* 61, no. 6 (March 15, 2000): 1605.

1. Name five significant differences between the Healthy People 2010 document and the Healthy People 2000 objectives.
2. What are the two major themes for the nation's health goals?
3. Name the ten leading health indicators described in Healthy People 2010.

Web Activity
Live Well Personal Wellness Assessment
http://wellness.uwsp.edu/Health_Service/

Sponsor University of Wisconsin—Steven's Point
Description This colorful and comprehensive site features 100 multiple-choice self-assessment questions encompassing ten dimensions of wellness. The site analyzes your overall state of health based on your composite score using a percentage scale for excellent, good, average, fair, and poor.
Available Activity

1. Take the self-assessment, which contains ten lifestyle questions in each of the following ten wellness dimensions: physical fitness, nutrition, self-care, drugs and driving, social environment, intellectual, occupational, spiritual, emotional awareness, and emotional control.

Web Work
1. From the University of Wisconsin–Stevens Point home page, click the services tab.
2. You will see a list of 3 interactive programs. Click on Live Well.
3. Honestly answer all of the ten multiple-choice questions describing your lifestyle, beliefs, and behaviors in each of the ten categories of wellness.

Helpful Hint
1. After answering all questions, click on the "Evaluate" button to receive your personalized results.

For additional Web activities, links, and suggested readings, visit our Health, Fitness, and Wellness Resource Center at http://health.wadsworth.com.

NOTES

1. U.S. Department of Health and Human Services, Centers for Disease Control and Prevention, National Center for Health Statistics, National Vital Statistics System: *Deaths, Final Data for 1998* 48:11 (July 24, 2000).

2. World Health Organization, Ch-1211 Geneva 27, Switzerland.

3. U.S. Dept. of Health and Human Services, Office on Smoking and Health, *The Health Consequences of Smoking* (Rockville, MD: DHHS [PHS] 84-50205, 1984), xii.

4. Jesse Williams.

5. Donald Ardell, *The History and Future of Wellness* (IA: Kendall Hunt, 1985).

6. Robert Moats Miller, *Preacher, Pastor, Prophet* (NY: Oxford University Press, 1988).

7. Norman Cousins, *Head First: The Biology of Hope* (NY: E. P. Dutton, 1989).

8. Bernie Siegel, *The Complete Book of Cancer Prevention* (Emmaus, PA: Rodale Press, 1986).

9. James Hardison, *Let's Touch: How and Why To Do It* (NJ: Prentice Hall, 1980).

HEALTH ASSESSMENT

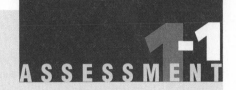

Name: _____ Date: _____ Grade: _____

Instructor: _____ Course: _____ Section: _____

Assessing mental health and stress is a complex task and difficult to do in limited space. The following assessment instruments represent a sampling of stress and mental-health indicators.

Self-Esteem Assessment

Write *a* in front of each statement that describes you and *b* in front of each statement that does not describe you.

_____ 1. People generally like me.
_____ 2. I am comfortable talking in class.
_____ 3. I like to do new things.
_____ 4. I give in easily.
_____ 5. I'm a failure.
_____ 6. I'm shy.
_____ 7. I have trouble making up my mind.
_____ 8. I'm popular with people at school.
_____ 9. My life is all mixed up.
_____ 10. I often feel upset at my home, room, or apartment.
_____ 11. I often wish I were like someone else.
_____ 12. I often worry.
_____ 13. I can be depended on.
_____ 14. I often express my views.
_____ 15. I think I am doing okay with my life.
_____ 16. I feel good about what I have accomplished recently.

Scoring/Interpretation

Determine how many matches you have with the following key. Total that number.

1. a	4. b	7. b	10. b	13. a	16. a
2. a	5. b	8. a	11. b	14. a	
3. a	6. b	9. b	12. b	15. a	

From the total number of matched, interpret as follows:

12–16 high self-esteem
8–11 moderately high self-esteem
4–7 moderately low self-esteem
0–3 low self-esteem

Depression Assessment

Indicate which of the following reflect what you do or how you feel. Indicate by marking an *X* in the space provided if it is like you.

_____ 1. I use drugs to relax or have fun.
_____ 2. I need to see a professional about how sad I feel.
_____ 3. I have trouble making it to class.
_____ 4. I think I would be better off dead.
_____ 5. My life seems hopeless.
_____ 6. I have thought through how I would kill myself.
_____ 7. People around me would be better off if I were gone.
_____ 8. I change my moods often.
_____ 9. I'm not interested in much anymore.
_____ 10. I can't seem to concentrate.
_____ 11. I feel unloved and unwanted.
_____ 12. I have a quick temper.
_____ 13. I feel guilty.
_____ 14. I take things too hard.
_____ 15. I have been thinking a lot about death lately.

Scoring/Interpretation

If you have marked number 2, 4, 5, 6, 7, or 11, you should talk with someone right away about your feelings and needs. You may want to talk to your instructor about where to go for help.

If you have marked any of the other responses (number 1, 3, or 8–13) in conjunction with number 15, then you should also talk with someone about how you feel.

If you have marked three or more of the remaining statements (number 1, 3, or 8–13), you also may want to seek help.

Assertiveness Assessment

Indicate what you would do in the following situations by circling *a*, *b*, or *c*.

1. A professor gives you a grade that is lower than you had expected.
   a. Ask the professor to recalculate the grade because you feel he or she is in error.
   b. Complain to the professor but accept the grade.
   c. Say nothing.
2. In a cafeteria line after waiting some time to get something to eat, a group of people recognize the person in front of you and crowd in line.
   a. Ask them to please move to the back of the line and wait like everyone else.
   b. Make a comment but not ask them to move back.
   c. Say nothing.
3. Someone near you is smoking in a nonsmoking section.
   a. Ask him or her to notice the no smoking sign and please put out the cigarette.
   b. Make a comment like, "Can't you read?" but don't ask him or her to put it out.
   c. Say nothing.
4. You have waited for ten minutes at a department secretary's office to get course information, and she is obviously making a personal call.
   a. Get her attention and say, "Can you help me?"
   b. Sigh heavily and give frustrated looks.
   c. Wait patiently.

Scoring/Interpretation

Assign the following number of points to each of your answers. Total your points.

a = 4   b = 2   c = 0

Interpret as follows:

12–16 assertive
6–11 moderately assertive
0–6 unassertive

Stress Index

To identify the types and degrees of stress you are experiencing, complete the following index. Circle the number that corresponds to your reaction to each statement. Total the numbers in each column and add them to arrive at a subtotal for each section.

	Always	Often	Sometimes	Rarely	Never
1. I get upset when I have to wait in lines.	5	4	3	2	1
2. I work by the clock to see how much I can get done in a short time.	5	4	3	2	1
3. I get upset if something takes too long.	5	4	3	2	1
4. I make almost every activity I do competitive with myself or others.	5	4	3	2	1
5. I feel guilty when I'm not working on something.	5	4	3	2	1

Section subtotal _____

	Always	Often	Sometimes	Rarely	Never
6. I get upset when I can't do something my way.	5	4	3	2	1
7. I get upset when my accomplishments depend on others' actions.	5	4	3	2	1
8. I get anxious when my plans become disrupted.	5	4	3	2	1
9. All good things are worth waiting for.	1	2	3	4	5
10. When I set a goal I can't reach, I simply alter it.	1	2	3	4	5

Section subtotal _____

	Always	Often	Sometimes	Rarely	Never
11. I have been given too much responsibility.	5	4	3	2	1
12. I get depressed when I think of everything I have to do.	5	4	3	2	1
13. People demand too much of me.	5	4	3	2	1
14. I often find myself without enough time to complete my work.	5	4	3	2	1
15. Sometimes I feel that my head is spinning, or I get confused because so much is happening.	5	4	3	2	1

Section subtotal _____

	Always	Often	Sometimes	Rarely	Never
16. I succeed in most things and try even when the task is difficult.	1	2	3	4	5
17. I am comfortable being with members of the opposite sex.	1	2	3	4	5
18. I am generally comfortable around teachers, bosses, and other superiors.	1	2	3	4	5
19. I prefer that others make decisions for me.	5	4	3	2	1
20. I don't think I have too much going for me.	5	4	3	2	1
21. I'm most relaxed when I'm busy.	5	4	3	2	1
22. I throw away old clothes, toys, and other mementos.	1	2	3	4	5
23. I enjoy being alone.	1	2	3	4	5
24. I feel the need to belong to a social group.	5	4	3	2	1
25. I get homesick easily.	5	4	3	2	1

Section subtotal _____

	Always	Often	Sometimes	Rarely	Never
26. I often feel my stomach knotting, my mouth getting dry, and my heart pounding when I get nervous.	5	4	3	2	1
27. When I get nervous, I can feel my muscles tense, my hands and fingers shake, and my voice become unsteady.	5	4	3	2	1
28. After a crisis I relive the experience over and over in my mind, even though it is resolved.	5	4	3	2	1
29. I know I must resolve a crisis or it will bother me for a long time.	5	4	3	2	1
30. When I'm nervous, I imagine the worst possible outcomes of the original crisis.	5	4	3	2	1

Section subtotal _____

TOTAL = _____

Scoring/Interpretation

By summing all the subtotals on the index, you estimate your overall susceptibility to stress based on social situation and personality. Interpret your score as follows:

100 or higher – High stress   50–99 – Moderate stress   49 or below – You are doing well for now; keep it up.

THE WELLNESS AND LONGEVITY POTENTIAL TEST

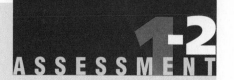

Name: _____ Date: _____ Grade: _____

Instructor: _____ Course: _____ Section: _____

Changeable Lifestyle Factors

1. Tobacco
(1 pipe = 2 cigarettes, 1 cigar = 3 cigarettes)

Never smoked	+20	
Quit smoking	+10	
Smoke up to one pack per day		−10
Smoke one to two packs per day		−20
Smoke more than two packs per day		−30

Pack-years smoked (number of packs smoked per day, times number of years smoked):

7–15	−5
16–25	−10
Over 25	−20

2. Alcohol
(1 beer or 1 glass of wine = 1.25 oz. alcohol)

1.25 oz. per day or less	+10	
Between 1.25 and 2.5 oz. per day		−4
−1 more for each additional 1.25 oz. per day		−__

3. Exercise
(20 min. or more moderate aerobic exercise)

3 or more times per week	+20	
2 times per week	+10	
No regular aerobic activity		−10
Work requires regular physical exertion or at least 2 miles walking per day	+3	
+1 more for each additional mile walked per day	+ __	

4. Weight

Maintain recommended weight for height	+5	
5–10 lbs. over recommended		−1
11–20 lbs. over recommended		−2
21–30 lbs. over recommended		−3
−1 more for each additional 10 lbs.		−__
Yo-yo dieting		−10

5. Nutrition

Eat a well-balanced diet	+3	
Do not eat a well-balanced diet		−3
Regularly eat meals at consistent times	+2	
Do not regularly eat meals at consistent times		−2
Snack or eat meals late at night		−2
Eat a balanced breakfast	+2	

Eat fish or poultry as primary protein source (totally replacing red meat)	+5	
Do not eat grains and fish as primary protein source		−2
Eat at least 5 servings of green leafy vegetables per week	+3	
Eat at least 5 servings of fresh fruit or juice	+3	
Try to avoid fats	+5	
Do not try to avoid fats		−5

For each of the following foods eaten 2 or more times per week:

Beef, veal, or pork	−1
Bacon or sausage	−1
Luncheon meat or hot dogs	−1
Fast food	−1
Fried food	−1
Processed food/TV dinners	−1
Eggs	−1
Cheese	−1
Butter	−1
Whole milk or cream	−1
Pastries, doughnuts, muffins	−1
Candy, chocolate	−1
Pretzels, potato chips	−1
Ice cream	−1

Eat some food every day that is high in fiber (whole-grain bread, fresh fruits and vegetables)	+3	
Do not eat some food every day that is high in fiber		−3
Take a daily multivitamin/mineral supplement	+10	
Women: Take a calcium supplement	+5	
Subscribe to health-related periodicals	+2	

Subtotal: _____ _____
               A   G

Fixed Factors

1. Gender

Male		−5
Female	+10	

2. Heredity

Any grandparent lived to be over 80	+5

This test was developed for the average healthy person. If you already have a serious health condition, such as heart disease, diabetes, cancer, or kidney disease, ask your physician for a health-risk assessment designed especially for you.

Average age all four grandparents lived to:

60–70	+5
71–80	+10
Over 80	+20

3. **Family history**

Either parent had stroke or heart
attack before age 50   −10

−5 for each family member (grandparent,
parent, sibling) who prior to age 65
has had any of the following:

Hypertension	−___
Cancer	−___
Heart disease	−___
Stroke	−___
Diabetes	−___
Other genetic diseases	−___

Subtotal B: ___ + ___

Partially Fixed Factors

1. **Family income**

0–$5,000	−10
$5,001–$14,000	−5
$14,001–$20,000	+1
+1 for each additional $10,000, up to $200,000	+ ___

2. **Education**

Some high school (or less)	−7
High school graduate	+2
College graduate	+5
Postgraduate or professional degree	+7

3. **Occupation**

Professional	+5
Self-employed	+6
In the health-care field	+3
Over 65 and still working	+5
Clerical or support	−3
Shift work	−5
Unemployed	−7
Possibility for career advancement	+5
Regularly in direct contact with pollutants, toxic waste, chemicals, radiation	−10

4. **Where you live**

Large urban area	−5
Near an industrial center	−7
Rural or farm area	+5
Area with air-pollution alerts	−5
Area where air pollution has curtailed normal daily activities	−7
High crime area	−3
Little or no crime area	+3
Home has tested positive for radon	−7

Total commuting time to and from work:

0–1/2 hour	+3
1/2 hour–1 hour	+0
−1 for each 1/2 hour over 1 hour	−___
Within 30 miles of major medical/trauma center	+3
No major medical/trauma center in area	−3

Subtotal C: ___ + ___

Changeable Health Status and Maintenance Factors

1. **Health status**

- Present overall physical health:

Excellent	+15
Good	+12
Fair	+5
Poor	−10

- Normal or low blood pressure   +5

High blood pressure	−10
Don't know	−5

- Low cholesterol (under 200)   +10

Moderate cholesterol (200–240)	+5
High cholesterol (over 240)	−10
Don't know	−5

- HDL cholesterol 29 or less   −25

30–36	−20
37–40	−5
41–45	+5
Over 45	+10
Don't know	−5

- Have medical insurance coverage   +10

Able to use physicians of your choice   +5

2. **Preventive and therapeutic measures**

Physical exams (every 3 to 4 years
before age 50, every 1 to 2 years
over 50)   +3

Women:

Yearly gynecological exam and Pap smear	+2
Monthly self breast exam	+2
Mammogram (35–50, every 3 years; over 50, every year)	+2
Smoke and use oral contraceptives	−5

Men:

Genital self-exam every 3 months	+2
Rectal or prostate exam (yearly after age 30)	+2

All:

Current on mumps, measles, rubella, diphtheria and tetanus immunizations	+2
Tested for hidden blood in stool (over 40, every 2 years; over 50, every year)	+2

If over age 50:

Yearly sigmoidoscopy of the
lower bowel   +2

All:

Regularly use sunscreen and avoid
excessive sun   +2

Actively involved in a life-extension,
prevention, or comprehensive
wellness program   +10

3. Accident control

Always wear seat belt as driver and
passenger   +7

Do not always wear seat belt as driver
and passenger   –5

Never drink and drive or ride with a driver
who has been drinking   +2

–10 for each arrest for drinking while
under the influence of alcohol in the
past 5 years   –__

–2 for every speeding ticket or accident in
the past year   –__

For each 10,000 miles per year driven
over 10,000 (national average)   –1

Primary car weighs more than 3,500 lbs.   +10

Subcompact   –5

Motorcycle   –10

–2 for every fight or attack you were
involved in, or witness to, in the
past year   –__

Smoke alarms in home   +1

Subtotal D: __ + __

Changeable Psychosocial Factors

Married or in long-term committed
relationship   +5

Satisfying sex life   +3

Children under 18 living at home   +3

For each 5-year period living alone   –1

No close friends   –10

+1 for each close friend (up to 5)   +__

+2 for each active membership in a
religious community or volunteer
organization (up to 4)   +__

Have a pet   +2

Regular daily routine   +10

No regular daily routine   –10

Hours of uninterrupted sleep per night:

Less than 5 hours   –5

5–8 hours   +5

8–10 hours   –7

–1 for each additional hour over 10   –__

Not consistent   –7

Regular work routine   +5

No regular work routine   –5

–2 for every 5 hours worked over
40 in a week   –__

Take a yearly vacation from work
(at least 6 days)   +5

Regularly use a stress-management
technique (yoga, meditation, music, etc.)   +3

Subtotal E: __ + __

Changeable Emotional Stress Factors

N = Never   R = Rarely   S = Sometimes
A = Always (or as much as possible)

	N	R	S	A
Generally happy	–2	–1	+1	+2
Have and enjoy time with family and friends	–2	–1	+1	+2
Feel in control of personal life and career	–2	–1	+1	+2
Live within financial means	–2	–1	+1	+2
Set goals and look for new challenges	–2	–1	+1	+2
Participate in creative outlet or hobby	–2	–1	+1	+2
Have and enjoy leisure time	–2	–1	+1	+2
Express feelings easily	–2	–1	+1	+2
Laugh easily	–2	–1	+1	+2
Expect good things to happen	–2	–1	+1	+2

	A	S	R	N
Anger easily	–2	–1	+1	+2
Critical of self	–2	–1	+1	+2
Critical of others	–2	–1	+1	+2
Lonely, even with others	–2	–1	+1	+2
Worry about things out of your control	–2	–1	+1	+2
Regret sacrifices made in life	–2	–1	+1	+2

Subtotal F: __ + __ + __ + __

Scoring

A+B+C+D+E+F = _____

(Subtotal, up to 200*)

Subtotal + G = Total

Divide total by 2. This gives your chance
(in %) of living to or beyond average life
expectancy of a person your age.

Total: _____ ÷ 2 =

_____ %

* If this number is higher than 200, use 200 as your subtotal. Maintain those healthy habits that allowed you to score much higher than the average person (around 50%) and try to turn any of the negatives in section G (e.g., smoking) into positives. You have the very best chance of living a long and healthy life, because these factors are totally in your control.

— Linda Addlespurger

If you scored 100%, congratulations. But don't rest on your laurels. Keep looking for ways to improve your good health. And if you didn't score as well as you would have liked, it's never too late to begin improving your longevity potential.

Interpretation and Conclusions

Based on the results of Assessments 1–1 and 1–2, indicate what you have learned about how your lifestyle habits are affecting your health and wellness. Do you feel that these assessments provide an accurate analysis of your lifestyle habits?

Please identify areas where you feel you can make improvements in your daily living habits that will be conducive to better health and wellness.

2 THE MIND-BODY CONNECTION

OBJECTIVES

- Describe the physiological manifestations of specific emotions.

- Define psychoneuro-immunology and its emphasis on links among the mind, the brain, and the immune system.

- Identify the connection between disease and personality.

- Describe the character-istics of the coronary-prone personality.

- Define the relaxed, cancer-prone, and distressed personalities.

- Explain the differences between anger and hostility and the health effects of each.

- Discuss the health effects of depression.

- List the warning signs of suicide and what to do to help someone who is considering suicide.

25

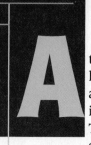

A GROWING BODY OF EVIDENCE indicates that virtually every illness known to modern humanity—from arthritis to migraine headaches, from the common cold to cancer—is influenced for good or bad by our emotions. To a profound extent, emotions affect our susceptibility to disease and our **immunity**. At least half of the leading causes of death among Americans (see Chapter 1) are related to behavioral factors. The way we react to what comes along in life can determine in great measure how we will react to the disease-causing organisms that we face. The feelings we have and the way we express them can either boost our immune system or weaken it.

Emotional health is a key part of total wellness. Most emotionally healthy people take care of themselves physically—they eat well, exercise, and get enough rest. They work to develop supportive personal relationships. In contrast, many people who are emotionally unhealthy are self-destructive. For example, they may abuse alcohol and other drugs or may overwork and not have balance in their lives.

The idea that emotional health and physical health are closely intertwined has received much national attention. Emotional health is so important that it affects what we do, who we meet, who we marry, how we look, how we feel, the course of our lives, and even how long we live.

Emotions cause physiological responses that can influence health. Certain parts of the brain are associated with specific emotions and specific hormone patterns. The release of certain hormones is associated with various emotional responses, and those hormones affect health. These responses may contribute to development of disease. Emotions have to be expressed somewhere, somehow. If they are suppressed repeatedly, and/or if a person feels conflict about controlling them, they often reveal themselves through physical symptoms.

These physiological responses may weaken the immune system over time. Negative emotional responses have been linked to a wide variety of conditions, including allergies, asthma, angina, heart disease, high blood pressure, arthritis, back pain, cancer, dental cavities, diabetes, gastric ulcers, insomnia, irritable bowel syndrome, and a variety of skin problems.

> What's really starting to be understood and documented about the mind-body connection is that there is a physiological effect for all our thoughts and feelings.
>
> —Mark Liponis, M.D.

> When people become seriously ill, they often "forget" what it is like to be physically healthy, and can no longer access a psychophysiological state of well-being.
>
> —Psychologist Joan Klagsbrun

THE SCIENCE OF PSYCHONEUROIMMUNOLOGY

The scientific investigation of how the brain affects the body's immune cells and how the immune system can be affected by behavior is called **psychoneuroimmunology**. In the 1970s, research indicated that the immune system could be "trained" to react in certain ways.[1] The resulting study of psychoneuroimmunology focuses on the links among the mind, the brain, and the immune system. As a science, it has received the endorsement of the National Institutes of Health. Research studies indicate that the mind-body connection is powerful, as shown below:[2]

- Positive emotions can help protect the heart.
- Among people with heart disease, pessimism is deadly but a healthy outlook is healing.
- Remaining calm during emotional conflict reduces the risk of heart attack.
- Anxiety and suppressed anger tripled the risk of premature death; depression boosted the risk of premature death eight times.

Today, research in this field is booming. A number of medical schools have already integrated psychoneuroimmunology into their curricula. Almost every important

POSITIVE EMOTIONS AND LAUGHTER

The late Norman Cousins, former editor of the **Saturday Review** and member of the UCLA medical faculty, twice intrigued the medical community and the public alike by overcoming usually fatal conditions—once a massive heart attack, and once an advanced case of a degenerative spinal disease. Cousins followed his physicians' regimen each time and also infused himself with vast doses of positive emotions and laughter. According to Cousins himself, he was healed not only by the miracle of modern medicine but also by the healing emotions of love, hope, faith, confidence, and a tremendous will to live.

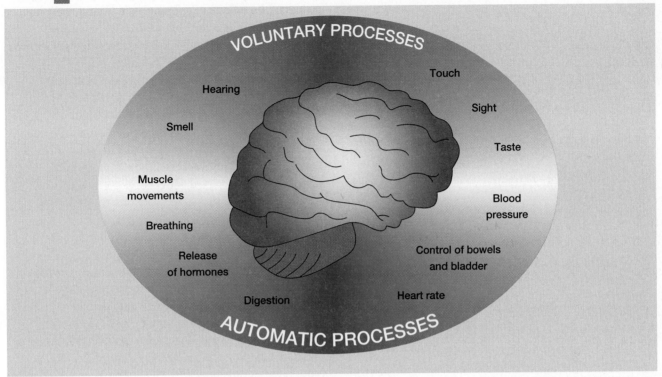

conference on immunology now includes at least one seminar on the relationship between the brain and the immune system, and an increasing number of physicians acknowledge that the way a patient thinks and feels can be a powerful determinant of physical health.

The Brain

The brain is a privileged organ. The heart supplies it with blood; the lungs supply it with oxygen; the intestines supply it with nutrients; and the kidneys remove poisons from its environment. It is the most important part of the nervous system. For the body to survive, the brain must be maintained. All other organs sacrifice to keep the brain alive and functioning when the entire body is under severe stress.

The brain directs nerve impulses that are carried throughout the body. It controls voluntary processes, such as the direction, strength, and coordination of muscle movements; the processes involved in smelling, touching, and seeing; and involuntary functions over which you have no conscious control. Among the latter are many automatic, vital functions in the body, such as breathing, heart rate, digestion, control of the bowels and bladder, blood pressure, and release of hormones. These functions are illustrated in Figure 2.1.

The brain is the cognitive center of the body, the place where ideas are generated, memory is stored, and emotions are experienced. The brain has a powerful influence over the body via the link between the emotions and the immune system. That link is extremely complex.

The emotions that the brain produces are a mixture of feelings and physical responses. Every time the brain manufactures an emotion, physical reactions accompany it. The brain's natural chemicals form literal communication links among the brain, its thought processes, and the cells of the body, including those of the immune system.

The Immune System

The immune system patrols and guards the body against attackers. This system consists of about a trillion cells called **lymphocytes** and about a hundred million trillion molecules called **antibodies**. The brain and the immune system are closely linked in a connection that allows the mind to influence both susceptibility and resistance to disease. A number of immune system cells—including those in the thymus gland, spleen, bone marrow, and lymph nodes—are laced with nerve cells.

Immunity The function that guards the body from invaders, both internal and external.

Psychoneuroimmunology (PNI) The scientific investigation of how the brain affects the body's immune cells and how the immune system can be affected by behavior.

Lymphocytes Specialized immune system cells.

Antibodies Substances produced by the white blood cells in response to an invading agent.

Cells of the immune system are equipped to respond to chemical signals from the central nervous system. For example, the surface of the lymphocytes contains receptors for a variety of central nervous system chemical messengers, such as catecholamines, prostaglandins, serotonin, endorphins, sex hormones, the thyroid hormone, and the growth hormone. Certain white blood cells possess the ability to receive messages from the brain.

Because of these receptors on the lymphocytes, physical and psychological stress alters the immune system. (Chapter 3 addresses the topic of stress.) Stress causes the body to release several powerful neuro-hormones that bind with the receptors on the lympho-cytes and suppress immune function. Corticosteroids, for example, have been found to be such powerful suppres-sors of the immune system that they are used widely to treat allergic conditions (such as asthma and hay fever) and **autoimmune disorders** (such as rheumatoid arthritis and rejection of transplanted organs). Other brain chemicals unleashed by the hypothalamus have equally profound effects on the immune system.

PERSONALITY AND HEALTH

Personality is the total physical, intellectual, and emotional structure of an individual, including abilities, interests, and attitudes. Personality is the way your habits, attitudes, and traits combine to make the person that is uniquely you. Because of your personality, you act in a similar way from one day to the next, and when you are placed in various situations, you still tend to act in a generally consistent way. Your personality, in essence, is the pattern of behavior that distinguishes you from everybody else. Personality depends partly on biology and genetics (the unique set of genes you inherited from your parents), but is also greatly affected by the family you grow up in, the environment that surrounds you, and the culture and subcultures that influence you.

The theory that personality affects health is, as world-renowned psychologist Hans Eysenck put it, a theory based on centuries of observations made by keen-eyed physicians.[3] The notion that a certain personality type leads to heart disease dates back more than 2,000 years to Hippocrates, and the belief that a certain personality is associated with cancer goes back several centuries. What is new is the scientific research that substantiates those notions.

However, this is not to say that people always bring illness on themselves. This viewpoint may lead to inhumanity and a lack of compassion for people who need it the most. Instead we can use this information to protect and preserve our health status.

Most people associate certain personalities with certain illnesses: Workaholics tend to have heart attacks. Worriers tend to get ulcers. People who get too uptight often have asthma attacks. In reality, can people be so neatly categorized? No. Yet, researchers have made tremendous strides in proving that personality does have an impact on health. They have found that the way we look at things, as determined by our personality, may contribute to illness or help keep us well.

Personality Types

Personality traits may be health-harming or health-enhancing.[4] Some researchers believe a specific combina-tion of personality traits may make a person susceptible to a general classification of disease conditions, not just a specific disease. Researchers categorize people into broad personality types to help determine if a person is more likely to become ill or stay well.[5] People generally are not exclusively one type but instead fluctuate between the traits of each personality.

THE CORONARY-PRONE PERSONALITY The most promi-nent in research has been the **Type A** or **coronary-prone personality**, characterized by a hard-driving and com-petitive person who is also hostile, angry, and suspicious.[6] The Type A pattern does not imply a stressful situation or distressed response, but refers to the behaviors of an individual who reacts to the environment with characteristic gestures, facial expressions, and pace, and who perceives daily events and stresses as challenges—all of which leads to an aggressive, time-urgent, im-patient, and more hostile style of living.

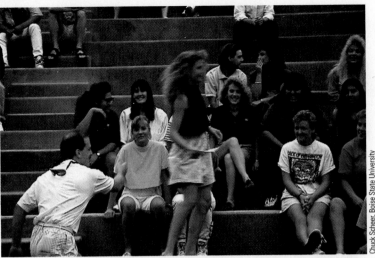
Research suggests that personality may play a role in health and wellness.

Although the Type A personality can result from a number of influences, including genetic and environmental factors, most prominent is a hostile, angry, nonsupportive family environment.

Type A has been dubbed the "hurry sickness." Type A personalities never seem to slow down. They[7]

- try to do two or more things simultaneously;
  - have a sense of time-urgency;
  - are impatient when waiting in lines or in traffic;
  - are involved in more car accidents;
- are extremely competitive and tend to keep score in even trivial situations;
- are aggressive;
  - make forceful, rapid, or "staccato" gestures;
  - have a loud voice and interrupt people;
  - eat and walk fast;
  - are insecure about their status;
  - are hard-driving and ambitious;
  - have a high need for achievement;
  - have a high level of job involvement; and
- sometimes harbor an unconscious drive to self-destruct.

These traits add up to joyless striving.

The Type A personality is in a chronic state of vigilant observation.[8] The hormones (particularly epinephrine and cortisol) that are released continually in the Type A person cause an increase in serum cholesterol and fat levels, leaching of blood platelets, overworking of the heart and arteries, excessive insulin secretion, and suppression of the immune system. The result is a higher risk for heart disease.

In one long-term study, researchers found that Type A personalities were more than twice as likely to develop heart disease; among those aged 39 to 49, the risk leaps to six times as high.[9] If a person with Type A personality also exhibits two other risk factors for heart disease (such as cigarette smoking or high blood pressure), that person's risk for developing coronary heart disease is eight times greater.[10]

One of the components of **hostility**—anger—has been shown to be a particular risk factor for heart disease. The Type A personality is increasingly being defined as a person who can't manage anger. Anger speeds up the heart and blood pressure. Suppressed anger is even more dangerous; the more often anger is suppressed, the higher the blood pressure.

The traits that are most detrimental to health, the most predictive of coronary disease, are the harmful Type A traits, a **toxic core** characterized by anger, cynicism, suspiciousness, and excessive self-involvement. Probably the most detrimental trait of the toxic core is free-floating hostility, a continuous state of anger that hovers quietly until some trivial incident causes it to erupt.

Fortunately, Type A behavior patterns can be modified to reduce disease risk. A group of Type A insurance representatives participated in behavior therapy targeted at reducing the negative effects of Type A actions. Results showed that the therapy significantly reduced the intensity of Type A behavior and its time urgency element.[11] See the box on the following page for ways to change a Type A personality.

Apparently a person can have many of the characteristics typically associated with Type A personality—such as competitive drive, an aggressive personality, and impatience—without running the risks of a heart attack as long as the person is not hostile. The hostility component is a more accurate predictor of coronary heart disease than the more general notion of Type A behavior.

Fortunately, not all components of the Type A personality are harmful to health. People do not have to slow down, as long as they are not driven by hostility. Those who have many of the Type A traits without the toxic core that harms health and who are positive and enthusiastic

Autoimmune disorder A condition in which the immune system attacks the body.

Personality The whole of a person's behavioral characteristics.

Type A personality Sometimes referred to as "hurry sickness," a person who is hard-driving and competitive and also is hostile, angry, and suspicious; sometimes referred to as coronary-prone behavior.

Coronary-prone personality A hard-driving, competitive person who is also hostile, angry, suspicious, and at increased risk for heart attack; sometimes referred to as Type A personality.

Hostility An ongoing accumulation of anger and irritation; a permanent, deep-seated type of anger that hovers quietly until some trivial incident causes it to erupt.

Toxic core Type A personality traits most detrimental to health: anger, cynicism, suspiciousness, and excessive self-involvement.

- Make a contract with yourself to slow down and take it easy. Put it in writing. Post it in a conspicuous spot, then stick to the terms you set up. Be specific. Abstracts ("I'm going to be less uptight") don't work.
- Work on only one or two things at a time. Wait until you change one habit before you tackle the next one.
- Eat more slowly, and eat only when you are relaxed and sitting down.
- If you smoke, quit.
- Cut down on your caffeine intake, because it increases the tendency to become irritated and agitated.
- Take regular breaks throughout the day, even as brief as 5 or 10 minutes, when you totally change what you're doing. Get up, stretch, get a drink of cool water, walk around for a few minutes.
- Work on fighting your impatience. If you're standing in line at the grocery store, study the interesting things people have in their carts instead of getting upset.
- Work on controlling hostility. Keep a written log. When do you flare up? What causes it? How do you feel at the time? What preceded it? Look for patterns and figure out what sets you off. Then do something about it. Either avoid the situations that cause you hostility or practice reacting to them in different ways.
- Plan some activities just for the fun of it. Load a picnic basket in the car and drive to the country with a friend. After a stressful physics class, stop at a theater and see a good comedy.
- Choose a role model, someone you know and admire who does not have a Type A personality. Observe the person carefully, then try out some techniques the person demonstrates.

- Simplify your life so you can learn to relax a little bit. Figure out which activities or commitments you can eliminate right now, then get rid of them.
- If morning is a problem time for you and you get too hurried, set your alarm clock half an hour earlier.
- Take time out during even the most hectic day to do something truly relaxing. Because you won't be used to it, you may have to work at it at first. Begin by listing things you'd really enjoy that would calm you. Include some things that take only a few minutes: Watch a sunset, lie out on the lawn at night and look at the stars, call an old friend and catch up on news, take a nap, sauté a pan of mushrooms and savor them slowly.
- If you're under a deadline, take short breaks. Stop and talk to someone for 5 minutes, take a short walk, or lie down with a cool cloth over your eyes for 10 minutes.
- Pay attention to what your own body clock is saying. You've probably noticed that every 90 minutes or so, you lose the ability to concentrate, get a little sleepy, and have a tendency to daydream. Instead of fighting the urge, put down your work and let your mind wander for a few minutes. Use the time to imagine and let your creativity run wild.
- Learn to treasure unplanned surprises: a friend dropping by unannounced, a hummingbird outside your window, a child's tightly clutched bouquet of wildflowers.
- Savor your relationships. Think about the people in your life. Relax with them and give yourself to them. Give up trying to control others, and resist the urge to end relationships that don't always go as you'd like them to.

possess characteristics that can be protective, not harmful.

| THE RELAXED PERSONALITY | The relaxed personality type has been named **Type B personality**, because it is opposite from the Type A personality. The Type B personality is characterized as relaxed, easy-going, noncompetitive, and laid back. Type B people have little or no hostility. They are not as driven as the Type A and do not strive as hard to reach goals. This personality type has been associated with low levels of heart disease.

| THE CANCER-PRONE PERSONALITY | The **Type C personality** also has been called the **cancer-prone personality**. A set of personality traits exist that can dispose a person

to cancer. These people show little emotion, are ambivalent toward self and others, and have not developed a close attachment with their parents.

Earliest research on this subject found that the patients with the fastest-growing tumors were consistently serious, overly cooperative, overly nice, overanxious, painfully sensitive, passive, and apologetic.[12] Furthermore, they had been that way all their lives. The patients with the slow-growing tumors, on the other hand, had developed a way of coping with life's stresses.

Other studies confirmed these findings. Researchers noticed a disturbing pattern in the personalities of patients with melanoma, a particularly virulent form of skin cancer. These patients were nice—too nice. They were passive about everything, including their cancer.[13]

The results of this and other research led to the term Type C personality. The hallmark of the cancer personality is the nonexpression of emotion. Even when these people are experiencing tremendous despair, they characteristically bottle it up. Although other people often describe cancer patients as kind, sweet, and benign, this sweetness is really a mask they wear to conceal their feelings of anger, hurt, and hostility.

In this area, as in almost all other areas of medical research, the findings are inconsistent. Not every study finds a link between cancer and personality, and a few have found no relationship at all between the two. Others find that personality may play a role in either—but not both—developing cancer or its progression once the disease is established. Even with these inconsistencies,

however, leading researchers believe that enough evidence of a link between cancer and personality is present for them to take a hard look at the possibility.

| **THE DISTRESSED PERSONALITY** | Another type of personality that increases mortality is the distressed personality or the **Type D personality**, which is characterized by negative emotions and social inhibition. People who think negatively and isolate themselves from others have a greater chance for heart disease and are more prone to depression.

The distressed personality has been associated with the development of or exacerbation of ulcers. This personality is characterized by excessive dependence on others, low levels of social support, excessive worry, annoyance, and fear of common situations or circumstances, as well as frequent crises. Whereas other people are able to "bend" with stress, distressed people tend to "break." People with this trait may have the same number of stressful situations as others, but distressed people perceive the situations as being far more negative than do other people.[14]

EMOTIONAL STATES THAT AFFECT HEALTH

An emotion is a felt tendency to move toward something assessed as favorable or away from something assessed as unfavorable. The terms "emotions" and "feelings" are often used interchangeably. Emotions are normal and healthy, but sometimes the way we handle our feelings is not healthy. This section presents some common emotions and discusses healthy ways to react to them.

Anger

Anger is usually a temporary emotion that combines physiological and emotional arousal. It can range in severity all the way from intense rage to "cool" anger that doesn't really involve arousal at all (and might be defined more accurately as an "attitude," such as resentment). Although the terms "anger" and "hostility" (described later) are often used interchangeably,

Type B personality A person who is easy-going and generally free of hostility, anger, and suspicion.

Type C personality An emotionally nonexpressive person who demonstrates ambivalence and is at increased risk for cancer; sometimes referred to as cancer-prone personality.

Cancer-prone personality An emotionally nonexpressive person who demonstrates ambivalence and is at increased risk for cancer; sometimes called Type C personality.

Type D personality A distressed personality characterized by negative emotions, social inhibition, and isolation.

Anger A feeling of extreme hostility, indignation, or exasperation; rage.

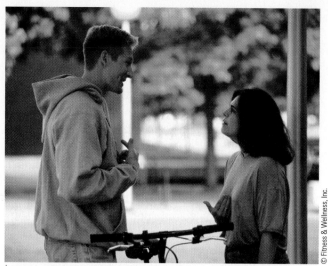
A person who is unable to manage anger is at particular risk for disease.

Mismanaged anger is perhaps the principal factor involved in predicting cardiovascular disease.[15] Volatile tempers are extremely dangerous. In a study of men, those who had difficulty controlling anger and who expressed anger in damaging ways had high blood pressure and high risk of heart disease. Another study showed that destructive ventilation of anger created problems including shame and guilt.[16] In addition, maladaptive responses to anger can result in hurtful or embarrassing behavior that is later regretted.[17]

Research also indicates a link between anger and cancer. The effect of anger on cancer may result from its effect on the immune system. In one study, volunteers were divided into two groups. One of the groups watched videos that produced feelings of caring and compassion; the other group were exposed to situations that resulted in anger and frustration. When their saliva was tested for signs of immune system activity, the people who had felt compassionate and caring had an increase in immunity. Those who had felt angry and frustrated had

they are not the same. Unlike anger, hostility is not a temporary emotion but, rather, an attitude expressed in aggressive behavior motivated by animosity and hatefulness.

To be healthy, people need to express anger appropriately, that is, at the right time and in a non-destructive manner. We need to confront the things that are making us angry and to work through the anger. Problems arise when anger is misdirected and when anger is expressed through miscommunication, emotional distancing, escalation of conflicts, rehearsing of grievances, assuming a hostile disposition, acquiring angry habits, making a bad situation worse, loss of self-esteem, and loss of the respect of others. Misdirected anger buries the real problem and creates more problems along the way.

> Expressing anger is healthy only if the expression itself is healthy.

Serious problems also result from suppressed anger. Bottling up anger can lead to many health consequences —among them heart disease, cancer, rheumatoid arthritis, hives, acne, psoriasis, peptic ulcer, epilepsy, migraine, and high blood pressure. Expressing anger is healthy, but it must be done in a way that does not cause damage or harm.

Chronic repression of anger has physical effects similar to those of chronic stress (see Chapter 3). One of the major physiological effects is the release of chemicals and hormones, principally adrenaline and noradrenaline, that affect proper heart functioning and the amount of constriction or dilation of the arteries. This situation is a large contributor to the development of arterial diseases.

PHYSIOLOGICAL REACTIONS ACCOMPANYING ANGER

This list includes physiological reactions to momentary and chronic anger. Monitor yourself for these symptoms. If anger is not managed, you may experience the effects of chronic anger.

Momentary Anger

changes in muscle tension	fatigue
scowling	jaws clenching
grinding of teeth	neck or jaw pain
glaring	ringing in the ears
clenching of fists	lower skin temperature
flushing	excessive sweating
goosebumps	skin redness
chills/shudders	hives
prickly sensations	itching
numbness	tension headache
choking	migraine headache
twitching	belching
sweating	hiccuping
losing self-control	diarrhea
feeling hot or cold	intestinal cramping

Chronic Anger

loss of appetite	peptic ulcers
frequent colds	chronic indigestion
acne	constipation

a drop in immunity that lasted for as long as 5 hours.[18] The angry, frustrated group also reported a variety of symptoms, including headaches, indigestion, muscle pain, and fatigue. The caring group reported feeling relaxation.

| Hostility |

Hostility comes from the Latin word *hostis*, which means "enemy." Simply stated, hostility is an ongoing accumulation of anger and irritation. It is a permanent kind of anger that shows itself in its response to trivial happenings. People experience real problems that warrant anger. But hostile people get equally angry about trivia and major injustices. Generally, a hostile person has an orientation toward hurting other people, either physically or verbally.

Hostile people typically have the following characteristics:[19]

- Even when they're smiling, they look uptight and tense; they appear ready to fight at a moment's notice.
- They have an intense need to win in sports and in games, even when other people are playing just for relaxation or fun.
- They are extremely sensitive to any perceived criticism against them but are loudly critical of others and of themselves.

- They argue incessantly, even over trivial issues. Every conversation becomes an angry debate, and they refuse to lose an argument.

Although almost everyone exhibits one or more of these traits occasionally, hostile people demonstrate them continuously. Life has become a sordid battle for them, and they charge into the fight armed with anger and irritation.

Through his research, Redford Williams has isolated what he believes to be the most harmful traits associated with hostility. These include cynical beliefs that others are inherently bad, selfish, mean, and not to be trusted; frequent angry feelings when these negative expectations are fulfilled; and overt expression of those angry feelings in aggressive acts directed toward others. The effects of hostility are especially devastating to the body for two reasons:

1. Hostility causes a continuous release of hormones that destroy health in a variety of ways.
2. Hostility weakens the branch of the nervous system designed to calm down the body after an emergency.

In essence, a hostile person goes throughout the entire day in a stressed condition. Many hostile people don't even get relief while sleeping: Stress hormones are secreted 24 hours a day.

Hostility (like stress or fear) causes the body to release of a sequence of stress hormones including epinephrine, norepinephrine, cortisol, prolactin, and testosterone. Blood pressure increases, the heart beats harder and faster, blood volume increases, blood moves from the skin and organs to the brain and muscles, the liver releases stored sugar, and breathing speeds up. Those reactions in themselves are not harmful if they happen only occasionally and if the body can use physical activity to dispel the chemicals. With hostility, neither is the case—the body is not allowed to recover from the stress. Hostility overcomes the body's built-in calming mechanism.

The autonomic nervous system has two main branches:

1. the "emergency branch," which pumps out hormones and prepares the body to respond in case of emergency, and
2. the "calming branch" (the parasympathetic branch), which switches off the hormones when the emergency is over. The calming branch soothes the body, preventing it from remaining in an aroused state too long, which can result in disease.

Hostility weakens the parasympathetic (calming) branch of the nervous system. The body therefore does

Hostility can be overcome. Here are some ways to do it:

- This may sound too simple, but when you realize you're feeling hostile, tell yourself to stop. You might have to shout it aloud at first. Later, as you get better at it, you can change to a silent command.

- Talk to yourself about how you're feeling. Evaluate the situation. Figure out why you're so upset. Decide whether your anger and hostility are justified. If they aren't, give them up. If they are (and in many cases they are), figure out another way to respond to the situation—one that won't fuel your fire.

- Don't let yourself get trampled. If your anger is justified, deal with it calmly and rationally. Stand up for yourself. Work to correct a wrong. If a classmate fails to recognize your contribution on an important project, for example, don't just blow up and seethe with hostility. Talk to the professor, set the record straight, and spell out what you did toward the project. Then confront your classmate calmly and express your feelings. Ask for a specific commitment (for instance, that he or she will explain to the professor what you did to help).

- Learn to trust other people. This might be hard at first, and, strange as it sounds, you might have to practice. Start with a minor situation in which you usually take control. Then let someone else be in charge. As you learn that others can be capable, you will gradually learn to trust other people more.

- Be tolerant and nonjudgmental of others. The source of anger and hostility is often our response to someone else. Put yourself in the other's shoes. Consider the situation from the other's point of view. Even if you still think you're right, you might gain empathy for that person that will allow you to deal with the situation free of hostility.

- Cut down on things that speed up your system, cause your body to churn out hormones, and lead to physical stress. These include sugar, caffeine, nicotine, and the hidden sources of caffeine such as soft drinks, chocolate, and many over-the-counter and prescription drugs.

- If all else fails, distract yourself. If you're caught in traffic, turn on the radio. Start singing. Visualize the last concert you went to. Do something to take your thoughts off the situation that is getting you riled up.

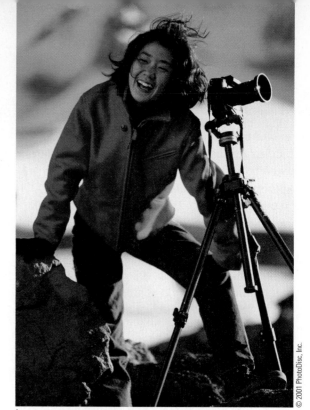

A positive level of self-esteem supports health.

© 2001 PhotoDisc, Inc.

not recover from the surge of stress hormones, calming does not occur, and the body remains in a state of prolonged, harmful arousal.

One of the most pronounced effects of hostility is heart disease. Hostility is now known to be an independent risk factor for coronary heart disease.[20] Heart-harming hostility is characterized by tendency toward anger, resentment, and suspicion. It is also marked by explosive and vigorous vocal mannerisms, competitiveness, impatience, and irritability.

Hostility has been shown to cause coronary blockages, coronary heart disease, and coronary death; to contribute significantly to a second heart attack; and to lead to the premature death of people with existing heart disease.[21] Hostility is also a significant factor in determining which heart attack patients will have a second heart attack. In addition, hostile people who seek revenge are much more likely to have another heart attack than hostile people who are less retributional. Assessment 2-2 covers the issue of hostility.

Perfectionism

Upholding high standards and striving to reach challenging goals are healthy behaviors. However, the compulsive pursuit of unrealistically high standards for yourself and those around you is unhealthy and has been labeled perfectionism.[22] One example of perfectionism is the student who begins exercising to improve her health, then finds herself exercising and dieting excessively in the pursuit of an ideal body.

Perfectionism can actually hinder academic and other performance. Some people who are perfectionistic have an obsessive attention to detail. A perfectionist may spend hours straightening out his desk but miss project deadlines. Procrastination often results from perfectionism.

TABLE 2.1 CHARACTERISTICS OF EMOTIONALLY HEALTHY PEOPLE VERSUS EMOTIONALLY UNHEALTHY PEOPLE

Emotionally Healthy People	Emotionally Unhealthy People
Have high self-esteem.	Have low self-esteem.
Are confident that their behavior is normal.	Guess at what normal behavior is.
Are honest.	Often lie when it would be just as easy to tell the truth.
Accept themselves.	Judge themselves without mercy.
Can have fun.	Have difficulty having fun.
Don't take themselves too seriously.	Take themselves very seriously.
Recognize that other people can enhance their lives but are not the sole source of their happiness.	Are certain their happiness hinges on others.
Can have intimate relationships.	Have unusual difficulty with intimate relationships.
Do not try to control things beyond their control.	Try to control things they cannot control.
Are able to affirm themselves.	Constantly seek approval and affirmation from others.
Communicate openly and assertively about their needs and wants.	Communicate indirectly and try to meet their needs using aggressiveness or manipulation.
Usually feel they are similar to other people.	Usually feel they are different from other people.
Take responsibility appropriately, but do not take too much responsibility for others.	Are super-responsible or super-irresponsible.
Give loyalty when it is appropriate and deserved.	Are extremely loyal, even when loyalty is undeserved.
Consider consequences before acting.	Act impulsively without considering consequences.
Deal with emotional pain by feeling it and expressing it.	Deal with emotional pain by resorting to addictions and compulsive behaviors.
Continue to mature mentally, emotionally, and spiritually throughout their lives.	Tend to remain immature; their mental, emotional, and spiritual growth is blocked.
Live with balance, not extremes.	Live lives that are punctuated by extremes.
Validate and acknowledge their observations, feelings, and reactions.	Invalidate and repress their observations, feelings, and reactions.
Attend to their physical and psychological needs.	Neglect their needs.
Disclose family problems when appropriate.	Hide family or other secrets.
Refuse to tolerate inappropriate behavior.	Have a high tolerance for inappropriate behavior.
Feel emotional pain; are able to grieve when they suffer.	Are unable to grieve losses to completion.
Cope with stress in positive ways, so are not prone to stress-related illnesses.	Are prone to stress-related illnesses.

Sources: Adapted from J. G. Woititz, *Adult Children of Alcoholics* (Deerfield Beach, FL: Health Communications, 1983); R. Hemfelt, F. Minirth, and P. Meier, *Love Is a Choice* (Nashville, TN: Thomas Nelson, 1989), pp. 9–16.

Some people put off projects because they fear they will make a mistake.

Perfectionism can hinder relationships with others. The fear of making a mistake might lead you to take so much time proofreading a paper that you neglect other important matters. For instance, if you rigidly hold others to unrealistic standards, you can project negative feelings when they fail to meet your expectations.

Self-Esteem

People who are emotionally healthy have high levels of self-esteem; they know and like themselves. Such people know they are not perfect, but they know how to cherish their positive qualities and are working to improve their negative traits. Table 2.1 lists characteristics of emotionally healthy and unhealthy people.

Self-esteem is so crucial for emotional health that some psychologists use attitudes toward the self as criteria for evaluating mental health.[23] Poor self-esteem is closely linked with alcoholism, drug abuse, crime and violence, child abuse, teenage pregnancy, prostitution, welfare dependency, and failure of children to learn. High self-esteem facilitates emotional growth and helps those around you. People who take care of themselves have more energy to offer their families, friends, and society.

Worry and Anxiety

Worry is a state in which we dwell on something so much it causes us to become apprehensive. **Anxiety** is the psychological and

Worry A state in which we dwell on something so much that we become apprehensive.

Anxiety A state of intense worry that is not grounded in reality.

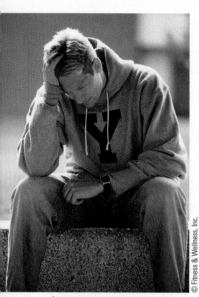

| Worry may trigger or increase the stress response. |

physiological response to worry. Anxiety causes physical changes, such as a racing pulse and fast breathing. Worry is the thinking part of anxiety.

Anxiety often translates into negative physical symptoms. These physical changes can impair the immune system and result in physical illness. Worry and anxiety have been shown to affect the heart and the circulatory system as a whole, causing irregular heartbeat, high blood pressure, and various abnormalities involving the arteries.[24] Strong connections exist among our thoughts and feelings and heart health.[25] Worry and anxiety can cause the body to produce the chemical acetylcholine, which causes the airways to contract and can result in asthma.

One specific kind of worry, uncertainty, has been shown to create a particularly devastating kind of stress. Uncertainty keeps a person in a constant state of semi-arousal, putting an extreme burden on the body's adaptive resources and resistance systems. The result is often disease, particularly gastrointestinal disease.

When worry and anxiety escalate, the outcome is **fear**. Fear causes the heart to race, the head to spin, the palms to sweat, the knees to buckle, and breathing to become labored. Fear causes the body to secrete adrenaline, which has a powerful effect on the heart. Both the rate and strength of heart contractions increase, and blood pressure rises. The body is stimulated in turn to release other hormones. If the fear is intense enough, all systems can be overloaded fatally.

| Depression |

Depression is much more than an occasional sad mood. Depression is characterized by a low energy state: the person feels apathetic, hopeless, and withdrawn from others. A depressed person does less and less, loses interest in people, abandons hobbies, and gives up in school or work. An estimated 10 to 14 million Americans suffer from depression at any given time.[26] To determine if you are depressed, see Assessment 2-3.

Depression is sometimes caused by the loss of something valued or someone important. It might occur in response to the death of a loved one, divorce, aging, diagnosis of serious illness, automobile accident, termination of employment, retirement, or children leaving home. Under those circumstances, feeling sad or discouraged is normal.

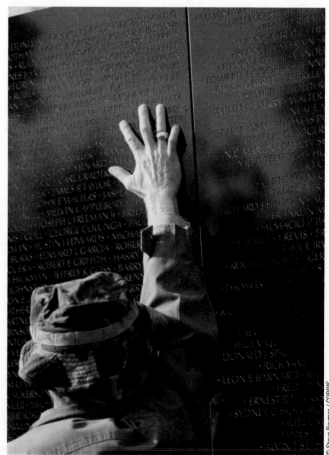

| To become free of pain, one may have to go through it. |

All losses evoke what is called the grief process. To maintain emotional health, it is beneficial to allow yourself to feel the pain and share your sadness with safe and supportive others. This permits completion of the grieving process and enables you to become free of it. If people do not learn how to complete this process, they accumulate lifetimes of unresolved grief. This is unhealthy.

Five stages of grief that people typically experience with loss are the following:

- Denial—"No, it can't be!"
- Anger—"Why me? I don't deserve this!"
- Bargaining—"I'll do anything; just let this not happen."
- Depression—withdrawal, loss of hope. "I'll never get over this."
- Acceptance—"I can make it."
- Hope for the future—"I can move on now."

Many people do not necessarily go through these stages in the sequence described. The grief process is different for everyone. However, anyone who represses such feelings associated with losses carries a heavy load of unresolved, lifelong grief in the form of chronic

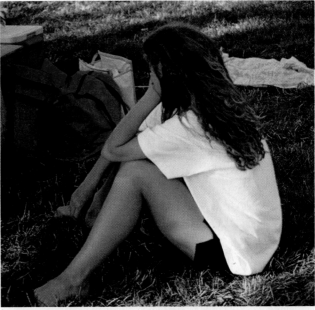

Depression can range from a mild case of the blues to severe clinical depression.

anxiety, tension, fear, anger, resentment, emptiness, confusion, or shame.[27] Learning to go through the pain is a way to be free of it.

In some cases depression is caused by biological factors—a chemical imbalance in the brain, a physical illness, a disturbance in the nervous system or neurotransmitters, or an injury involving brain tissue. These cases require medical attention; a variety of antidepressant drugs are available for treatment.[28]

Other characteristics of depression may not be as obvious but can have even more profound effects. During depression, the body undergoes hormonal and chemical changes similar to those of stress. However, the mechanisms that normally regulate the stress response fail in depressed people. In addition to having high levels of the hormones usually associated with stress, depressed people have significantly lower levels of three important brain chemicals—norepinephrine, dopamine, and serotonin, the chemicals that make us feel good.

Depression can increase mortality in some obvious ways. Severe depression, for example, can lead to suicide. Most people who commit suicide suffer from deep despair, loneliness, and hopelessness. They feel that their lives are completely out of their control and that the only way they can regain control is to take their lives. Suicide among young people is an epidemic problem. Signs of depression that may warn of impending suicide include:

- Withdrawal from friends; cessation of hobbies and activities.

HEART DISEASE AND DEPRESSION

Each year in the United States, mild or major depression affects 50 percent of the people who survive a heart attack, and up to 40 percent of the nation's 350,000 heart-bypass patients.

Until recently, few doctors treated their patients' minds after they treated their hearts. It's now known that patients who aren't treated for depression are at far greater risk for a second heart attack and death.

At highest risk for post-cardiac depression are women (who often outlive their husbands and have to face illness alone), people with a history of depression, and people who are socially isolated or recently bereaved.

Memory loss—a common but temporary side effect of heart surgery—also can trigger depression. Symptoms to watch for include lethargy, sleeplessness, and weight changes.

Source: National Institutes of Health, Hope Heart Institute.

Fear A state of escalated worry and apprehension that causes distinct physical and emotional reactions.

HOW TO RELIEVE DEPRESSION

If your depression is caused by biological factors, you need medical help. If your depression is mild or your physician rules out biological factors, try these coping measures:

- Start by admitting you are depressed, then try to figure out why. Once you have identified a cause, you might be able to eliminate it.
- As much as you can, stick to your normal routine. Change, even positive change, is a source of stress and can intensify depression.
- If you can, plan some quiet times each day when you can relax, pamper yourself, do something you enjoy, or just get away from stresses you might feel. If you've been feeling depressed for a while, you might start by actually making a list of things you'd like to do: Read the newest book on the best-selling list, take a watercolor class, travel to a new area.
- Find a confidant, someone you can talk to about your feelings. If you're lucky, you'll find someone who will listen without judging or giving advice. Whatever you do, don't choose another depressed person as your confidant. You'll only end up dragging each other down.
- Do something you're good at: Write an essay for a literary magazine, enter a local bicycle race, volunteer to play the piano at a local retirement center, ask your landlord if you can plant flowers around your apartment building. You'll get an immediate boost.
- Get regular exercise. Studies have shown that exercise is one of the best ways to conquer depression. Exercise causes the body to produce endorphins, natural painkillers that result in a "high" for people who exercise longer than 30 minutes. Plan an activity you enjoy, something you can do regardless of the weather, and something for which you have the equipment.
- Whatever you do, don't try to get rid of depression by using alcohol or drugs. They only make things worse.

- Slackening of interest in schoolwork and decline in grades.
- Not caring what happens, good or bad; passive behaviors.
- Feeling bad about oneself, pessimistic, and helpless.
- Ceasing to groom oneself or care for one's room, possessions, or clothes.
- Ceasing to meet responsibilities (pay bills, return phone calls, or answer the phone).
- Changes in eating or sleeping habits, alcohol or drug use.

- Abrupt changes in personality; aggressive, hostile behavior or impulsiveness; sudden mood swings.
- Anxiety at times of separation.
- Inability to concentrate.
- Refusal to leave the room or the bed.
- Obsession with death; a death wish.

To help someone if you suspect an imminent suicide attempt, take the person seriously and get involved. Don't wait to see what develops, because tomorrow may be too late. Do not be afraid to ask outright if the person is planning suicide. The two most important actions to take if a person seems on the verge of making a suicide attempt are

- Phone a suicide hotline or crisis intervention center immediately. They will be able to help. Dial 911, the operator, or the police.
- Stay with the person until help arrives.

In addition to the increased risk of suicide among depressed people, depression can shorten life in other ways. Studies of depressed people show that people who are depressed have significantly higher mortality rates than people who are not depressed.[29] Depression can become a potent risk factor in determining whether a person will die sooner than expected, either of natural causes or of underlying disease.

Depression consistently predicts poor health outcomes.[30] A relationship appears to exists between depression and self-rated physical health. People who are depressed tend to believe their physical health is poor, even when physical exams show no clinically-defined illness.[31]

Depression impairs the immune system in a variety of ways, one of the most significant being its impact on the immune cells that assist the body in its surveillance against tumors and its resistance to viral disease. Natural killer cell activity is impaired in people who are depressed, and the more severe the depression, the greater this impairment.

Other components of the immune system are crippled by depression as well. Depression causes a striking reduction in white blood cells, an upset in the ratio of helper and suppressor cells, and overall suppression of immune function.

The hormones triggered by depression—especially cortisol and norepinephrine—have significant damaging effects on the heart. Norepinephrine speeds up heart rate, encourages blood clotting (which can

> Depression is one of the most common complications of heart disease.

lead to heart attack), increases the level of harmful cholesterol in the blood, and impairs the heart's ability to adapt when demands increase. The cortisol that is produced during depression leads to a particularly dangerous kind of irregular heartbeat and encourages fat storage around the abdomen (another risk factor for heart disease). Depression increases the risk of heart disease and worsens the outcomes for people who already have heart disease.[32]

As the relationships between depression and heart disease become more clear, physicians are beginning to recognize the importance of treating depression with cognitive therapy.[33] They increasingly recommend behavioral counseling to reduce heart disease risk, improve quality of life, and increase survival.

HARDINESS

Certain groups of people enjoy remarkably good health and longevity. One of the most important concepts in staying well is **hardiness**. The personality traits of hardiness are the "three Cs": commitment, control, and challenge.

> Two big causes of stress are unrealistic expectations we place on ourselves and unrealistic expectations we place on others.

Commitment entails a commitment to yourself, your work, your family, and the other important values in your life. This is not a fleeting involvement, but a deep and enduring interest. People who are committed are involved with their work and their families, possess a

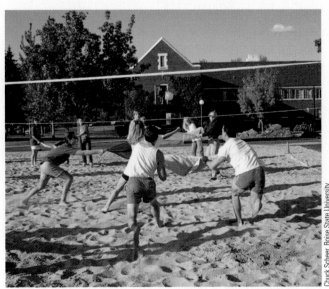

Chuck Scheer, Boise State University

Hardy people are characterized by "three Cs": commitment, control, and challenge.

belief that their lives have meaning, and have a pervasive sense of direction in their lives.

Control is a belief that one can influence the aversiveness of an event. It is a belief that you can cushion the hurtful impact of a situation by the way you look at it and react to it. The kind of control that keeps a person healthy is the opposite of helplessness. It is the firm belief that you can influence how you will react and the willingness to act on that basis. It is the refusal to be victimized.

Control does not mean controlling your environment, your circumstances, or other people. That kind of an attitude leads to illness, not health. The control that keeps you healthy is a belief that you can control yourself and your reactions to what life hands you.

People with this trait cope with problems in a direct

Hardiness A set of personality traits marked by commitment, control, and challenge.

> **One of the biggest foes of human happiness is boredom.**

manner. When faced with difficulties, they use active strategies to either change the way they think about a problem or attempt to resolve the issues by dealing directly with a problem.[34] The healthiest students approach problem-solving with a sense of control instead of passivity.[35] People who believe they have little or no control over their health and their lives are less likely to take positive actions and are more likely to be depressed and anxious. The healthiest and hardiest people are those who focus on what they can control and ignore the rest. They believe every problem has a solution through skill, planning, and diligent attention to detail.

Challenge means the ability to see change as an opportunity for growth and excitement. Excitement is critical, because boredom puts people at a high risk for disease. People who are challenged constructively are healthier. One of the biggest foes of human happiness is boredom.

A person who is not healthy and hardy views change with helplessness and alienation. A healthy, hardy person, in contrast, faces change with confidence, self-determination, eagerness, and excitement. Change becomes an eagerly sought-after challenge, not a threat.

All of these characteristics come into play when illness threatens. Illness is often preceded by a series of events. First, a person perceives a distressing life situation. For whatever reason, he or she is not able to resolve the distressing situation effectively. As a result, the person feels helpless and anxious. Those feelings of helplessness weaken the immune system and resistance to disease, and the person becomes more vulnerable to disease-causing agents that are always in the environment.

The traits of a disease-resistant personality, which includes the 3Cs, interrupt this cycle and, therefore, help prevent illness. This personality trait has also been labeled emotional intelligence. Emotionally intelligent people remain positive, even under adverse circumstances.[36] Healthy people and ill people view things in entirely different ways. For example, healthy people tend to maintain reasonable personal control in their lives. If a problem crops up, they look for resources and try out solutions. If one doesn't work, they try another one. People who are frequently ill, on the other hand, leave decisions up to others and try to get other people to solve their problems. Their approach tends to be passive.

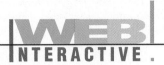
WEB INTERACTIVE.

WEB ACTIVITIES

■ **Dr. Koop—Mental Health Site** This comprehensive site features reliable information on a variety of mental health topics, including depression, stress, attention deficit disorder, phobias, post-traumatic stress disorder, medications, as well as interactive self-assessment tools for depression and stress.
http://www.drkoop.com/wellness/mental_health

■ **World Health Organization Mental Health** This comprehensive site features a wealth of information on mental and neurological topics. Some of the topics include global statistical information on depression, suicide, and women's mental health.
http://www.who.int/mental_health

■ **The Mind-Body Connection: Granny Was Right** This interesting site, sponsored by the University of Rochester Medical Center, describes research involving the physiological link between the mind and the body.
http://www.rochester.edu/pr/Review/V59N3/feature2.html

■ **Do You have a "Type A" Personality?** This site features 17 questions designed to determine if you have characteristics of a "Type A" personality.
http://www.queendom.com/typea2.html

InfoTrac
You can find additional readings related to wellness via InfoTrac College Edition, an on-line library of more than 900 journals and publications. Follow the instructions for accessing InfoTrac that came packaged with your textbook, then search for articles using a key word search.

Suggested Reading Alan Doris, Klaus Ebmeier, and Polash Shajahan, "Depressive Illness," *The Lancet* 354, no. 9187 (Oct. 16, 1999): 1369.

1. What constitutes depressive symptoms that are pathological?
2. Describe the relative contributions of genetics and environment in relation to the cause and pathophysiology of major depressive illness.
3. In the treatment of depression, what are some of the pharmacologic and alternative forms of therapy?

Web Activity

Depression Screening Test

http://www.depression-screening.org/index.htm

Sponsor National Mental Health Association

Description This interactive site features a series of confidential multiple-choice questions designed to assess whether you are suffering from depression.

Available Activities Review the following site features:

1. A confidential depression screening test
2. Several links dealing with depression, including depression symptoms and treatments, "Depression can affect anyone" link, personal stories, education and advocacy opportunities, as well as sources of help

Web Work

1. From the home page, click on the violet box entitled "Confidential Screening Test."
2. Honestly answer the series of ten multiple-choice questions.
3. Once the questionnaire is completed, the site automatically provides you with a personal analysis

and recommendations if your answers suggest that you might be suffering from clinical depression.

Helpful Hints

1. This site's strong disclaimer informs the user that on-line screening tests are *not* intended to provide a diagnosis for clinical depression, but they *may* help identify any depressive symptoms and determine whether a further evaluation by a medical or mental health professional is necessary. As with any other illness, you should see your doctor if you think you might have symptoms of depression.
2. After completing the test and receiving your recommendations, you should also click on the "Follow-up Survey" link to answer a question regarding what you plan to do with these results. Choices include calling 911 or seeking professional help.

For additional Web activities, links, and suggested readings, visit our Health, Fitness, and Wellness Resource Center at http://health.wadsworth.com.

NOTES

1. R. Ader et al., "Behaviorally Conditioned Immunosuppression," *Psychosomatic Medicine* 37 (1975).
2. "Research Documents the Mind-Body Connection," *Canyon Ranch Roundup* 17 (June/July 1997): 1.
3. "Health's Character," *Psychology Today* (December 1988): 28; Hans J. Eysenck, "Personality, Stress, and Cancer: Prediction and Prophylaxis," *British Journal of Medical Psychology* 61 (March 1988): 57–75.
4. I. Deary et al., "Personality Traits and Personality Disorders," *British Journal of Psychology* 89 (November 1998): 647.
5. "Is Personality Related to Illness? Cluster Profiles of Aggregated Data," *Advances* 3 (Spring 1986): 4–15.
6. J. Denollet et al., "Personality as Independent Predictor of Long-Term Mortality in Patients with Coronary Heart Disease," *The Lancet* 347 (February 17, 1996): 417–421.

7. L. Karlberg et al., "Is There a Connection Between Car Accidents, Near Accidents, and Type A Drivers?," *Behavioral Medicine* 24 (Fall 1998): 99; N. Koivula et al., "Type A/B Behavior Pattern and Athletic Participation: Attitudes and Actual Behavior," *Journal of Sport Behavior* 21 (June 1998): 148–166.
8. *The Trusting Heart: Great News About Type A Behavior* (New York: Times Books, Division of Random House, 1989).
9. R. M. Sunin, "The Cardiac Stress Management Program for Type A Patients," *Cardiac Rehabilitation* 5 (1975): 13–15.
10. M. Angell, "Disease as a Reflection of the Psyche," *New England Journal of Medicine* 312 (1985): 1570–1572.
11. A. Moller et al., "Effects of a Group Rational-Emotive Behavior Therapy Program on the Type A Behavior Pattern," *Psychological Reports* 78 (June 1996): 947–961.

12. S. Locke and D. Colligan, *The Healer Within: The New Medicine of Mind and Body* (New York: E. P. Dutton, 1986).
13. "Is There an Ulcer Personality?" *The Wellness Newsletter*, (July 1987): 2; The Editors of Prevention Magazine, *Take Control of Your Life: A Complete Guide to Stress Relief* (Emmaus, PA: Rodale Press, 1988).
14. See note 13.
15. I. Kawachi et al., "A Prospective Study of Anger and Coronary Heart Disease. The Normative Aging Study," *Circulation* 94 (November 1, 1996): 2090–2095.
16. J. Tangney et al., "Relation of Shame and Guilt to Constructive Versus Destructive Responses to Anger Across the Lifespan," *Journal of Personality and Social Psychology* 70 (April 1996): 797–809.
17. R. DeRubeis et al., "Medications Versus Cognitive Behavior Therapy for Severely Depressed Outpatients: Mega-Analysis of Four Randomized Comparisons," *American Journal of Psychiatry* 156 (July 1999): 1007–1013.

18. G. Rein et al., "The Physiological and Psychological Effects of Compassion and Anger," *Journal of Advancement in Medicine* 8 (1995): 87–105.

19. J. Arenofsky, "Anger: How to Cool It," *Current Health 2*, no. 22 (February 1996): 16–17.

20. C. E. Thoresen, "The Hostility Habit: A Serious Health Problem?" *Healthline* (April 1984): 5.

21. "Hostility, Anger, and Heart Disease," *Drug Therapy* (August 1986): 43.

22. M. Antony, "Being Perfect Can be Very Dangerous to Your Health," *Health* (December 1999): 3–4.

23. B.J. Mushinski-Fulk, Training Positive Attitudes: "I Tried Hard and Did Well," *Journal of School Health* (March 1991): 141–142.

24. "Hearts and Minds, Part I," *Harvard Mental Health Letter* 14 (July 1997): 1–3.

25. "What Triggers Heart Trouble?," *Harvard Heart Letter* 6 (July 1996): 5–6.

26. K. Wells et al., "Impact of Disseminating Quality Improvement Programs for Depression in Managed Primary Care: A Randomized Controlled Trial," *The Journal of the American Medical Association* 283 (January 12, 2000): 212–218.

27. N. Eisenberg, "Emotion, Regulation, and Moral Development," *Annual Review of Psychology* (Annual 2000): 665–675.

28. J. Stephenson, "Treating Depression," *The Journal of the American Medical Association* 281 (May 19, 1999): 1784.

29. "Heart Disease: The Mind-Body Connection," *Johns Hopkins Medical Letter* (July 1997): 4.

30. M. Whooley et al., "Depression, Falls, and Risk of Fracture in Older Women," *Archives of Internal Medicine* 159 (March 8, 1999): 484–490.

31. C. Leibson et al., "The Role of Depression in the Association Between Self-Related Physical Health and Clinically Defined Illness," *The Gerontologist* 39 (June 1999): 291–298.

32. "Heart Disease: The Mind-Body Connection," *Johns Hopkins Medical Letter* (July 1997): 5.

33. F. Lesperance et al., "Negative Emotions and Coronary Heart Disease: Getting to the Heart of the Matter," *The Lancet* 347 (February 17, 1996): 414–415.

34. L. Lengua et al., "Self-regulation as a Moderator of the Relation Between Coping and Symptomatology in Children of Divorce," *Journal of Abnormal Child Psychology* 24 (December 1996): 681–701.

35. C. Magai, "Personality Change in Adulthood: Loci of Change and the Role of Interpersonal Process," *International Journal of Aging and Human Development* 49 (December 1999): 339–352.

36. J. O'Neil, "On Emotional Intelligence: A Conversation with Daniel Goleman," *Educational Leadership* 54 (September 1996): 6–11.

DO YOU CULTIVATE EMOTIONAL WELL-BEING?

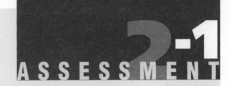

Name: _____ Date: _____ Grade: _____

Instructor: _____ Course: _____ Section: _____

Try answering these questions to get an idea. Don't take your score too seriously; this is just for fun.

1. I spend time doing work that I enjoy.
   a. almost always
   b. sometimes
   c. almost never

2. I find it easy to relax.
   a. almost always
   b. sometimes
   c. almost never

3. In my spare time, I participate in activities that I enjoy.
   a. almost always
   b. sometimes
   c. almost never

4. When I am about to be in a stressful situation, I realize it ahead of time, and I prepare for it.
   a. almost always
   b. sometimes
   c. almost never.

5. I handle anger:
   a. by expressing it in ways that hurt neither myself nor other people
   b. by bottling it up so that no one knows I'm angry
   c. I never am angry, or I express my anger aggressively

6. I participate with group organizations such as school, sports, church, or community activities.
   a. quite often
   b. very seldom
   c. never

7. I find it easy to express my feelings.
   a. almost always
   b. sometimes
   c. almost never

8. I can talk to close friends, relatives, or others about personal matters.
   a. almost always
   b. sometimes
   c. almost never

9. When I need help with personal matters, I seek it out.
   a. almost always
   b. sometimes
   c. almost never

10. When I am under stress, I make extra sure to exercise regularly, to work off my tension.
    a. almost always
    b. sometimes
    c. almost never

For each *a* answer, give yourself 2 points; for each *b* answer, give yourself 1 point; for each *c* answer, give yourself 0 points. A score of 18 to 20 is excellent; 16 or 17 is very good; 14 or 15 is good; and 13 or below means that you need improvement.

Source: Adapted from U.S. Department of Health and Human Services, *Health Style*, HHS publication no. (PHS) 81-50155, 1981 (a self-test distributed by National Health Information Clearinghouse).

HOSTILITY COULD HARM YOUR HEART

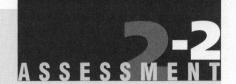

Name: _____   Date: _____   Grade: _____

Instructor: _____   Course: _____   Section: _____

Experts now conclude that feelings of hostility increase your risk of heart disease. Dr. Redford Williams, Duke University Medical Center, has designed a questionnaire to help you determine whether you have a hostile personality. Circle the answer that most closely fits how you would respond to the given situation:

1. A teen-ager drives by my yard blasting the car stereo:

   A. I begin to understand why teen-agers can't hear.
   B. I can feel my blood pressure starting to rise.

2. A boyfriend/girlfriend calls at the last minute "too tired to go out tonight." I'm stuck with two $15 tickets:

   A. I find someone else to go with.
   B. I tell my friend how inconsiderate he/she is.

3. Waiting in the express checkout line at the supermarket where a sign says "No More Than 10 Items Please":

   A. I pick up a magazine and pass the time.
   B. I glance to see if anyone has more than 10 items.

4. Most homeless people in large cities:

   A. Are down and out because they lack ambition.
   B. Are victims of illness or some other misfortune.

5. At times when I've been very angry with someone:

   A. I was able to stop short of hitting him/her.
   B. I have, on occasion, hit or shoved him/her.

6. When I am stuck in a traffic jam:

   A. I am usually not particularly upset.
   B. I quickly start to feel irritated and annoyed.

7. When there's a really important job to be done:

   A. I prefer to do it myself.
   B. I am apt to call on my friends to help.

8. The cars ahead of me start to slow and stop as they approach a curve:

   A. I assume there is a construction site ahead.
   B. I assume someone ahead had a fender-bender.

9. An elevator stops too long above where I'm waiting:

   A. I soon start to feel irritated and annoyed.
   B. I start planning the rest of my day.

10. When a friend or co-worker disagrees with me:

    A. I try to explain my position more clearly.
    B. I am apt to get into an argument with him or her.

11. When I was really angry in the past:

    A. I have never thrown things or slammed a door.
    B. I've sometimes thrown things or slammed a door.

12. Someone bumps into me in a store:

    A. I pass it off as an accident.
    B. I feel irritated at their clumsiness.

13. When my spouse/significant other is fixing a meal:

    A. I keep an eye out to make sure nothing burns.
    B. I talk about my day or read the paper.

14. Someone is hogging the conversation at a party:

    A. I look for an opportunity to put him/her down.
    B. I soon move to another group.

15. In most arguments:

    A. I am the angrier one.
    B. The other person is angrier than I am.

Score one point for each of these answers: 1. B, 2. B, 3. B, 4. A, 5. B, 6. B, 7. A, 8. B, 9. A, 10. B, 11. B, 12. B, 13. A, 14. A, 15. A. If you scored 4 or more points you may be hostile. Questions 1, 6, 9, 12, and 15 reflect anger. Questions 2, 5, 10, 11, and 14 reflect aggression. Questions 3, 4, 7, 8, and 13 reflect cynicism. If you scored 2 points in any category, you should work on that area of your personality.

From Redford B. Williams and Virginia Williams, *Anger Kills: 17 Strategies*. Copyright © 1993 by Redford B. Williams, M.D., and Virginia Williams, Ph.D. Reprinted by permission of Times Books, a division of Random House, Inc.

HOW WELL DO YOU EXPRESS RESENTMENTS?

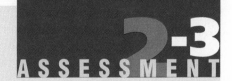

Name: _____   Date: _____   Grade: _____

Instructor: _____   Course: _____   Section: _____

This is a measure of how assertive or aggressive you are. (Some items may not apply to you. Try to imagine that they do.)

1. Your mother has emphasized that she wants you with the family at six o'clock today. At five o'clock, a friend invites you to a get-together you can't refuse. You:
   a. Go with your friend, stay through six, and explain to your mother later.
   b. Call your mother and tell her that you will be going with your friend.
   c. Complain to your mother that she is too demanding, but stay home.
   d. Tell your friend you can't go, and say nothing to your mother.

2. Several of your friends and you studied together for a test. All of your friends got good grades. You wrote the same kinds of answers on the test but got a low grade. You think your work was just as good as theirs. You:
   a. Write an anonymous note to the instructor's supervisor saying that the test grades are obviously unfair.
   b. Take your test to the instructor and ask why your grade was low.
   c. Complain to all your friends, and say nothing to the instructor.
   d. Keep your mouth shut so that the instructor won't be even more unfair to you the next time.

3. You have just cleaned up the kitchen area. The next person puts a greasy frying pan on the countertop and starts to leave. You:
   a. Wait until you are alone, and then put the greasy frying pan between the bedsheets, where the person will be sure to find it.
   b. Tell the person, "Please wash your frying pan before you leave."
   c. Make a general remark about inconsiderate people who leave dirty dishes for others to clean.
   d. Say nothing, and wash it yourself later.

4. You are on your first date with someone you have admired from a distance for a long time. At the end of the evening, the other person gets much more sexual than you want to be. You:
   a. Back off, and leave as quickly as you can without saying anything.
   b. Tell the other person that things are going too far for you.
   c. Keep pulling away, and let the other person guess the message.
   d. Say nothing and go along, because you want to date the person again.

5. You get home with a newly bought bag of groceries, only to find that the chicken you bought is already spoiled in the package. You:
   a. Storm back into the store and make a scene, so that all the other customers will know you were sold some rotten chicken.
   b. Go back to the store, ask to see the manager, and explain that the chicken you just bought is spoiled.
   c. Never shop in that store again.
   d. Do nothing.

6. You are in your room, studying for a big exam. Your neighbor is playing the stereo loudly. You:
   a. Knock on your neighbor's door, walk in, and switch off the stereo.
   b. Ask your neighbor to turn down the volume, and explain why.
   c. Go someplace else to study, and never speak to your neighbor again.
   d. Give up and stop trying to study.

7. Your friends like horror movies, but you don't enjoy them at all. Your friends are making plans to see the latest horror movie this Saturday night. You:
   a. Tell them you think horror movies are for mental midgets, and you're not going.
   b. Tell them you don't enjoy horror movies and ask if they'd consider another movie.
   c. Go to the movie and afterward make some humorous negative remarks about it, hoping they will get the message.
   d. Stay home Saturday night.

8. You occasionally babysit for Mrs. Harper's three children. Lately she has been making excuses when it comes time to pay you. You:
   a. Tell her that you're fed up and that you won't babysit for her anymore.
   b. Tell her that it's inconvenient for you to be paid late.
   c. Decide you won't work for her again.
   d. Say nothing.

9. You and your friend are in a record store together, and you see your friend slip a cassette into a coat pocket. You:
   a. Grab the cassette, put it back on the shelf, and threaten to turn your friend in.

CHAPTER 2: THE MIND-BODY CONNECTION   **47**

b. Tell your friend how you feel about shoplifting and recommend replacing the cassette.

c. Say nothing, but resolve never to go shopping with your friend again.

d. Act as if nothing has happened.

10. Your parents have given you some money to spend on clothes, and they have told you exactly what they want you to buy. You need clothes, but you disagree with the style they are urging on you. You:

a. Buy what you want, and tell them they are way out of touch with today's styles.

b. Tell them how you'd rather spend the money and why it's important to you.

c. Buy what they want you to have, and try to trade it for something else latter.

d. Buy what they want you to have, wear it, and thank them for it.

Scoring

Give yourself 10 points for each *a* answer, 8 for each *b*, 6 for each *c*, and 4 for each *d*. Add them up. If you scored:

85 to 100—You have no trouble asserting yourself, but your behavior borders on aggressiveness. You know what you want, but you have to give more thought to how you go about getting it.

70 to 84—You have a good sense of what you want, and you speak your mind. You are assertive.

45 to 69—You need to practice voicing your opinions and speaking up for your rights.

Below 45—You almost never voice an opinion. You may be building up some resentments. Start practicing assertiveness—be honest with yourself and direct with others.

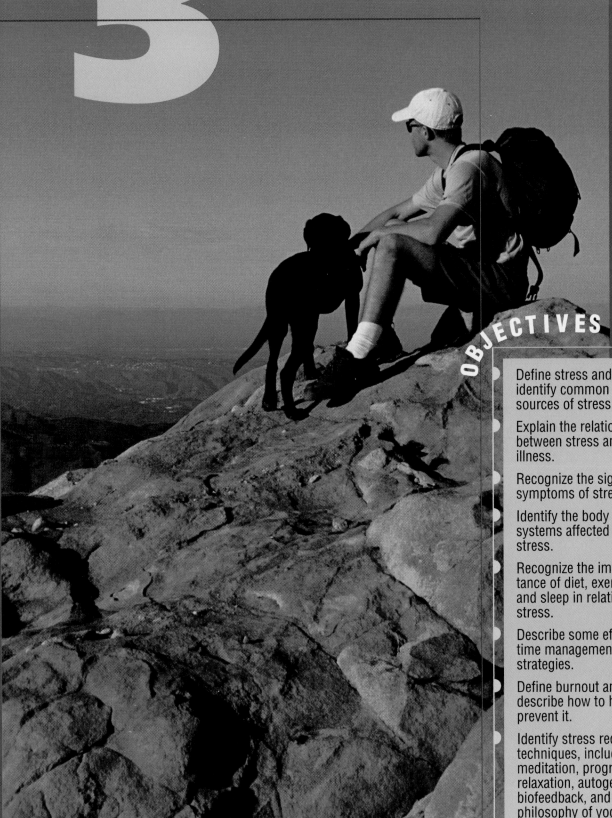

3 STRESS AND HEALTH

OBJECTIVES

- Define stress and identify common sources of stress.

- Explain the relationship between stress and illness.

- Recognize the signs and symptoms of stress.

- Identify the body systems affected by stress.

- Recognize the importance of diet, exercise, and sleep in relation to stress.

- Describe some effective time management strategies.

- Define burnout and describe how to help prevent it.

- Identify stress reduction techniques, including meditation, progressive relaxation, autogenics, biofeedback, and the philosophy of yoga.

49

THE WORD "STRESS" is widely used. What do you mean when you say you're stressed? Some people feel stressed from their surroundings, such as being exposed to extreme heat or cold, noise, pollution, or overcrowding. Stress means different things to different people, and what causes stress for one person may not stress someone else. Stressors can be physical (such as fatigue or a bacterial infection), emotional (such as pent-up anger or hostility), social (such as rejection or embarrassment), intellectual (such as confusion), and spiritual (such as guilt).

Stress is caused by **stressors**, or demands that require us to adapt. **Stress** is the combination of a stressor (anything that makes us adapt) and our response to the stressor. Stress can arise from situations that are happy (such as the birth of a baby) or sad (such as the death of a loved one). Stress is not the same as frustration, anxiety, or conflict, though it can lead to all of those emotions.

Stress is a biological response to demands made upon an individual. Scientifically speaking, stress is any challenge to homeostasis, or the body's internal sense of balance. Stress is a biological and biochemical process that begins in the brain and spreads through the autonomic nervous system, causing the release of hormones.

Stress can be altered by perceptions and attitude. For example, when confronted by the stress of an upcoming final exam in a difficult class, you may react either by becoming extremely anxious and unable to study (becoming distressed) or by welcoming the challenge by studying twice as long and enlisting the help of study companions (experiencing eustress).

Dr. Hans Selye, the father of stress research,[1] was the first to explore the notion of "desirable" stress, the stress that keeps life interesting and provides opportunity for growth (such as marriage, birth, new job, new

friends, or an exciting vacation). This kind of stress, which he termed **eustress**, is the physiological stress that is essential for maintaining life (such as the churning of the digestive tract and the rhythmic contractions of the heart). **Distress**, on the other hand, is negative. It results from stressors that are too intense or that persist for a long period of time.

Challenges can be stressful—and beneficial.

© 2001 PhotoDisc, Inc.

SIGNS AND SYMPTOMS OF STRESS

Cardiovascular
- Pounding of the heart
- Racing of the heart
- High blood pressure
- Irregular heartbeat
- Chest pain
- Cold, sweaty hands

Mental
- Inability to concentrate
- Lack of creativity
- Loss of memory
- Low self-esteem

Respiratory
- Shortness of breath
- Rapid breathing
- Asthma attacks

Sleep Disorders
- Insomnia
- Fatigue
- Nightmares

Emotional
- Nervousness
- Unexplained fearfulness
- Anxiety
- Emotional instability
- Impulsive behavior
- Difficulty in completing tasks
- Changes in eating/smoking/drinking
- Increased dependence on drugs
- Irritability
- Depression
- Forgetfulness
- Severe mood swings
- Tearfulness
- Urge to hide

Skin
- Acne
- Excessive dryness of skin
- Rashes
- Excessive perspiration

Gastrointestinal
- Dryness of the mouth and throat
- Difficulty swallowing
- Grinding of the teeth
- Indigestion
- Nausea or queasiness
- Vomiting
- Loss of appetite
- Excessive appetite
- Diarrhea or constipation
- Abdominal pain
- Increased cravings
- Frequent urination

Musculoskeletal
- Twitching or shakiness
- Neck or back pain
- Headache, including migraine
- Stiffness of the muscles

Stress occurs as a result of stressors and how we react to their demands. The way we perceive stress drives how it affects us. Some stress promotes curiosity and exploration. Stress can be challenging, stimulating, and rewarding.

SOURCES OF STRESS

Stress results from our experience of and reaction to stressors. College students experience a variety of stressors. Some researchers believe that the college years may be the most stressful in one's life. The most common kinds of pressures experienced by students include[2]

- Pressures to achieve. Students may create their own pressure, if they have high internal standards. Or students may feel pressure from parents and teachers to perform according to their high expectations.
- Financial burdens. Many students have to work while earning their degrees. These students have to balance employers' expectations with academic goals. For those with families to support, the stress is even more intense.
- Family stressors. Students who experience specific family stressors such as divorce of parents, health problems of a family member, or family conflict are burdened with stress.[3]
- Living adjustments. Many students are living away from home, usually for the first time, and have not established a network of social support, which is crucial for coping.
- Social pressure. Students are confronted with choices regarding alcohol, drug use, and sexuality. The current epidemic of sexually transmitted diseases adds even more pressures. Figure 3.1 illustrates these and other stressors.

Assessment 3-1 may help you identify specific things that are causing stress in your life. Assessments 3-2 and 3-3 can provide you with more information about how stress affects you.

WHAT MAKES PEOPLE THE MOST NERVOUS?

1. Making a speech
2. Getting married
3. Getting divorced
4. Going to the dentist

Source: Bernice Kanner, Are You Normal?.

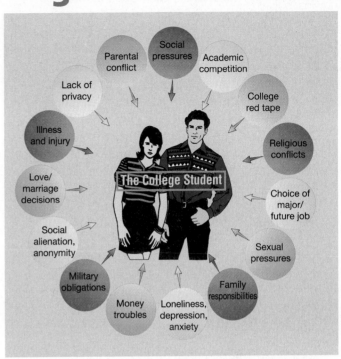

FIGURE 3.1 STRESSORS IN THE LIVES OF STUDENTS.

Organisms that challenge the body are physical sources of stress. Infection by bacteria, viruses, parasites, fungi, and protozoa can cause stress. So can fever, pain, trauma, injury, and deformity. Alcohol and other drugs can stress the body. These physical stressors can interfere with the body's ability to recover.

The environment itself can be a source of stress. Temperature, humidity, and weather extremes cause stress. So do pollutants in the air and water. Noise itself can be a significant source of environmental stress; the stress response is triggered by noise over 85 decibels (a loud television, garbage disposal, motorcycle, lawn mower, vacuum cleaner). Something as simple as being in a room that is too hot or too cold can cause stress. More dramatic examples of environmental stress include catastrophic events like severe storms, long-term drought, famine, fires, earthquakes, tornadoes, hurricanes, floods, or war.

Other stressors are emotional and social. One of the most common sources of stress is **conflict**, which occurs

Stressor Any situation or event that makes us adapt or adjust.

Stress An automatic biological response to stressors, or demands made on an individual; the result of any event or condition that requires adaptation.

Eustress Positive, desirable stress.

Distress Negative stress, usually consisting of too much stress in a short time, chronic stress over a prolonged time, or a combination of stressors.

Conflict The stress that results from two opposing and incompatible goals, demands, or needs.

when we are faced with incompatible needs, demands, motives, opportunities, or goals.[4] Some of the most pervasive stressors are daily **hassles**—the seemingly minor, irritating annoyances that happen every day, such as losing the car keys, getting stuck in a slow grocery-store line, waking up to a miserable snowstorm, being kept waiting for an appointment, having unexpected company drop in, or getting stuck in traffic.[5] These seemingly trivial problems may actually be more damaging to health and wellness than major stressors, partly because they occur frequently, and the net effect of an accumulation of daily hassles can be inability to cope.

Some factors make stressors more tolerable. Being able to exert even a small amount of control over a stressor and believing the outcome will be positive reduces the impact of a stressor.[6] Being able to predict an event with certainty also makes it less stressful. In contrast, knowing a stressor could occur but being in a state of uncertainty and lacking control increases the stress response.[7] One study showed that people who perceived that they had a high level of control over their situation showed an enhanced immune response when compared with subjects who perceived a low level of control.[8]

Factors on the job have been recognized as significant sources of stress.[9] Stressors in the workplace can include

- physical demands, such as uncomfortable seating, extremes in temperature, inadequate lighting;
- role demands, such as conflict or ambiguity in an employee's role;
- conflict between work and family;
- interpersonal demands, such as an abrasive boss, passive leaders, or abusive co-workers; and

- task demands, such as repetition, too few or too many changes, job insecurity, or overload.

Work overload is a huge source of stress and some employers are seeking ways to help their employees cope with stress.[10]

Although some stress can be beneficial, unmanaged stressful demands can arouse anxiety, which in turn often causes mental and physical harm, as the next sections describe.

STRESS AND DISEASE

Stress has been shown to affect almost all body systems. It can result in cardiovascular disease, neuromuscular disorders, respiratory and allergic ailments, immunologic disorders, gastrointestinal disturbances, skin conditions, dental problems, and a host of other disorders. Because most diseases are caused by a combination of factors, stress is a factor in the onset of disease.[11] Stress has been shown to be a major factor in a number of disease conditions, including the following:

- Cardiovascular diseases. Certainly cigarette smoking and obesity are risk factors for heart disease, however, stress seems to play a significant role in heart disease because of the specific effects it has on the cardiovascular system (discussed later in this chapter).[12] Stress causes an increase in blood cholesterol, blood pressure, and stroke.[13] Coronary artery disease and congestive heart failure both are partly caused or aggravated by stress.[14]
- Gastrointestinal diseases. Though many ulcers (especially in the stomach) are caused by bacteria, some ulcers are related to stress. Stress impairs the gastrointestinal tract, resulting in diarrhea, constipation, and ulcerative colitis (deterioration of the membranes lining the colon). Stress can alter our

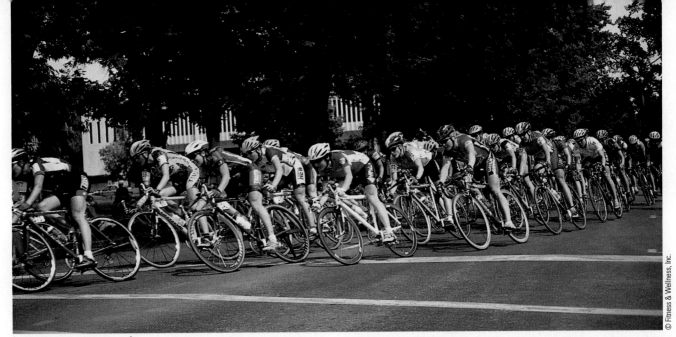

| Some stress is positive. |

eating patterns, causing severe loss of appetite in some people and eating disorders or obesity in others.

- Musculoskeletal disorders. One of the most common results of stress is the tension headache, caused by chronic tension in the muscles of the scalp and neck. Another type of headache—the migraine, in which the blood vessels of the scalp become dilated and exert extreme pressure—also is caused by stress. Other musculoskeletal disorders associated with stress include rheumatoid arthritis, chronic muscle tension, low back pain,[15] and temporomandibular joint (TMJ) syndrome, which interferes with chewing.
- Respiratory distress. Stress may induce shortness of breath and rapid breathing. Also, asthma and hay fever, both allergic reactions, are linked strongly to stress.[16] Significant emotional stress can precipitate an attack even in the absence of the allergen.

Stress also is a factor in a number of skin conditions (such as hives, eczema, and psoriasis), metabolic disorders (such as thyroid malfunctions and diabetes), menstrual irregularity, and gout. Some researchers find convincing evidence that stress plays a significant role in the development of some cancers.

HOW THE BODY REACTS TO STRESS

In an ideal state, the body enjoys **homeostasis**, a physiological state of balance in which all systems function smoothly. When the body becomes stressed and homeostasis is disrupted, the body goes through an adaptive response in an effort to reestablish homeostasis. Regardless of the source of stress, the body undergoes the same **fight-or-flight response** primitive people experienced when facing physical threats in their environment. This response consists of a series of physiological changes that occur in succession to enable people confronted with physical harm to face their enemies or run for their life.

Although society has become more civilized, our bodies have not. A student with communication anxiety giving an oral presentation in front of a class has the same physiological response as a person who faces physical danger. The stress response, termed the **general adaptation syndrome**, occurs in three general stages: alarm, resistance, and recovery or exhaustion (see Figure 3.2).

Alarm

The **alarm** stage of the stress response begins when a person is faced with a stressor.

> Regardless of its source, the stressor itself is only part of what causes stress. Your reaction to the stressor determines whether stress exists and how intense it is.

Hassles Seemingly minor, irritating, everyday annoyances that increase the level of stress.

Homeostasis A stable sense of physiological balance wherein all of the body's systems are functioning normally.

Fight-or-flight response A series of rapid-fire physical reactions to stress that provides maximum physical readiness to face threats in the environment.

General adaptation syndrome A three-stage attempt of the body to react and adapt to stressors that disrupt its normal balance.

Alarm The first stage of the general adaptation syndrome, characterized by the release of stress hormones.

FIGURE 3.2 THE STRESS RESPONSE MAY END IN EITHER RECOVERY OR EXHAUSTION.

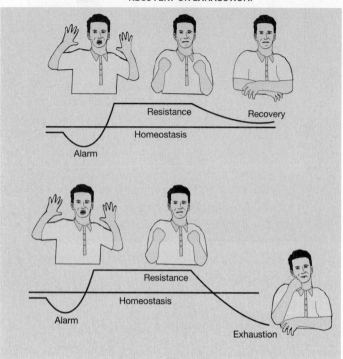

Following an initial emotional reaction, physical reactions follow rapidly: The brain triggers an immediate response from the autonomic nervous system (the branch of the nervous system that regulates body functions we cannot consciously control). All body systems mobilize and prepare for defense. Manifestations of the alarm reaction are depicted in Figure 3.3.

The mouth gets dry, and the palms get sweaty. Air sacs in the lungs dilate and breathing rate increases, infusing the blood with oxygen. Adrenaline and other hormones are pumped throughout the body, speeding the heart to deliver oxygen-rich blood to the muscles. Digestion is delayed so the much-needed blood is not diverted to the stomach. The liver releases glucose, which the muscles use as fuel. The muscles get tense, prepared for a workout. The senses—sight, hearing, smell, and taste—become acute, ready to identify any "danger." The brain releases endorphins to relieve pain.

If stress is prolonged, further changes occur during the alarm stage. A hormone released by the pituitary gland causes the adrenal glands to release cortisol. As a result, more stored nutrients are made available to the body for energy.

FIGURE 3.3 THE ALARM REACTION.

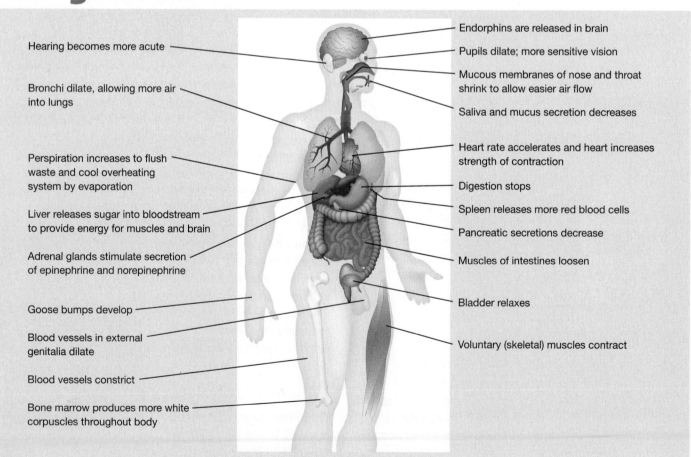

HOW STRESS HORMONES AFFECT THE BODY

- Speed up the heart
- Increase the amount of blood the heart pumps
- Increase fats in the blood
- Increase blood cholesterol levels
- Reduce the white blood cell count
- Decrease production of lymphocytes
- Deplete protein stored in the body
- Raise body core temperature

Resistance

The **resistance** stage of the stress response begins almost immediately after the alarm stage begins. During resistance, the body intensifies the physical changes of the alarm stage in anticipation of the perceived challenge. The adrenal glands continue to release adrenaline, the thyroid pumps out thyroid hormones, and the hypothalamus continues to release endorphins. More glucose and cholesterol are released into the bloodstream, providing both instant energy and endurance. Heart and breathing rates increase to boost the supply of oxygen to the body. The blood thickens. More than 1,400 known physiochemical reactions occur during the alarm and resistance stages of the stress response.

The resistance stage of the stress response is ideally suited to meeting the challenges of short-term stress. Simply stated, the body tries to adapt or meet the challenge so it can later return to the balance (homeostasis) that existed before the stress occurred.

This reaction is designed to cope with physical threats. The body is prepared for energy to be expended physically. However, our body experiences the same physical response when confronted with psychological stressors. Consider what happens if you experience alarm and resistance, but you take no physical action. The body prepares for exercise, that is, it mobilizes its resources (blood sugar, fats, and hormones) but doesn't use them. Your muscles are tense and your blood is rich with fuels that can accumulate and damage your heart. This state of chronic arousal can cause damage.

If the stressful situation is short-term and subsides, the body is able to adapt and return to a state of balance or recovery. If the stress becomes chronic, however, the body eventually loses its ability to adapt and becomes exhausted.

> The threats you face today are seldom physical, but the stress reaction is physical.

Recovery or Exhaustion

Although most people experience the alarm and resistance stages of the stress response frequently, the final stage of the stress response varies. Hopefully, the stressor leaves you before your resources run out, and the **recovery** period arrives. You relax and recuperate. Normal functioning resumes, needed repairs take place, fuel stores are refilled, and you become ready for the next round of excitement. If you remain in a stressful state for too long, however, your resources may become depleted. People with chronic stress experience the **exhaustion** stage, in which the body's resources are depleted and its adaptive abilities are lost. Many of the events of the alarm stage occur again as the body attempts to adjust to higher levels of stress, but the resulting wear and tear compromise the immune system and injure body systems and organs—which can lead to illness. The exhaustion stage is when long-term effects of stress set in.

HOW STRESS AFFECTS THE BODY SYSTEMS

Repeated episodes of the fight-or-flight response can impair specific body systems. The next sections describe how excessive stress can damage the digestive system, the cardiovascular system, and the immune system.

Stress affects every aspect of the gastrointestinal system. When someone is stressed, the mouth produces less saliva. The regular rhythmic contractions of the esophagus are disrupted, making swallowing difficult. The stomach slows down. Stress causes the stomach to secrete more hydrochloric acid and thins the gastric mucus that normally protects the stomach lining, which can cause ulcers. The liver releases excess glucose, and the pancreas can become chronically inflamed. Increased hydrochloric acid and disruption of normal peristaltic (rhythmic) action in the intestinal tract lead to duodenal ulcers and chronic diarrhea or constipation.

Excess stress affects the cardiovascular system, resulting in increased heart rate, damaged blood vessels, high blood pressure, and a boost in serum cholesterol levels, all of which lead to an increased risk of cardiovascular disease. The heart itself beats more forcefully and pumps a

Resistance The second stage of the general adaptation syndrome, characterized by meeting the perceived challenge.

Recovery The return to homeostasis after a stressful event.

Exhaustion The final stage of the general adaptation syndrome, characterized by depletion of the body's resources and loss of adaptive abilities.

greater volume of blood during stress; severe shock can cause the heart to stop. Research efforts have shown a strong link between stress and all kinds of cardiovascular disease, including deaths attributed to cardiovascular disease. Stress can cause blood pressure to rise, resulting in permanent hypertension if stress persists over time.

For people with existing heart disease, mental stress may be just as hard on the heart as is intense physical exertion. Stress causes blood vessels to constrict instead of expand, reducing the amount of blood that can be circulated. Stress causes the body to release cholesterol into the bloodstream. When the bloodstream carries too much cholesterol or other fats, fatty deposits build up on the walls of the coronary arteries, narrowing them and restricting blood flow to the heart. If the arteries eventually become clogged, blood flow to a certain part of the heart stops, that part of the heart muscle dies, and the victim has a heart attack. As part of the fight-or-flight reaction (the alarm stage of the stress response), the blood thickens. As a result, it coagulates more easily. Blood platelets build up along fatty deposits in the coronary arteries, worsening existing arteriosclerosis.

Perhaps the greatest effect of stress is on the immune system. The condition of the person exposed to a microorganism determines whether the person will develop illness. Stress compromises the immune system,

STRESS, THE IMMUNE SYSTEM, AND DISEASE

Conditions caused or aggravated by stress include the following, among others:

- heart disease
- arteriosclerosis
- atherosclerosis
- high blood pressure
- coronary thrombosis
- stroke
- angina
- respiratory ailments
- ulcers
- irritable bowel syndrome
- ulcerative colitis
- gastritis
- pancreatitis
- diabetes
- migraine headache
- myasthenia gravis

- epileptic attacks
- chronic backache
- kidney disease
- chronic tuberculosis
- allergies
- rheumatoid arthritis
- psoriasis
- eczema
- cold sores
- shingles
- hives
- asthma
- Raynaud's disease
- multiple sclerosis
- cancer
- endocrine and auto-immune problems

making the body less capable of fighting disease and infection.[17] Stress can also severely hinder the immune response.[18] Simply stated, stress suppresses the immune system's ability to produce and maintain lymphocytes (the white blood cells necessary for killing infection) and natural killer cells (the specialized cells that seek out and destroy foreign invaders), both crucial in the fight against infection and disease. Stress impairs the key players in immunity, from the body's levels of interferon to the organs (such as the thymus) vital to immune system functioning.

Also, stress increases the risk of suffering allergic reactions, contracting infectious diseases, and developing autoimmune diseases such as rheumatoid arthritis. Stress suppresses the body's production of T lympho-cytes, the immune cells that fight bacterial and viral infections, fungi, and cancer cells. Stress also worsens existing infections. People with existing infections who have high stress levels experience accelerated disease progression.[19]

STRESS AND HEART ATTACKS

Five times more people than usual had fatal heart attacks the day Los Angeles had its last big earthquake. On the day of the quake—January 17, 1994—24 people ages 45 to 92 died of cardiac arrest. Only three of these people were doing something strenuous (such as running from a shaking building) when they died.

Researchers estimate that some sort of outside trigger, such as emotional stress, touches off about 40 percent of all heart attack deaths. In the case of the L.A. quake, the whole population was simultaneously exposed to enormous stress.

Sudden stress can stop blood circulation in three ways:

1. It can send the heart into unorganized quivering.
2. It can break open a piece of fatty plaque so a clot forms in an artery.
3. It can cause an artery to go into spasms.

People who maintain healthy weight, avoid cigarettes, exercise regularly, and maintain healthy blood pressure and blood cholesterol levels are less at the mercy of stress.

Source: New England Journal of Medicine, 334:7.

RESILIENCY

People who can withstand extreme stress without suffering the negative consequences have been said to be resilient or hardy. The hardiness concept (described in

Chapter 2) includes the three Cs: commitment, control, and challenge. All three contribute to a healthier response to stress.

COPING WITH STRESS

Some people turn to unhealthy behaviors to cope with stress. For example, some people may use tobacco, alcohol, or other drugs in attempt to relieve stress. These behaviors are unhealthy in themselves, and they only mask the cause of the stress. Successful coping strategies provide long-term solutions to stressful problems without harming the body. Assessment 3-4 addresses your stress management skills.

Just as each individual reacts differently to stress,[20] each individual has **adaptation energy stores**, the physical, mental, and emotional reserves that enable us to cope with stress. Researchers think these stores occur in two layers: a deep layer surrounded by a superficial layer. The energy stores in the superficial layer are used first and are easy for the body to access. These reserves can be replaced through positive health behaviors. The deep energy stores seem to be determined in part by heredity. They cannot be replaced, and when they are spent, the body dies.

Coping with stress successfully allows you to replenish adaptation energy stores. It prepares you to deal with stress. People who are educated about stress management strategies are better able to cope than those who are not, and people who maintain strong programs of personal wellness during ordinary life are best able to withstand crises when they arise. Eating well, sleeping well, being physically active, cultivating daily joy and laughter, and cultivating spiritual health can help you maintain your ability to cope successfully with stress. This section describes strategies to bolster your ability to withstand stress.

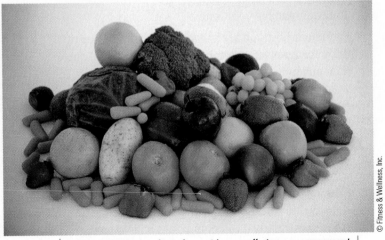

| Proper nutrition is a key element in overall stress management. |

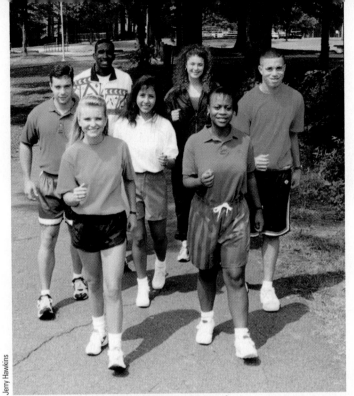

An active lifestyle buffers the effects of stress.

Diet and Physical Activity

Consuming a balanced diet containing foods low in fat and high in fiber will help you physically cope with stress. A balanced diet follows the guidelines in the food guide pyramid. Most of your calories should come from complex carbohydrates: grains, pastas, vegetables, and fruits. (See Chapter 8 for more information about nutrition.)

Physical activity decreases the intensity of stress, lessens its effects, reduces the time needed to recover from stress, and even minimizes the physiological reactions of the stress response.[21] An active lifestyle reduces the risk of getting sick, even for those under severe or chronic stress. Exercise reduces hostility, improves mental acuity, increases energy, eases muscle tension, and floods the system with endorphins.

If you have not been exercising, start slowly. If you try too much at first, you are more likely to get injured or, at least, stiff and sore. The resulting discouragement might keep you from exercising at all. If you are just starting out, take it easy. Try 10 to 15 minutes at a time, then extend the session as you get more conditioned. (Information on developing and implementing an active lifestyle and a regular exercise program is provided in Chapter 7.)

Adequate Sleep

Sleep is essential to coping with stress. If you've had your

Adaptation energy stores
Reserves of physical, mental, and emotional energy that give us the ability to cope with stress.

rest, it's easier to face almost anything. Sleep offers other, not-so-obvious benefits, too, including the relaxation so important to minimizing the effects of the stress response.

If you're feeling fatigued, try the following strategies:

- Try to establish a sleep pattern. Go to bed at about the same time every night and wake up at the same time every morning instead of skimping on sleep during the week and sleeping until noon on weekends.

> One in three Americans say they have "sleep problems."

- If you really need to, take a short nap during the day; 20 minutes is optimal. Less than that doesn't give you enough sleep, and more than that can make you sluggish.
- If you're having trouble falling asleep at night, don't nap during the afternoon, eat a light dinner, and avoid caffeine after 6 P.M.
- Use your bedroom only for sleeping. Don't watch television, study, or do work in bed. You need to associate your bed and your bedroom with sleep.
- Most people need 6 to 8 hours of sleep a night to function well and feel refreshed, but that requirement can vary from one person to another. To discover how much sleep you really need, go to sleep at the same time every night, then sleep until you wake up. It will take a couple of weeks to determine what you need. Once you've figured it out, discipline yourself and set a goal to get the rest you need.

SLEEP STEALERS

- Stress
- Depression
- Alcohol
- Nicotine
- Caffeine
- Exercising too close to bedtime
- Going to bed/getting up at differing times
- Shift work
- Jet lag
- Bed partner with sleep problems
- Bedroom that's too hot/too cold/too noisy/too bright
- Arthritis, hormonal shifts (e.g., menopause), asthma, sleep apnea, pain
- Medications (side effect)

Source: National Sleep Foundation.

Positive Attitude

A positive attitude is a valuable component in stress management. For many, it involves **reframing** thoughts. Reframing entails changing the way you look at things, learning to be an optimist instead of a pessimist. The way you think reduces the negative effects of stress and increases your resilience.[22] To help reframe your own thinking,

- Listen carefully to the words you use to describe yourself and your situation. Are they positive or negative? Listen for a few weeks. Then, if you need to, use different phrases and descriptions.
- Role play, either by yourself or with a friend. Start by relating a stressful situation you have experienced lately; tell how you reacted. Then come up with some different ways in which you could have reacted to the situation. If you're role playing with a friend, ask for feedback or suggestions. Next, imagine some plausible stressful situations and outline how you'd handle them. Concentrate on positive responses.
- For one week, look for the good in every person and every situation you encounter. This can be tough, but you always can find something! This kind of exercise is like conditioning your attitudes. Before long, it can become a habit.
- Avoid words that signal defeat: always, never, should have, ought to. Replace them with more benign choices. Instead of saying, "I always fail quizzes in class," say, "I'm sometimes unprepared when the teacher springs a quiz on us."

Effective Time Management

One of the leading sources of stress is simply too much to do in too little time. We are living in a fast-paced society, and the mere speed at which we move can be a significant stressor. Learning to manage the time you have can alleviate stress and reduce anxiety.

To better manage your time,

- Figure out how you are spending your time: Keep a diary for 2 weeks. You might be stunned to find out how much time you are spending on the phone or watching television programs. You cannot outline realistic goals until you know what you are currently doing.
- Try to figure out your peak performance time. Are you a "morning person," or do you get your second wind when most people are quitting for the day? Plan your most demanding tasks—studying, working —for the time you are at your peak. If you have to take a particularly challenging class and you are generally sluggish in the morning, see if you can

schedule it for the afternoon or find out if it is offered at night.

- Before you schedule anything else on your daily calendar, schedule time for a break. Plan several periods to do what you want—soak in a hot tub, read a good book, watch a football game on TV, or talk to a friend. Knowing you can look forward to a few breaks can help you face the stressful periods of your day more easily.
- Learn to prioritize. Not every demand is a top priority. You usually can split tasks into those that are essential, important, and unimportant or trivial. Spend your time and attention on the ones that are essential and important.
- Attack tasks one at a time. If you are faced with a number of demands, do not try to accomplish everything at once. Instead, decide on a course of action that lets you move through the list calmly. Limit the number of interruptions you have, but do not schedule yourself so tightly that a few interruptions throw you off completely.
- Learn to realistically judge how long a task will take. Most people underestimate by about 50%, so get into the habit of adding 50% to the time you think it will take. Once you learn how to estimate the time different tasks take realistically, you can stop overcrowding your day.
- If some things do not require your personal attention, delegate them to someone else.
- Before you go to bed each night, write down your schedule for the next day. Think through what has to be done—classes you need to attend, your part-time job, a commitment at the community crisis center. Prioritize. Figure out which are most important and make the time for those. Include times for leisure.
- Set challenging, yet realistic goals. Write them down and break them up into chunks you can accomplish more readily. Keep track of your progress and reward yourself for a job well done.
- Do not feel guilty if you have to say "no" to a request. You can do only so much in a single day. If you start to get overwhelmed, back off. Going to the movies with a few friends might be fun, but not if it means you'll have to stay up half the night to study for an exam.
- The ability to say "no" contributes in another way to stress management: Your stress level diminishes when you can feel good about expressing yourself and satisfying your own needs (assertive behavior). Stress increases when you deny your own needs or wishes to satisfy someone else (this is nonassertive behavior) or try to get your own way at the expense of someone else (this is aggressive behavior).

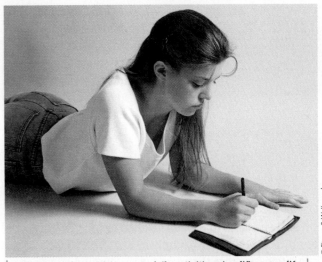

Planning and prioritizing your daily activities simplifies your life.

Burnout Prevention

Stress—especially chronic stress—can lead to **burnout**, a state of physical and mental exhaustion with few remaining resources.[23] Accompanying physical symptoms may include headache, indigestion, fatigue, and muscle soreness. Mental symptoms might be depression, resentment, apathy, inability to cope, or loss of enjoyment in life.[24] A quiz on burnout is Assessment 3-5.

> Another name for stress is change and too much change, even if it's positive, can translate into stress.

To prevent burnout,

- Surround yourself with a strong network of social support. Have at least one friend in whom you can confide.
- Distract yourself from your routine by developing a new interest, trying a new hobby, or volunteering for something new. Two hours a week telling animated stories to a group of captivated preschoolers at the local library might be just what you need to get a fresh perspective on things.
- Take the time to have fun. With all the demands of everyday life, a person can get bogged down in things that aren't always enjoyable. Go fly a kite, wade in a ditch, or have a picnic in the middle of a downtown park. Aim for fun, silly things you can laugh over at least once a day. Laughter has been shown to actually strengthen the immune system.

Reframing Changing the way you look at things.

Burnout A state of physical and mental exhaustion in which few resources remain.

• If you've got a strenu-
ous class load, take a
class just for fun. Go
for something you
have always wanted
to do—maybe a water-
color class or bowling.

RELAXATION TECHNIQUES

One of the best and most immediate ways of breaking the
stress response is to use a relaxation technique. This may
be any one of a host of techniques that bring on the
relaxation response to counteract the harmful effects of
unmanaged stress.

Invoking the relaxation response not only reduces the
negative effects of stress, but it also gives you a more
positive mental outlook, eases anxiety, and brings on a
sense of control (essential to overcoming the negative
aspects of stress). Regular relaxation exercises can reduce
stress, increase resistance to stress-induced illness,
minimize the symptoms of illness (such as headache),
lower your blood pressure, and alleviate pain.

Some relaxation exercises are based on deep
relaxation, with its myriad benefits, and others (such as
deep breathing or a quick massage) reduce immediate
stress and are a good way of leading into more extensive
relaxation exercises. As with physical exercise, learning
about various relaxation exercises takes some time.
Before you decide which ones to try, you should consider
your likes and dislikes, your personality, and your
situation. You can learn some techniques on your own,
and you will need some training for others. The
techniques discussed below are meditation, prayer,
progressive relaxation, deep breathing techniques,
autogenics, biofeedback training, and yoga. A little
research will help you find others.

A note of caution: If you are taking medication for
high blood pressure, heart conditions, diabetes, epilepsy,
or psychological conditions, consult with your health care
practitioner before you begin practicing relaxation techniques. These exercises can cause physiological changes.

Meditation

Simply stated, **meditation** is an exercise in which you
control your thoughts and thus affect certain body
processes.[25] Meditation is recognized as one of the most
effective ways to reduce stress. It requires total
concentration and prevents mental distraction, drifting
attention, and unfocused thoughts.

LAUGHTER AS MEDICINE

The benefits of laughter are many. It lowers blood pressure,
increases muscle flexibility, and triggers a flood of beta
endorphins, the brain's natural compounds that induce
euphoria.

Laughter's most profound effects are on the immune
system. Gamma-interferon, a disease-fighting protein, rises
with laughter—as do B-cells, which produce disease-
destroying antibodies, and T-cells, which orchestrate the
immune response.

Laughter also shuts off the flow of stress hormones, the
fight-or-flight compounds that come into play during times of
stress, hostility, and rage.

Stress hormones suppress the immune system, raise
blood pressure, and increase the number of platelets, which
can cause fatal blockages in the arteries.

The average child laughs hundreds of times a day. The
average adult laughs a dozen times. We need to find these
lost laughs—and use them to our advantage.

Sources: Lee Berk, M.D. and Stanley Tan, M.D., American Association for
Therapeutic Humor; Loma Linda University.

The meditator focuses exclusively on a specific
thought or object. Heartbeat and breathing slow down,
blood pressure drops (often for 12 to 24 hours after the
meditative period), and the body's metabolism slows,
decreasing its need for oxygen and other nutrients. As the
person becomes relaxed, blood flow to the arms and legs
increases, which helps to ease muscle tension. Laboratory
studies have shown that people who meditate have fewer
blood lactates, the enzymes associated with stress and
anxiety.

Meditation has psychological benefits, too. It lessens
anxiety, produces better sleep, and promotes less fear,
fewer phobias, greater internal locus of control, and more
positive mental health. Meditation also has helped people
stop drug abuse and cigarette smoking.

To be effective, meditation has to be done in a
comfortable position in a quiet place, free of distractions.
No specific posture is required for meditation, but because
the physiological processes of meditation are different
from those of sleep, meditators often sit so they will not
fall asleep during meditation.

The goal of meditation is relaxation, which involves
diverting blood to the arms and legs. After a meal, blood
pools in the abdomen, where it is used to help digestion.
Therefore, it's best to meditate before you eat. Also, avoid
using any stimulants, including tobacco and caffeine,

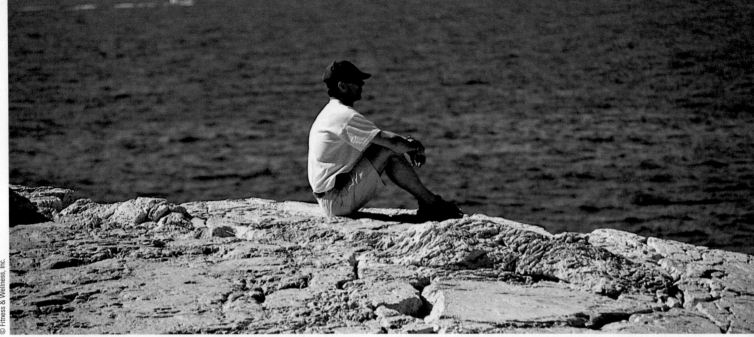

| Meditation is an effective stress reduction technique. |

before you meditate, because they can interfere with relaxation.

For maximum effect, experts recommend meditating 20 minutes at a time, twice during the day. The procedure is as follows:

1. Find a quiet room as free from distraction as possible. Lighting and temperature are a matter of individual preference. Just make sure you're comfortable. Turn off the phone. Alert others that you don't want to be disturbed. (At first, it's important to have quiet surroundings; later, after you've practiced for a while, you will be able to meditate in almost any situation.)
2. Loosen your clothing if it is tight, especially at the wrists, neck, and waist. Get in the most comfortable position you can, in a chair or on a couch. Some recommend a straight-backed chair to prevent you from falling asleep. Place your feet flat on the floor and rest your hands in your lap.
3. Inhale slowly and deeply through your nose, hold your breath briefly, then exhale slowly. As you begin to breathe deeply, let the tension flow out of your body. Do not force it or concentrate on it. Just let it happen.
4. If you are concentrating on an unchanging object, close your eyes partially so the object appears blurred. Softly focus on it without bringing in any of the sharp details. Gradually focus all your attention on that object. Do not let any other thoughts invade your meditation.
5. Continue meditating for approximately 20 minutes. Do not worry about the exact time. You will probably have to work up to it at first. Learning to sit still for 20 minutes at a time takes a lot of practice, especially

when you are focusing so intensely on a single object or phrase.
6. When you are finished meditating, give yourself time—at least several minutes—to readjust. Open your eyes, focus on various objects around the room, and return gradually to your normal rate and pattern of breathing. While still seated, stretch your arms, legs, back, shoulders, and neck. Finally, stand up slowly.

It is important to let your body readjust after meditating. If you stand up too soon or too quickly, you may get dizzy, because your heart rate and blood pressure drop during meditation.

| Prayer |

Some people use prayer with meditation and claim that either prayer alone or the combination of prayer and meditation enhances the effectiveness of stress management. Prayer involves communicating spiritually. When people pray, they seek help for problems and situations. By obtaining spiritual assistance, they reduce their perceptions of stress. (Prayer is discussed in greater detail in Chapter 5.)

| Progressive Relaxation |

Progressive relaxation is a technique for physically relaxing the nerves and

Meditation A mental exercise to help gain control over thoughts.

Progressive relaxation A method of reducing stress that consists of tensing, then relaxing, small muscle groups.

muscles. Practitioners learn how to recognize muscle tension and how to differentiate it from muscle relaxation. This three-step technique is simple: You first contract (tense) a small muscle group, then relax the muscle group, and finally concentrate on how different the two sensations feel.

Progressive relaxation helps relieve tension headache, migraine headache, back pain, and other conditions related to muscle tension. It even has been shown to relax the smooth, or involuntary, muscles (like those in blood vessels and the digestive tract). It also has been shown to reduce anxiety, relieve depression, and improve sleep patterns.

Progressive relaxation is simple. In essence, you contract, then relax the muscles of the body, progressing from one group of muscles to another. You can design your own routine—working from your head to your toes, for example, or from your feet to your head—as long as all major groups in the body are involved eventually. When you start doing progressive relaxation, you should first tense the muscles as hard as you can, then relax them. Once you become practiced, you can relax the muscles easily and effortlessly without having to first contract them.

Unlike meditation, in which you should not think about what is happening to your body, progressive relaxation requires you to concentrate on what is happening to your muscles. For the best results, you have to be acutely aware of the relaxed condition of your body.

Regardless of your individual routine, the following steps apply:

1. Take off your shoes and loosen any restrictive clothing. Stretch out on the floor on your back in the most comfortable position possible. Support your neck with a small pillow. If you need it, put a pillow under your knees. Close your eyes and rotate your ankles outward. Depending on which helps you relax best, either put your arms at your sides or rest your hands on your abdomen. You need to be completely relaxed before you start.
2. First tense, then relax, each muscle group. (Make sure you move to all major muscle groups in the body.) Don't forget your face—including your forehead, eyes, nose, mouth, cheeks, and tongue.
3. As you move to each muscle group, contract the muscles as tightly as you can and hold the contraction for 20 or 30 seconds. If you experience pain or cramping, release the contraction immediately.
4. Concentrate on the dramatic difference in feeling between a tensed muscle and a relaxed one. With practice, you'll be able to achieve relaxation without first tensing the muscle.

Breathing Techniques

Breathing exercises also can be an antidote to stress. These exercises have been used for centuries in the Orient and India as a means to develop better mental, physical, and emotional stamina. Breathing exercises can be learned in only a few minutes and require considerably less time than other forms of stress management.

In breathing exercises, the person concentrates on "breathing away" the tension and inhaling fresh oxygen to the entire body. To be effective, the breathing must be so deep that the belly is expanded with each breath—a sign that the diaphragm is being expanded.

Following is an example breathing exercise:

1. Lie in a comfortable position on your back, with your hands placed lightly over your lower abdomen.
2. Keeping your eyes open, imagine a balloon lying beneath your hands.
3. Begin to slowly inhale through your nose, concentrating on the warm air entering your nose and slowly filling the balloon. You should be able to feel your lower abdomen rise as you breathe in. When the "balloon" is full (this should take 3 to 4 seconds initially), pause for a second, then slowly exhale to empty the balloon, feeling your chest and abdomen relaxing.
4. Repeat the entire process two or three times.
5. When finished, sit quietly for a few minutes before rising. If you feel dizzy at any point, stop the procedure.[26]

Autogenics

Similar to progressive relaxation, **autogenics** is self-induced relaxation that causes all major muscle groups in the body to feel relaxed, heavy, and warm. It begins with a routine that relaxes all the major muscles (much like that of progressive relaxation), followed by imagery (vivid mental visualization) that extends the relaxed state. It is a form of self-hypnosis that is recognized as an effective relaxation technique for managing stress.

Autogenics and meditation both result in relaxation, but they do it in different ways. In meditation, you first relax the mind, which causes the body to relax. In autogenics, you first relax the body, which causes the mind to relax.

The general sensations resulting from autogenics are feelings of warmth and heaviness, especially in the arms and legs, caused by dilation of blood vessels and relaxation of muscles. Autogenics and the associated imagery reduce heartbeat and breathing rates, ease muscle tension, and increase the brainwaves associated with deep relaxation. Autogenics can help relieve migraine headache, tension headache, low back pain, and asthma and can improve high blood pressure. Autogenics also can relieve anxiety, reduce depression, increase resistance to stress, and increase pain tolerance.

Autogenics requires time, motivation, commitment, and practice. Commercial tapes are available to guide you through the relaxation exercises. You also can make your own tape or simply repeat the phrases aloud as you move through the exercises. As with progressive relaxation, you can design your own routine.

1. In a quiet room with mild temperature, free of distractions, sit in the most comfortable position you can. Experts recommend sitting in a straight-backed but comfortable chair with your feet flat on the floor, your head hanging loosely forward, your eyes closed, and your hands in your lap with your palms turned upward. Loosen any restrictive clothing.
2. Imagine you have just had a strenuous workout. You might begin with your legs. As you inhale and exhale deeply and slowly, repeat, "My legs are so tired. My legs are so heavy. My legs are very heavy and warm." As you repeat these phrases, feel the heaviness and warmth in your legs. With practice, your legs should become so heavy and relaxed that you can lift them only with considerable struggle.
3. Move to other muscle groups—buttocks, abdomen, chest, arms, shoulders, and so on. You even might imagine your internal organs, such as your stomach and your heart, relaxed and warm.
4. Concentrate on how cool your forehead feels. For you to feel refreshed and alert, your forehead must feel cool.
5. Once your entire body is relaxed, visualize an image that you find relaxing. It might be waves lapping against a sandy beach, a cloud drifting lazily across the afternoon sky, an eagle soaring silently across a ravine. The image is different for everyone, but it should lead you to total relaxation.

For the greatest benefit, experts recommend that you practice twice a day for 10 minutes at a time. As with other kinds of relaxation exercises, autogenics requires practice, starting out slowly, then working up to a 10-minute period of visualization and relaxation.

┃BIOFEEDBACK TRAINING

Essentially, **biofeedback** training is a method of measuring physiological functions you are not normally aware of (such as skin temperature and blood pressure) and then training yourself to control those functions. It has three basic stages:

1. Measuring the physiological function,
2. Converting the measurement into something meaningful, and
3. Feeding back the information.

Unlike some other forms of relaxation exercises, you can't learn biofeedback training on your own. It requires that you be monitored by extremely sensitive equipment, then taught to regulate your own physiological responses. Biofeedback training is valuable as a stress management technique, because it allows you to control your body's responses to stress. Most people can learn effective biofeedback techniques in a few sessions from a trained therapist.

Within a few sessions, most people are able to competently control physiological effects of stress such as higher blood pressure, increasing heart rate, and muscle contraction. An obvious disadvantage is the necessity of using expensive machinery and trained therapists. Most people, however, quickly gain the ability to control their own physiological responses without the biofeedback machinery.

┃ Yoga ┃

Yoga, an ancient exercise technique known to induce calm and invigorate the mind, has been shown in scientific studies to reduce the biological effects of stress. Yoga is an excellent exercise for improving muscular strength, flexibility, and endurance. It consists of precise postures done in a specific sequence combined with an exact breathing rhythm designed to reduce tension and inflexibility.

There are many different styles of yoga, which comes from a Sanskrit word meaning union. The most common type of yoga used in the western world is hatha yoga, which involves stretching exercises to induce relaxation.

The yoga postures are difficult and complex and require training and practice. Few people can assume the postures at first, and you may not be able to complete the sequence properly for as long as 3 months. The goal of yoga is relaxation, so you should not force positions that make you tense or could cause injury.

A number of good yoga instruction books and videotapes are on the market, and yoga classes are taught

Autogenics A relaxation technique in which the person is trained, with the aid of specialized equipment, to relax all major muscle groups through a form of self-hypnosis, followed by imagery.

Biofeedback A relaxation technique that involves measuring and controlling physiological functions.

Yoga An exercise technique involving stretching, used to relieve stress and induce calm.

throughout the United States. Most experts recommend practicing yoga for 15 to 45 minutes a day in a place free of distraction. Many people sign up for classes, where they actually perform yoga daily.

CHECKMATE FOR STRESS

Like improving your game of chess, you can develop strategies to put stress in check. You don't want to eliminate stress completely. Research reveals that minimal or moderate stress enhances immunity.[27] Too little stress leaves you feeling restless, bored, unhappy, and tired. Conversely, with too much stress, you feel exhausted, irritable, and burned out. Just the right amount of stress can help you feel energetic, creative, happy, and productive. The key is to achieve the middle ground.

Three more techniques for coping are the following:

1. Situational reconstruction: When a stressful event occurs, replay it in your mind to gain understanding and pinpoint where the anxiety is coming from. If you have had an argument, what contribution did you make? What did the other person do? Next, get some perspective by imagining both how the situation could get worse and how it could get better. Finally, ask yourself what you could do to increase the likelihood of it getting better and put your answer into action.

2. Focusing: If you cannot get your imagination going in the first exercise, the situation may be evoking emotions you are not acknowledging. For example, you assume you are angry when, in fact, you are frightened. In this case, let your body cue you in. Focus on your center, the chest-abdomen area, and ask yourself, "What is it about this situation that stands in the way of my feeling good?" If you come up with an answer that seems familiar, put it aside, refocus, and ask the question again. When an unexpected thought or feeling pops into your mind, that's probably the information you've been burying. Acknowledge it and try the first step again.

3. Compensatory self-improvement: When you can't think of anything you could do to make the situation better, you may be confronting something you cannot change. If this is the case, accept the reality gracefully without falling into bitterness and self-pity. One way to do this is by choosing another problem related to the first one and work on that instead. Rather than

TIPS FOR ACTION

SOME COPING STRATEGIES

The following strategies are designed to reduce the amount and extent of stress in your life, not to cause you more stress. To reach that goal,

- Don't try to incorporate too many strategies at once. Changing old habits and developing new ways of dealing with things require time. If you take on too much at once, you'll end up feeling frustrated and stressed. Another name for stress is change, and too much change, even if it's positive, can translate into stress.
- Before you decide on the strategies you want to use, consider your own strengths and skills. Think about what you would enjoy. Assess what kind of social support you'll have. Those kinds of considerations can help you choose the most workable and pleasant strategies for you.
- Keep in mind that what works for you won't necessarily work for someone else—and won't even work for you in all situations. Be flexible, be willing to change your coping strategies, and never stop assessing.
- Do not expect a single coping strategy to provide you with enough coping power. Several coping strategies will be required to do the trick.
- Realize that you will not be able to change or control some things. The death of a family member, the diagnosis of a serious illness, the loss of property in a crime—these are examples of things you can't change. The best strategy here is to accept what has happened and determine to move on in a positive way.
- Recognize that even negative stress can have a positive outcome if you meet it head-on and use it as an opportunity for learning and growth. Even a stressful situation can give you insight or help you become more prudent.

feeling victimized or overwhelmed, say to yourself, "I may not be able to fix everything, but I can improve some things."

In short, start with yourself. There are few situations that cannot be improved by working on your own personal changes. For example, try seeking greater understanding by identifying with the people who are causing you the stress. In this way they become human again and are no longer monsters. They'll also be more likely to listen to you and to help find a solution that will ease your stress.

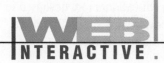

WEB ACTIVITIES

■ **Stress Management: A Review of Principles** is presented by Wesley E. Sime, Ph.D., M.P.H., professor of Health and Human Performance at the University of Nebraska—Lincoln. This on-line series of lectures on stress management education features information on the psychobiology of stress and relaxation as well as pathophysiology of stress.
http://www.unl.edu/stress/mgmt

■ **Access Health Stress Guide** This site features a series of professional articles on all aspects of stress and how prolonged stress can affect your health, including information on common stress symptoms and management tips.
http://www.accenthealth.com/stress/stressguide.html

■ **Stress: Who Has Time For It?** A visually appealing site that describes the symptoms of stress and how to manage your daily stress.
http://health4teens.org/stress

■ **Exercise Can Help Control Stress** This site, sponsored by the American Council on Exercise, lists several ways to help manage stress through regular exercise.
http://www.acefitness.org/fitfacts/fitfacts_display.cfm?itemid=51

■ **Are You Under Stress?** Take this comprehensive stress questionnaire to find out how well you are handling stress in your life. The tool assesses eight key stress warning signs: anger, perfectionism, time-urgency, disappointment, negative mood, under-achievement, tension, and physical problems.
http://www.thriveonline.com/serenity/stress/smq.index.html

InfoTrac
You can find additional readings related to wellness via InfoTrac College Edition, an on-line library of more than 900 journals and publications. Follow the instructions for accessing InfoTrac that came packaged with your text-book, then search for articles using a key word search.

Suggested Reading Edward P. Sarafino and Maureen Ewing, "The Hassles Assessment Scale for Students in College: Measuring the Frequency and Unpleasantness of and Dwelling on Stressful Events,"

Journal of American College Health 48, no. 2 (Sept. 1999): 75.

1. What are the two types of stressors that are assessed using the self-report methods as described in the article?
2. Hassles Assessment Scale for Students in College (HASS/Col) provides an opportunity for the participants to rate each of the stressful events in what three categories?
3. Describe how the HASS/Col instrument can be used as a research tool as well as for counseling.

Web Activity
Stress Assess
http://wellness.uwsp.edu/Health_Service/services/stress

Sponsor National Wellness Institute at the University of Wisconsin—Steven's Point

Description This is a three-part on-line educational tool developed by the National Wellness Institute at the University of Wisconsin—Steven's Point. This question-naire is designed to increase your knowledge about stress and features separate evaluations for stress sources, distress symptoms, and stress-balancing strategies. Based on these results, you will learn healthy strategies to better manage your specific stressors.

Available Activities Select from the following three evaluations:

1. *Stress Sources* Helps you evaluate the sources of stress in your life. Each stage of life is accompanied by its own unique stress sources: family, social, individual, environment, work, and college. This assessment measures the various sources of stress in your life at the current time.
2. *Distress Symptoms* Helps you to identify what your symptoms of stress are. When answering the questions, you select your symptoms and signs of distress (feelings, behaviors, body reactions).
3. *Stress-Balancing Strategies* Provides you with information to help you handle stress.

Web Work
1. From the home page, click on the "Stress Sources" link first. Answer these questions honestly to determine your major stressors.
2. Upon completion of the "Stress Sources" evaluation, click on the "Distress Symptoms" link from the home page to help you identify your symptoms of stress. Answer the demographic information and then the questions in the "Distress Symptoms" section using the pull-down menu.

3. Complete the questions for the "Signs of Distress" section for all three areas (feelings, behaviors, and body reactions). When you're finished, click on the "Perform Your Stress Assessment" button to obtain your results for this section.

4. Repeat these directions for the other two evaluations available at this site.

Helpful Hint

1. "Stress Assess" is an educational tool designed to enhance your knowledge about stress. It is not a clinical instrument or diagnostic tool.

For additional Web activities, links, and suggested readings, visit our Health, Fitness, and Wellness Resource Center at http://health.wadsworth.com.

NOTES

1. R. R. Ross and E. M. Altmaier, *Intervention in Occupational Stress* (London: Sage Publications, 1994).

2. J. Silberg, "The Influence of Genetic Factors and Life Stress on Depression Among Adolescent Girls," *The Journal of the American Medical Association* 281 (1999): 1970–1975.

3. R. Forehand et al., "Cumulative Risk Across Family Stressors: Short- and Long-term Effects for Adolescents," *Journal of Abnormal Child Psychology* 26 (1998): 119–128.

4. R. C. Kessler et al., "Social Support, Depressed Mood, and Adjustment to Stress: A Genetic Epidemiological Investigation," *Journal of Personality and Social Psychology* 62 (1992): 257–272.

5. K. Doner, "Heal Your Angry Heart," *American Health* 15 (1996): 74–77.

6. L. S. Kim et al., "Locus of Control as a Stress Moderator and Mediator in Children of Divorce," *Journal of Abnormal Child Psychology* 25 (1997): 145–155.

7. J. J. Hurrell Jr., "Editorial: Are You Certain?—Uncertainty, Health, and Safety in Contemporary Work," *American Journal of Public Health* 88 (1998): 1012–1013.

8. J. F. Brosschot et al., "Experimental Stress and Immunological Reactivity: A Closer Look at Perceived Uncontrollability," *Psychosomatic Medicine* 60 (1998): 359–361.

9. M. F. Dollard et al., "Predicting Work Stress Compensation Claims and Return to Work in Welfare Workers," *Journal of Occupational Health Psychology* 4 (1999): 279–287.

10. C. A. Beatty, "The Stress of Managerial and Professional Women: Is the Price Too High?," *Journal of Organizational Behavior* 17 (1996): 233–251; J. Von Onciul, "Stress at Work," *British Medical Journal* 313 (1996): 745–748.

11. S. Stewart-Brown, "Emotional Wellbeing and its Relation to Health: Physical Disease May Well Result From Emotional Distress," *British Medical Journal* 317 (1998): 1608–1609.

12. R. J. Benschop et al., "Cardiovascular and Immune Responses to Acute Psychological Stress in Young and Old Women: A Meta-Analysis," *Psychosomatic Medicine* 60 (1998): 290–296.

13. D. S. Krantz et al., "Effects of Mental Stress in Patients with Coronary Artery Disease: Evidence and Clinical Implications," *The Journal of the American Medical Association* 283 (2000): 1800–1802.

14. E. C. Suarez et al., "Neuroendocrine, Cardiovascular, and Emotional Responses of Hostile Men: The Role of Interpersonal Challenge," *Psychosomatic Medicine* 60 (1998): 78–88.

15. A. Feyer et al., "The Role of Physical and Psychological Factors in Occupational Low Back Pain: A Prospective Cohort Study," *Occupational and Environmental Medicine* 57 (2000): 116–120.

16. R. J. Wright et al., "Review of Psychosocial Stress and Asthma: An Integrated Biopsychosocial Approach," *Thorax* 53 (1998): 1066–1074.

17. R. Glaser et al., "Stress-Induced Immunomodulation: Implications for Infectious Diseases?," *The Journal of the American Medical Association* 281 (1999): 2268–2270.

18. T. Kushnir et al., "Science, Prevention, and Practice: V. Meeting the Needs of Care Givers: Concurrent: Individual: Managing Stress and Burnout at Work: A Cognitive Group Intervention Program for Directors of Day-Care Centers," *Pediatrics* 94 (1994): 1074–1077.

19. J. Leserman et al., "Progression to AIDS: The Effects of Stress, Depressive Symptoms, and Social Support," *Psychosomatic Medicine* 61 (1999): 397–406.

20. A. V. Horwitz et al., "The Use of Multiple Outcomes in Stress Research: A Case Study of Gender Differences in Responses to Marital Dissolution," *The Journal of Health and Social Behavior* 37 (1996): 278–291.

21. S. J. Campbell, "Maxed Out? Mellow Out with These Personal Stress Management Strategies," *American Journal of Maternal/Child Nursing* 21 (1996): 123–127.

22. N. E. Adler et al., "Additional Validation of a Scale to Assess Positive States of Mind," *Psychosomatic Medicine* 60 (1998): 26–32.

23. S. R. O'Brien, "Staff Wellness Program Promotes Quality Care," *American Journal of Nursing* 98 (1998): 16B–16D.

24. P. Nolan, "A Measurement Tool for Assessing Stress Among Mental Health Nurses," *Nursing Standard* 9 (1995): 36–39.

25. J. Graham, "Meditation for Type A's: Even the Restless Can Chill Out With This New Spin on an Ancient Practice," *Women's Sports and Fitness* 19 (1997): 76–77.

26. D. A. Girdano, G. S. Everly, and D. Dusek, *Controlling Stress and Tension*, 3d ed. (Englewood Cliffs, NJ: Prentice Hall, 1990).

27. M. May, "Skin-deep Stress," *American Scientist* 84 (1996): 224–225.

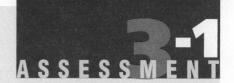

SCORING YOUR STRESS:
A TEST TO PINPOINT WHAT'S EATING YOU

Name: _____   Date: _____   Grade: _____

Instructor: _____   Course: _____   Section: _____

How Stressed Are You?

The answer depends in part on what's going on in your life. But it also depends on some other factors—like what your *attitudes* are about those events and how much control you feel over what happens.

The first step in managing stress, of course, is to *identify* it—and the test below will help you do just that. It's simple: Read each question, then circle the number that most closely describes your situation or attitude. If you're completely neutral, circle **5**; if a question doesn't apply to you at all, skip it.

Ready?

Sharpen your pencil and go to work:

1 How often do you suffer stress-related physical symptoms, such as headaches, jaw pain, neck pain, back pain, indigestion, abdominal pain, diarrhea, loss of appetite, excessive perspiration, fatigue, or a pounding in your chest?

Rarely or never   Every day

1   2   3   4   5   6   7   8   9   10

2 Do you wash your hands before you eat?

Always   Rarely or never

1   2   3   4   5   6   7   8   9   10

3 Do you take measures to keep your food safe, such as cooking it adequately, storing it properly, and avoiding obvious contaminants?

Almost always   Rarely or never

1   2   3   4   5   6   7   8   9   10

4 How often do you eat fresh fruits, fresh vegetables, whole grains, and foods high in fiber?

Every day   Rarely or never

1   2   3   4   5   6   7   8   9   10

5 How often do you eat high fat or high-sugar foods—including candy, pastry, soft drinks, and food from fast-food restaurants?

Occasionally   Every day

1   2   3   4   5   6   7   8   9   10

6 How often do you exercise?

Every day   Rarely or never

1   2   3   4   5   6   7   8   9   10

7 How many hours of sleep do you get each day?

Eight or more   Less than four

1   2   3   4   5   6   7   8   9   10

8 How many cups of coffee or caffeinated soft drinks do you drink each day?

None   Five or more

1   2   3   4   5   6   7   8   9   10

9 How often do you use alcohol, tobacco, over-the-counter drugs, or prescription drugs to relieve stress?

Never   Every day

  1   2   3   4   5   6   7   8   9   10

10 If you have a relationship with a significant other, how would you describe that relationship?

Mutually satisfying in many ways   Marked by jealousy or insecurity

  1   2   3   4   5   6   7   8   9   10

11 How do you feel when you have to say "no" to a request for your time, energy, talents, or money?

Confident and at ease   Anxious and guilt-ridden

  1   2   3   4   5   6   7   8   9   10

12 How would you characterize your support system?

Broad-based, many sources   Limited or no sources

  1   2   3   4   5   6   7   8   9   10

13 What kinds of friendships do you have?

At least several close friends/confidants   No close friends

  1   2   3   4   5   6   7   8   9   10

14 What do you do if you have a problem you can't solve on your own?

Seek help immediately   Suffer on my own

  1   2   3   4   5   6   7   8   9   10

15 How many major changes (such as entering or ending an intimate relationship, the death of a family member, a change in your financial status, moving, starting a new job, a change in sleeping habits, a change in living conditions, or a change in the number of arguments you have with roommates) have occurred in your life during the last year?

None   Many

  1   2   3   4   5   6   7   8   9   10

16 How do you react when confronted with a problem or stressful situation?

Put it aside to gain perspective,   Feel overwhelmed
then focus on solutions   or panic-stricken

  1   2   3   4   5   6   7   8   9   10

17 How often do you "retreat" temporarily when you start to feel overwhelmed by stress?

Most of the time   Never

  1   2   3   4   5   6   7   8   9   10

18 How do you normally feel at the end of the day?

I got the important things done   I didn't accomplish anything

  1   2   3   4   5   6   7   8   9   10

19 How many hassles do you have in a typical day?

A few   A lot

  1   2   3   4   5   6   7   8   9   10

20 How much noise are you exposed to every day?

Not very much   Most of the day is noisy

  1   2   3   4   5   6   7   8   9   10

21 How comfortable is your environment? (Consider temperature extremes, humidity, crowding, and environmental pollutants.)

Very comfortable   Very uncomfortable

    1   2   3   4   5   6   7   8   9   10

22 Overall, how satisfying is your life?

Very satisfying   Very disappointing

    1   2   3   4   5   6   7   8   9   10

Scoring

Time to take a look at your stress level. This exercise will tell you two things: First, it will indicate your general stress level. Then it will help pinpoint the specific things that are causing you stress.

First, total up your score by adding every number you circled. Now divide it by the number of questions you answered. This is one test on which you don't want a high score: The closer your average creeps toward 10, the higher your stress level is likely to be. (By the way, it's important to average your stress score this way; a high level of stress in a few areas won't cause your general stress level to skyrocket.)

Next, go back and isolate what's causing you problems. Look back through your responses. Find those in which you circled a number higher than 5. Simple—you've found your problem areas.

Finally, determine some stress-busting strategies.

HOW STRESSED ARE YOU?

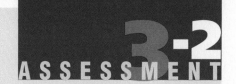

Name: Date: Grade:

Instructor: Course: Section:

To find out your stress level, take the "stress scale"—a test developed by University of Washington researchers Thomas Holmes and Richard Rahe. The test rates life events known to produce stress. Check off the events that have happened to you in the past year. Add them up. If you score 300 or more, you are at highest risk of developing stress-induced disease.

Stress	Points	Stress	Points
1. Death of spouse	100	24. Trouble with in-laws	29
2. Divorce	73	25. Outstanding personal achievement	28
3. Marital separation	65	26. Spouse beginning or stopping work	26
4. Jail term	63	27. Beginning or ending school	26
5. Death of close family member	63	28. Change in living conditions	25
6. Personal injury or illness	53	29. Revision of personal habits	24
7. Marriage	50	30. Trouble with boss	23
8. Fired from job	47	31. Change in work hours or conditions	20
9. Marital reconciliation	45	32. Change in residence	20
10. Retirement	45	33. Change in schools	20
11. Change in health of family member	44	34. Change in recreation	19
12. Pregnancy	40	35. Change in worship activities at church or temple	19
13. Sexual difficulties	39	36. Change in social activities	18
14. Gain of new family member	39	37. Mortgage or loan less than $10,000	17
15. Business readjustment	39	38. Change in sleeping habits	16
16. Change in financial state	38	39. Change in number of family get-togethers	15
17. Death of close friend	37	40. Change in eating habits	15
18. Change to different line of work	36	41. Vacation	13
19. Change in number of arguments with spouse	35	42. Christmas	12
20. Mortgage over $10,000	31	43. Minor violation of the law	11
21. Foreclosure of mortgage or loan	30		
22. Change in responsibilities at work	29	**Total Points**	
23. Son or daughter leaving home	29		

TAKE YOUR STRESS TEMPERATURE

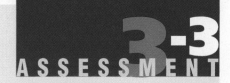

Name: _____ Date: _____ Grade: _____

Instructor: _____ Course: _____ Section: _____

How Stressed Are You?

Let's play 20 questions. Check "yes" or "no" for the following:

	YES	NO
1. Do you prefer to do everything yourself rather than let people help you?	☐	☐
2. For you, is there only one right way to do things?	☐	☐
3. Do you find it hard to make decisions?	☐	☐
4. Do you forget to laugh?	☐	☐
5. Do you never have time to daydream?	☐	☐
6. Is it important to you that everyone likes you?	☐	☐
7. When little things go wrong, does it ruin your whole day?	☐	☐
8. Do you constantly feel exhausted?	☐	☐
9. Have you had problems with insomnia?	☐	☐
10. Do you grind your teeth?	☐	☐
11. In the last year, have you had three or more illnesses that could have been triggered by stress—headaches, diarrhea, colds, flus?	☐	☐
12. Do you hate it when the plan changes?	☐	☐
13. Do you get upset when you have to wait in line?	☐	☐
14. Are you easily bored?	☐	☐
15. Do you find it hard to say no?	☐	☐
16. Do you hate the shape your body is in but can't seem to do anything about changing it?	☐	☐
17. Does your life feel out of control?	☐	☐
18. Are you resentful that so many people make demands on your time?	☐	☐
19. Have you moved, broken up with a boyfriend/girlfriend, lost a parent, or gone through any other big changes in the last year?	☐	☐
20. Was the last time you had a vacation over a year ago?	☐	☐

Count one point for each "yes." The closer your total is to 20, the higher your stress level. If you rate 10 or above, be sure you do *something* because, with this level of stress in your life, you have a high risk of getting sick unless you learn to manage it.

Reprinted with permission from Elizabeth Somer, M.A.R.D., *Food & Mood*, 1999.

STRESS MANAGEMENT SKILLS: WHAT DO YOU DO?

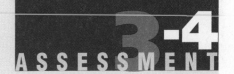

Name: Date: Grade:

Instructor: Course: Section:

For each skill, circle the number that corresponds to your typical skill use.

I use the following skills . . .	Never	Rarely	Occasionally	Regularly
Personal Management Skills: Organizing Yourself				
Valuing: Investing self appropriately	1	2	3	4
Planning: Moving toward goals	1	2	3	4
Commitment: Saying yes and sticking to it	1	2	3	4
Time Use: Setting priorities	1	2	3	4
Pacing: Controlling the tempo	1	2	3	4
Relationship Skills: Changing the Scene				
Contact: Reaching out	1	2	3	4
Listening: Tuning in to others	1	2	3	4
Assertiveness: Saying no	1	2	3	4
Fight: Standing your ground	1	2	3	4
Flight: Leaving the scene	1	2	3	4
Nest-Building: Creating a home	1	2	3	4
Outlook Skills: Changing Your Mind				
Relabeling: Turning a spade into a diamond	1	2	3	4
Surrendering: Saying goodbye	1	2	3	4
Faith: Accepting your limits	1	2	3	4
Imagination: Laughing, creativity	1	2	3	4
Whispering: Talking nicely to oneself	1	2	3	4
Physical Stamina: Building Your Strength				
Exercise: Fine-tuning your body	1	2	3	4
Nourishment: Feeding your body	1	2	3	4
Gentleness: Wearing kid gloves	1	2	3	4
Relaxation: Cruising in neutral	1	2	3	4

Look down the column of 1s. These are your underdeveloped skills. Underline the ones you would like to use more often. **Look at the column of 4s.** These are probably your skills of habit. Mark those you tend to overuse. Which three individual coping skills do you use most often? For what kinds of stressors? As you identify your pattern of skill use, what insights and observations strike you?

Reprinted with permission from Donald A. Tubesing, *Kicking Your Stress Habits*, copyright 1981, 1989. Published by Whole Person Associates Inc., 210 West Michigan, Duluth, MN 55802, (218) 727-0500.

BURNOUT QUIZ

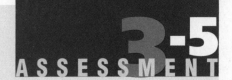

Name: _____   Date: _____   Grade: ____

Instructor: _____   Course: _____   Section: ____

Take a look at all three aspects of your life—career/school, personal, and relationships—and ask yourself the following questions. If the answer is an emphatic *yes*, score 5 points. If it's definitely no, give yourself 0 points. If you're in between, score 1 to 4 points, depending on your level of discomfort.

Score

1. I feel more negative than positive lately. ☐

2. I feel more fatigued than energetic. ☐

3. I work harder and harder and accomplish less and less. ☐

4. Joy is elusive, and I'm often invaded by a sadness I can't explain. ☐

5. I'm increasingly irritable and choosing not to be with people. ☐

6. I suffer from physical complaints (legs feel heavy, backache, headache, lingering colds). ☐

7. I'm unable to laugh at a joke about myself. ☐

8. I feel a loss of self-esteem, confidence, and can-do attitude. ☐

9. Sex seems like more trouble than it's worth. ☐

10. I'm increasingly judgmental, short-tempered, and disappointed in the people around me. ☐

Total Points ☐

SCORING

0–15:	You're doing fine.
16–25:	Oops! There are things you should be watching.
26–35:	You're a candidate for burnout.
36–45:	You're burning out.
46 and over:	Take special note. There are distinct threats to your health and well-being.

Reprinted with permission from Elizabeth Somer, M.A.R.D., *Food & Mood*, 1999.

4 SOCIAL SUPPORT AND HEALTH

THE CLAIM THAT SOCIAL SUPPORT is important to health is not new. What is new is the collection of hard evidence that supports this claim—proof positive that social support is related to positive health practices and can indeed protect people from a wide variety of diseases.[1]

People with positive social ties—regardless of their source—live longer than people who are isolated.[2] People who are isolated are at greater risk of dying early from a number of causes.[3] Being isolated contributes to higher rates of alcoholism, arthritis, depression, heart disease, suicide, and other problems.[4] People who have close-knit networks of positive personal ties with other people seem to be better equipped for avoiding disease, maintain higher levels of health, and in general deal more successfully with life's difficulties.

SOCIAL SUPPORT DEFINED

Social support consists of the resources that other people provide. It includes a person's perception that he or she can rely on other people for help with problems or in times of crisis. It is giving and receiving help from others; it refers to the type, source, number, and quality of resources in one's social network. A social network refers to the durability, intensity, and frequency of social contacts. Social relationships, an important part of social support, includes the presence, number, and type of relationships.

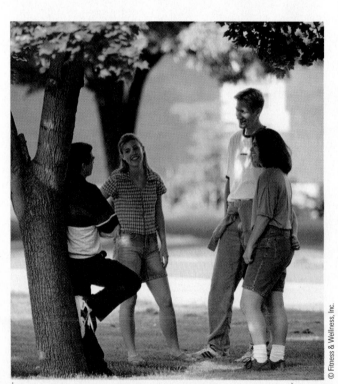

A network of social support can enhance and protect health.

© Fitness & Wellness, Inc.

Four types of social support are important:

- **Instrumental support** is when the resource a social network provides comes in the form of tangible aid, such as lending you money, running an errand for you, or giving you a ride to class when your car is being repaired.
- **Emotional support** provides affection, understanding, acceptance, and respect.
- **Informational support** is when a person provides you with direct information, such as which classes to take, where to go to sign up for a club, and so on.
- **Appraisal support** involves providing you with advice and direction. People who provide this type of support are helpful when you are trying to make a decision.

Do you have people who help you with each of these four aspects of social support?

BENEFITS OF SOCIAL SUPPORT

Social support not only reduces mortality but is key to protecting health as well. The number and strength of an individual's close relationships are related closely to that individual's health and longevity. People who have frequent interactions with others and a variety of relationships usually have better health outcomes. People who have six or more different types of relationships are less likely to experience stress and its negative effects.

Another important aspect of social support is having feelings of connectedness and of being part of a community. The most significant predictor against violence, stress, suicide, and substance abuse are feelings of connectedness at home and in school. Individuals who lack the comfort of another human being may very well lack one of nature's most powerful antidotes to stress.[5] Dr. James Lynch, a social support researcher, remarked:

> Happy relationships depend not on finding the right person, but on being the right person.
> —Eric Butterworth

> The mandate to love your neighbor as you love yourself is not just a moral mandate. It's a physiological mandate. Caring is biological. One thing you get from caring for others is you're not lonely; and the more connected you are to life, the healthier you are.[6]

Nearly 3,000 adults in Tecumseh, Michigan, were the subjects of one long-term study.[7] At the beginning of the

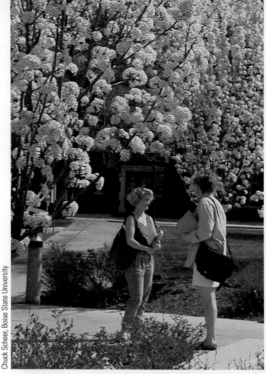

Social ties play an important role in good health.

RELATIONSHIPS FEND OFF COLDS

Loners are four times more likely to come down with a cold than people rich in relationships. This is the conclusion of a study probing the mind-body connection. The study strengthens the notion that an active network of family, friends, neighbors, and even co-workers can bolster resistance to disease, perhaps by activating the immune system.

"This is the first time that anyone has directly linked personal relationships with an immunologically relevant disease outcome," said Janice Kiecolt-Glaser, clinical psychologist at the Ohio State University Medical Center.

The researchers who conducted the study, led by psychologist Sheldon Cohen of Carnegie Mellon University in Pittsburgh, cannot explain precisely why socially deprived people were comparatively worse at warding off a cold virus.

Source: "Relationships Fend Off Colds, Study Finds," *Los Angeles Times*, June 25, 1997.

study, each adult was given a thorough physical examination to rule out any existing illness that would force a person to become isolated. Researchers then watched these people closely for the next 10 years, making special note of their social relationships and group activities. Those who were socially involved were found to have optimal positive health status. When social ties were interrupted or broken, the incidence of disease increased significantly. The researchers concluded that interrupted social ties seemed to actually suppress the body's immune system. The study called close personal relationships a safety net and said that people without this safety net were most vulnerable to a wide variety of diseases.

Social support is important not only to physical health but also to attitude. A study of 60 women living alone in the central Appalachian area showed that the stronger the social support, the better their attitudes. And those with the best attitudes also had enhanced physical health status.[8] Another study showed that a perceived lack of social support was strongly related to depression, poorer health, and a lower quality of life.[9]

If we want to live longer, happier lives, we need to surround ourselves with at least a few good people as friends and confidants. These people must be

> If we want to live longer, we need to surround ourselves with at least a few good people as friends and confidants.

FINDING A SUPPORT GROUP

You can locate a support group through your physician, psychologist, or health-care worker; through local chapters of national organizations; or through newspaper ads. To determine if a group is right for you:

- Attend one of its meetings; check out who is there and whether you feel welcome and free to participate.
- Decide whether you feel free to express your own ideas and thoughts. A good group should provide for open discussion without judgment or criticism.
- You should leave the group feeling uplifted and helped. If you do not, the group probably is not for you.

positive and encouraging in order to provide benefits. Do the people you socialize with help you feel good about yourself? Do your social networks provide you with a sense of belonging and intimacy? Do you feel more competent and confident from your social interactions?

TOUCH: A CRUCIAL ASPECT OF SOCIAL SUPPORT

As important as social support is to health, perhaps one of its most powerful components is also one of its simplest: People who appropriately touch others and receive welcome physical

Social support The network of support that people provide to each other, including instrumental, emotional, informational, and appraisal support.

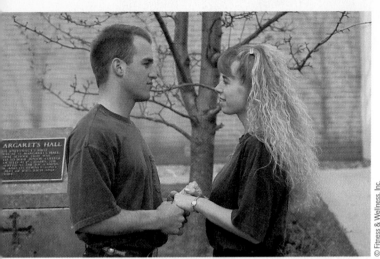

Appropriate touch is an important form of social support.

© Fitness & Wellness, Inc.

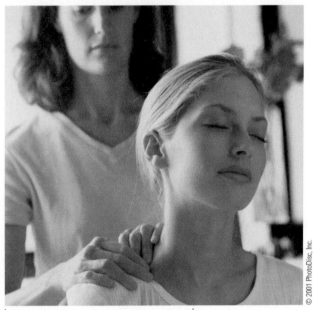

A therapeutic touch can hasten healing.

© 2001 PhotoDisc, Inc.

touch seem to enjoy the positive health benefits. People who enjoy regular, satisfying touch—a pat on the back, a hug—enjoy health benefits as a result. The good health that emanates from touch is both psychological and physical.

To achieve the benefits of stress reduction and physical and emotional healing, some people obtain therapeutic massage. The physical touch can hasten healing and provide other emotional and physical health benefits. It also helps to reduce stress and fatigue and enhances relaxation.

LONELINESS AND HEALTH

Loneliness has been characterized as an unpleasant experience that occurs when a person's network of social relationships is significantly deficient in either quality or quantity. Loneliness is an unwelcome feeling of lack or loss of companionship. It is undesirable and personal.

What one person may consider acceptable solitude may for another be anguish. Loneliness is not necessarily a consequence of living alone. Almost a fourth of Americans who live alone claim that they do not feel lonely.[10] On the other hand, loneliness can exist even when we are surrounded by people. Loneliness is less related to the number of people in our lives than our satisfaction with those relationships. Loneliness sets in when our relationships do not meet our needs or when a positive relationship becomes negative.

Feelings of loneliness are worse when the lonely person is surrounded by people who do not seem to be lonely, such as people who seem to have interpersonal attachments. Loneliness is also felt more keenly when the lonely person has low self-esteem. And, loneliness can stem from lack of attachment to someone else, or from a sense of not belonging to a community. Factors related to loneliness include negative attitude and feelings of boredom.

Loneliness carries with it a risk for health problems.[11] Loneliness, and the stress that accompanies it, have been connected not only to premature death but also to a host of physical and mental disorders. Loneliness is a significant risk factor for minor conditions such as colds and serious illnesses such as heart disease.[12] People who are not lonely have a better chance of staying healthy or recovering from disease than people who are lonely.[13]

Loneliness is a more prevalent and serious problem among adolescents than any other age group.[14] As loneliness increases, so do psychological and physical problems. One study showed that, among adolescents, loneliness correlated strongly with introspection, a poor perception of health, and a number of physical symptoms

LANDMARK STUDY ON SOCIAL SUPPORT

Dr. David Spiegel conducted a landmark study of women whose breast cancer had metastasized. One group was given counseling and social support in addition to the proper medical care. The comparison group of women received only the appropriate medical care without the counseling or peer support. The latter group reported more pain and did not live as long as the group that had received social support from friends and family.

Source: Bill Moyers, **Healing and the Mind** (New York: Doubleday, 1993): 157.

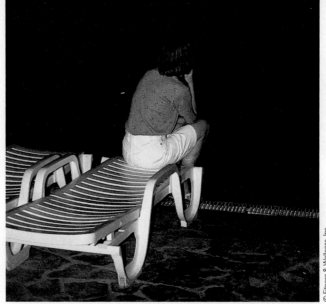

Loneliness may increase the risk of disease and health problems.

including headaches, nausea, sleep disorders, and eating disorders. Adolescent girls had more health problems related to loneliness than did adolescent boys.[15] In addition to identifying loneliness, people can take actions to alleviate it.[16]

The Importance of Good Friends

Close friendships clearly buffer stress and help overcome the unwanted effects of loneliness. Friendship involves certain attitudes that may in themselves help boost health. Friends enjoy trust, respect, and acceptance. A good friend accepts you as you are, without trying to make you change or become a different person. Friends support and help each other, act in the other's best interests, and respect what is important to the other. Friends share feelings and experiences with each other that they don't share with other people. And, despite occasional annoyances, friends enjoy each other most of the time.

Friends contribute to health by meeting needs and providing social support. In some cases, friends may be closer confidants than family members. Confiding in

> I find there is a quality to being alone that is incredibly precious. Life rushes back into the void, richer, more vivid, fuller than before. It is as if in parting one did actually lose an arm. And then, like starfish, one grows it anew; one is whole again, complete and round—more whole, even, than before, when the other people had pieces of one.
>
> —Anne Morrow Lindbergh

another person—having a confidant with whom you can share personal information—forges a powerful and lasting bond and can provide many health benefits. However, some risks are involved in sharing sensitive information with a friend. You may want to consider the following before you begin to confide in someone:

- Realize that sharing information about sensitive issues may strain the friendship. In most cases, confiding in someone helps the two of you grow closer. Your friend, however, might feel threatened or hurt by what you say, and this could change the nature of the relationship.

- Recognize that disclosing your past traumas may be difficult or uncomfortable for the listener. If the information you divulge is upsetting, the listener may be so burdened by what you say that he or she, in turn, may need to tell someone else.

- Understand that what you say and how you say it depends on how your confidant reacts to you. In the best possible situation, your friend will allow you to express your feelings and frustrations without judging or criticizing you.

- Realize that you might have a selfish motive for sharing information that is hurtful to someone. A surprising number of people confide out of revenge ("You hurt me, so I'm going to hurt you.") Revenge, anger, and hurt are not constructive reasons for disclosing certain information.

- Recognize that there might be a better way to solve a problem than by disclosing specific information. You might be able to take direct action, for example. If so, do it. Don't spend your time and energies

Loneliness A condition that occurs when a person's network of social relationships is significantly deficient in either quality or quantity.

discussing grievances in a hurtful manner.

- Before disclosing specific information, ask yourself three questions: Is it true, Is it hurtful, and Is it necessary? If you can answer these questions in ways that reflect sincere motives for sharing information, then it is probably wise to speak to a friend about it.

Enriching Your Support Network

Having a strong social network is a stress-reducing, health-enhancing situation. If your social connections are weak, consider investing time and energy into building your support network. Although it may seem like a burden in today's fast-paced society, the health benefits make it a wise investment of time. Assessment 4-1 can help you assess your friendship qualities.

Enriching your existing friendships is one way to enhance your support network. Experts recognize the importance of connecting with others by phone, mail, and email, but stress that it is also vitally important to spend time with people in person. Face-to-face interactions provide benefits that cannot be obtained by talking on the phone or communicating on the Internet. Non-verbal communication and physical touch are often parts of connecting in person that enrich relationships.

Another way to enhance your social support is to emphasize diversity in your social interactions. Have a variety of different types of friends: some with whom you enjoy deep conversations, others with whom you enjoy light conversation and a casual movie. Seek friendships with people who have similar interests. You can meet people in classes or clubs that focus on computers, poetry, or sports activities.

Establishing rituals for connecting is another valuable way to enhance a support network. Getting together on a regular basis to play golf, play cards, watch a movie, or celebrate birthdays are possible rituals. Seeking ways to build and maintain these rituals can enhance friendships.

Become more involved in positive relationships and less involved in negative relationships. Some relationships are energizing and validating, others are exhausting and unpleasant. People tend to gravitate toward relationships that enhance their self-esteem, however, some people keep in touch with at least one person they do not particularly like—often out of habit or obligation or because they cannot think of a way to end the relationship. Having people around to talk with and relate to is positive for health only if the quality of those relationships is positive.[17] One way to tell if a relationship is health-enhancing is to observe whether you feel better or worse after you've spent time with a particular friend. If a person repeatedly leaves you feeling worse than before the visit, this is likely to be a negative person. Reducing the time involved with negative people and increasing your involvement with positive people will have a beneficial effect on your social network and your health.

Another way to enrich a social network during a crisis or when coping with a difficult situation is to join a support group. These groups provide support from people facing the same or similar problems. This activity can be reassuring and healing. Being involved in a support group can lower psychological stress, reduce depression, and raise self-esteem. Support groups provide emotional and informational support. Members share their feelings and experiences and provide coping strategies. Some support groups enlist experts to talk about related topics.

The Importance of Pets

Comfort does not have to come only from people. Pets fulfill a variety of needs for their human owners. They provide a chance for interaction with another living being and fulfill the same emotional needs. Pets can meet our need to provide care to another and our desire to feel loved. As anyone who owns a pet knows, pets also give affection in return.

Pet ownership has a positive effect on the physical health of pet owners.[18] Pet ownership provides enhanced well-being and a type of social support. Owning a pet may require you to be more physically active than you would

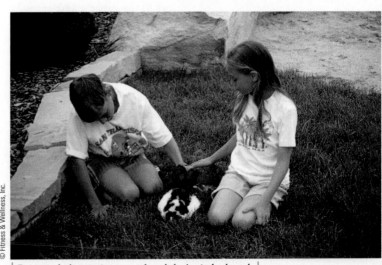

© Fitness & Wellness, Inc.

| Pets can help meet our need and desire to be loved. |

not be otherwise; for example, caring for a pet may require you to take walks.

Even though the health benefits of pets are obvious, that does not mean you should rush into pet ownership without weighing the pros and cons. Owning a pet requires a tremendous commitment, and you have to be in a position to handle it before you take on the care of a pet.

What is the downside to owning a pet? An important issue to consider before getting a pet is the fact that pets cost money. There's the initial expense of purchasing the pet, plus bills for food and veterinary expenses (inoculations, neutering or spaying, and inevitable illnesses). Added to those are the expenses of licensing your pet and purchasing any related paraphernalia, such as food bowls, cages, or leashes. Pets also can ruin carpets and furniture, dig up flowers or shrubs, and damage other personal items. Replacing these items can be costly as well.

Another common problem is some pets are difficult to housebreak. You can overcome this by purchasing a pet that is housebroken already, but you should expect some minor accidents as the pet adjusts to its new surroundings.

A pet can interfere with your independence. If you have a dog, for example, and want to travel for a week, you have to take the dog with you or pay for boarding the dog at a kennel or for someone to come to your home and care for the dog every day. You can overcome this problem by selecting another type of pet such as a mouse, hampster, or a bird. Smaller pets can also provide affection.

Another issue of concern is that caring for pets can generate anxiety if they are injured or get ill. Pets also die eventually, which means a period of bereavement as you grieve the loss of your pet.

Even considering the responsibilities involved, owning a pet has great advantages. In addition to the health benefits already discussed, pet ownership can bring the following benefits:

- Pets bring cheerfulness, play, and laughter to your life. Watching a healthy pet play is entertaining and enjoyable.
- Pets help boost your self-esteem. After a hard day away from home, when all the world seems to be against you, a greeting from your pet can make you feel loved.
- Pets can provide physical touch. Caressing a purring cat or a friendly dog can be soothing and comforting, and may lower blood pressure.
- If you choose a pet that needs exercise, your own exercise will increase, too. You're the one who has to walk the dog twice a day.
- Some pets, such as watchdogs, can contribute to your safety.

TIPS FOR ACTION — CHOOSING THE RIGHT PET

Pets provide rewards, but they also require attention! Carefully consider your schedule and the demands on your time before you choose a pet. You can expect the following from these pets:

- Birds, fish, hamsters, guinea pigs. These and other similar pets require much less time and direct care than dogs and cats. You have to make sure they have food and you have to clean their cages or bowls. Although these kinds of pets require less care, they also provide less intense interaction.
- Cats. Cats require more care than the pets listed above, but less care than dogs. You can leave a large amount of water and dry food if you need to be gone for extended periods, and a cat will do just fine. You also can train cats to use an indoor litter box, so cats can adapt to staying indoors. Cats preen themselves, so they do not need grooming and do not require you to provide exercise. Cats can adjust to even a small apartment. Even though they provide interaction, they also can be independent.
- Dogs. Dogs offer the most intense interaction and also require the most care. They must be fed at the same time each day, must be exercised twice a day, and must be groomed several times a month. Larger dogs need plenty of space for exercise, and you must clean up after dogs.

MARRIAGE AND HEALTH

A good marriage can help protect people from illness and disease, help them recover more quickly if they do get sick, and even help people live longer. Divorced people and those who are unhappily married don't fare nearly as well in terms of health and long life.

What does "happily married" mean? Research suggests the following:[19]

1. The partners find their prime source of joy in each other, but they maintain separate identities. They are independent; they have outside interests and hobbies that don't depend on their partner.
2. They are generous and giving out of love, not because they expect repayment or are keeping score.
3. The partners enjoy a healthy and satisfying sexual relationship.
4. The partners address conflict in a constructive way. For people in a healthy marriage, verbalizing issues of conflict offers a chance to air feelings and frustrations without implying that the other person is wrong or at fault. They resolve issues without harming each other.

5. The partners communicate with each other openly and honestly. There's a risk in it, but experts claim the benefits are worth the risk if the communication is constructive.
6. The two partners in the marriage trust each other. Even after a misunderstanding, closeness can be reestablished if both work at it.
7. Both partners talk about their future together, a future they plan to share because they want to. They may dream about a house on the beach, a vacation to Europe, or a having a child. This kind of planning and talking indicates that both people intend to share their futures together.

| Health Hazards of Divorce |

In the United States, more than half of all marriages end in divorce. The U.S. divorce rate almost doubled between 1965 and 1995. The parents of more than 1 million children divorce in the United States each year.

> Marriage is our last, best chance to grow up.
> —Joseph Barth

A number of factors lead to divorce in today's society. Consider the following:

- Divorces are easier to obtain today than ever before. Many states have no-fault divorces, in which one partner does not have to prove the other is to blame. In some states, "do-it-yourself divorce kits" enable couples to split property, and even custody of children, without the assistance of an attorney.
- The negative social stigma attached to people who divorce no longer exists.
- Many people enter marriage without the proper preparation. The resulting unrealistic expectations can make adjustment to marriage extremely difficult. An amazing number of couples think they should never argue, for example, when in reality constructive fighting is a characteristic of a healthy relationship. As a result, they abandon the marriage when they begin fighting.
- A large percentage of married women work outside the home, making them less financially dependent on their husbands and thus making divorce a less devastating option.

Perhaps because of the emotional repercussions, divorce seems to pose particular health hazards. Men and women who are separated or divorced have poorer physical health than do comparable widowed, married, or single adults.[20] Of all these groups, divorced people have

FACTORS LEADING TO A HAPPY MARRIAGE

Your attitudes about marriage and the person you choose to marry determine how happy you'll be. Your marriage is more likely to be happy if you both want the marriage to succeed and you share the following attitudes about marriage with your partner:

- Marriage is a long-term commitment ("We're in this for good").
- Marriage is a spiritual, sanctified institution between two people.

Your chances for marital happiness are highest if you marry

- Your best friend.
- Someone you genuinely like as a person.
- Someone who grows more interesting to you as time goes on.
- Someone who shares your basic dreams, goals, and aspirations.

more medical complaints, chronic medical conditions, and overall disability, than people who are married.

People who are divorced and who are legally separated from their mates experience more mental and physical illness than those who are married. Psychologically, divorced people are more likely to experience depression, alcoholism, traffic accidents, accidental death, psychiatric problems, suicide, and homicide. Physically, divorced people have higher rates of cancer, heart disease, diabetes, pneumonia, and high blood pressure than do married, single, or widowed persons.

Divorce actually can compromise the immune system, which helps explain why illness and death rates are higher among divorced people. This is especially apparent the first year following divorce. A study of divorced or separated women during the first year following divorce or separation showed that they had poor cellular immune function, and reduced ability to fight disease with responsive lymphocytes.[21]

One reason divorce compromises health is related to social support. Being married provides built-in important social networks, economic ties, and instrumental support. People who are divorced often have to work harder to build these social networks.

Children of divorce suffer the most profoundly.[22] Divorce is one of the most disruptive of all life events for children, and it leads to changes in their biological health. Children almost universally experience divorce as a profound personal, familial, and social loss. In addition to health problems, most children involved in divorce suffer emotional and behavioral changes that also can harm health. Divorce is particularly damaging to a child's emotional and physical health if it involves a geographical move.

While divorce impairs health, being unhappily married may also have a negative effect on health status. Repeated marital conflict can harm health. Actual physical damage occurs during any conflict caused by feelings of anger. Marital conflict can generate an immediate increase in blood pressure. Over the long term, repeated issues of conflict can result in a much higher risk for all kinds of illness and reduced functioning of the immune system. Interactions characterized by hostility, sarcasm, and blame (refusing to take responsibility and demeaning the other partner) seem to be the most damaging.

Positive health benefits are experienced by those who are happily married. The health benefits of marriage result from a number of factors: good integration into the community, social support, the tendency to eat more regular and nutritionally balanced meals, and higher economic status. However, marriage is not necessary for positive health—single people are also able to achieve the health benefits that result from social support.

> The great secret of a successful marriage is to treat all disasters as incidents and none of the incidents as disasters.
>
> —Harold Nicholson

FAMILIES AND HEALTH

A family is a group that shares common goals and values and works together to achieve those goals. A family may be a dual-career family, a single-parent family, or a "bi-nuclear family" (in which the father and mother no longer live together but both provide a place for the children). What goes on in a family—the relationships between its members—can have a profound effect on the health and longevity of each member.

How children are perceived in the family can have great impact on their health and even on their physical growth. An emotionally healthy family supports emotionally healthy development.[23] Conversely, a weak or unhealthy family exhibiting abnormal, impaired, or incomplete functioning impairs the emotional health and self-esteem of family members.

All families occasionally express some degree of problem. Families are neither perfectly healthy or total unhealthy. Unhealthy or dysfunctional family dynamics both cause and result from several conditions:[24]

- Alcoholism and other chemical addictions, chronic mental illnesses, or disabling physical illnesses;
- Dependence on, or obsession with, people who have such conditions; or
- Physical or sexual child abuse.

When these conditions persist, parents are not able to meet their children's emotional needs consistently. The more severe the dysfunction, the more emotional damage to the children. Table 4.1 describes characteristics of functional versus dysfunctional families.

People from dysfunctional families bear a painful legacy of confusion, fear, anger, and hurt. Then, because they instinctively seek what is familiar, even if it is unpleasant, they tend to repeat the patterns they have learned. When developing relationships, they choose people who will interact with them in the same unhealthy ways that their families of origin did. Each person from a dysfunctional family is at high risk of either marrying someone with alcoholism (or another such condition), or repeating a life of addictions, or both.

In general, people from dysfunctional or weak families tend to have poor health outcomes. Families that are weak in structure and support produce children who will have more disease symptoms, impaired physical health, and weakened emotional health.[25] Just as weak or stressed families can contribute to illness, strong families can contribute to good health and long lives.

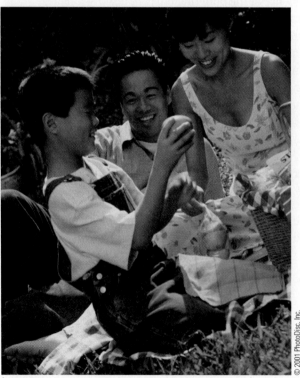

| A strong family contributes to a long and healthy life. |

TABLE 4.1 CHARACTERISTICS OF A FUNCTIONAL VERSUS A DYSFUNCTIONAL FAMILY

Functional Family	Dysfunctional Family
Establishes rules for the sake of functioning cooperatively that are appropriate, consistent, and reasonably flexible.	Establishes rules for control's sake that are rigid and arbitrary.
Encourages its members to develop well-rounded personalities with many facets.	Establishes rigid roles for each member: For example, one is always the scapegoat, one is unnoticed, one is overly responsible, and one is the family clown.
Accepts its problems and treats them as factual.	Has deep, dark secrets that no one may ever disclose (alcoholism, infidelity, or other).
Welcomes outsiders into the system.	Resists allowing outsiders to enter the system.
Typically has members who are relaxed and have a sense of humor.	Has members who are usually serious and tense.
Permits members the right to personal privacy, so that they can develop a sense of self.	Permits members no personal privacy, so that they have difficulty defining themselves as individuals.
Fosters a spontaneous "sense of family," so that members feel free to leave and reenter the system.	Enforces loyalty to the family; members must always act as part of the system.
Allows and resolves conflict between members.	Denies and ignores conflict between members.
Continually changes.	Resists change.
Has spontaneous loyalty and a sense of wholeness.	Has no real unity; is fragmented.

Individuals in healthy families have lower stress levels, fewer illnesses, and the enhanced ability to recover from illness and disease much more rapidly than those in unhealthy families. A strong family helps an individual cope with stress, reducing the risk of illness and disease. Evidence of the buffering effect of healthy families abounds. People in strong families recover more quickly from surgery, tend to follow medical instructions, maintain treatment recommendations, take prescribed medications, and recover more quickly with fewer complications. People in strong families also tend to manage chronic illness better. They tend to live longer than people in weak families.

Should You Have Children?

Should your family include children? Answering this question depends on you, your partner, your lifestyle, and your goals. Before you decide whether to have children, do the following:

- Talk openly and honestly with your partner. Is your relationship healthy? Do you both want a child? If one partner wants a child and the other does not, problems could result.
- Discuss your parenting philosophies. You should share similar views about discipline and techniques for correcting and guiding children. What about

religion? Do you share the same religious views? If not, in which church will the child be reared?

- Consider why you want to have a child. A positive reason is to share your life with someone and to share your love. However, having a child to help to realize an unfulfilled goal or dream is not healthy. Other unhealthy reasons for having a child include being pressured by your spouse or other people or hoping the child will make you happy or take care of you.
- Consider your lifestyle carefully. If you're both working, do you both want to keep working after you have a child? How will that affect you? If one of you decides to quit, can you pay the bills on one income? If you both decide to keep working, can you afford day care, and how will you make those arrangements? If you're going to school, will having a child interfere with your educational goals? Are you ready to give up the freedom and independence that is necessary for making a commitment to a child?
- Assess your personal characteristics. How do you express yourself when you're angry? Would you be likely to become violent with a child? Are you a person who gives love easily? Can you share? Do you enjoy teaching other people? Do you get along with your parents and your brothers and sisters? Most important, do you like children? If you've been miserable around children, you might need to take a hard look at your own decision to become a parent.

12 WAYS TO BUILD STRONG FAMILY VALUES

1. Eat together as a family as often as possible, including several full family dinners a week. Involve everyone (for example, younger children can set the table and older ones can clear up).
2. Hold weekly gatherings to plan family activities, trips, and vacations and to discuss immediate and persistent problems.
3. Schedule daily stress-reduction periods when the entire household is quiet—no TV or CDs. According to your family values, read, meditate, pray, exercise, or whatever works for your family.
4. Volunteer time and talent to worthy causes in the church or community.
5. Participate in school. Become involved with teachers and administrators. Help with after-school and summer programs.
6. Do recreational activities as a family. Take walks or bike rides together.
7. Make or build things together. Share creative activities, and let children take the lead in some of these. Go for accomplishment, not perfection.
8. Take organized trips to sporting events, concerts, local fairs. Include everyone.
9. Bring children to work on occasion to let them see their parents' life away from home.
10. At least once a year, travel away from home. Discuss vacation ideas with children.
11. Limit TV watching. Watch TV with children, monitor what they watch, and discuss what they see.
12. Stay involved. Keep informed about community and national issues that concern you and your children. Let children know your concerns and opinions, and listen to theirs.

Copyright by Dr. Benjamin Spock, **A Better World for Children** (New York: National Press Books, 1994); excerpted from the **Denver Post**.

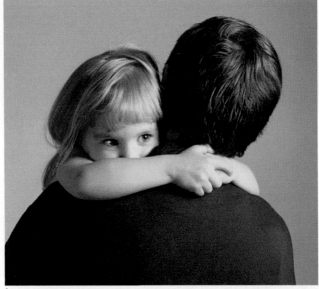

The decision to have a child should be made with deliberate thought and care.

HOW TO DEVELOP PARENTING SKILLS

If you're thinking about becoming a parent, parent education is available—and well worth the effort. You'll find out ahead of time what to expect, how to react, and how you can best build a healthy relationship between you and your child. To find a parent education course, check the following:

- Local public schools
- Local churches or synagogues
- Local community centers
- Local institutions offering adult education courses, including school districts and local colleges
- YMCA
- Your physician or health care provider

SOCIAL SUPPORT AND GRIEF

Social support is needed to help people cope with loss and deal with **grief**. For more than 2,000 years, people have recognized that grief can make people sick. Even longer ago, philosophers and physicians knew that grief alone could kill. Today, loss and the grief that follows it are recognized precursors to distress, depression, and disease. Loss has been implicated in premature death.

Losses range from minor disappointments to situations that pose major discouragement. Some types of loss are especially devastating. Losing a loved one is the most difficult loss to endure. Parents who lose their children suffer deeply, as do children who lose their parents. The loss of loved ones through death, separation, or divorce is emotionally devastating and can result in health problems. The untimely loss of loved ones is associated with both physical and psychological illness.

Bereavement is a special kind of grief. The intense and pivotal grief involved in

Grief The overwhelming sorrow that follows a loss.

Bereavement The process of "disbonding" from someone who played an important role in one's life and is now gone.

WHAT'S "NORMAL" GRIEF?

When you experience a loss significant enough to cause grief, you can expect the following:

- For the first few days, you'll be in a state of shock and denial. It probably will be difficult to accept the loss, and you're likely to feel numb. You'll probably cry a lot during this time, too, which usually lasts about 3 days.
- For the next 2 or 3 months, you'll go through a series of emotions—including anger. You may "bargain" with God, offering all kinds of things in exchange for what was lost. You'll feel sad, tearful, and preoccupied. You may have vivid memories of the lost person and may even sense his or her presence. You may lose your appetite, as well as interest in things you used to enjoy. These feelings generally peak about a month after the loss and usually last for 3 or 4 months but can last as long as a year.
- Within a year after the loss, you'll be able to resume your ordinary activities and will be able to generate happy memories about the lost person. You'll feel sad less often and finally will be able to resolve the loss within yourself.

PROTECTING YOUR IMMUNE SYSTEM WHILE YOU GRIEVE

To keep your immune system in shape,

- Get plenty of rest. Take naps if you need them and try to maintain your normal sleep pattern at night.
- Eat a balanced diet: three solid meals a day with choices from all four food groups. When you feel hungry between meals, eat low-fat snacks high in complex carbohydrates.
- Get plenty of fluids, but avoid those that contain alcohol or caffeine. Both alcohol and caffeine increase dehydration.
- Exercise regularly. Choose an activity you enjoy and do it for at least half an hour at least three times a week. Bicycling, walking, and swimming are good choices.

Above all, stay connected to other people! Social support is especially important during grief to keep your immune system healthy.

bereavement has been shown to pose significant health risks, ranging all the way from immune system disorders to sudden deaths and increased death rates from all causes.[26]

Experiencing grief is necessary for healing. For grief to progress "normally," a person needs to pass through the stages described in Chapter 2 (page 37). Grieving is hard work, and recovery can take several months. People who don't go through the stages of grieving can get stuck in a stage and experience what professionals call "abnormal grief." The result can be serious illness and premature death. Having a strong support network can help people pass through the stages of grief.

Grieving requires a tremendous amount of emotional and physical energy. Positive support systems can provide understanding, love, and comfort during times of loss. When a grieving person is ready, friends can help the person get back into activities they enjoy. A support network can help the person get through the grief process and move on.

The best protection for the bereaved is good social support, strong religious beliefs, rituals, and a conviction that one can control the bereavement.[27] These factors all increase the odds of good health and long life.[28]

> The human spirit has an innate ability to bounce back from loss and despair.

COPING WITH LOSS

- Try to keep things in your life as close to the status quo as possible. Avoid things that could cause additional stress right now, such as a new job, a vacation, or moving to a new residence.
- Postpone decisions that can wait until later. You'll be thinking more clearly and won't be reacting under duress.
- Keep in touch with other people. Social support is especially important now. Let other people express their concern and help you out.
- Avoid the temptation to use drugs or alcohol to ease your feelings of grief; they only make things worse.
- Believe in yourself and your ability to recover. You have the right to go through the stages of grief, so don't be too hard on yourself.

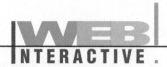

WEB ACTIVITIES

■ **Friends' Health Connection** This site is sponsored by the Friends' Health Connection—a nonprofit organization that connects people who have or have overcome the same disease, illness, disability, or injury—to provide a medium for mutual support. Participants are matched based upon a number of criteria including age, health problems, symptoms, lifestyle effects, tests and surgeries, attitude, occupation, hobbies, and interests. People of all ages participate, and their health problems range from the most common to very rare disorders. There is also an opportunity for networking friends and family members.
http://www.48friend.org

■ **Relationship Skills and Heart Disease: A New Frontier** This site is based on a lecture presented by Martin Sullivan, M.D., a cardiologist at Duke University. He describes the following "relationship risk factors" for cardiac disease: social isolation, sleep disorder and depression, hostility, repression of emotion, work stress, loss of meaning, and low affiliation/high power.
http://www.smartmarriages.com/healthyheart.html

InfoTrac
You can find additional readings related to wellness via InfoTrac College Edition, an on-line library of more than 900 journals and publications. Follow the instructions for accessing InfoTrac that came packaged with your textbook, then search for articles using a key word search.

Suggested Reading Kathleen P. Pittman, Judith L. Wold, Astrid H. Wilson, Carolyn Huff, and Sharon Williams, "Community Connections: Promoting Family Health," *Family and Community Health* 23, no. 2 (July 2000): 72.

1. Who do most adolescents consider their most reliable source of critical health information?
2. Describe the multidimensional model, PCAP, that provided the framework for the development of the partnership between the College of Health and Human Sciences at Georgia State University, a major urban university, and M. L. King Middle School, an inner-city middle school.
3. What was the mission of the partnership?

Web Activity
"Go Ask Alice"
http://www.goaskalice.columbia.edu

Sponsor Columbia University Health Education Department, a division of the University Health Service.

Description This site, sponsored by Columbia University Health Education Department, features a large interactive question-and-answer site. It contains its own search engine. The mission of "Go Ask Alice!" is to provide factual and nonjudgmental information written by health educators and health practitioners to assist readers' decision-making about their physical, emotional, sexual, and spiritual health.

Available Activity

1. Search the archives of more than 1,800 previously answered questions in the following six health disciplines: general health, fitness and nutrition, sexuality, relationships, sexual health, and alcohol and other drugs.

Web Work
1. From the home page, click on "Relationships."
2. Scroll down to read the different categories of questions, including general relationship "stuff"; gay, lesbian, bisexual, and nonconsensual relationships; talking with parents; friendship; roommate rumblings; miscellaneous.
3. Read the description of each question found on the links. When you see a question that interests you, simply click on that link.
4. Repeat this procedure for each question whose answer you would like to view.

Helpful Hints
1. "Go Ask Alice!" provides health information only and should not be viewed as providing personalized medical advice or diagnoses. You should consult with a qualified health care provider if you have specific symptoms or concerns. "Go Ask Alice!" does not respond immediately to your questions. Not all questions are answered.
2. Return to this site regularly to view new questions and answers on a variety of health topics of special interest to college students and young adults. Questions and answers on this site are updated weekly.

For additional Web activities, links, and suggested readings, visit our Health, Fitness and Wellness Resource Center at http://health.wadsworth.com.

NOTES

1. N. E. Mahon et al., "Social Support and Positive Health Practices in Young Adults. Loneliness as a Mediating Variable," *Clinical Nursing Research* 7 (1998): 292–308.

2. L. F. Berkman, "The Role of Social Relations in Health Promotion," *Psychosomatic Medicine* 57 (1995): 245–254.

3. M. A. Lewis et al., "Social Control in Personal Relationships: Impact on Health Behaviors and Psychological Distress," *Health Psychology* 18 (1999): 63–71.

4. "This Season: Make Friends with Good Health," *Consumer Reports on Health* (1999).

5. *The Broken Heart: The Medical Consequences of Loneliness* (New York: Basic Books, 1977).

6. B. Q. Hafen and K. J. Frandsen, *In People Who Need People Are the Healthiest People: The Importance of Relationships* (Provo, UT: Behavioral Health Associates).

7. See Note 6.

8. J. M. Collins et al., "Functional Health, Social Support, and Morale of Older Women Living Alone in Appalachia," *Journal of Women & Aging* 6 (1994): 39–51.

9. J. T. Newsom et al., "Social Support as a Mediator in the Relation Between Functional Status and Quality of Life in Older Adults," *Psychology and Aging* 11 (1996): 34–44.

10. B. Blai, "Health Consequences of Loneliness: A Review of the Literature," *Journal of the American College Health Association* (1989): 162.

11. A. Forbes, "Loneliness," *British Medical Journal* 313 (1996): 352–354.

12. J. Geller et al., "Loneliness as a Predictor of Hospital Emergency Department Use," *Journal of Family Practice* 48 (1999): 801–803.

13. M. A. R. Tijhuis et al., "Changes in and Factors Related to Loneliness in Older Men. The Zutphen Elderly Study," *Age and Aging* 28 (1999): 491–495.

14. N. E. Mahon et al., "Loneliness and Health-Related Variables in Young Adults," *Perceptual and Motor Skills* 85 (1997): 800–802.

15. N. E. Mahon et al., "Health Consequences of Loneliness in Adolescents," *Research in Nursing and Health* 16 (1993): 23–31.

16. N. E. Mahon, A. Yarcheski, and T. J. Yarcheski, "Social Support and Positive Health Practices in Young Adults. Loneliness as a Mediating Variable," *Clinical Nursing Research* 7 (3): 292–308, 1998 Aug.

17. D. Vandervoort, "Quality of Social Support in Mental and Physical Health," *Current Psychology* 18 (1999): 205–214.

18. P. Raina et al., "Influence of Companion Animals on the Physical and Psychological Health of Older People: An Analysis of a One-Year Longitudinal Study," *Journal of the American Geriatrics Society* 47 (1999): 323–329.

19. Editors of *Prevention* Magazine, *Positive Living and Health: The Complete Guide to Brain/Body Healing and Mental Empowerment* (Emmaus, PA: Rodale Press, 1990).

20. X. S. Ren, "Marital Status and Quality of Relationships: The Impact on Health Perception," *Social Science and Medicine* 44 (1997): 2241–2249.

21. B. R. Sarason, I. G. Sarason, and G. R. Pierce, *Social Support: An Interactional View* (New York: John Wiley and Sons, 1990).

22. R. E. Emery et al., "Delinquent Behavior, Future Divorce or Nonmarital Childbearing, and Externalizing Behavior Among Offspring: A 14-Year Prospective Study," *Journal of Family Psychology* 13 (1999): 568–579.

23. S. S. Mull, "Help for the Children of Alcoholics," *Health Education* (September/October 1990): 42.

24. C. L. Whitfield, *Healing the Child Within* (Deerfield Beach, FL: Health Communications, 1987): 25–53.

25. G. R. Parkerson Jr. et al., "Associations Among Family Support, Family Stress, and Personal Functional Health Status," *Journal of Clinical Epidemiology* 42 (1989).

26. B. R. Hayslip et al., "Selective Attrition Effects in Bereavement Research: A Three-Year Longitudinal Analysis," *The Journal of Death and Dying* 38 (1998): 21.

27. E. Hallowell, "Strong Relationships Really Do Help Ensure Good Health," *Health* (2000): 3–4.

28. C. F. Mendes de Leon et al., "Social Networks and Disability Transitions Across Eight Intervals of Yearly Data in the New Haven EPESE," *Journal of Gerontology* 54B (1999): S162–S172; R. Williams et al., "Improving Your Relationships Will Improve Your Health," *Health* (1999): 13–14.

DO YOU HAVE THE QUALITIES OF FRIENDSHIP?

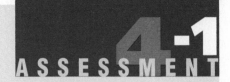

Name: _____   Date: _____   Grade: _____

Instructor: _____   Course: _____   Section: _____

Friendship is a two-way business. To make friends, you have to be a friend. The better friend you are, the more friends you are likely to have. This questionnaire lists some of the qualities of friendship.

Check "yes" or "no" to the questions. Then look at the scoring key at the end.

YES   NO

1. Are people able to depend on you to keep your word?

2. Can they rely on you to respect their confidences?

3. Do you keep the friends you make?

4. Do you often put yourself to trouble and inconvenience to oblige other people?

5. Suppose they want to do something you are not particularly keen on. Would you go along with them and do what they want to do?

6. Are you quick to pay your share of the expenses?

7. Are you generous with your praise and appreciation?

8. Do you show affection when you feel it?

9. Is it easy for you to forgive and forget?

10. Do you readily give people the benefit of the doubt and make allowances?

11. In a sharp difference of opinion, would you speak first?

12. Do you own up when you are wrong and say you are sorry?

13. You may like somebody very much, but would you feel the same if he or she were to become unpopular?

14. Are you quick off the mark to give sympathy and practical help when people need it?

15. Do you like to see others praised and fussed over?

16. Can you agree to differ and stay on the best of terms?

17. Are you an attentive and sympathetic listener?

18. Are you always the same, not full of welcome today and too busy to bother tomorrow?

19. Do you mind people having other friends and interests that you do not share?

20. Can you say you are much more interested in other people than in yourself?

Scoring

Count 5 points for every "yes." A score of 70 or over is good, and 60–70 is satisfactory. Under 60 is not satisfactory. You are not likely to be a good friend. Usually, when we are like this, we're wrapped up in ourselves. We like only the individuals who notice us and make a fuss over us and dislike anybody who is not interested in us or who will not do what we want. If you desire to be a good friend, you will have to be more interested in other people than in yourself and put them first.

Adapted from Singer Communications, Inc., Anaheim, California. Used by permission.

5 PERCEPTIONS, THE SPIRIT, AND HEALTH

OBJECTIVES

- Define explanatory style and explain the differences between a pessimistic style and an optimistic style, as well as their effects on health.

- Explain the differences between an internal health locus of control and an external health locus of control.

- Describe the connection between self-esteem and health.

- Explain how to protect health with a fighting spirit.

- Describe the connection between spirituality and health, including the power of prayer, forgiveness, faith, and contentment.

- Describe the altruistic personality and the health benefits of volunteerism.

- Contrast the health effects of hope versus hopelessness.

95

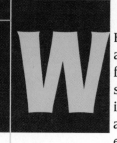

WHEN PEOPLE THINK ABOUT HEALTH and ways to be healthy, they usually first think about nutrition, exercise, and stress reduction and overlook other very important aspects of health—those of attitude and spirituality. This chapter explains spiritual concepts and how attitude and spirituality influence health. The first aspect of this area is related to attitude and perceptions.

The habitual manner in which people explain the things that happen to them is their **explanatory style**. It is a way of thinking when all other factors are equal and when there are no clear-cut right and wrong answers. The contrasting explanatory styles are pessimism and optimism.

> An optimist may see a light where there is none, but why must the pessimist always run to blow it out?
>
> —Michel de Saint-Pierre

People with a pessimistic explanatory style interpret events negatively; people with an optimistic explanatory style interpret events in a positive light—every cloud has a silver lining.

The pessimistic explanatory style can be identified by three thought patterns, which may appear during conversation:

1. Assuming a problem is never-ending, being convinced it will never go away.
2. Believing a problem is global—that it applies in every situation instead of being an isolated incident.
3. Internalizing everything ("It's my fault"), destructively assigning blame to self or others.

Explanatory style can be a potent predictor of physical health. It affects both emotional and physical well-being. In the emotional arena, a negative explanatory style can lead to anxiety, depression, guilt, anger, or hostility. In the physical realm, a negative explanatory style can interfere with the healing process.

A pessimistic explanatory style can delay healing time and worsen the course of illness in several major diseases. For example, it can affect the circulatory system and general outlook for people with coronary heart disease. Blood flow actually changes as thoughts, feelings, and attitudes change. People with a pessimistic explanatory style have a higher risk of developing heart disease.

Studies of explanatory style verify that a negative explanatory style also compromises immunity. Blood samples taken from people with a negative explanatory style revealed suppressed immune function, a low ratio of helper/suppressor T-cells, and fewer lymphocytes (the cells responsible for waging war against disease or infection).[1]

In contrast, an optimistic style tends to increase the strength of the immune system. An optimistic explanatory style and the positive attitude it fosters can also enhance the ability to resist infections, allergies, autoimmunities, and even cancer. Dr. Bernie Siegel, who helps patients change their explanatory style and resolve stress and conflict in their lives, says a change in explanatory style has been accompanied by remarkable changes in the course of disease.[2] He maintains that an optimistic explanatory style and the positive emotions it embraces—such as love, acceptance, and forgiveness—stimulate the body's healing systems.

Optimism is a trait that people can cultivate. To assess your optimism, see Assessment 5-1. To boost your own optimism, try the following:

- Before you start to change your attitudes, surround yourself with people who care about you and can help you. Ideally, they are optimistic people. When you surround yourself with optimists, you begin to "catch" their attitude. Tell others you want to change and solicit their help and suggestions.
- Learn to genuinely like other people. Look for their good qualities and respect their differences.
- Realize that changing your explanatory style is a big commitment. In essence, it is a change in lifestyle. You did not develop your explanatory style overnight, and you will not be able to change it overnight, either. Be patient with yourself and expect some hard work. Get past the inevitable setbacks and disappointments. Look at these as challenges and do not let them deter you.
- Set small, attainable goals, then reward yourself richly when you meet those goals. Celebrate your accomplishments.
- Look beyond yourself. The world does not revolve around you. Get involved in helping others to expand your horizons.
- Guard against exaggeration. An argument with a friend does not mean the friendship is collapsing. One poor exam score does not mean your college career is doomed. Do not blow things out of proportion.
- Avoid generalization. Just because you experience one disappointment does not mean that nothing ever turns out right. Recount and embrace your past successes and the good things that have happened to you.
- Face your problems head-on. Develop strategies for solving them instead of trying to escape them.
- Above all, have fun. Learn to laugh at yourself, to relax, to enjoy and respect yourself.

HEALTH LOCUS OF CONTROL

Our **health locus of control** is determined by the extent to which we believe that our behavior affects our health status. Control does not mean that we need to control everything around us, such as other people or our circumstances. Control does mean how much we believe our actions can affect a situation. We can choose how to react and respond.

> If the theme song of the external is "Cast Your Fate to the Winds," the theme song of the internal is "I Did It My Way."
>
> —Philip Rice

Each person's health locus of control lies somewhere along a continuum. At one end of the continuum shown in Figure 5.1 is the **external locus of control**. At the opposite end is the **internal locus of control**. People with an external locus of control believe the things that happen to them are unrelated to their own behavior and, therefore, are beyond their control. People with an internal locus of control, in contrast, believe that events are a consequence of their personal actions and, thus, potentially can be controlled.

As a whole, people with a greater sense of internal control have fewer illnesses because they usually practice healthier behaviors. In addition, an internal locus of control has a significant influence over the body's release of hormones, which has been found to be a powerful determinant of health.[3] Following are three of the hormones influenced by a lack of control:

1. Serotonin, which regulates moods, relieves pain, and helps control the release of the pain-killing endorphins;
2. Dopamine, largely responsible for a sense of reward and pleasure; and
3. Norepinephrine, which, when depleted, causes depression.

When people perceive that they have little control, the levels of corticosteroids in their bloodstream rise. The corticosteroids, released by the body during stress, have a

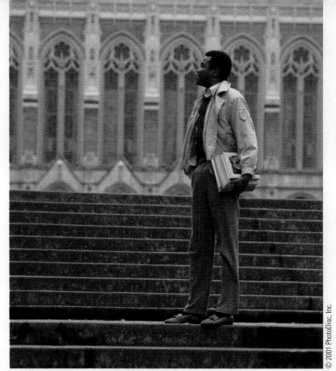

Attaining a goal affirms an internal locus of control.

variety of negative physical effects. They lower the body's resistance to disease and suppress the body's manufacture of the three hormones above, making lack of control a two-edged sword. A sense of lack of control may impair health status more than a high level of stress.

People in stressful situations who believe they have some control over their situations experience less of the physiological damage normally associated with stress. Internal locus of control functions as a buffer against stress.

SELF-ESTEEM

Self-esteem is a way of viewing and assessing yourself. Positive self-esteem is a sense of feeling good about one's capabilities, goals, accomplishments, place in the world, and relationship to others. People with high self-esteem respect themselves. Self-esteem is a powerful determinant of health

Explanatory style The way people perceive the events in their lives, from an optimistic or a pessimistic perspective.

Health locus of control The extent to which a person believes his or her behavior affects their health status.

External locus of control One's prevailing belief that the things that happen are unrelated to one's own behavior.

Internal locus of control One's prevailing belief that events are a consequence of one's own actions and, thus, potentially can be controlled.

Self-esteem A sense of positive self-regard and self-respect.

FIGURE 5.1 CONTINUUM OF LOCUS OF CONTROL.

LOCUS OF CONTROL

External ←———— CONTINUUM ————→ Internal

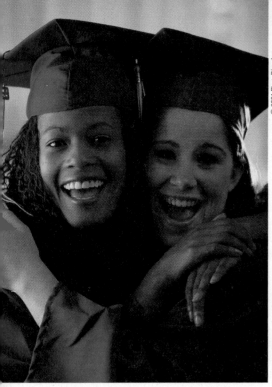
Self-esteem can enhance mental and physical health.

behavior and, therefore, of health status. Self-esteem might be called the blueprint for behavior.

Healthy self-esteem is one of the best things a person can develop for overall health, both mental and physical. A good, strong sense of self can boost the immune system, protect against disease, and aid in healing.

> We can secure other people's approval if we do right and try hard; but our own is worth a hundred of it.
> —Mark Twain

Whether people get sick—and how long they stay that way—may depend in part on the strength of their self-esteem. For example, low self-esteem worsens chronic pain. The higher the self-esteem, the more rapid the recovery. If we have strong self-esteem, the outlook is good. If our self-esteem is poor, however, our health can decline in direct proportion, as our attitude and negative perceptions worsen.

Belief in oneself is one of the most powerful weapons people have to protect health and live longer, more satisfying lives. It has a dramatic and positive impact on wellness, and we can work to harness it to our advantage. To assess your views about yourself, see Assessment 5-2.

To boost your self-esteem,

- Use **affirmations**. Prepare a list of your positive traits. Boost your sense of esteem by saying positive things about you to yourself, such as, "I'm honest and open in expressing my feelings." Write some affirmations of your own and use them every day.
- List the traits you would like to have or experience. Construct the statements as if you were already enjoying those situations, beginning each sentence with "I am . . . ". For example: "I am feeling great about doing well in my classes," or "I am enjoying the opportunity to meet new people." Visualize each situation and get in the habit of repeating this process several times a day.
- When your "internal critic"—the negative inner voice we all have—starts putting you down, tune it out. Force yourself to think of a situation that you handled well or to recall something about yourself that you're especially proud of. Assessment 5-3 can provide you with insight about your thought patterns.

> What wise people and grandmothers have always known is that the way you feel about yourself, your attitudes, beliefs, values, have a great deal to do with your health and well-being.
> —Madeline Gershwin

A FIGHTING SPIRIT

A **fighting spirit** involves the healthy expression of emotions, whether they are negative or positive. At the other extreme is hopelessness, a surrender to despair. In between these are attitudes of indecision and stoic acceptance, as shown in Figure 5.2.

Fighting spirit can play a major role in recovery from disease. People with a fighting spirit accept their disease diagnosis, adopt an optimistic attitude filled with faith, seek information about how to help themselves, and are determined to fight the disease.

A fighting spirit may be the underlying factor in what is called **spontaneous remission** from incurable illness. More and more physicians believe that the phenomenon is real and that the patient is the key in spontaneous remission. They believe the patient's attitude, especially the presence of a fighting spirit, is responsible for victory over disease. Fighters are not stronger or more capable than others—they simply do not give up as easily. They enjoy better health and live longer, even when physicians and laboratory tests say they should not.

Specific factors bolster a fighting spirit and promote survival.[4] A fighting spirit makes a person take charge.

FIGURE **5.2**   CONTINUUM SHOWING ATTITUDES TOWARD SERIOUS ILLNESS.

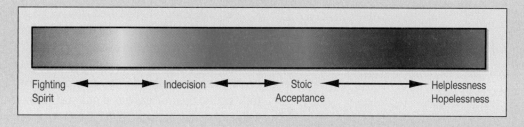

Fighting
Spirit ←——————→ Indecision ←——————→ Stoic
Acceptance ←——————→ Helplessness
Hopelessness

CASE STUDY OF A FIGHTING SPIRIT

In discussing the power of a fighting spirit, psychoneuro-immunology pioneer Dr. George Solomon told the story of a Harvard professor who had been stricken with cancer; he had lesions in his head, lungs, and liver. Nonetheless, the professor continued teaching his classes, reassuring his friends and students.

Solomon says of the professor, "It was thrilling to see how powerful the fighting spirit can be. For most of a year, he battled that cancer. And he won. The most important thing he had to teach us came not out of his medical lectures but out of his own experience and example. He won against all the odds—against the predictions of the specialists and against the reports based on sophisticated technology."

What the professor taught all around him was, in essence, that if we are willing to fight, we can win.

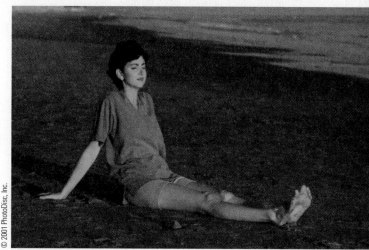

© 2001 PhotoDisc, Inc.

Spirituality entails a belief in a power higher than oneself.

Fighters are intrinsically different from people who give up, and their health status reflects those differences.

SPIRITUALITY

Spirituality is an integral part of being human. The word "spirituality" itself is derived from the Latin word for breath, or that which gives life to or animates a person. It connotes what is at the center of one's life.[5] Spirituality includes belief in and a person's relationship with a higher being.[6]

Spirituality enhances meaning and purpose in life. Spirituality is a personal value system regarding the way people approach life. It is a dimension of a person that encompasses one's relationship with self, others, and a higher power, and it is manifested through creative expressions, familiar rituals, meaningful work, and religious practices. Spirituality involves finding meaning in life and even in death.

People have spiritual needs. They need to make sense of their particular situations, to find meaning and purpose in their days, relationships, and life. People need to feel connected. They need approval and they need to know that their lives have been of worth to themselves, their families, friends, and communities. People need hope, meaning in life, and forgiveness.[7] They need to know that they are loved and that others care for them and find them worthwhile. For many people, these spiritual needs are met through a relationship with God and their religious beliefs.[8]

Spiritual health includes the ability to discover and articulate our own basic purpose in life and to learn how to experience love, joy, peace, and fulfillment. It is the experience of helping ourselves and others achieve full potential.[9] Through the spiritual dimension, we emphasize our connectedness to others.

Affirmations Positive statements that help reinforce the positive aspects of personality and experience.

Fighting spirit Determination; the open expression of emotions, whether negative or positive.

Spontaneous remission Inexplicable recovery from incurable illness.

Spiritual health Dimension of health related to a person's moral or religious nature; a relationship with a higher being.

People with spiritual health display specific traits. They

- Search for deep meaning and purpose in life
- Live in accordance with values
- Participate in religious rituals
- Experience consistent contentment with life
- Express hope in life and after death
- Express feelings of being loved by others and by God
- Seek good in others
- Trust God with the outcome of situations in which they have no control
- Express hope and creativity
- Forgive others and express feelings of forgiveness from God

Adapted from F. M. Highfield and C. Carson, "Spiritual Needs of the Patients: Are They Recognized? *Cancer Nursing* 6 (1983):187–192.

| Spirituality Enhances Health Status |

The cultivation of spiritual health—which is a process or journey, not an endpoint—can enhance physical, mental, and emotional health, sometimes in dramatic ways. One study indicated that many professionally successful men and women have strong spiritual values and beliefs in spite of having suffered major psychological or physical traumas.[10] Researchers indicated that the subjects' spirituality enabled them to handle crises and develop effective styles of coping with life crises.

> Psychiatrists no longer dismiss out of hand the importance of religious faith in recovery from emotional illness and the healing power of forgiveness; there is a recognition of the connection between prayer and healing. A strong faith can have a profound effect on our lifestyles and outlook in terms of health.
>
> —George Gallup, Jr.

Spirituality seems to buffer stress. People with a deep sense of spirituality are not defeated by crises; they have traits of hardiness that protect them from negative effects of stress.[11] Spirituality helps people interpret crises in a growth-producing way. As a result, they are able to use trials, and even illness, as a means of spiritual growth. Even when disease claims a life, spirituality can make the experience one of positive growth.

Not everyone will be cured from disease. At some time or another, everyone will die. Nevertheless, people who are busy living, who are trying to make positive changes in their lives, experience growth even in the face of serious illness. People who face disease with that attitude define their disease as a gift, a challenge, a wake-up call, and a new beginning. They take it as an opportunity to fully experience life until they die.

Twenty years ago, the field of medicine ignored spirituality, at least formally. At most, a medical doctor might call a hospital chaplain. Although a spiritual dimension of the human being is a widely accepted aspect of health, the medical profession had given little attention to nurturing the spirit.[12] Today things have changed. At least 40 U.S. medical schools have integrated spirituality education into their required curricula.[13]

Religion and spirituality are increasingly viewed as important for patient recovery and quality of life. A recent survey of family physicians found that 99 percent believed that religious beliefs can help the healing process.[14] Spirituality is an important source of hope for patients struggling with recovery from illnesses.[15] It is one of the most important coping mechanisms. Patients receive strength and comfort from spirituality, and this improves recovery outcomes.

Medical physicians are being encouraged to learn about patients' religious and spiritual beliefs and to address these issues when a patient needs spiritual support.[16] The question being asked by today's health care providers is not whether spirituality has health benefits, but how these benefits can be obtained. Three reasons to include spirituality in healing are the following:

1. Hope is a crucial element in psychological adjustment,
2. Emotional strength is important in healing to achieve an energized mental state, and
3. Emotional support is necessary during healing.

| Prayer |

Prayer is communication with a higher power. It sometimes includes asking for guidance, wisdom, and strength. Prayer signals a commitment to a set of moral and ethical values. It is a signpost of our spirituality, at the core of most personal and spiritual experiences.

Prayer has powerful beneficial physiological effects on the body. In a national survey of family physicians, 94 percent stated that they believed that personal prayer or other spiritual practices can aid medical treatment and improve healing.[17]

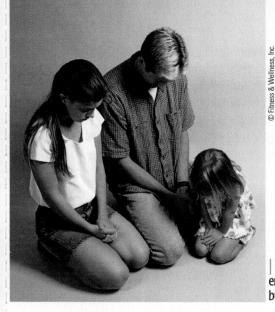

© Fitness & Wellness, Inc.

| Sincere prayer can enhance health and buffer stress. |

| Contentment |

Contentment means feeling satisfaction, being pleased, or experiencing happiness. Many people in today's society feel chronically dissatisfied with life. They suffer from emptiness and unhappiness. In response to this emptiness, some people look to external sources for fulfillment —a better job, more money, more things—in other words, materialism. Others may seek wealth, popularity, and sometimes superficial highs. Often this pursuit only leads to short-lived episodes of fleeting happiness. But most people truly long for enduring contentment: a deep-down, soul-satisfying peace and contentment.

People who truly reach this kind of contentment do not depend on life circumstance. They develop inner harmony through spirituality and learn to cultivate contentment by understanding that they are totally loved and accepted by their higher power. Their faith and practice of prayer and simple living lead to an enduring contentment.

Another important aspect of contentment is gratitude. People who are appreciative and thankful are truly happy. Gratitude involves appreciating what you have and not longing for what you do not have. To become consistently contented, practice being grateful. Focus on the positive aspects of your life.

Researchers who study prayer test its effectiveness by the same methodical scrutiny used in traditional trials. They have found that prayer accelerates healing and other positive health outcomes.[18] Prayer can reduce or prevent despair; it prepares the mind to be responsive to treatment. It effectively induces the **relaxation response**, which is important in medical treatment and health status.

Prayer can exert a powerful benefit on people even when they do not know prayers are being offered in their behalf. One study organized a group of people around the country to pray daily for 192 coronary care unit patients at a hospital without telling the patients that anyone was praying for them. A separate group of 201 patients had no one assigned to pray for them. The praying continued for 10 months. The patients who were prayed for had significantly fewer complications while they were in the coronary care unit.[19] Another well-designed study found that remote intercessory prayer was associated with enhanced healing and recovery of heart patients.[20] Researchers advised that prayer be considered an effective adjunct to standard medical care. Critical review of this study stated that the remote effects of prayer should not be discounted, even if the mechanism involved is not completely understood.[21]

> Large majorities of Americans say that prayer is an important part of their lives, that they believe that miracles are performed by the power of God, and that they are sometimes conscious of the presence of God.
>
> —Pollster George Gallup, Jr.

| Forgiveness |

Essential to a spiritual nature is **forgiveness**. Forgiving means not holding wrongs against people and not seeking revenge when others have hurt you. To forgive is to give up the desire to punish or to pardon for wrongdoing. If you forgive someone, you do not hold hard feelings toward that person. It means accepting the core of every human being and giving them the gift of not judging them. It involves releasing resentment.

To understand the health benefits of forgiveness, we can examine what happens when we do not forgive. When we choose to hold hard feelings toward someone and feed anger and resentment, we suffer mentally and physically. The body releases hormones that cause the heart to pound, blood pressure to rise, muscles to contract, and abdominal pain to develop. If the situation continues unchecked, gastric ulcers, gastritis, or irritable bowel syndrome can result. People who refuse to forgive harbor resentment and bitterness. A negative, bitter attitude is harmful emotionally and physically.

People with spirituality are often more willing to forgive

Relaxation response
The body's ability to enter a scientifically defined state of relaxation.

Forgiveness The ability to release from the mind all past hurts and failures, all sense of guilt and loss.

LEARNING TO FORGIVE

For day-to-day mishaps—a roommate offended you, you were served cold food in a restaurant—you can learn to forgive, and it may be easier than you think.

- Start practicing forgiveness of minor infractions, things that are easy to forgive. Once you've learned the technique, it's easier to transfer to more difficult problems.
- Set aside a "forgiveness hour." For that hour, forgive everything that happens, even the things you do. Expand it to a "forgiveness day." Realize how great you feel to forgive someone instead of lugging around a burden of grudges and hard feelings.
- Take a hard look at the way you judge others. Your own judgment, not the actions of someone else, is often what makes forgiveness difficult. Make it a policy to reserve judgment until you have all the facts. Better yet, make a hard-and-fast rule to postpone all judgments for one year. (Chances are good that you will have forgotten the whole thing by then.)
- Don't say you've "forgiven" someone, then tell your roommates what happened. Forgiving entails forgetting.
- Learn to forgive yourself. If you have to, say it aloud ("I forgive myself for cutting class and not being up front with the professor"). Learn from your mistakes and turn them into positives instead of using them as ammunition against yourself forever.

others because they have experienced forgiveness. When people experience forgiveness, anger and resentment dissolve. Healing occurs through forgiveness.

| Religious Attendance |

Religion refers to the spiritual experience as part of an organized system of beliefs, practices, and knowledge.[22] Religion is an expression of spirituality. Religion refers to the ritual and practices that people utilize to express their relationship with God.[23]

People with active religious faith and people who are strongly affiliated with a place of worship generally enjoy better health. A six-year study conducted at Duke University of almost 4,000 older people found that people who attended religious services once a week or more lived longer than people who did not attend.[24] Another study showed that people who attended church at least once a week lived 7 years longer than people who never attended.[25] People who attended church frequently

reported greater social support, less depression, and better health practices. They also had less anxiety, less substance abuse, fewer strokes, lower blood pressure, and overall enhanced well-being.

One study showed that people who attended church weekly and prayed or studied the Bible at least daily had consistently lower blood pressure and recovered from depression more quickly than others.[26] Religious patients also had more thorough recoveries from depression. Attending religious services is likely to improve social support, self-esteem, and coping skills. Lack of religious involvement is considered a risk factor for poorer health.[27]

Even though no one knows precisely how religious participation protects health, probable reasons have been advanced:

- Many religious services prescribe behavior that prevents illness or assists in the treatment of illness and discourage behavior that is harmful to health.
- Places of worship provide social support that can reduce loneliness, and they offer support groups for people in times of need.
- Most religions place strong emphasis on marriage and the family, both of which have health benefits.
- People who attend religious services are more likely to pray and be prayed for, and prayer benefits health.
- Religious people sometimes have a strong sense of self-esteem and control, as well as a deep sense of spiritual well-being. One study found a strong association between religion and well-being that is consistent throughout life.[28]
- Places of worship promote positive approaches toward illness, pain, or disability, which can influence the outcome of disease. People with chronic disabling conditions, such as heart disease and diabetes, are less likely to become depressed if they use religion (such as prayer, faith, and spiritual reading) to adapt to stress.
- Religious faith and activity improve coping skills and generally give people a value system that helps them prioritize in times of indecision.

| Altruism |

One aspect of spirituality is **altruism**, a selfless giving to other people out of genuine concern without expecting something in return. It is an unselfish devotion to the interests and welfare of others. People who are altruistic are self-sacrificing for the benefit of others. During a selfless career, physician and philosopher Albert Schweitzer proclaimed that true happiness is to be found only by serving others.

The ability to put another's needs above one's own also seems to contribute to a longer and healthier life.

CHARACTERISTICS OF VOLUNTEERS

A true volunteer has the following characteristics:

- The helper actually connects with people (that is, makes one-on-one contact). Writing out a check to a charity doesn't provide the same health benefits as working for a few hours at the local food bank.
- The helper has a desire to help.
- The helper likes what he or she is doing.
- The helper is consistent (the greatest health benefits have been reaped by those who do regular volunteer work at least once a week).
- The helper gives freely, not out of a sense of obligation. A person who swings a hammer on low-income housing because of her desire to see better housing for the poor will have better health benefits than a person who cleans up litter along the interstate as part of court-enforced community service requirements.
- The volunteer work is part of a balance in the helper's life. If volunteer work begins to interfere with school, work, or family obligations, the helper may have more, not fewer, health problems.

GUIDELINES FOR VOLUNTEERS

To guard against burnout, volunteers should adhere to the following guidelines:

- Don't try to do too much. A good goal is roughly 2 hours of volunteer work a week. If you have a tight schedule, just an hour a week may be advisable.
- Do something you enjoy and something you'd feel comfortable doing. A suicide hotline may be begging for volunteers, but if that kind of work makes you extremely uncomfortable, another volunteer option would be better.
- Realize that any line of work, volunteer or paid, has occasional setbacks or bad experiences, but that plenty of good happens in the meantime.
- Realize that you are not responsible for anyone else. You can't keep a person from committing suicide or an addict from returning to cocaine. You can provide help and support, but the responsibility is up to the person being helped.
- Get out of any situation that isn't right for you; look for something else. Just because the other volunteers seem to be doing well and enjoying themselves, it doesn't mean this specific situation is the best one for everybody.

Doing good for others benefits the nervous system and the immune system. Whereas stress can undermine the immune system, the positive emotions related to altruism help stabilize the immune system against the normal immunosuppressing effects of stress.

What makes a person altruistic? Some believe it is instinctive, others believe it is learned from the value systems and behaviors of people you are close to. Growing numbers believe that altruism is a capacity everyone shares to some extent. Anyone can develop altruism. Some believe in an altruistic "personality" that enables them to reach out to others. Most altruistic people[29]

- do not regard others as inferiors;
- have a positive view of people in general;
- value human relationships more than money;
- are concerned about others' welfare;
- believe that ethical values should be applied universally;
- believe in the right of innocent people to be free from persecution;
- have a healthy perspective about themselves;
- take personal responsibility for how other people are doing;
- are "connected" to others;
- have a profound commitment to caring; and

- believe they can control events and shape their own destiny but are willing to risk failure.

Background and family values help determine the altruistic personality. Altruists are usually raised in families that are warm and nurturing. The emotional self-acceptance and compassion for others that is developed in such an environment encourages people to be generous, creative, playful, and relaxed. Altruistic people often engage in volunteer work. People who engage in volunteer work have better health, visit the doctor less often, and have fewer medical complaints than others.[30]

To help others, you can volunteer. Places that need volunteers include schools, churches, synagogues, homeless shelters, food pantries, thrift shops, libraries, zoos, animal shelters, museums, hospitals, and nursing homes. The best volunteer opportunities

- provide a regular schedule and a specific description of what the volunteers are expected to do;
- provide personal contact with the people the volunteers are going to help;

Religion The system of how to know God; system of belief and worship.

Altruism The act of giving of oneself out of a genuine concern for other people; unselfish devotion to the interests and welfare of others.

In the early 1960s, Bruce Randolph was almost 60 years old and nearly broke when he headed to Denver to be near his son. He began his little barbecue restaurant out of a house, using his mother's "secret" sauce recipe. Four years later, he started a holiday meal tradition, feeding a few hundred people out of the back of a truck.

By the time he died in 1994, he was a household name in Denver. "Daddy Bruce" was the only name he needed. Annually for 30 years, he organized giant Thanksgiving dinners for thousands of needy people who had nowhere else to go for the holiday. His philanthropy didn't end there. He often served free meals on Christmas and on his birthday. He collected and distributed clothing for the poor, and he organized Easter egg hunts in the park for children.

After his death at age 93, a street was named in his honor. A handpainted sign on the closed restaurant reads, "It is more blessed to give than to receive." No one would argue that one of Daddy Bruce's secrets to a long life was altruism, a giving spirit.

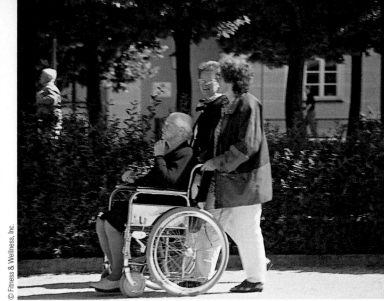

Altruism enhances health and well-being.

© Fitness & Wellness, Inc.

- utilize skills the volunteers have already or train them for something they'd like to be able to do;
- fall within volunteers' area of interest (it's easier to stick with the volunteer work if it's something they really enjoy doing); and
- expect a reasonable commitment—2 hours a week is a good goal.

Before making a commitment, the prospective volunteer should explore what is available in the area, visit the facilities, watch what goes on, then narrow the choices. Before signing up for volunteer work, the volunteer should obtain as much information as possible and not be afraid to ask questions. This will enable the prospective volunteer to find the most satisfying outlet for altruism.

Volunteering to help others can bring tremendous health benefits. However, if people overextend themselves or get involved in an activity that is not compatible, they may get burned out and run the risk of getting sick instead of protecting their health.

Another way to express altruism is through random acts of kindness. This involves doing something for another person that will make their day easier or better in some way. For one person, this might include paying a bridge toll for the next driver. Another person might see that an unknown person's parking meter has expired and deposit a few quarters. Acts of kindness that are performed without the other person knowing offer the highest reward to the giver.

Faith

Faith is belief in something that is unseen. It is believing and trusting without proof. To have faith is to have confidence that things will work out for the best. Faith is the belief and trust in a higher power.

Faithfulness is a positive trait to cultivate. A faithful person is loyal and honest. Being faithful means being worthy of trust, doing one's duty, and keeping one's promise. A faithful person is reliable and dependable.

Personal belief gives us an unseen power that enables us to do what seems impossible, even to facilitate healing. History is replete with examples of people who have benefited from the healing power of faith. It has relieved headaches, reduced angina pains, controlled hypertension, overcome insomnia, prevented hyperventilation attacks, alleviated backaches, enhanced cancer treatment, controlled panic attacks, reduced cholesterol levels, lowered overall stress, and alleviated symptoms of anxiety, including nausea, vomiting, diarrhea, and constipation.

A good example of faith's power over physiological processes is its beneficial influence on blood pressure. Devoutly faithful groups of people tend to have lower blood pressure than others who lack this quality.[31]

The power of faith is apparent in the healing process. Faith is a hidden ingredient in Western medicine and in

> Faith is an excitement and an enthusiasm: it is a condition of intellectual magnificence to which we must cling as a treasure, and not squander in the small coin of empty words.
>
> —George Sand

every traditional system of healing. Many illnesses can be treated more successfully if the patient believes in a cure.[32]

| Hope |

Hope is a feeling that what one desires will happen. It is positive expectation or anticipation. Hope benefits health and the human body. Spirituality is a key element of hope.[33] Interpersonal connectedness and purpose in life, along with religious practice, have been shown to foster hope in terminally ill people.[34] Spiritual behaviors are hope-inspiring and can transcend suffering associated with illness.[35]

Medical history is replete with examples of "terminal" patients who, awash with hope, defied all medical odds. Some lived months or years longer than predicted. Some were able to remain symptom-free and enjoy comfort for the last period of their lives. Some lived and were healed. More and more, physicians are finding that hope is a powerful tool in their work with patients.

Hope is an active way of coping with threatening situations by focusing on the positive. No matter how dark or grim a situation may appear, optimistic people are able to extract the positive aspects and concentrate on them. They fill their minds with hopeful scenarios, stories with happy endings, or positive outcomes.

Hope has a powerful influence on physical health and well-being. It can bring not only enhanced health but a longer life as well. Dr. Elisabeth Kübler-Ross, whose work with dying patients revolutionized the medical profession, stressed the importance of hope. Even though they cannot hope for a cure, she said, patients can hope for enriched relationships, freedom from pain, dignity and peace.

If hope can influence health profoundly for the better, its opposite—**hopelessness**—can have the opposite effect. Hopelessness is marked by negative future expectations and the belief that the future holds nothing good or positive. It also is characterized by the inability to reach a desired goal, futility in planning for goals, and a lack of motivation to use constructive action to gain control of life. People who feel hopeless usually feel despondent, desperate, and despairing; they feel they have lost control and are helpless about what the future holds.

One physician gives a poignant example of what happens when hope is lost.[36] She remembers a 55-year-old woman who was admitted to the hospital with a cancerous lesion in her lung. She was an energetic woman, who was vigorous and friendly. She even assisted in work on the hospital floor, helping to pass the meal trays and running minor errands. The staff came to love her.

When the woman underwent biopsy, it revealed a deadly cancer that already had invaded the lymph nodes. The surgeons could not remove it, so they closed the incision. The next day a group of residents and interns surrounded her bed. One of them looked down and said, "Well, it's cancer, and we couldn't really resect it, so we just opened and closed."

The patient kept repeating the question, "Opened and closed?" As the intern nodded and repeatedly confirmed the procedure, she finally asked, "You mean you left the cancer in there?" "Yes," he replied. She closed her eyes and told the interns she was tired. They left the room.

The woman died that night. The autopsy revealed no specific cause of death, just the cancer—but it had been there for months. Her physician believed that she died because all hope had been taken away from her.

An attitude of hope is not just a mental state; it causes specific electrochemical changes in the body that benefits not only the strength of the immune system but the workings of individual organs in the body as well. Hope is tremendous expectation, and expectation can have powerful influence over the human body. Hope is so powerful and so real that it can even influence the outcome of supposedly terminal and irreversible diseases, such as cancer. People often recover when their prognoses were negative.

In summary, attitude, spirituality, self-esteem, contentment, altruism, hope, faith, love, and a strong will to live can not only extend length of life, but can also enhance quality of life. As we learn to appreciate our uniqueness as human beings, we find we have the opportunity to experience full growth even under the grimmest circumstances. The length of our lives provides only a technical measurement of how long we live. Far more important than how long we live is the way we embrace each day and experience an abundant and meaningful life.

> Hope is the essential ingredient. Without it, patients find no reason for struggling to survive; without it, we find it easy to give up and stay in bed.
>
> —journalist Natalie Davis Springarn

Faith Belief and trust in God, God's promises, or religion.

Hope To desire and expect optimism; positive anticipation and expectation.

Hopelessness A mental state marked by negative expectations about the future; despairing.

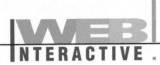

WEB ACTIVITIES

■ **Resources for Improving Self-Esteem, Self-Confidence, Self-Acceptance** This site features links to a variety of resources, including on-line articles and books. The site also links to several self-assessment tests to provide you an opportunity to measure your self-esteem.
http://www.webheights.net/lovethyself/home.htm

■ **ABC's of Personal Growth** This is a self-help improvement site featuring psychology tests/quizzes on self-esteem and spiritual health, as well as educational articles about love, sex, violence, parenting, E-IQ test/quiz, self-esteem, dieting/weight loss, happiness, wellness, and mental health.
http://www.helpself.com

■ **Optimism/Pessimism Test** This site, sponsored by the award-winning QueenDom.com mental health Internet site, features an 18-question multiple-choice inventory designed to determine whether you have an optimistic or pessimistic viewpoint.
http://www.queendom.com/tests/eng/optim_frm.html

■ **Spirituality and Health** This site consists of a series of articles dealing with spiritual health, including interviews with the Dalai Lama and Bernie Siegel, M.D.
http://fire.he.net/~sandh/life/xlif.html

■ **Exploring Practical Spirituality** This site, inspired by Mary Baker Eddy's *Science and Health with Key to the Scriptures*, features several links dealing with spirituality, including wellness, self-identity, relationships, career, and current events.
http://www.spirituality.com

InfoTrac

You can find additional readings related to wellness via InfoTrac College Edition, an on-line library of more than 900 journals and publications. Follow the instructions for accessing InfoTrac that came packaged with your textbook, then search for articles using a key word search.

Suggested Reading Linda L. Barnes, Gregory A. Plotnikoff, Kenneth Fox, and Sarah Pendleton, "Spirituality, Religion, and Pediatrics: Intersecting Worlds of Healing," *Pediatrics* 16, no. 4 (Oct. 2000): 899.

1. Describe the different stages of James Fowler's faith-development theory.

2. How does spirituality and religion affect child development and improve self-esteem?
3. List several examples of how religious engagement can contribute to children's pursuit of health-promoting and preventive health behaviors.

Web Activity
The Soul-Body Connection: Spirituality and Well-being Check-up
http://www.spiritualityhealth.com/check/inspirit/kintro.html

Sponsor Jared Kass, Ph.D., professor of Counseling and Psychology and director of the Study Project on Well-Being, Graduate School of Arts and Social Sciences, Lesley College, Cambridge Massachusetts.

Description This site features an easy-to-complete self-assessment questionnaire to determine your level of spirituality and how you can achieve greater personal fulfillment in the midst of a stressful life.

Available Activities This site features a three-part questionnaire to determine your level of spirituality and stress management, including

1. Questions in Part I determine your spiritual experience.
2. Part II questions determine your sense of wellness and include assessment of your energy level, goals, sources of stress, hopefulness, love, and life satisfaction.
3. Part III questions assess your stress load and how you respond to stress from the following areas: health, work, relationships, finances, daily hassles, and lifestyle choices.

Web Work
1. From the home page, click on the "Start the Tests" link. Answer all questions by clicking on the appropriate radio button.
2. Answer the questions in Part I, "Your Spiritual Experience."
3. Complete the 13 questions in the spiritual experiences table.
4. Answer the 32 questions in Part II, "Your Sense of Well-being," which immediately follows the Part I table.
5. Answer the questions in Part III, which immediately follows the Part II questions.
6. Once you have answered all questions, click on the "I'm finished" button to obtain your evaluation. You also have the opportunity to go back to change your answers if you choose.

For additional Web activities, links, and suggested readings, visit our Health, Fitness, and Wellness Resource Center at http://health.wadsworth.com.

NOTES

1. Leslie Kaman-Siege et al., "Explanatory Style and Cell-Mediated Immunity in Elderly Men and Women," *Health Psychology* 10 (1991): 229–235.

2. "Mind Over Cancer: An Exclusive Interview with Yale Surgeon Dr. Bernie Siegel," *Prevention* (March 1988): 59–64.

3. *Head First: The Biology of Hope* (New York: E. P. Dutton, 1989).

4. S. Fishman, "Absolutely, Positively, Refusing to Die," *Longevity* (September 1990): 69.

5. M. B. Dombeck, "Dream-telling: A Means of Spiritual Awareness," *Holistic Nursing Practice* 9 (1995): 37–47.

6. P. Fryback et al., "Spirituality and People with Potentially Fatal Diagnoses," *Nursing Forum* 34 (1999): 13–17.

7. K. Wright, "Professional, Ethical, and Legal Implications for Spiritual Care in Nursing," *Image: Journal of Nursing Scholarship* 30 (1998): 81–83.

8. G. Laukhug et al., "Spirituality: The Missing Link," *Journal of Neuroscience Nursing* 30 (1998): 60–67.

9. C. Marwick, "Should Physicians Prescribe Prayer for Health? Spiritual Aspects of Well-Being Considered," *Journal of the American Medical Association* 273 (May 24/31, 1995): 1561.

10. "The Spirit of Health," *Journal of the Institute for the Advancement of Health* 5 (1988): 4.

11. J. Pace et al., "Correlates of Spiritual Well-Being in Terminally Ill Persons with AIDS and Terminally Ill Persons with Cancer," *Journal of the Association of Nurses in AIDS Care* 8 (1997): 31–42.

12. M. C. Leetun, "Wellness Spirituality in the Older Adult: Assessment and Intervention Protocol," *The Nurse Practitioner* 21 (1996): 60–65.

13. Jan Ziegler, "Spirituality Returns to the Fold in Medical Practice," *Journal of the National Cancer Institute* 90 (1998): 1255–1254.

14. M. L. Albert, "Spirituality and Healing in Medicine," *HealthInform: Essential Information on Alternative Health Care* 4 (1999): 7.

15. D. O'Neill et al., "Spirituality and Chronic Illness," *Image: Journal of Nursing Scholarship* 30 (1998): 275–280.

16. M. Mitka, "Getting Religion Seen as Help in Being Well," *The Journal of the American Medical Association* 280 (1998): 1896.

17. "Meditation and Prayer Facilitate Healing Hope," *HealthInform: Essential Information on Alternative Health Care* 4 (1999): 1.

18. S. L. Johnston, "Prayer and Healing," *Paraplegia News* 53 (1999): 23.

19. "Does Prayer Help Patients?" *MD* (December 1986): 35; B. Justice, *Who Gets Sick: Thinking and Health*, (Houston: Peak Press, 1987).

20. W. Harris et al., "A Randomized, Controlled Trial of the Effects of Remote, Intercessory Prayer on Outcomes in Patients Admitted to the Coronary Care Unit," *Archives of Internal Medicine* 159 (1999): 2273–2278.

21. L. Dossey, "Prayer and Medical Science: A Commentary on the Prayer Study by Harris et al. and a Response to Critics," *Archives of Internal Medicine* 160 (2000).

22. H. G. Koenig et al., "Religion and Well-Being in Later Life," *Gerontologist* 28 (1988): 18–27.

23. S. Pehler, "Children's Spiritual Response: Validation of the Nursing Diagnosis Spiritual Distress," *Nursing Diagnosis* 8 (1997): 55–66.

24. H. Koenig et al., "Does Religious Attendance Prolong Survival? A Six-Year Follow-Up Study of 3,968 Older Adults," *Journal of Gerontology* 54A (1999): M370–M376.

25. R. A. Hummer et al., "Religious Involvement and U.S. Adult Mortality," *Demography* 36 (1999): 273–285.

26. "Therapeutic Efficacy of Prayer," *Archives of Internal Medicine* 160 (2000).

27. C. Marwick, "Should Physicians Prescribe Prayer for Health? Spiritual Aspects of Well-Being Considered," *Journal of the American Medical Association* 273 (May 24/31, 1995): 1562.

28. J. S. Levin et al., "Religious Effects on Health Status and Life Satisfaction Among Black Americans," *Journal of Gerontology* 50B (1995): S154–S163.

29. "The Altruistic Personality: Rescuers of Jews in Nazi Europe" (New York: Macmillan/Free Press, 1988).

30. A. Luks with P. Payne, *The Healing Power of Doing Good: The Health and Spiritual Benefits of Helping Others* (New York: Ballantine Books, 1991).

31. S. Long, "Extend Your Hand, Extend Your Life," *Longevity* (March 1989): 18.

32. See note 31.

33. J. Kylma et al., "Hope in Nursing Research: A Meta-Analysis of the Ontological and Epistemological Foundations of Research on Hope," *Journal of Advanced Nursing* 25 (1997): 364–371.

34. K. Herth, "Fostering Hope in Terminally-Ill People," *Journal of Advanced Nursing* 15 (1990): 1250–1259.

35. J. F. Miller, "Hope-Inspiring Strategies of the Critically Ill," *Applied Nursing Research* 2 (1989): 23–29.

36. "The Importance of Hope," *Western Journal of Medicine* 150 (May 1989): 609.

THE LIFE ORIENTATION TEST: ARE YOU AN OPTIMIST?

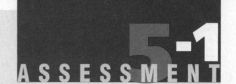

Name: _____   Date: _____   Grade: _____

Instructor: _____   Course: _____   Section: _____

In the following spaces, write how much you agree with each of the items, using the following scale:

4 = strongly agree   3 = agree   2 = neutral   1 = disagree   0 = strongly disagree

1. In uncertain times, I usually expect the best.

2. If something can go wrong for me, it will.

3. I always look on the bright side of things.

4. I'm always optimistic about my future.

5. I hardly ever expect things to go my way.

6. Things never work out the way I want them to.

7. I'm a believer in the idea that "every cloud has a silver lining."

8. I rarely count on good things happening to me.

How to Score

For items 2, 5, 6, and 8, you will need to reverse the numbers. For example, if you strongly agree with statement 8, "I rarely count on good things happening to me," change your score from 4 to 0. Now total up your score.

Interpreting Your Results

This test has been used to demonstrate a relationship between an optimistic or a pessimistic outlook and physical well-being. When college students completed this test 4 weeks before final exams, the optimists (with 20 points and over) reported far fewer health problems. The pessimists complained of more dizziness, fatigue, sore muscles, and coughs.

HOW DO YOU FEEL ABOUT YOURSELF?

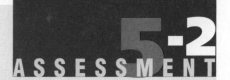

Name:	**Date:**	**Grade:**
Instructor:	**Course:**	**Section:**

This scale is designed to help you understand your self-image. Positive attitudes toward oneself are important components of maturation and emotional well-being.

Self-image aspect	Strongly agree	Agree	Disagree	Strongly disagree
1. I feel that I'm a person of worth, at least on an equal plane with others.	A	B	C	D
2. I feel that I have a number of good qualities.	A	B	C	D
3. All in all, I am inclined to feel that I am a failure.	A	B	C	D
4. I am able to do things as well as most other people.	A	B	C	D
5. I feel I do not have as much to be proud of as others.	A	B	C	D
6. I take a positive attitude toward myself.	A	B	C	D
7. On the whole, I am satisfied with myself.	A	B	C	D
8. I wish I could have more respect for myself.	A	B	C	D
9. I certainly feel useless at times.	A	B	C	D
10. At times I think I am no good at all.	A	B	C	D

How to Score

Use the following table to determine the number of points to assign to each of your answers. To determine your total score, add up all the numbers that match the letter (A, B, C, or D) you circled for each statement.

Statement	A	B	C	D
1.	4	3	2	1
2.	4	3	2	1
3.	1	2	3	4
4.	4	3	2	1
5.	1	2	3	4
6.	4	3	2	1
7.	4	3	2	1
8.	1	2	3	4
9.	1	2	3	4
10.	1	2	3	4

Total: _____ This is your self-esteem score.

Interpreting Your Score

Classify your score in the appropriate score range.

Score range	Current self-esteem level
Less than 20	Low self-esteem
20–29	Below-average self-esteem
30–34	Above-average self-esteem
35–39	High self-esteem
40	Highest self-esteem

The higher your score, the more positive your self-esteem.

High self-esteem means that individuals respect themselves, consider themselves worthy, but do not necessarily consider themselves better than others. They do not feel themselves to be the ultimate in perfection; on the contrary, they recognize their limitations and expect to grow and improve.

Self-esteem is the most important variable in regard to human development and maturation. It is the master key that can open the door to the actualization of an individual's human potential.

From M. Rosenberg, *Society and the Adolescent Self-Image* (Hanover, NH: Wesleyan University Press, 1986). Used by permission.

— SUMMARY STATEMENT —
Workshop On
Physical Activity and Public Health

Sponsored By:
U. S. Centers for Disease Control and Prevention
and
American College of Sports Medicine

In Cooperation with the President's Council on Physical Fitness and Sports

Regular physical activity is an important component of a healthy lifestyle — preventing disease and enhancing health and quality of life. A persuasive body of scientific evidence, which has accumulated over the past several decades, indicates that regular, moderate-intensity physical activity confers substantial health benefits. Because of this evidence, the U.S. Public Health Service has identified increased physical activity as a priority in Healthy People 2000, our national health objectives for the year 2000.

A primary benefit of regular physical activity is protection against coronary heart disease. In addition, physical activity appears to provide some protection against several other chronic diseases such as adult-onset diabetes, hypertension, certain cancers, osteoporosis, and depression. Furthermore, on average, physically active people outlive inactive people, even if they start their activity late in life. It is estimated that more than 250,000 deaths per year in the U.S. can be attributed to lack of regular physical activity, a number comparable to the deaths attributed to other chronic disease risk factors such as obesity, high blood pressure, and elevated blood cholesterol.

Despite the recognized value of physical activity, few Americans are regularly active. Only 22% of adults engage in leisure time physical activity at the level recommended for health benefits in Healthy People 2000. Fully 24% of adult Americans are completely sedentary and are badly in need of more physical activity. The remaining 54% are inadequately active and they too would benefit from more physical activity. Participation in regular physical activity appears to have gradually increased during the 1960s, 1970s, and early 1980s, but has plateaued in recent years. Among ethnic minority populations, older persons, and those with lower incomes or levels of education, participation in regular physical activity has remained consistently low.

Why are so few Americans physically active? Perhaps one answer is that previous public health efforts to promote physical activity have overemphasized the importance of high-intensity exercise. The current low rate of participation may be explained, in part, by the perception of many people that they must engage in vigorous, continuous exercise to reap health benefits. Actually the scientific evidence clearly demonstrates that regular, moderate-intensity physical activity provides substantial health benefits. A group of experts brought together by the U.S. Centers for Disease Control and Prevention (CDC) and the American College of Sports Medicine (ACSM) reviewed the pertinent scientific evidence and formulated the following recommendation:

Every American adult should accumulate 30 minutes or more of moderate-intensity physical activity over the course of most days of the week. Incorporating more activity into the daily routine is an effective way to improve health. Activities that can contribute to the 30-minute total include walking up stairs (instead of taking the elevator), gardening, raking leaves, dancing, and walking part or all of the way to or from work. The recommended 30 minutes of physical activity may also come from planned exercise or recreation such as jogging, playing tennis, swimming, and cycling. One specific way to meet the standard is to walk two miles briskly.

Because most adult Americans fail to meet this recommended level of moderate-intensity physical activity, almost all should strive to increase their participation in moderate or vigorous physical activity. Persons who currently do not engage in regular physical activity should begin by incorporating a few minutes of increased activity into their day, building up gradually to 30 minutes of additional physical activity. Those who are irregularly active should strive to adopt a more consistent pattern of activity. Regular participation in physical activities that develop and maintain muscular strength and joint flexibility is also recommended.

This recommendation has been developed to emphasize the important health benefits of moderate physical activity. But recognizing the benefits of physical activity is only part of the solution to this important public health problem. Today's high-tech society entices people to be inactive. Cars, television, and labor-saving devices have profoundly changed the way many people perform their jobs, take care of their homes, and use their leisure time. Furthermore, our surroundings often present significant barriers to participation in physical activity. Walking to the corner store proves difficult if there are no sidewalks; riding a bicycle to work is not an option unless safe bike lanes or paths are available.

Many Americans will not change their lifestyles until the environmental and social barriers to physical activity are reduced or eliminated. Individuals can help to overcome these barriers by modifying their own lifestyles and by encouraging family members and friends to become more active. In addition, local, state, and federal public health agencies; recreation boards; school groups; professional organizations; and fitness and sports organizations should work together to disseminate this critical public health message and to promote national, community, worksite, and school programs that help Americans become more physically active.

The American College of Sports Medicine and the U.S. Centers for Disease Control and Prevention, in cooperation
with the President's Council on Physical Fitness and Sports, released this statement July 29, 1993, at the National Press Club in Washington, D.C.

TABLE 6.1 PERCENT OF TOTAL U.S. ADULT POPULATION THAT REGULARLY PARTICIPATES IN PHYSICAL ACTIVITY

	Moderate Intensity*	High Intensity**
Overall	20%	14%
By Gender		
Men	21	13
Women	19	16
By Ethnicity		
White	21	15
African American	15	9
Hispanic American	20	12

* A minimum of 5 days per week for at least 30 minutes per session.

** At least 3 days per week for a minimum of 20 minutes.U.S. Department of Health and Human *Services, Physical Activity and Health: A Report of the Surgeon General* (Atlanta: Centers for Disease Control and Prevention, National Center for Chronic Disease Prevention and Health Promotion, 1996).

Furthermore, the number of people who are not physically active is more than twice the number who suffer from hypertension, have high cholesterol, or smoke cigarettes. This report became a call to action nationwide. Regular **moderate physical activity** can prevent premature death, unnecessary illness, and disability. It also can help control health care costs and help to maintain a high quality of life into old age.

The report states that regular moderate physical activity provides substantial benefits in health and well-being for the vast majority of people who are not physically active. Among these benefits are significantly reduced risks for developing or dying from heart disease, diabetes, colon cancer, and high blood pressure. Regular physical activity also is important for the health of muscles, bones, and joints, and it seems to reduce symptoms of depression and anxiety, improve mood, and enhance the ability to perform daily tasks throughout life. Individuals who are already moderately active can achieve greater health benefits by increasing the amount of physical activity.

In the report, moderate physical activity has been defined as physical activity that uses 150 calories of energy per day or 1000 calories per week. People should strive to achieve at least 30 minutes of physical activity per day most days of the week. Examples of moderate physical activity are walking, cycling, playing basketball or volleyball, swimming, performing water aerobics, dancing fast, pushing a stroller, raking leaves, shoveling snow, washing or waxing a car by hand, washing windows or floors, and even gardening.

active at all. Further, almost half of all people between 12 and 21 years of age are not vigorously active on a regular basis. The report also stated that physical inactivity is more prevalent in

1. Women than men
2. African Americans and Hispanics than whites
3. Older than younger adults
4. Less-affluent than more-affluent people
5. More-educated than less-educated adults

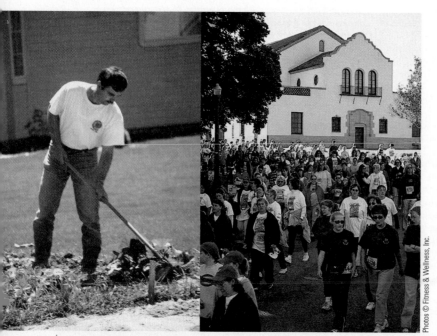

The U.S. Surgeon General has determined that moderate-intensity physical activity is beneficial to health and well-being.

Photos © Fitness & Wellness, Inc.

FITNESS AND HEALTH

Several significant research studies linking physical activity habits and mortality rates have shown a decrease in premature mortality rates among physically active people. A study conducted by Dr. Ralph Paffenbarger and his colleagues involving 16,936 Harvard alumni showed that, as the amount of weekly physical activity increased, the risk of cardiovascular deaths decreased.[5] The greatest decrease in cardiovascular deaths was observed among alumni who used in excess of 2,000 calories per week through physical activity (see Figure 6.2).

Another major study, conducted by Dr. Steve Blair and his associates, upheld the findings of the Harvard alumni study.[6] Based on data from 13,344 people who were followed over an average of 8 years, the results confirmed that the level of cardiorespiratory fitness

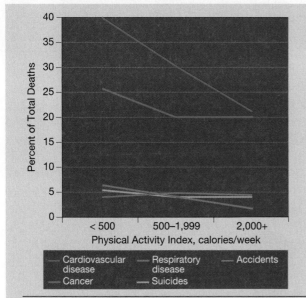

FIGURE 6.2 DEATH RATES ACCORDING TO PHYSICAL ACTIVITY INDEX.

Percent of Total Deaths

Physical Activity Index, calories/week

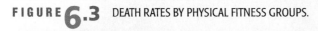

- Cardiovascular disease
- Cancer
- Respiratory disease
- Suicides
- Accidents

From R. S. Paffenbarger, R. T. Hyde, A. L. Wing, and C. H. Steinmetz, "A Natural History of Athleticism on Cardiovascular Health," by *Journal of the American Medical Association* 252 (1984): 491–495.

Based on 10,000 man-years of observation. One person-year indicates one person followed up 1 year later.

FIGURE 6.3 DEATH RATES BY PHYSICAL FITNESS GROUPS.

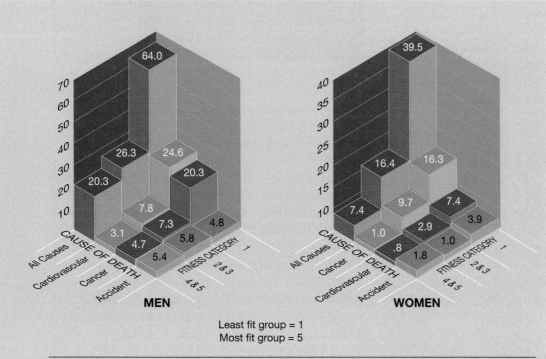

MEN

WOMEN

Least fit group = 1
Most fit group = 5

Note: Study included 13,344 people, followed for 10,000 person-years 1970–1985. One person-year indicates one person followed up 1 year later.

Based on data from S. N. Blair, H. W. Kohl III, R. S. Paffenbarger, Jr., D. G. Clark, K. H. Cooper, and L. W. Gibbons, "Physical Fitness and All-Cause Mortality: A Prospective Study of Healthy Men and Women," *Journal of the American Medical Association* 262 (1989), 2395–2401.

is related to mortality from all causes. In essence, the higher the level of cardiorespiratory fitness, the longer the life (see Figure 6.3). Death rates from all causes for the least-fit (group 1) men was 3.4 times higher than it was for the most-fit men. For the least-fit women, the death rate was 4.6 times higher than it was for the most-fit women.

The same study reported a much lower rate of premature deaths even at the moderate-fitness levels most adults can achieve. Even greater protection was attained when a higher fitness level was combined with elimination of other risk factors such as hypertension, high cholesterol, cigarette smoking, and excessive body fat.

Additional research that looked at changes in fitness and mortality found a substantial (44 percent) reduction in mortality risk when people abandoned a sedentary lifestyle and became moderately fit.[7] The lowest death rate was found in people who were fit and remained fit, and the highest rate was found in men who remained unfit (see Figure 6.4).

Subsequent research published in 1995 substantiated the previous findings and also indicated that primarily vigorous activities are associated with greater longevity.[8]

Vigorous activity was defined as any activity that requires a MET* level equal to or greater than 6 METs (21 ml/kg/min—see Health Fitness Standards, p. 122). Examples of vigorous activities used in the later study

*One MET is the energy expenditure at rest, or approximately 3.5 ml/kg/min; 6 or more METs represents exercising at an oxygen uptake (VO_2) equal to or greater than 6 times the resting energy requirement.

Moderate-intensity physical activity Physical activity that uses 150 calories of energy per day or 1,000 calories per week.

Vigorous activity Any activity that requires a MET level equal to or greater than 6 METs (21 ml/kg/min).

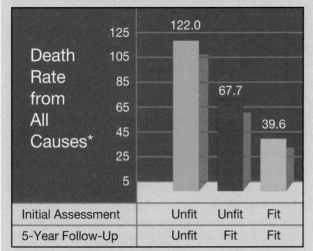

Death Rate from All Causes*			
	122.0	67.7	39.6
Initial Assessment	Unfit	Unfit	Fit
5-Year Follow-Up	Unfit	Fit	Fit

* Death rate per 10,000 man-years observation. Based on data from "Changes in Physical Fitness and All-Cause Mortality: A Prospective Study of Healthy Men," *Journal of the American Medical Association* 273 (1995): 1193–1198.

Source: S. N. Blair, H. W. Kohl III, C. E. Barlow, R. S. Paffenbarger, Jr., L. W. Gibbons, and C. A. Macera, "Changes in Physical Fitness and All-Cause Mortality: A Prospective Study of Healthy and Unhealthy Men," *Journal of the American Medical Association* 273 (1995): 1193–1198.

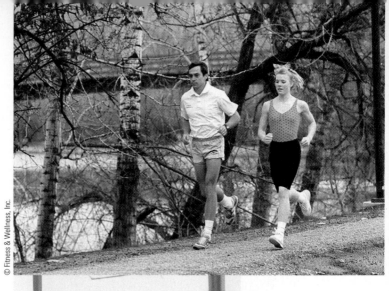

© Fitness & Wellness, Inc.

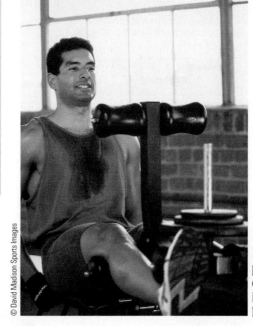

© David Madison Sports Images

| Regular participation in a lifetime exercise program increases quality of life and longevity. |

include brisk walking, jogging, swimming laps, squash, racquetball, tennis, and shoveling snow. The results also indicated that vigorous exercise is as important as not smoking and maintaining recommended weight.

The results of all these studies indicate clearly that fitness improves health, wellness, and longevity. If people are able to do vigorous exercise, it is preferable because it is most clearly associated with longer life.

IMPACT OF PHYSICAL FITNESS

Most people exercise because it improves their personal appearance and makes them feel good about themselves. The greatest benefit of all, however, is that physically fit individuals enjoy a better quality of life. These people live life to its fullest potential, with fewer health problems than inactive individuals (who may also indulge in other negative lifestyle patterns).

| Health Care Costs |

The economic impact of sedentary living can leave a strong impression on a nation's economy. As the need for physical exertion in Western countries decreased steadily during the last century, health care expenditures increased dramatically. Health care costs in the United States rose from $12 billion in 1950 to $1.035 trillion in 1996.

At the present rate of escalation, health care expenditures are estimated at $1.6 trillion in the year 2002. This figure represents about 18 percent of the gross national product (GNP), and it is projected to reach about 37 percent by the year 2030. In terms of yearly health care costs per person, the United States spends more per person, $3,724, than any other nation in the world. The next closest country, Switzerland, spends $2,644 per year. Yearly health care costs in Canada ($1,836) are less than half the costs in the United States.

| Programs in the Workplace |

Strong scientific evidence now links participation in fitness and wellness programs not only to better health but also to lower medical costs and higher job productivity. Most of this research is being conducted and reported by organizations that already have implemented fitness or wellness programs.

As a result of the recent staggering rise in medical costs, many organizations are beginning to realize that keeping employees healthy costs less than treating them once they are sick. A survey by the American Institute for Preventive Medicine found that large corporations are reaping health-cost savings by implementing health promotion programs.[9] A sample return on investment per dollar spent is provided in Figure 6.5. Containing the costs of health care through fitness and wellness programs has become a major issue for many U.S. organizations.

Another reason some organizations are offering wellness programs to their employees—overlooked by many because it does not seem to affect the bottom line directly—is simply top management concern for employees' physical well-being. Regardless of whether the program lowers medical costs, wellness programs help individuals feel better about themselves and improve their quality of life.

In addition to the financial and physical benefits, some corporations are offering health promotion programs as an incentive to attract, hire, and retain employees. Many executives believe that an on-site health promotion program is the best fringe benefit they can offer at their company. Young executives are looking for organizations such as these, not only for the added health benefits but also because the head corporate officers are showing an attitude of concern and care.

PRE-EXERCISE SCREENING AND GOALS

Even though exercise testing and participation are relatively safe for most apparently healthy individuals under age 40, the reaction of the cardiovascular system to more-intense levels of physical activity cannot always be predicted. Consequently, people face a small but real risk of some bodily changes during exercise testing or participation. These changes may include abnormal blood pressure, irregular heart rhythm, fainting, and, rarely, a heart attack or cardiac arrest.

Before you start an exercise program or participate in any exercise testing, you should fill out the Physical Activity Readiness Questionnaire (PAR-Q) in Assessment 6-1. This questionnaire, developed by the Ministry of Health in British Columbia, Canada, is used widely in the United States and Canada as a screening instrument prior to fitness testing.

If your answer to any of the PAR-Q questions is positive, you should consult a physician before participating in fitness testing or a fitness program. Exercise testing or participation is not advised under some of the conditions listed in the questionnaire and may require a stress electrocardiogram (ECG) test (see Chapter 11). If you have any questions regarding your current health status, you should consult your doctor before initiating, continuing, or increasing your level of physical activity.

As you work through this chapter and assess the various components of fitness, you will be able to develop a fitness profile. When you obtain the information pertaining to each component of fitness, you can enter your results on the profile found in Assessment 6-2.

FIGURE 6.5 HEALTH-CARE COST SAVINGS BY SELECTED CORPORATIONS PER DOLLAR SPENT ON HEALTH PROMOTION PROGRAMS.

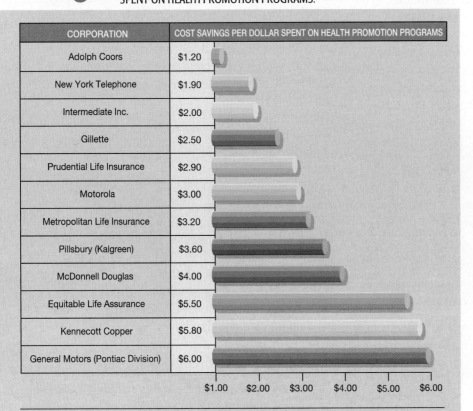

CORPORATION	COST SAVINGS PER DOLLAR SPENT ON HEALTH PROMOTION PROGRAMS
Adolph Coors	$1.20
New York Telephone	$1.90
Intermediate Inc.	$2.00
Gillette	$2.50
Prudential Life Insurance	$2.90
Motorola	$3.00
Metropolitan Life Insurance	$3.20
Pillsbury (Kalgreen)	$3.60
McDonnell Douglas	$4.00
Equitable Life Assurance	$5.50
Kennecott Copper	$5.80
General Motors (Pontiac Division)	$6.00

Source: 1991 Survey by the American Institute for Preventive Medicine, Southfield, Michigan.

Once the results for each component have been established, either with your instructor's help or using your own judgment, you can set your own target goals to achieve over the next 10 to 14 weeks. You then may proceed with an exercise program as outlined in Chapter 7. Following 8 to 12 weeks of exercise training, you should retest each component to assess your improvements in physical fitness.

PHYSICAL FITNESS

Physical fitness has been defined in several ways and has meant different things to different people. Perhaps the most comprehensive definition has been given by the American Medical Association, which defined physical fitness as the general capacity to adapt and respond favorably to physical effort. This implies that individuals are physically fit when they can meet the ordinary and the unusual demands of daily life safely and effectively, without being overly fatigued, and still have energy left for leisure and recreational activities.

As the fitness concept gained ground at the end of the 20th century, it became clear that a battery of tests was necessary to assess overall fitness because several specific components contribute to it.

Most authorities agree that physical fitness can be subdivided into health-related and motor skill–related fitness. As illustrated in Figure 6.6, the four fitness components, from a health point of view, are cardiorespiratory (aerobic) endurance, muscular strength and endurance, muscular flexibility, and body composition.

FIGURE **6.6** HEALTH-RELATED COMPONENTS OF PHYSICAL FITNESS.

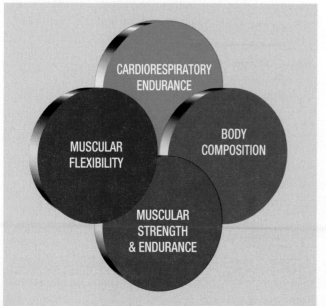

The first three components of health-related fitness are discussed in this chapter. Body composition is discussed in Chapter 9.

The motor skill–related components of fitness are identified mostly with athletics. Motor skill–related fitness encompasses agility, balance, coordination, power, reaction time, and speed. Although these components are important in achieving success in athletics, they are not crucial for developing better health.

In terms of health and wellness, the main emphasis of fitness programs should be placed on the health-related components, and that is the focus of the fitness information in this book.

FITNESS STANDARDS

A meaningful debate has arisen over determining sound age- and gender-related fitness standards for the general U.S. population. Two standards have started to develop in this regard: a health fitness standard (criterion-referenced) and a physical fitness standard.

Health Fitness Standards

As illustrated in Figure 6.7, although fitness (see VO_{2max} discussion on page 124) improvements with a moderate aerobic activity program are not as notable, significant health benefits are reaped with such a program. Only slightly better health benefits are obtained with a more intense exercise program. Benefits include a reduction in blood lipids, lower blood pressure, decreased risk for diabetes, weight loss, stress release, and lower risk for disease, including cardiovascular diseases and cancer, and a lower risk for premature mortality.

The health fitness standards proposed here are based on epidemiological data linking minimum fitness values to disease prevention and health. Attaining the health fitness standards requires only moderate amounts of physical activity. For example, a 2-mile walk in less than 30 minutes, five to six times per week, seems to be sufficient to achieve the health fitness standard for cardiorespiratory endurance.

> Attaining the health fitness standards requires only moderate amounts of physical activity.

Physical Fitness Standards

Physical fitness standards are set higher than the health fitness norms and require a more vigorous exercise program. Many experts believe that people who meet the

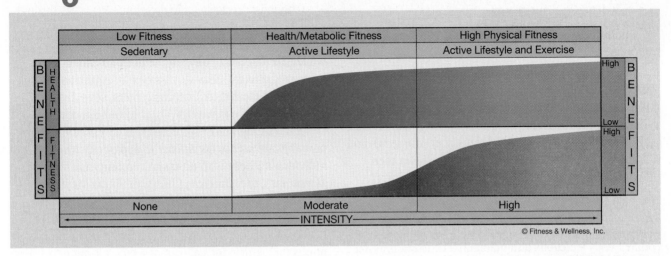

	Low Fitness	Health/Metabolic Fitness	High Physical Fitness
	Sedentary	Active Lifestyle	Active Lifestyle and Exercise

BENEFITS — HEALTH FITNESS — BENEFITS

High / Low / High / Low

| None | Moderate | High |

INTENSITY

© Fitness & Wellness, Inc.

criteria of "good" physical fitness should be able to do moderate to vigorous physical activity without undue fatigue and to maintain this capability throughout life. In this context, physically fit people of all ages will have the freedom to enjoy most of life's daily and recreational activities to their fullest potential. Current health fitness standards may not be enough to achieve these objectives.

Sound physical fitness gives the individual a degree of independence throughout life that many people in North America no longer enjoy. Most older people should be able to carry out activities similar to those conducted in their youth, though not with the same intensity. A person does not have to be a championship athlete, but activities such as changing a tire, chopping wood, climbing several flights of stairs, playing a game of basketball or soccer, mountain biking, walking several miles around a lake, and hiking through a national park do require more than the current "average fitness" level of the American people.

In this book, fitness standards for cardiorespiratory endurance, strength, flexibility, and body composition provide both a health fitness standard and a physical fitness standard. You will have to decide your own objectives. If the main objective of a fitness program is to lower the risk of disease, attaining the health fitness standards may be enough. If you want to participate in more vigorous fitness activities, achieving a high physical fitness standard is recommended.

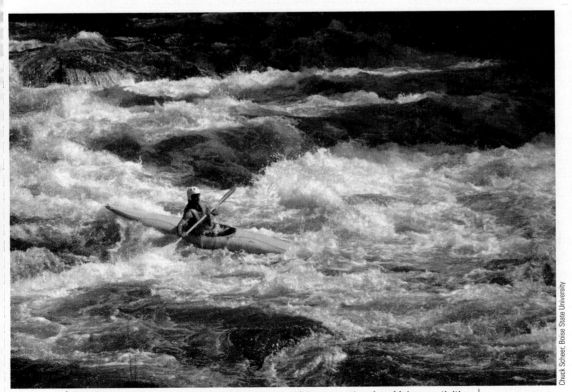

Chuck Scheer, Boise State University

| A high level of fitness is needed to enjoy many of life's recreational and leisure activities. |

Physical fitness The general capacity to adapt and respond favorably to physical effort.

ASSESSMENT OF CARDIORESPIRATORY ENDURANCE

Cardiorespiratory endurance has been defined as the ability of the lungs, heart, and blood vessels to deliver adequate amounts of oxygen to the cells to meet the demands of prolonged physical activity. As you breathe, part of the oxygen in the air is taken up in your lungs and transported in the blood to your heart. The heart then pumps the oxygenated blood through your circulatory system to all organs and tissues of your body. At the cellular level, oxygen is used to convert food substrates, primarily carbohydrates and fats, into energy necessary to conduct body functions and maintain a constant internal equilibrium.

Cardiorespiratory endurance is measured in terms of the maximal amount of oxygen the body is able to utilize per minute of physical activity, called **maximal oxygen uptake**, or VO_{2max}. VO_{2max} commonly is expressed in milliliters of oxygen per kilogram of body weight per minute (ml/kg/min). Individual values can range from about 10 ml/kg/min in cardiac patients to approximately 80 to 90 ml/kg/min in world-class runners and cross-country skiers.

Data from the research study presented in Figure 6.3 indicate that VO_{2max} values of 35 and 32.5 ml/kg/min for men and women, respectively, may be sufficient to lower the risk for all causes of mortality significantly. Although greater improvements in fitness yield a slightly lower risk for premature death, the largest drop is seen between the least fit (group 1) and the moderately fit (groups 2 and 3). Therefore, the 35 and 32.5 ml/kg/min values could be selected as the health fitness standards.

During physical exertion, a greater amount of energy is needed. As a result, the heart, lungs, and blood vessels have to deliver more oxygen to the cells. During prolonged exercise, an individual with a high level of cardiorespiratory endurance is able to deliver the required amount of oxygen to the tissues quite easily. The cardiorespiratory system of a person with a low level of endurance has to work much harder, because the heart has to pump more often to supply the same amount of oxygen to the tissues and, consequently, fatigues faster. A higher capacity to deliver and utilize oxygen (oxygen uptake), then, indicates a more efficient cardiorespiratory system.

A sound cardiorespiratory endurance program greatly enhances health. With the exception of older adults, cardiorespiratory endurance is the single most important component of health-related physical fitness. Certain levels of muscular strength and flexibility are necessary in daily activities to lead a normal life. Even so, a person can get by without a lot of strength and flexibility but cannot do without a good cardiorespiratory system.

The most precise way to determine VO_{2max} is through **open circuit indirect calorimetry** (also called "direct gas analysis"). This is done using a metabolic cart through which the amount of oxygen the body consumes can be measured directly. Because this type of equipment is not available in most health/fitness centers, several alternative methods of estimating VO_{2max} have been developed.

Even though most cardiorespiratory endurance tests probably are safe to administer to apparently healthy individuals (those with no major coronary risk factors or symptoms), the American College of Sports Medicine recommends that a physician be present for any **maximal exercise test** on apparently healthy men over age 45 and women over age 55.[10] A maximal test is any test that requires the participant's all-out or nearly all-out effort. For submaximal exercise tests, a physician should be present when testing higher risk/symptomatic individuals or diseased people, regardless of the participant's current age.

Two exercise tests frequently used to assess cardiorespiratory fitness are the 1.5-Mile Run test and the 1.0-Mile Walk test. Depending on fitness level and personal preference, you may choose either or both of these. The running test is recommended for individuals who exercise regularly, whereas the walking test is preferred for those who have not yet initiated an exercise program. Because these are field tests to estimate VO_{2max}, each test will not necessarily yield exactly the same results. To make valid comparisons, the same test should be used for pre- and post-assessments.

The 1.5-Mile Run Test

The 1.5-Mile Run test is used most frequently to predict cardiorespiratory fitness. VO_{2max} is estimated based on the time required to run (or walk) a 1.5-mile course (see Table 6.2).

The only equipment necessary to conduct this test is a stopwatch and a 440-yard track (6 laps to complete the 1.5 miles) or a premeasured 1.5-mile course. A person should be cautious prior to doing the 1.5-mile run. Because the objective of this test is to cover the distance in the shortest time, it is considered a maximal exercise test. Therefore, its use should be limited to conditioned individuals who have been cleared for exercise. The 1.5-Mile Run test is not recommended for unconditioned beginners, men over age 40 and women over age 50 without proper medical clearance, symptomatic individuals, and those with known disease or coronary heart disease risk factors. Unconditioned individuals should participate in at least 6 weeks of aerobic training before taking this test.

TABLE 6.2 ESTIMATED MAXIMAL OXYGEN UPTAKE (VO$_{2max}$) IN ML/KG/MIN FOR THE 1.5-MILE RUN TEST

Time	VO$_{2max}$ (ml/kg/min)	Time	VO$_{2max}$ (ml/kg/min)	Time	VO$_{2max}$ (ml/kg/min)	Time	VO$_{2max}$ (ml/kg/min)
6:10	80.0	9:30	54.7	12:50	39.2	16:10	30.5
6:20	79.0	9:40	53.5	13:00	38.6	16:20	30.2
6:30	77.9	9:50	52.3	13:10	38.1	16:30	29.8
6:40	76.7	10:00	51.1	13:20	37.8	16:40	29.5
6:50	75.5	10:10	50.4	13:30	37.2	16:50	29.1
7:00	74.0	10:20	49.5	13:40	36.8	17:00	28.9
7:10	72.6	10:30	48.6	13:50	36.3	17:10	28.5
7:20	71.3	10:40	48.0	14:00	35.9	17:20	28.3
7:30	69.9	10:50	47.4	14:10	35.5	17:30	28.0
7:40	68.3	11:00	46.6	14:20	35.1	17:40	27.7
7:50	66.8	11:10	45.8	14:30	34.7	17:50	27.4
8:00	65.2	11:20	45.1	14:40	34.3	18:00	27.1
8:10	63.9	11:30	44.4	14:50	34.0	18:10	26.8
8:20	62.5	11:40	43.7	15:00	33.6	18:20	26.6
8:30	61.2	11:50	43.2	15:10	33.1	18:30	26.3
8:40	60.2	12:00	42.3	15:20	32.7	18:40	26.0
8:50	59.1	12:10	41.7	15:30	32.2	18:50	25.7
9:00	58.1	12:20	41.0	15:40	31.8	19:00	25.4
9:10	56.9	12:30	40.4	15:50	31.4		
9:20	55.9	12:40	39.8	16:00	30.9		

Adapted from K. H. Cooper, "A Means of Assessing Maximal Oxygen Intake" *Journal of the American Medical Association* 203 (1968): 201–204; M. L. Pollock et al., *Health and Fitness Through Physical Activity,* (New York: John Wiley and Sons, 1978), and J. H. Wilmore, *Training for Sport and Activity* (Boston: Allyn and Bacon, 1982).

Before the actual run, you should warm up properly by doing some stretching exercises, walking, and slow jogging. Equally important, at the end of the 1.5-mile run, you should cool down by walking slowly or jogging another 3 to 5 minutes. You should not sit or lie down after the test. If any unusual symptoms arise during the run, the test should be terminated immediately, and you should cool down through slow jogging or walking. You may retake the test following 6 weeks of aerobic training.

Table 6.2 can be consulted to find the estimated VO$_{2max}$. The corresponding fitness categories based on VO$_{2max}$ are found in Table 6.3. You can record the results of

Cardiorespiratory endurance The ability of the lungs, heart, and blood vessels to deliver adequate amounts of oxygen to the cells to meet the demands of prolonged physical activity.

Maximal oxygen uptake (VO$_{2max}$) The maximum amount of oxygen the body is able to utilize per minute of physical activity, commonly expressed in ml/kg/min. The best indicator of cardiorespiratory or aerobic fitness.

Aerobic capacity The maximal amount of oxygen the human body is able to utilize per minute of physical activity (also see maximal oxygen uptake).

Open circuit indirect calorimetry (direct gas analysis) The most precise way to determine VO$_{2max}$ using a metabolic cart to measure the amount of oxygen consumed by the body.

Maximal exercise test Any test that requires the participant's all-out or nearly all-out effort.

TABLE 6.3 CARDIORESPIRATORY FITNESS CLASSIFICATION ACCORDING TO MAXIMAL OXYGEN UPTAKE (VO$_{2max}$) IN ml/kg/min

Gender	Age	Fitness Classification (in ml/kg/min)				
		Poor	Fair	Average	Good	Excellent
Men	<29	<24.9	25–33.9	34–43.9	44–52.9	>53
	30–39	<22.9	23–30.9	31–41.9	42–49.9	>50
	40–49	<19.9	20–26.9	27–38.9	39–44.9	>45
	50–59	<17.9	18–24.9	25–37.9	38–42.9	>43
	60–69	<15.9	16–22.9	23–35.9	36–40.9	>41
Women	<29	<23.9	24–30.9	31–38.9	39–48.9	>49
	30–39	<19.9	20–27.9	28–36.9	37–44.9	>45
	40–49	<16.9	17–24.9	25–34.9	35–41.9	>42
	50–59	<14.9	15–21.9	22–33.9	34–39.9	>40
	60–69	<12.9	13–20.9	21–32.9	33–36.9	>37

■ Health fitness standard   ■ High physical fitness standard

your 1.5-Mile Run test in the fitness profile in Assessment 6-2.

The 1.0-Mile Walk Test[11]

For the walking test, either a 440-yard track (4 laps to a mile) or a premeasured 1.0-mile course can be used. A stopwatch is required to determine total walking time and exercise heart rate. Prior to the walk, you have to know your body weight in pounds.

You should walk the 1.0-mile course at a brisk pace in such a way that your exercise heart rate at the end of the test is above 120 beats per minute. At the end of the 1.0-Mile Walk, walking time is checked and the pulse is counted immediately for 10 seconds.

You can take your pulse on the wrist by placing two fingers over the radial artery (inside of the wrist near the base of the thumb) or over the carotid artery (in the neck just below the jaw next to the voice box). Next, the 10-second pulse count is multiplied by 6 to obtain the exercise heart rate in beats per minute (bpm).

Now the walking time is converted from minutes and seconds to whole-minute units. Because each minute has 60 seconds, the seconds are divided by 60 to obtain the fraction of a minute. For instance, a walking time of 12 minutes and 15 seconds equals 12 + (15 ÷ 60) or 12.25 minutes.

To obtain the estimated VO_{2max} in ml/kg/min for the 1.0-Mile Walk test, plug your values into the following equation:

$$VO_{2max} = 88.768 - (0.0957 \times W) + (8.892 \times G) - (1.4537 \times T) - (0.1194 \times HR)$$

Where:

W = weight in pounds
G = gender (use 0 for women and 1 for men)
T = total time for the mile walk in minutes
HR = exercise heart rate in beats per minute at the end of the mile walk

For example, a woman who weighs 140 pounds completed the mile walk in 14 minutes and 39 seconds with an exercise heart rate of 148 beats per minute. The estimated VO_{2max} is:

W = 140 lbs
G = 0 (female gender = 0)
T = 14:39 = 14 + (39 ÷ 60) = 14.65 min
HR = 148 bpm

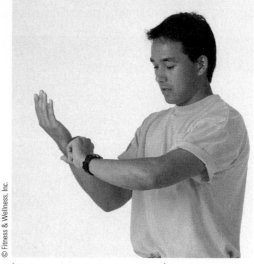

Pulse taken at the radial artery.

© Fitness & Wellness, Inc.

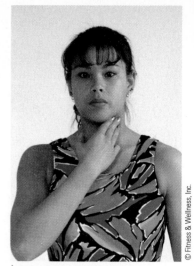

Pulse taken at the carotid artery.

© Fitness & Wellness, Inc.

$$VO_{2max} = 88.768 - (0.0957 \times 140) + (8.892 \times 0) - (1.4537 \times 14.65) - (0.1194 \times 148)$$
$$VO_{2max} = 36.4 \text{ ml/kg/min}$$

As with the 1.5-Mile Run test, the fitness categories based on VO_{2max} are found in Table 6.3. The cardiorespiratory fitness test results can be recorded in Assessment 6-2.

ASSESSMENT OF MUSCULAR STRENGTH AND ENDURANCE

Strength, a basic component of fitness and wellness, is crucial for optimal performance in daily activities, such as walking, running, lifting and carrying objects, doing housework, and even enjoying recreational activities. Strength also is of great value in improving posture, personal appearance, and self-image; in developing sports skills; and in meeting certain emergencies in life.

From a health standpoint, strength helps to maintain muscle tissue and a higher resting metabolism (see Chapter 10), facilitates weight loss and weight control, decreases the risk for injury, helps to prevent and correct chronic low back pain, and is thought to help with childbearing and delivery.

An important adaptation to strength training is that with time the heart rate and blood pressure response to lifting a heavy resistance decreases. This adaptation reduces the demands on the cardiovascular system when performing activities such as carrying a child, the groceries, or a suitcase.

Adequate strength is especially critical in maintaining functional independent living in advanced age. Many older adults lack sufficient strength to move about and perform simple tasks of daily living, such as being able to stand up or get out of bed without help, walk up a flight of stairs, or lift and carry small objects. Additional information on strength training and older adults is presented in Chapter 7, page 148.

Strength Versus Endurance

The difference between muscular strength and muscular endurance has to be clarified. Although these components are interrelated, they have a basic difference: Strength is the ability to exert maximum force against resistance; endurance is the ability of a muscle to exert submaximal force repeatedly over a period of time.

Muscular endurance (also referred to as localized muscular endurance) depends to a large extent on muscular strength. Weak muscles cannot repeat an action several times or sustain it for a long time. Strength tests and training programs have been designed to measure and develop absolute muscular strength, muscular endurance, or a combination of both.

Muscular strength is usually determined by the maximal amount of resistance—**one repetition maximum**, or 1 RM—that an individual is able to lift in a single effort. This assessment gives a good measure of absolute strength, but it does require a considerable amount of time, because the 1 RM is determined through trial and error.

For example, the strength of the chest muscles is frequently measured with the bench press exercise. If the individual has not trained with weights, he or she may try 100 pounds and lift this resistance quite easily. Then 50 pounds are added, but the person fails to lift the resistance. The resistance then is decreased by 10 or 20 pounds, and finally, after several trials, the 1 RM is established. Fatigue also becomes a factor, because by the time the 1 RM is established, several maximal, or near-maximal attempts have been performed already.

Muscular endurance is commonly determined by the number of repetitions an individual can perform against a submaximal resistance, such as lifting 80 pounds 20 times. It also can be determined by the length of time a given contraction is sustained—for example, how long a chin-up can be maintained.

Muscular Endurance Tests

Muscular strength and endurance both are required to enjoy a good quality of life. Because muscular endurance depends to a large extent on muscular strength, a muscular endurance test has been selected to determine strength.

Three exercises that assess the endurance of the upper body, lower body, and abdominal muscle groups have been selected for the muscular endurance test. A stopwatch, a metronome, a bench or gymnasium bleacher 16¼ inches high, and a partner are needed to administer the three following tests: bench-jump, modified-dip (men) or modified push-up (women), and bent-leg curl-up (or abdominal crunch for individuals prone to low-back pain).

BENCH-JUMP Using a bench or gymnasium bleacher 16¼ inches high, attempt to jump up onto and down off of the bench as many times as possible in a 1-minute period. If you cannot jump the full minute, step up and down. A repetition is counted each time both feet return to the floor.

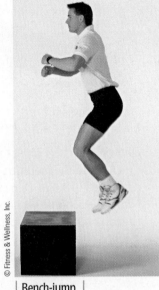

© Fitness & Wellness, Inc.

| Bench-jump. |

MODIFIED DIP This upper-body exercise is performed by men only. Using the same bench or gymnasium bleacher 16¼ inches high, place the hands on the bench with the fingers pointing forward. Have a partner hold your feet in front of you. Your hips should be bent at approximately 90°. Lower your body by flexing your elbows until the elbows are bent at a 90° angle, and then return to the starting position. A repetition does not count if your elbows do not reach 90°. Perform the repetitions to a two-step cadence (down-up), regulated with a metronome set at 56 beats per minute. Perform as many continuous repetitions as possible. The test is terminated if you fail to follow the metronome cadence.

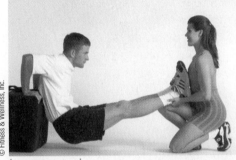

© Fitness & Wellness, Inc.

| Modified dip. |

Muscular endurance The ability of a muscle to exert submaximal force repeatedly over a period of time.

Muscular strength The ability to exert maximum force against resistance.

One repetition maximum (1 RM) The maximal amount of resistance (weight) that an individual is able to lift in a single effort.

MODIFIED PUSH-UP | Women are to perform this exercise instead of the modified dip exercise. Lie face-down on the floor, bend your knees (raise feet up in the air), and place your hands on the floor by your shoulders with your fingers pointing forward. The lower body will be supported at the knees (rather than the feet) throughout the test. The objective is to raise and lower the upper body by fully extending and flexing the elbows. The chest must touch the floor on each repetition.

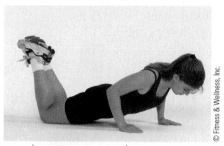

| Modified push-up. |

As with the modified dip exercise, the repetitions are performed to a two-step cadence (up-down) regulated with a metronome set at 56 beats per minute. Perform as many continuous repetitions as possible. The test is stopped when you can't do any more repetitions or you can no longer follow the metronome cadence.

BENT-LEG CURL-UP | Lie face-up on the floor and bend both legs at the knees at about 100° (see bent-leg curl-up photo). Your feet should be on the floor, and you must hold them in place yourself throughout the test. Cross the arms in front of your chest, each hand on the opposite shoulder. Now raise the head off the floor, placing the chin against your chest. This is the starting and finishing position for each curl-up. The back of the head may not come in contact with the floor, the hands cannot be removed from the shoulders, nor may the feet or hips be raised off the floor at any time during the test. The test is terminated if any of these four conditions occur.

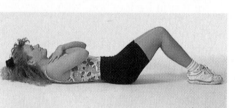

| Bent-leg curl-up. |

When you curl up, you must bring your upper body to an upright position before going back down. The repetitions are performed to a two-step cadence (up-down) regulated with the metronome set at 40 beats per minute. For this exercise, you should allow a brief practice period of 10 to 15 seconds to familiarize yourself with the cadence. The up movement is initiated with the first beat, then you must wait for the next beat to initiate the down movement; one repetition is accomplished every two beats of the metronome. Count as many repetitions as you are able to perform following the proper cadence. This test is also terminated if you fail to maintain the appropriate cadence or if you accomplish 100 repetitions. Have your partner check the angle at the knees throughout the test to make sure the 100° angle is maintained as closely as possible.

ABDOMINAL CRUNCH | This test is very difficult to perform correctly. Individuals often gain an unfair advantage by bending the elbows, shrugging the shoulders, or sliding the body during the test.[12] Test results are not valid unless the test procedure and the exercise form are monitored carefully.[13] Further, a large upper body mass and lack of spinal flexibility make it impossible or difficult for some individuals to reach the full range of motion required during the abdominal crunch.[14] This test, therefore, should be used only by individuals who, because of back pain or risk for low back injury, cannot perform the bent-leg curl-up test.

To administer the test, tape a 3½ × 30-inch strip of cardboard onto the floor (for this test you may also use a Crunch-Ster Curl-Up Tester *). Lie face-up on the floor with your knees bent at approximately 100° and legs slightly apart (see abdominal crunch photos). Both feet should be on the floor, and you must hold them in place yourself throughout the test. Straighten your arms and place them on the floor alongside the trunk with the palms down and the fingers fully extended. The fingertips of both hands should barely touch the closest edge of the cardboard. Bring your head off the floor until the chin is 1 to 2 inches away from your chest. Your head should remain in this position during the entire test (do not move the head by flexing or extending the neck). You are

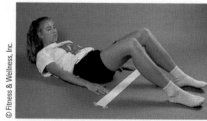

| Abdominal crunch—the fingertips of both hands should barely touch the closest edge of the cardboard. |

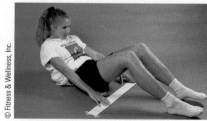

| Abdominal crunch—as you curl up, slide the fingers over the cardboard until the fingertips reach the far edge of the board. |

* Available from Novel Products Figure Finder Collection, P.O. Box 408, Rockton, IL 61072-0408, (800) 624-4888.

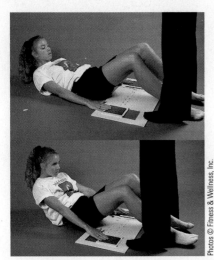

Abdominal crunches using a Crunch-Ster Curl-Up Tester.

now ready to begin the test.

The repetitions are performed to a two-step cadence (up-down) regulated with a metronome set at 60 beats per minute. As you curl up, slide the fingers over the cardboard until the fingertips reach the far edge (3½ inches) of the board, then return to the starting position.

Allow a brief practice period of 5 to 10 seconds to familiarize yourself with the cadence. The up movement is initiated with the first beat, and the down movement with the next beat. One repetition is accomplished every two beats of the metronome. Count as many repetitions as you are able to perform following the proper cadence. You may not count a repetition if the fingertips fail to reach the distant edge of the cardboard.

The test is terminated if (a) you fail to maintain the appropriate cadence, (b) your heels come off the floor, (c) your chin is not kept close to the chest, (d) you accomplish 100 repetitions, or (e) you can no longer perform the test. Have your partner check the angle at the knees throughout the test to make sure that the 100° angle is maintained as closely as possible.

Look up the percentile rank based on the number of repetitions performed on each test and the respective strength fitness categories in Table 6.4. Record this information in Assessment 6-2.

ASSESSMENT OF MUSCULAR FLEXIBILITY

Flexibility is defined as the ability of a joint to move freely through its full range of motion. Sports medicine specialists believe that many muscular/skeletal problems and injuries, especially in adults, may be related to a lack of flexibility. Improving and maintaining good range of motion in the joints throughout life enhances the quality of life.

Because flexibility is joint-specific—good flexibility in one joint does not necessarily indicate the same is true in other joints—two tests are used to obtain an indication of current flexibility levels: the

Flexibility The ability of a joint to move freely through its full range of motion.

TABLE 6.4 PERCENTILE RANKS AND FITNESS STANDARDS FOR THE MUSCULAR ENDURANCE TESTS

Percentile Rank	MEN Bench Jump	MEN Modified Dip	MEN Bent-leg Curl-up	MEN Abdominal Crunch*	WOMEN Bench Jump	WOMEN Modified Push-up	WOMEN Bent-leg Curl-up	WOMEN Abdominal Crunch*	Fitness Classification
99	66	54	100	100	58	95	100	100	
95	63	50	81	100	54	70	100	100	Excellent
90	62	38	65	100	52	50	97	69	
80	58	32	51	66	48	41	77	49	Good
70	57	30	44	45	44	38	57	37	
60	56	27	31	38	42	33	45	34	Average
50	54	26	28	33	39	30	37	31	
40	51	23	25	29	38	28	28	27	Fair
30	48	20	22	26	36	25	22	24	
20	47	17	17	22	32	21	17	21	
10	40	11	10	18	28	18	9	15	Poor
5	34	7	3	16	26	15	4	0	

▊ High physical fitness standard   ▊ Health fitness standard

* Use this exercise only if you are unable to perform a bent-leg curl-up because of back pain or risk of lower back injury.

Improving and maintaining good range of motion in the joints throughout life enhances functional independence.

Modified Sit-and-Reach and the Total Body Rotation tests. Before doing any flexibility testing, participants should warm up properly with a few stretching exercises. Assistance from another person is necessary to administer both tests.

| Modified Sit-and-Reach Test |

To administer the Modified Sit-and-Reach test, you'll need an Acuflex I* flexibility tester or you may design your own equipment by placing a yardstick on top of a box 12 inches high. To perform the test, remove your shoes and sit on the floor with your hips, back, and head against a wall. Fully extend your legs with the bottom of your feet placed against the box (see starting position for the Modified Sit-and-Reach Test photo).

Position one hand on top of the other and reach forward as far as possible without letting your head or back come off the wall. The person assisting with the test then should slide the reach indicator (or yardstick) until the zero (end) point of the scale touches your fingers. He or she then must hold the indicator firmly in place throughout the rest of the test.

* Available from Novel Products Figure Finder Collection, P.O. Box 408, Rockton, IL 61072-0408, (800) 624-4888.

Your head and back now can come off the wall, and you should gradually reach forward as far as possible on the indicator, holding the final position at least 2 seconds. Be sure that, during the test, you keep the back of your knees flat against the floor.

Two trials are necessary and the average of the two scores, each recorded to the nearest half inch, is used as the final test score. Flexibility fitness categories for this test are provided in Table 6.5.

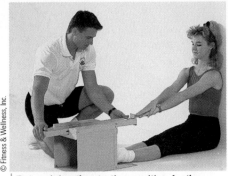

Determining the starting position for the Modified Sit-and-Reach Test.

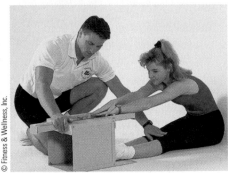

Modified Sit-and-Reach Test.

| Total Body Rotation Test |

An Acuflex II* flexibility tester or a measuring scale with a sliding panel is needed to administer this test. The Acuflex II or scale is placed on the wall at shoulder height

TABLE 6.5 PERCENTILE RANKS AND FITNESS STANDARDS FOR THE MODIFIED SIT-AND-REACH TEST

MEN						WOMEN					
Percentile Rank	Age Category				Fitness Category	Percentile Rank	Age Category				Fitness Category
	<18	19–35	36–49	>50			<18	19–35	36–49	>50	
99	20.8	20.1	18.9	16.2		99	22.6	21.0	19.8	17.2	
95	19.6	18.9	18.2	15.8	Excellent	95	19.5	19.3	19.2	15.7	Excellent
90	18.2	17.2	16.1	15.0		90	18.7	17.9	17.4	15.0	
80	17.8	17.0	14.6	13.3	Good	80	17.8	16.7	16.2	14.2	Good
70	16.0	15.8	13.9	12.3		70	16.5	16.2	15.2	13.6	
60	15.2	15.0	13.4	11.5	Average	60	16.0	15.8	14.5	12.3	Average
50	14.5	14.4	12.6	10.2		50	15.2	14.8	13.5	11.1	
40	14.0	13.5	11.6	9.7	Fair	40	14.5	14.5	12.8	10.1	Fair
30	13.4	13.0	10.8	9.3		30	13.7	13.7	12.2	9.2	
20	11.8	11.6	9.9	8.8		20	12.6	12.6	11.0	8.3	
10	9.5	9.2	8.3	7.8	Poor	10	11.4	10.1	9.7	7.5	Poor
05	8.4	7.9	7.0	7.2		05	9.4	8.1	8.5	3.7	
01	7.2	7.0	5.1	4.0		01	6.5	2.6	2.0	1.5	

■ High physical fitness standard   ■ Health fitness standard

and should be adjustable to accommodate individual differences in height.

If you need to build your own scale, use two measuring tapes, each at least 30 inches long, and glue them above and below the sliding panel, centered at the 15-inch mark. Place one tape upside down, so the 1-inch ends are opposite each other. If no sliding panel is available, simply tape the measuring tapes onto a wall so the panel is at your shoulder height. Also, draw a line centered on the 15-inch marks on the floor, as shown in the photo below.

Stand sideways, an arm's length away from the wall, your feet straight ahead, slightly separated, and your toes right up to the corresponding line drawn on the floor. Hold out the arm opposite to the wall horizontally from your body, making a fist with your hand. The Acuflex II, measuring scale, or tapes should be shoulder height at this time. Rotate your trunk, moving the extended arm backward and so it makes contact with the panel (as shown in the photo). Gradually slide the panel forward as far as possible. If no panel is available, slide your fist alongside the tapes as far as possible. Hold the final position for at least 2 seconds.

Your hand should be positioned with the little finger side forward during the entire sliding movement. It is crucial to have the proper hand position. Many people attempt to open the hand or push with extended fingers or slide the panel with the knuckles, none of which is an acceptable test procedure. During the test, the knees can be slightly bent, but the feet cannot be moved; they always must point straight forward. The body must be kept as straight (vertical) as possible.

Conduct the test on either the right or the left side of the body. You are allowed two trials on the selected side. The farthest point reached, measured to the nearest half inch and held for at least 2 seconds, is recorded. The average of the two trials becomes the final test score. Flexibility fitness categories for the test are provided in Table 6.6.

After obtaining your flexibility scores, record your percentile ranks and flexibility fitness categories in the fitness profile provided in Assessment 6-2.

EXERCISE PRESCRIPTION

Upon completing the health-related fitness assessment, Chapter 7 will help you learn how to develop and implement your own exercise programs for cardio-respiratory endurance, muscular strength, and muscular flexibility. In Chapter 9 you also will learn how to assess your body composition (the fourth component of health-related fitness) and compute your recommended body weight based on your current percent body fat. Guidelines for a weight management program are provided in Chapter 10.

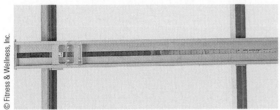
Acuflex II measuring device for the Total Body Rotation test.

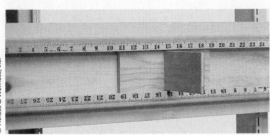
Homemade measuring device for the Total Body Rotation test.

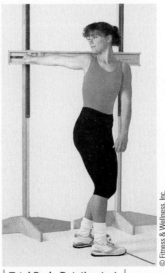
Total Body Rotation test.

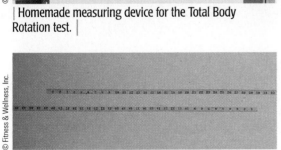
Measuring tapes for the Total Body Rotation test.

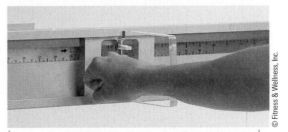
Proper hand position for the Total Body Rotation test.

TABLE 6.6 PERCENTILE RANKS AND FITNESS STANDARDS FOR THE TOTAL BODY ROTATION TEST

	Percentile Rank	Left Rotation				Right Rotation				Fitness Category
		<18	19–35	36–49	>50	<18	19–35	36–49	>50	
Men	99	29.1	28.0	26.6	21.0	28.2	27.8	25.2	22.2	Excellent
	95	26.6	24.8	24.5	20.0	25.5	25.6	23.8	20.7	
	90	25.0	23.6	23.0	17.7	24.3	24.1	22.5	19.3	
	80	22.0	22.0	21.2	15.5	22.7	22.3	21.0	16.3	Good
	70	20.9	20.3	20.4	14.7	21.3	20.7	18.7	15.7	
	60	19.9	19.3	18.7	13.9	19.8	19.0	17.3	14.7	Average
	50	18.6	18.0	16.7	12.7	19.0	17.2	16.3	12.3	
	40	17.0	16.8	15.3	11.7	17.3	16.3	14.7	11.5	Fair
	30	14.9	15.0	14.8	10.3	15.1	15.0	13.3	10.7	
	20	13.8	13.3	13.7	9.5	12.9	13.3	11.2	8.7	Poor
	10	10.8	10.5	10.8	4.3	10.8	11.3	8.0	2.7	
	05	8.5	8.9	8.8	0.3	8.1	8.3	5.5	0.3	
	01	3.4	1.7	5.1	0.0	6.6	2.9	2.0	0.0	
Women	99	29.3	28.6	27.1	23.0	29.6	29.4	27.1	21.7	Excellent
	95	26.8	24.8	25.3	21.4	27.6	25.3	25.9	19.7	
	90	25.5	23.0	23.4	20.5	25.8	23.0	21.3	19.0	
	80	23.8	21.5	20.2	19.1	23.7	20.8	19.6	17.9	Good
	70	21.8	20.5	18.6	17.3	22.0	19.3	17.3	16.8	
	60	20.5	19.3	17.7	16.0	20.8	18.0	16.5	15.6	Average
	50	19.5	18.0	16.4	14.8	19.5	17.3	14.6	14.0	
	40	18.5	17.2	14.8	13.7	18.3	16.0	13.1	12.8	Fair
	30	17.1	15.7	13.6	10.0	16.3	15.2	11.7	8.5	
	20	16.0	15.2	11.6	6.3	14.5	14.0	9.8	3.9	Poor
	10	12.8	13.6	8.5	3.0	12.4	11.1	6.1	2.2	
	05	11.1	7.3	6.8	0.7	10.2	8.8	4.0	1.1	
	01	8.9	5.3	4.3	0.0	8.9	3.2	2.8	0.0	

■ High physical fitness standard   ■ Health fitness standard

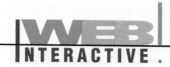

INTERACTIVE.

WEB ACTIVITIES

■ **Rate Your Own Fitness Level** This is an interactive fitness assessment measuring aerobic endurance, body composition, flexibility, and muscular strength/ endurance for abdominal and upper body muscles, developed by Texas Tech University. What is your personal best? Take the challenge and find out.
http://www.dce.ttu.edu/courses/phys_ed/fittest.htm

■ **American Council of Exercise Cardiovascular Fitness Facts** This site features information about a variety of cardiovascular forms of exercise, including walking, running, jumping rope, swimming, spin- ning, cross-training, interval training, and others.
http://www.acefitness.org/fitfacts/fitfacts_list.cfm#1

■ **The Internet Fitness Resource** This site contains information on a variety of fitness topics, including a Fitness Trainer site, as well as information on aerobics, lifting, and nutrition.
http://sickbay.com/netsweat

■ **Aerobics and Fitness Association of America** This interactive site features "Exercise Gets Personal™" where you can create a customized exercise program that compiles activities you select, geared to your current level of fitness activity. Exercises include aerobics, muscular conditioning, and flexibility with descriptions and precautions for each activity.
http://www.afaa.com

InfoTrac
You can find additional readings related to wellness via InfoTrac College Edition, an on-line library of more than 900 journals and publications. Follow the instructions for accessing InfoTrac that came packaged with your text- book, then search for articles using a key word search.

Suggested Reading Avery Comarow, "Keep Fit for Life by Matching Your Training to Your Age," *U.S. News & World Report* 29, no. 12 (Sept. 25, 2000): 62.

1. According to the American College of Sports Medicine (ACSM), what are the three types of exercises necessary for a lifetime physical fitness regimen?
2. What is the special focus for fitness in someone between the ages of 20 and 40? Specifically what

type of exercise accounts for the 86 percent increase in the rate of injuries in men ages 25 to 44?
3. Physiologically, what happens to people after the age of 40, and what can one do to reverse this tendency? What should be the focus of a sound physical fitness program for the 40- to 60-year-old population?

Web Activity
Shape Up America
http://www.shapeup.org

Sponsor Former U.S. Surgeon General Dr. C. Everett Koop in partnership with industry and non-profit organizations.

Description This interactive site will provide you with an excellent assessment of your level of physical fitness. It offers a battery of physical fitness assessments, including activity level, strength, flexibility, and an aerobic fitness test. You get started by entering your weight, height, age, and gender and then taking a quick screen test to assess your physical readiness for physical activity. Your final results in each of these areas will be based on your personal data.

Available Activities This site contains five different self-assessments, each designed to provide you with reliable fitness and nutrition information. The interactive activities include:

1. PAR-Q test
2. Activity Level Assessment to determine whether your daily level of activity is Sedentary, Light, Moderate, Heavy, or Very Heavy
3. Flexibility Test to assess your range of movement
4. Muscular Strength and Endurance Test to assess the strength of the muscles in your upper body
5. Two tests for aerobic fitness

Web Work
1. From the home page, click on "Fitness Center" link.
2. Then, click on the "Assessment" link.
3. First, click on the "Take the PAR-Q Test" link to begin the self-assessment questionnaire to measure your readiness for physical activity.
4. Click on the radio button "Yes" or "No" that corre- sponds to the answers to each of the seven questions. Once completed, click on the "Continue" button.
5. The assessment will provide you with your results concerning your ability to participate in physical activity. Then, click on the "Return to the Assessment Main Page" link to continue with the other four assessments listed in the "Available Activities" above.

Helpful hints

1. The information gathered from the results on these assessment tests will be used in other parts of the Fitness Center on this Web site. Therefore, you must complete the PAR-Q Test first.

For additional Web activities, links, and suggested readings, visit our Health, Fitness, and Wellness Resource Center at http://health.wadsworth.com.

NOTES

1. U.S. Centers for Disease Control and Prevention and American College of Sports Medicine, "Summary Statement: Workshop on Physical Activity and Public Health," *Sports Medicine Bulletin* 28:4, p. 7.

2. National Institutes of Health, Consensus Development Conference Statement, "Physical Activity and Cardiovascular Health," Washington, DC, December 18–20, 1995.

3. See note 2.

4. U.S. Department of Health and Human Services, *Physical Activity and Health: A Report of the Surgeon General*, Atlanta: U.S. Department of Health and Human Services, Centers for Disease Control and Prevention, National Center for Chronic Disease Prevention and Health Promotion, 1996.

5. R. S. Paffenbarger, Jr., R. T. Hyde, A. L. Wing, and C. H. Steinmetz, "A Natural History of Athleticism and Cardiovascular Health," *Journal of the American Medical Association* 252 (1984): 491–495.

6. S. N. Blair, H. W. Kohl III, R. S. Paffenbarger, Jr., D. G. Clark, K. H. Cooper, and L. W. Gibbons, "Physical Fitness and All-Cause Mortality: A Prospective Study of Healthy Men and Women," *Journal of the American Medical Association* 262 (1989): 2395–2401.

7. S. N. Blair, H. W. Kohl III, C. E. Barlow, R. S. Paffenbarger, Jr., L. W. Gibbons, and C. A. Macera, "Changes in Physical Fitness and All-Cause Mortality: A Prospective Study of Healthy and Unhealthy Men," *Journal of the American Medical Association* 273 (1995): 1193–1198.

8. I. Lee, C. Hsieh, and R. S. Paffenbarger, Jr., "Exercise Intensity and Longevity in Men: The Harvard Alumni Health Study," *Journal of the American Medical Association* 273 (1995): 1179–1184.

9. R. C. Chadbourne, "Fit for Hire," *Fitness Management* 12, no. 2 (1996): 28–30.

10. American College of Sports Medicine, *Guidelines for Exercise Testing and Prescription* (Philadelphia: Lea & Febiger, 2000).

11. F. A. Dolgener, L. D. Hensley, J. J. Marsh, and J. K. Fjelstul, "Validation of the Rockport Fitness Walking Test in College Males and Females," *Research Quarterly for Exercise and Sport* 65 (1994): 152–158.

12. R. A. Faulkner, E. J. Sprigings, A. McQuarrie, and R. D. Bell, "A Partial Curl-Up Protocol for Adults Based on Analysis of Two Procedures," *Canadian Journal of Sports Science* 14 (1989): 135–141;

 P. A. Macfarlane, "Out with the Sit-Up, in with the Curl-Up!" *Journal of Physical Education, Recreation, and Dance* 64 (1993): 62–66;

 D. Knudson and D. Johnston, "Validity and Reliability of a Bench Trunk-Curl-Up Test of Abdominal Endurance," *Journal of Strength and Conditioning Research* 9 (1995): 165–169.

13. R. Kjorstad. "Validity of Two Field Tests of Abdominal Strength and Muscular Endurance," unpublished master's thesis, Boise State University, 1997;

 G. L. Hall, R. K. Hetzler, D. Perrin, and A. Weltman, "Relationship of Timed Sit-Up Tests to Isokinetic Abdominal Strength," *Research Quarterly for Exercise and Sport* 63 (1992): 80–84.

14. L. D. Robertson and H. Magnusdottir, "Evaluation of Criteria Associated with Abdominal Fitness Testing," *Research Quarterly for Exercise and Sport* 58 (1987): 355—359;

 See also Macfarlane, note 12.

PHYSICAL ACTIVITY
READINESS QUESTIONNAIRE (PAR-Q)

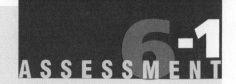

Name: _____ Date: _____ Grade: _____

Instructor: _____ Course: _____ Section: _____

Necessary Lab Equipment:
None required.

Objective:
To determine safety of exercise participation.

Regular physical activity is fun and healthy, and increasingly more people are starting to become more active every day. Being more active is very safe for most people. However, some people should check with their doctor before they start becoming much more physically active.

If you are planning to become much more physically active than you are now, start by answering the seven questions in the box below. If you are between the ages of 15 and 69, the PAR-Q will tell you if you should check with your doctor before you start. If you are over 69 years of age, and you are not used to being very active, check with your doctor.

Common sense is your best guide when you answer these questions. Please read the questions carefully and answer each one honestly: check YES or NO.

YES	NO	
☐	☐	1. Has a doctor ever said that you have a heart condition *and* that you should only do physical activity recommended by a doctor?
☐	☐	2. Do you feel pain in your chest when you do physical activity?
☐	☐	3. In the past month, have you had chest pain when you were not doing physical activity?
☐	☐	4. Do you lose your balance because of dizziness or do you ever lose consciousness?
☐	☐	5. Do you have a bone or joint problem that could be made worse by a change in your physical activity?
☐	☐	6. Is your doctor currently prescribing drugs (for example, water pills) for your blood pressure or heart condition?
☐	☐	7. Do you know of *any other reason* why you should not do physical activity?

If you answered

YES to one or more questions

Talk with your doctor by phone or in person BEFORE you start becoming much more physically active or BEFORE you have a fitness appraisal. Tell your doctor about the PAR-Q and which questions you answered YES.

- You may be able to do any activity you want—as long as you start slowly and build up gradually. Or, you may need to restrict your activities to those which are safe for you. Talk with your doctor about the kinds of activities you wish to participate in and follow his/her advice.
- Find out which community programs are safe and helpful for you.

NO to all questions

If you answered NO honestly to *all* PAR-Q questions, you can be reasonably sure that you can:

- start becoming much more physically active—begin slowly and build up gradually. This is the safest and easiest way to go.
- take part in a fitness appraisal—this is an excellent way to determine your basic fitness so that you can plan the best way for you to live actively.

Delay becoming much more active:

- if you are not feeling well because of a temporary illness such as a cold or a fever—wait until you feel better; or
- if you are or may be pregnant—talk to your doctor before you start becoming more active.

Please note: If your health changes so that you then answer YES to any of the above questions, tell your fitness or health professional. Ask whether you should change your physical activity plan.

Informed Use of the PAR-Q: The Canadian Society for Exercise Physiology, Health Canada, and their agents assume no liability for persons who undertake physical activity, and if in doubt after completing this questionnaire, consult your doctor prior to physical activity.

> You are encouraged to copy the PAR-Q but only if you use the entire form

Note: If the Par-Q is being given to a person before he or she participates in a physical activity program or a fitness appraisal, this section may be used for legal or administrative purposes.

I have read, understood and completed this questionnaire. Any questions I had were answered to my full satisfaction.

Name _____

Signature _____ Date _____

Signature of Parent _____ Witness _____
or Guardian (for participants under the age of majority)

© Canadian Society for Exercise Physiology Supported by: [🍁] Health Santé
Société canadienne de physiologie de l'exercice Canada Canada

Exercise Participation

Do you feel that it is safe for you to proceed with an exercise program? Explain any concerns or limitations that you may have regarding your safe participation in a comprehensive exercise program (which will include exercises to improve cardiorespiratory endurance, muscular strength and endurance, and muscular flexibility).

_____
_____
_____
_____
_____
_____
_____
_____

In a few words, describe your previous experiences with sports participation, whether you have taken part in a structured exercise program, and express your own feelings about exercise participation.

_____
_____
_____
_____
_____
_____
_____
_____
_____
_____
_____
_____
_____
_____
_____

PHYSICAL FITNESS PROFILE

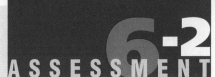

Name: Date: Grade:

Instructor: Course: Section:

Age: Male or Female: M / F   Body Weight:

Necessary Lab Equipment:

Pre-measured 1.5-mile or 1.0 mile course, 16¼ inch bench, stopwatch, metronome, equipment for abdominal crunches, modified sit-and-reach box (Acuflex I), and total body rotation scale (Acuflex II).

Lab Preparation:

Wear appropriate exercise clothing, including a good pair of athletic (jogging/walking) shoes. Avoid strenuous physical activity for 36 hours prior to this lab.

Objective:

To assess your current level of cardiorespiratory endurance, muscular strength endurance, and muscular flexibility fitness.

PRE-TEST

Fitness Component	Test Data	Test Results	Fitness Classification
Cardiorespiratory Endurance	Time	VO_{2max}	
1.5-Mile Run	:	.	
	Time		
1.0-Mile Walk	:		
	Heart Rate	VO_{2max}	
		.	
Muscular Strength / Endurance	Reps	Percentile	
Bench Jumps			
Chair Dips or Modified Push-Ups			
Bent-Leg Curl-Ups or Abdominal Crunches			
Muscular Flexibility	Inches	Percentile	
Modified Sit-and-Reach			
Body Rotation (R/L)			

POST-TEST

Fitness Component	Test Data	Test Results	Fitness Classification
Cardiovascular Endurance	Time	VO$_{2max}$	
1.5-Mile Run	___ : ___	___ . ___	___
1.0-Mile Walk	Time ___ : ___		
	Heart Rate ___	VO$_{2max}$ ___ . ___	___
Muscular Strength / Endurance	Reps	Percentile	
Bench Jumps	___	___	___
Chair Dips / Modified Push-Ups	___	___	___
Bent-Leg Curl-Ups or Abdominal Crunches	___	___	___
Muscular Flexibility	Inches	Percentile	
Modified Sit-and-Reach	___	___	___
Body Rotation (R/L)	___	___	___

What I Learned and Where Do I Go From Here

Based on the results of your cardiorespiratory endurance test(s), muscular strength endurance, and muscular flexibility tests, interpret how these results relate to your present level of daily physical activity or exercise habits.

_____

_____

_____

_____

Please indicate the fitness components that you would like to improve, the fitness category that you wish to achieve by the end of the term, and what do you intend to do to achieve your goal(s).

_____

_____

_____

_____

EXERCISE PRESCRIPTION FOR WELLNESS

- Understand the benefits of an active lifestyle.

- Define aerobic and anaerobic exercise.

- Learn the guidelines for cardiorespiratory, strength, and flexibility exercise prescription.

- Recognize the different types of muscle fibers.

- Understand the progressive overload principle for strength development.

- Clarify misconceptions related to exercise training programs.

- Become familiar with concepts for injury prevention and treatment.

- Identify stages of change during the process of behavior modification.

- Learn the role of goal setting in the process of change.

- Learn basic skills to enhance motivation and exercise adherence.

A MOST INSPIRING STORY illustrating what fitness can do for a person's health and well-being is that of George Snell from Sandy, Utah. At age 45, Snell weighed approximately 400 pounds, his blood pressure was 220/180, he was blind because of undiagnosed diabetes, and his blood glucose level was 487. Snell had determined to do something about his physical and medical condition, so he started a weight management program along with a walking/jogging program.

After about 8 months on this program, Snell had lost almost 200 pounds, his eyesight had returned, his glucose level was down to 67, and he was taken off medication. Two months later, less than 10 months after initiating his personal exercise program, he completed his first marathon, a running course of 26.2 miles.

There is no drug in current or prospective use that holds as much promise for sustained health as a lifetime program of physical exercise.[1] Results of epidemiological research have established that a physically active lifestyle and participation in a lifetime exercise program greatly contribute to good health (see Chapter 6). Nonetheless, many individuals who are active and exercise regularly find, when they take a battery of fitness tests, that they may not be as conditioned as they thought they were. Although these individuals may be exercising regularly, they most likely are not following the basic principles for exercise prescription and, therefore, are not reaping the full benefits of their activity and exercise programs.

A key principle in exercise prescription is that all programs must be individualized to obtain optimal results. Our bodies are not all alike, and fitness levels and needs vary among individuals. The information presented in this chapter provides the necessary guidelines to write a personalized cardiorespiratory endurance, muscular strength or endurance, and muscular flexibility exercise program that promotes and maintains good health and fitness. Information on weight control to achieve and maintain recommended body weight and body composition, a key component of good physical fitness, is given in Chapters 9 and 10.

LIFESTYLE DETERMINES CARDIORESPIRATORY HEALTH

Physical activity is no longer a natural part of our existence. If we need to go to a store only a couple of blocks away, most people drive their cars and then spend a couple of minutes driving around the parking lot to find a spot 10 yards closer to the store's entrance. We do not even have to carry out the groceries any more. A

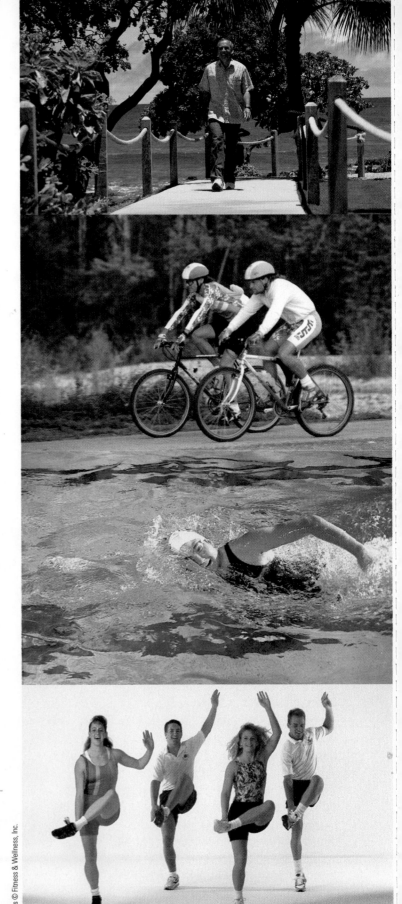

Photos © Fitness & Wellness, Inc.

Aerobic exercise requires oxygen to supply the energy needed to carry out the activity.

youngster working at the store usually takes them out in a cart and places them in your vehicle. During a normal visit to a multilevel shopping mall, almost everyone chooses to ride the escalators instead of taking the stairs. Automobiles, elevators, escalators, telephones, intercoms, remote controls, and electric garage door openers—all are modern-day commodities that minimize body movement and effort.

One of the most detrimental effects of modern-day technology has been an increase in chronic conditions related to this lack of physical activity. Some examples are hypertension, heart disease, chronic low back pain, and obesity. These conditions also are called **hypokinetic diseases**. "Hypo" means low or little, and "kinetic" denotes motion.

Lack of adequate physical activity is a reality of modern life that most people no longer can avoid, but to enjoy modern-day commodities and still expect to live life to its fullest, a personalized lifetime exercise program must become part of daily living. Based on current estimates, more than 60 percent of adults do not achieve the recommended amount of physical activity, and 25 percent are not physically active at all.[2]

CARDIORESPIRATORY ENDURANCE

Cardiorespiratory endurance refers to the ability of the lungs, heart, and blood vessels to deliver adequate amounts of oxygen to the cells to meet the demands of prolonged physical activity. Because the body uses oxygen to convert food (carbohydrates and fats) into energy, a greater capacity to deliver and utilize oxygen (referred to as oxygen uptake or VO_2) indicates a more efficient cardiorespiratory system.

Cardiorespiratory endurance activities also are called aerobic exercise. The word **aerobic** means "with oxygen." Whenever an activity requires oxygen to produce energy, it is considered an aerobic exercise. Examples of cardio-respiratory or aerobic exercise are walking, jogging, swimming, cycling, cross-country skiing, water aerobics, rope skipping, and aerobic workouts.

Anaerobic activities, on the other hand, are carried out "without oxygen." The intensity of anaerobic exercise is so high that oxygen is not utilized to produce energy. Because energy production is limited without oxygen, these activities can be carried out for only short periods (2 to 3 minutes). The higher the intensity of the activity, the shorter the duration of the anaerobic activity.

Activities such as the 100-, 200-, and 400-meter dash in track and field, the 100-meter in swimming, gymnastics routines, and weight training are good examples

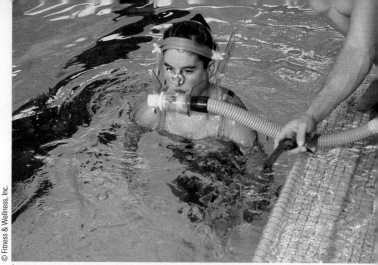

Physical work capacity, measured through an oxygen uptake test, increases with aerobic training.

of anaerobic activities. Anaerobic activities will not contribute much to development of the cardiorespiratory system. Only aerobic activities will enhance cardio-respiratory endurance.

Significance of Cardiorespiratory Endurance

Aerobic exercise is especially important in preventing coronary heart disease. A poorly conditioned heart that has to pump more often just to keep a person alive is subject to more wear and tear than a well-conditioned heart. In situations that place strenuous demands on the heart, such as doing yard work, lifting heavy objects or weights, or running to catch a train, the unconditioned heart may not be able to sustain the strain. In addition, regular participation in cardiorespiratory endurance activities helps achieve and maintain recommended body weight, the fourth component of health-related physical fitness.

Everyone who initiates a cardiorespiratory or aerobic exercise program can expect a number of physiological adaptations from training. Among the most significant adaptations are

1. **A higher maximal oxygen uptake (VO_{2max}).** The amount of oxygen the body is able to use during physical activity significantly increases. This allows the individual to exercise longer and at a higher rate before becoming fatigued.

   Small increases in VO_{2max} can be observed in as few as 2 to 3 weeks of

Hypokinetic disease Condition associated with a lack of physical activity (for example, hypertension, coronary heart disease, obesity, and diabetes).

Aerobic exercise Exercise that requires oxygen to produce the necessary energy (ATP) to carry out the activity.

Anaerobic activity Activity that does not require oxygen to produce the necessary energy (ATP) to carry out the activity.

aerobic training. Depending on the initial fitness level, VO_{2max} may rise as much as 30 percent, although higher increases have been reported in people with very low initial levels of fitness.

2. **An increase in the oxygen-carrying capacity of the blood.** As a result of training, the red blood cell count goes up. Red blood cells contain hemoglobin, which transports oxygen in the blood.

3. **A decrease in resting heart rate and an increase in cardiac muscle strength.** During resting conditions, the heart ejects between 5 and 6 liters of blood per minute (a liter is slightly larger than a quart). This amount of blood, also referred to as **cardiac output**, meets the energy demands in the resting state.

   Like any other muscle, the heart responds to training by gaining strength and size. As the heart gets stronger, the muscle can produce a more forceful contraction. A stronger contraction causes a greater ejection of blood with each beat (that is, it increases stroke volume), yielding a lower heart rate. This reduction in heart rate also allows the heart to rest longer between beats.

   Resting heart rates frequently decrease 10 to 20 beats per minute (bpm) after only 6 to 8 weeks of training. A reduction of 20 bpm saves the heart about 10,483,200 beats per year. The average heart beats between 70 and 80 bpm. Resting heart rates in highly trained athletes frequently are around 45 bpm.

4. **A lower heart rate at given workloads.** When compared with untrained individuals, a trained person has a lower heart rate response to a given task, because of higher efficiency of the cardio-respiratory system. Following several weeks of training, the heart's response to a given workload (let's say a 10-minute mile) is a much lower heart rate compared with the response when training first started.

5. **An increase in the number and size of the mitochondria.** All energy necessary for cell function is produced in the mitochondria. As their size and number increase, so does the potential to produce energy for muscular work.

6. **An increase in the number of functional capillaries.** These smaller vessels allow for the exchange of oxygen and carbon dioxide between the blood and the cells. As more vessels open up, more gas exchange can take place, thereby decreasing the onset of fatigue during prolonged exercise. This increase in capillaries also speeds up the rate at which waste products of cell metabolism can be removed. Increased capillarization also is seen in the heart, which enhances the oxygen delivery capacity to the heart muscle itself.

7. **Faster recovery time.** Trained individuals have a faster recovery time following exercise. A fit system is able to more rapidly restore any internal equilibrium disrupted during exercise.

8. **A decrease in blood pressure and blood lipids.** A regular aerobic exercise program will result in lower blood pressure and reduced cholesterol and triglycerides (these two fats are linked to the formation of the atherosclerotic plaque, which obstructs the arteries). This reduction lowers the risk for coronary heart disease (see Chapter 11). High blood pressure also is a leading risk factor for strokes.

9. **An increase in fat-burning enzymes.** Fat is lost primarily by burning it in muscle. As the concentration of these enzymes increases with aerobic training, so does the ability to burn fat.

Guidelines for Cardiorespiratory Exercise Prescription

To develop the cardiorespiratory system, the heart muscle has to be overloaded like any other muscle in the human body. Just as the biceps muscle in the upper arm is developed through strength-training exercises, the heart muscle also has to be exercised to increase in size, strength, and efficiency. To better understand how the cardiorespiratory system can be developed, we have to be familiar with the four basic principles of intensity, mode, duration, and frequency of exercise. These principles are discussed separately in this section, and Figure 7.1 summarizes the cardiorespiratory exercise prescription guidelines according to the American College of Sports Medicine (ACSM), the world's leading sports medicine organization.[3]

The ACSM recommends that a medical exam and a diagnostic exercise stress test or stress ECG be administered prior to vigorous exercise by apparently healthy men over age 45 and women over 55.[4] Vigorous exercise has been defined as an exercise intensity above 60 percent of VO_{2max}. This intensity is the equivalent of exercise that provides a "substantial challenge" to the participant or one that cannot be maintained for 20 continuous minutes.

INTENSITY OF EXERCISE | When people try to develop their cardiorespiratory system, the **intensity of exercise** perhaps is the most commonly ignored factor. This principle refers to how high the heart rate needs to be during exercise to improve cardiorespiratory endurance.

Muscles have to be overloaded to a given point for them to develop. Whereas the training stimulus to develop the biceps muscle can be accomplished with curl-up exercises, the stimulus for the cardiorespiratory

FIGURE 7.1 CARDIORESPIRATORY EXERCISE PRESCRIPTION GUIDELINES.

Activity:	Aerobic (examples: walking, jogging, cycling, swimming, aerobics, racquetball, soccer, stair climbing)
Intensity:	55/65%–90% of maximal heart rate
Duration:	20–60 minutes of continuous aerobic activity
Frequency:	3 to 5 days per week

From American College of Sports Medicine, "The Recommended Quantity and Quality of Exercise for Developing and Maintaining Cardiorespiratory and Muscular Fitness in Healthy Adults," *Medicine and Science in Sports and Exercise* 30 (1998): 975–991.

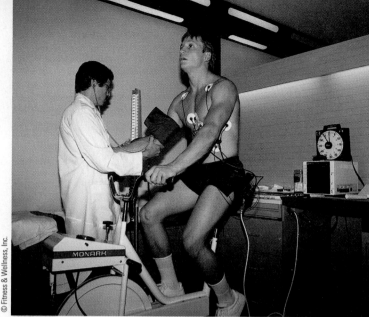

Exercise stress electrocardiogram test (stress ECG).

system is provided by making the heart pump at a higher rate for a certain period of time. Research has shown that cardiorespiratory development occurs when you work at between 55/65–90 percent of your **maximal heart rate**. The lower intensity, 55–65 percent, is recommended for beginners and people with health problems that have been cleared for exercise by a physician. The higher rate (65 to 90 percent) is for healthy people who have gone through the proper conditioning program.

Exercise intensity can be calculated easily and training can be monitored by checking your pulse. Use the following procedure to determine the intensity of exercise or your cardiorespiratory training zone.

1. Estimate the maximal heart rate (MHR). The maximal heart rate depends on the person's age and can be estimated according to the following formula:

   MHR = 220 minus age (220 − age)

2. Calculate the training intensities (TI) at 55 percent, 65 percent, and 90 percent. Multiply MHR by 55 percent, 65 percent, and 90 percent, respectively. For example, the 55 percent, 65 percent, and 90 percent training intensities for a 20-year-old person are

   MHR: 220 − 20 = 200 beats per minute (bpm)
   55% TI = (200 × .55) = 110 bpm
   65% TI = (200 × .65) = 130 bpm
   90% TI = (200 × .90) = 180 bpm
   Cardiorespiratory training zone: 110 to 180 bpm

According to your present age, you also may look up your cardiorespiratory training zone in Table 7.1. The training zone indicates that whenever you exercise to improve your cardiorespiratory system, you should maintain your heart rate between the 55 and 90 percent training intensities to obtain adequate development.

If you have been physically inactive and the objective is to attain the high physical fitness standard (see Chapter 6), you should train around the 55 to 65 percent intensity during the first 4 to 6 weeks of the exercise program. After the first few weeks, you can exercise between 65 and 90 percent training intensity.

Monitor your exercise heart rate regularly during exercise to make sure you are training in the correct zone. Wait until you are about 5 minutes into the exercise session before taking your first rate. When checking exercise heart rate, count your pulse for 10 seconds. Next, multiply the 10-second count by 6 to obtain the rate in beats per minute. Exercise heart rate will remain at the same level for about 15 seconds following exercise. After 15 seconds, heart rate will drop rapidly. Do not hesitate to stop during your exercise bout to check your pulse. If the rate is too low, increase the intensity of exercise. If the rate is too high, slow down.

HEALTH VERSUS FITNESS INTENSITIES To develop your cardiorespiratory system, you do not have to exercise above the 90 percent rate. From a fitness standpoint, training above this percentage will not yield extra benefits and actually may be unsafe for some people.

For unconditioned people and older adults, cardiorespiratory training should be conducted at about the 55 to 65 percent rate. This lower rate is recommended to reduce potential problems associated with high-intensity exercise.

Training benefits obtained by exercising at the 55 to 65

Cardiac output Amount of blood ejected by the heart in 1 minute.

Resting heart rate Heart rate after a person has been sitting quietly for 15–20 minutes.

Intensity of exercise In cardiorespiratory exercise, how hard a person has to exercise to improve or maintain fitness.

Maximal heart rate (MHR) Highest heart rate for a person, primarily related to age.

TABLE 7.1 RECOMMENDED CARDIORESPIRATORY EXERCISE INTENSITIES

Age	Estimated Max HR*	55% HR Intensity	65% HR Intensity	90% HR Intensity
15	205	113	133	185
20	200	110	130	180
25	195	107	127	176
30	190	105	124	171
35	185	102	120	167
40	180	99	117	162
45	175	96	114	158
50	170	94	111	153
55	165	91	107	149
60	160	88	104	144
65	155	85	101	140
70	150	83	98	135
75	145	80	94	131

*HR = Heart Rate

FIGURE 7.2 RATE OF PERCEIVED EXERTION SCALE.

6	
7	Very, very light
8	
9	Very light
10	
11	Fairly light
12	
13	Somewhat hard
14	
15	Hard
16	
17	Very hard
18	
19	Very, very hard
20	

From Gunnar Borg, "Perceived Exertion: A Note on History and Methods," *Medicine and Science in Sports and Exercise* (1983): 90–93.

percent training intensity may place a person only in an average or "moderately fit" category (see Table 6.3 in Chapter 6). Even though it is not an excellent cardio-respiratory fitness rating, exercising at this lower intensity does significantly decrease the risk for cardio-vascular mortality (a health fitness criterion) and other chronic diseases. An excellent fitness rating is obtained by exercising closer to the 90 percent threshold.

RATE OF PERCEIVED EXERTION Many people do not check their heart rate during exercise, so an alternative method of prescribing intensity of exercise can be used. This method uses a **rate of perceived exertion (RPE)**, scale developed by Gunnar Borg.[5] Using the scale in Figure 7.2, a person subjectively rates the perceived exertion or difficulty of exercise when training in the appropriate target zone. The exercise heart rate then is associated with the corresponding RPE value.

If the training intensity requires a heart rate between 130 and 170 bpm, for example, this is associated with training between "somewhat hard" and "very hard" (13 and 17 on the scale). Some individuals, however, may perceive less exertion than others when training in the correct zone. Therefore, you should associate your own inner perception of the task with the phrases given on the scale. You then may proceed to exercise at that rate of perceived exertion.

Whether you monitor the intensity of exercise by checking your pulse or using the rate of perceived exertion, changes in normal exercise conditions affect the training zone. For example, exercising on a hot or humid day or at high altitude increases the heart rate response

to a given task. Therefore, the intensity of your exercise may have to be adjusted.

MODE OF EXERCISE The **mode of exercise** that develops the cardiorespiratory system has to be aerobic in nature. Once you have established your cardiorespiratory training zone, any activity or combination of activities that will get your heart rate up to that training zone and keep it there for as long as you exercise will produce adequate development.

Examples of aerobic activities are walking, jogging, aerobics, swimming, water aerobics, cross-country skiing, rope skipping, cycling, racquetball, stair climbing, and stationary running or cycling. Most of these activities can be used for either moderate- or high-intensity programs. Additional moderate-intensity activities include garden-ing; mowing the lawn (with a push mower); house cleaning; pushing a stroller; washing a car; raking leaves; or playing golf, tennis, or volleyball.

The activity you choose should be based on your personal preferences, what you enjoy doing most, and your physical limitations. Different activities may affect the amount of strength or flexibility developed, but as far as the cardiorespiratory system is concerned, the heart doesn't know whether you are walking, swimming, or cycling. All the heart knows is that it has to pump at a certain rate, and as long as that rate is in the desired range, cardiorespiratory development will take place.

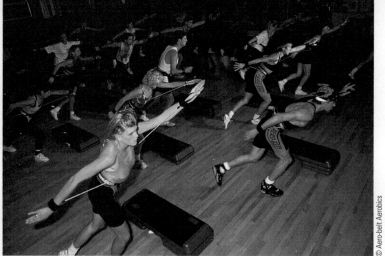

The greater the number of muscle groups involved during aerobic exercise, the greater the benefits.

© Aero-belt Aerobics

| **DURATION OF EXERCISE** | The general recommendation is that a person should train between 20 and 60 minutes per session. **Duration** is based on how intensely a person trains. If the training is done at around 90 percent intensity, 20 minutes are sufficient. At 65 percent intensity, a person should train at least 30 minutes. As mentioned, unconditioned people and older adults should train at lower percentages; therefore, the activity should be carried for a longer duration.

Although most experts recommend 20 to 30 minutes of aerobic exercise per session, research indicates that three 10-minute exercise sessions per day (separated by at least 4 hours), at approximately 70 percent of maximal heart rate, also produce training benefits.[6] Increases in VO_{2max} with this program were not as large (only 57 percent) as those in a group performing a continuous 30-minute bout of exercise per day, but the researchers concluded that "moderate-intensity" exercise training, conducted for 10 minutes three times per day, benefits the cardiorespiratory system. The results of this study are meaningful because people often mention lack of time as the reason for not taking part in an exercise program. Many think they must exercise at least 20 minutes to get any benefits at all. Even though 20 to 60 minutes are recommended, short, intermittent bouts of exercise also are beneficial to the cardiorespiratory system.

The training session always should include a 5-minute warm-up and a 5-minute cool-down period (see Figure 7.3). The warm-up should consist of general **calisthenics**, stretching exercises, or exercising at a lower intensity level than the actual target zone. To cool down, the intensity of exercise is gradually decreased. Abruptly stopping causes blood to pool in the exercised body parts, diminishing the return of blood to the heart. A decreased blood return can cause dizziness and faintness or even bring on cardiac abnormalities.

| **FREQUENCY OF EXERCISE** | In terms of **frequency of exercise**, research indicates that a person should engage in aerobic exercise three to five times per week.[7] Any training beyond 5 days per week produces only minimal improvements in cardiorespiratory capacity (VO_{2max}).

For people on a weight-loss program, 45- to 60-minute exercise sessions of moderate intensity, conducted 5 or 6 days a week, are recommended. Longer exercise sessions increase caloric expenditure for faster weight reduction (see Chapter 10).

Ideally, a person should engage in physical activity six to seven times per week. To reap maximum benefits of physical activity, a person needs to exercise a minimum of three times per week in the appropriate target zone for high fitness maintenance and three to four additional times per week in moderate-intensity activities to enjoy the full benefits of health fitness. As indicated in the Surgeon General's report on physical activity and health,[8] people should strive to attain at least 30 minutes of physical activity per day most days of the week.

| Physical Activity and Diabetes |

According to the Centers for Disease Control and Prevention, there are 10.3 million reported diabetics in the United States and an additional 5.4 million undiagnosed cases. There are two types of diabetes: Type I, or insulin-dependent diabetes (IDDM), and Type II, or non-insulin-dependent diabetes (NIDDM). In Type I, found primarily in young people, the pancreas produces little or no insulin. With Type II, the pancreas may not produce enough insulin or the cells become insulin-resistant, thereby keeping glucose from entering the cell. Type II accounts for over 90 percent of all diabetes cases, and it occurs mainly in adults over 40 who are also overweight.

If you are a diabetic, consult your physician before you start exercising. You may not be able to start until your diabetes is under control. Never exercise alone and use a bracelet that identifies your condition. If you take insulin, the amount and timing of each dose may need to be regulated with your physician. If you inject insulin, inject it over a muscle that won't be exercised and then wait one hour before exercising. For Type I diabetics, it is recommended that you ingest 15 to 30 grams of carbohydrate during each 30

Rate of perceived exertion (RPE) A perception scale to monitor or interpret the intensity of aerobic exercise.

Mode of exercise Form of exercise.

Duration of exercise How long a person exercises.

Calisthenics The exercise of muscles for the purpose of gaining health, strength, and grace of form and movement.

Frequency of exercise How often a person engages in an exercise session.

FIGURE **7.3** TYPICAL CARDIORESPIRATORY TRAINING PATTERN.

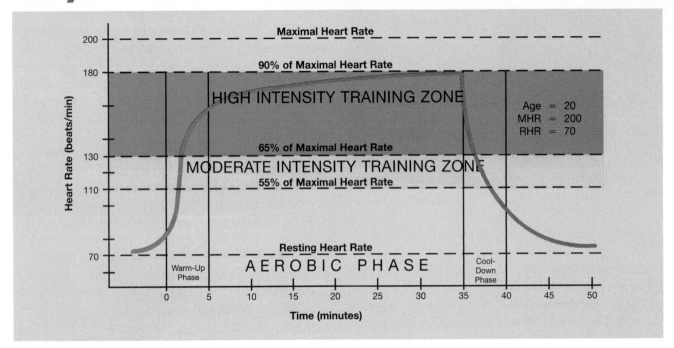

minutes of intense exercise and follow it with a carbohydrate snack after exercise.

Both types of diabetes improve with exercise, although the results are more notable in patients with Type II diabetes. Exercise usually lowers blood sugar and helps the body use food more effectively. The degree to which blood glucose level can be controlled in overweight Type II diabetics appears to be directly related to how long and how hard a person exercises. Normal or near-normal blood glucose levels can be achieved through a proper exercise program.

As with any fitness program, the exercise must be done on a regular basis to be effective against diabetes. The benefit of a single exercise bout on blood glucose level is highest between 12 and 24 hours following exercise. These benefits are completely lost within 72 hours after exercise. Thus, regular participation is crucial to derive ongoing benefits. In terms of fitness, all diabetic patients can achieve higher fitness levels and reductions in weight, blood pressure, and total cholesterol and triglycerides.

According to the ACSM, the following guidelines should be followed by diabetic patients to make the exercise program safe and derive the best benefits:[9]

- Burn a minimum of 1,000 calories per week through your exercise program.
- Exercise at a low–to-moderate intensity (55 to 65 percent of MHR). Start your program with 10 to 15 minutes per session, on at least 3 nonconsecutive days, but preferably exercise 5 days per week. Gradually increase the time you exercise to 30 minutes until you achieve your goal of at least 1,000 weekly calories. Diabetic individuals with a weight problem should build up to daily physical activity for 60 minutes per session.
- Choose an activity that you enjoy doing and stay with it. As you select your activity, be aware of your condition. For example, if you have lost sensation in your feet, swimming or stationary cycling is better than walking or jogging from an injury prevention point of view.
- Check blood glucose levels before and after exercise. If you are on insulin or diabetes medication, monitor blood glucose regularly and check it at least twice before exercise.
- Schedule your exercise 1 to 3 hours after a meal and avoid exercise when your insulin is peaking.
- Be ready to treat low blood sugar with a fast-acting source of sugar, such as juice or raisins.
- Discontinue exercise immediately if you feel that a reaction is about to occur. Check your blood glucose level and treat the condition as needed.
- When you exercise outdoors, always do so with someone who knows what to do in a diabetes-related emergency.
- Strength training twice per week, using 8 to 10 exercises with a minimum of one set of 10 to 15

repetitions to near-fatigue is also recommended for individuals with diabetes.

Maintaining Cardiorespiratory Fitness

A decrease in cardiorespiratory fitness has been observed in as little as 2 weeks of nontraining. Depending on the length of participation in the aerobic program, complete loss of training benefits is seen between 3 and 8 months after discontinuing the program. After an aerobic conditioning program, a person must continue a regular training program to maintain cardiorespiratory fitness.

The key to maintaining fitness seems to be the intensity of training.[10] Even though the duration and frequency of training may be reduced, VO_{2max} does not decline as long as the proper intensity is maintained. Three 20-minute training sessions per week, on nonconsecutive days, maintains cardiorespiratory fitness as long as the heart rate is in the appropriate target zone.

Personal Cardiorespiratory Exercise Prescription

Having learned the basic principles of cardiorespiratory exercise prescription, you can proceed to Assessment 7-1 at the end of this chapter and fill out your own prescription. If you have not been exercising regularly, you could go ahead and attempt to train five or six times a week for 30 minutes at a time. You may find this discouraging, however, and may drop out before getting too far because you probably will develop some muscle soreness and stiffness and possibly incur minor injuries. Muscle soreness and stiffness and the risk for injuries can be lessened or eliminated by progressively increasing the intensity, duration, and frequency of exercise.

Once you have determined your exercise prescription, the difficult part begins: starting and sticking to a lifetime exercise program. Although you may be motivated after reading the benefits to be gained from physical activity, lifelong dedication and perseverance are necessary to reap and maintain good fitness.

The first few weeks are probably the most difficult, but where there's a will, there's a way. Once you begin to see positive changes, it won't be as hard. Soon you will develop a habit for exercise that will be deeply satisfying and will bring about a sense of self-accomplishment.

MUSCULAR STRENGTH

An adequate level of strength is an important component of good physical fitness. The two forms of strength, as defined in Chapter 6, are muscular strength and muscular endurance. Muscular strength is the ability to exert maximum force against resistance; muscular endurance is the ability of a muscle to exert submaximal force repeatedly over a period of time. For example, a person may have the muscular strength to lift 100 pounds once but may not have the muscular endurance to lift 60 pounds 20 times.

Over the years it has been well-documented that the capacity of muscle cells to exert force increases and decreases according to the demands placed upon the muscular system. If muscle cells are overloaded beyond their normal use, such as in strength-training programs, the cells increase in size (**hypertrophy**) and strength. If the demands placed on the muscle cells decrease, such as in sedentary living or required rest because of illness or injury, the cells decrease in size (**atrophy**) and lose strength.

Significance of Strength

Strength is important for optimal performance in daily tasks and recreational activities, to improve personal appearance and self-image, to lessen the risk of injury, and to cope with emergency situations in life. Adequate strength levels also contribute to weight control and enhanced overall health and well-being.

Perhaps one of the most significant benefits of maintaining a good strength level is its relationship to human **metabolism**. Metabolism is defined as all energy and material transformations that occur within living cells.

A primary result of a strength-training program is an increase in muscle mass or size (lean body mass), known as muscle hypertrophy. Muscle tissue uses energy even at rest, whereas fatty tissue uses very little energy (that is, few calories) and may be considered metabolically inert.

As muscle size increases, so does the **resting metabolism,** or the amount of energy (expressed in calories) an individual requires during resting conditions to sustain proper cell function. Even small increases in muscle mass may affect resting metabolism. In one study, a group of inactive older adults between the ages of 56 and 86 who participated in a 12-week strength-training program increased lean body mass by about three pounds, lost about four pounds of fat, and increased their resting metabolic rate by almost 7 percent.[11]

Hypertrophy An increase in the size of the cell (for example, muscle hypertrophy).

Atrophy Decrease in size of a cell.

Metabolism All energy and material transformations that occur within living cells necessary to sustain life.

Resting metabolism The amount of energy (expressed in milliliters of oxygen per minute or in total calories per day) an individual requires during resting conditions to sustain proper body function.

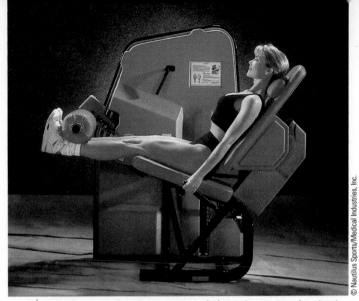

A regular strength-training program helps to increase and maintain a higher resting metabolic rate.

Each additional pound of muscle tissue is estimated to increase resting metabolism by approximately 35 calories per day.[12] All other factors being equal, if two individuals at 150 pounds have different amounts of muscle mass—let's say 5 pounds—the one with the greater muscle mass will have a higher resting metabolic rate. A higher metabolic rate indicates that this person can afford to eat more calories without gaining weight—because the calories are used to maintain the additional muscle tissue.

Loss of lean tissue is thought to be the main reason for the decrease in metabolism as people grow older. Contrary to some beliefs, metabolism does not have to slow down significantly with aging. We slow down. Lean body mass declines with sedentary living, which, in turn, slows down the resting metabolic rate. If people continue eating at the same rate, body fat increases. The average decrease in resting metabolism for a 60-year-old individual is about 300 to 400 calories per day, compared with a 25-year-old person. Hence, participating in a strength-training program is a means of preventing and reducing obesity.

One of the most common misconceptions about physical fitness relates to women and strength training. Because of the increase in muscle mass commonly seen in men, some women think strength-training programs are counterproductive because they, too, will develop large muscles. Although the quality of muscle in men and women is the same, endocrinological differences will not allow women to achieve the same amount of muscle hypertrophy (size) as men. Men also have more muscle fibers, and because of the male sex-specific hormones, each fiber has a greater potential for hypertrophy.

As more women participate in sports, the myth that strength training for women leads to larger muscle size has waned. In recent years, better body appearance has become the rule rather than the exception for women who participate in strength-training programs. Some of the most attractive women movie stars and many beauty pageant participants train with weights to further improve their personal image.

Another benefit of strength training, accentuated even more when combined with aerobic exercise, is a decrease in adipose (fatty) tissue. Research has shown that the decrease in fatty tissue often is greater than the amount of muscle hypertrophy gained through strength training. Therefore, losing inches but not body weight is a typical outcome.

Because muscle tissue is more dense than fatty tissue, and despite the fact that inches are being lost, people, especially women, often become discouraged because they cannot readily see the results on the scale. This discouragement can be offset easily by regularly determining body composition to monitor changes in percent body fat rather than simply measuring total body weight changes.

Adequate strength levels are especially critical in older age. Functional independence, or the physical capacity to meet ordinary and unexpected demands of daily life safely and effectively, is to a large extent dependent on a person's strength level.

Older adults with good strength enjoy greater freedom of movement and functionality than their inactive counterparts. Simple daily tasks such as getting out of bed, getting in and out of a tub, doing household chores, climbing a flight of stairs, and crossing a street safely are greatly enhanced through a strength-training program.

Research has shown that older adults can increase their strength levels, but the amount of muscle hypertrophy achieved decreases with age. Strength gains as high as 200 percent have been found in previously inactive adults over age 90.[13] Suddenly, many of these individuals, previously dependent on others, can perform most of life's daily tasks without restrictions or functional dependence.

Guidelines for Strength Development

Because muscular strength and endurance are important in developing and maintaining overall fitness and well-being, the principles necessary to develop a strength-training program have to be followed, as in the prescription of cardiorespiratory exercise. These principles are built around mode, resistance, sets, and frequency of training. Before discussing these principles, the concepts of progressive overload and specificity of training are explained.

PROGRESSIVE OVERLOAD PRINCIPLE | Strength gains are achieved in two ways: (a) through greater ability of individual muscle fibers to get a stronger contraction, and (b) by recruiting a greater proportion of the total available fibers for each contraction. These two factors combine in the **progressive overload principle**. This principle states that, for strength to improve, the demands placed on the muscle must be increased systematically and progressively over a period of time, and the resistance must be of a magnitude significant enough to cause physiologic adaptation. In simpler terms, just like all other organs and systems of the human body, muscles have to be taxed beyond their accustomed loads to increase in physical capacity.

SPECIFICITY OF TRAINING | The principle of **specificity of training** states that, for a muscle to increase in strength or endurance, only a training program for that express purpose will obtain the desired effects. In like manner, to increase static (isometric) versus dynamic strength, an individual must use static, instead of dynamic, training procedures to achieve the desired results.

MODE OF TRAINING | Two basic types of training methods are used to improve strength: **isometric** and **dynamic** (previously known as isotonic). Isometric training refers to a muscle contraction producing little or no movement, such as pushing or pulling against immovable objects. Dynamic training refers to a muscle contraction with movement, such as lifting an object over the head. Generally, the mode of training an individual uses depends mainly on the type of equipment available and the specific objective the training program is attempting to accomplish.

Isometric training does not require much equipment. It was commonly used in the 1950s and 1960s, but its popularity has waned. Because strength gains with isometric training are specific to the angle of muscle contraction, this type of training is most beneficial in a sport such as gymnastics, which requires regular static contractions during routines. Thus it has limited applications for overall health fitness.

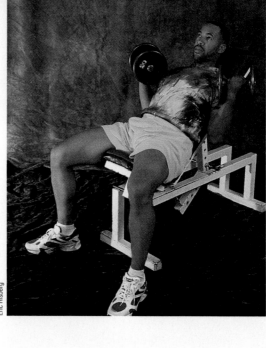
Eric Risberg

| Dynamic training. |

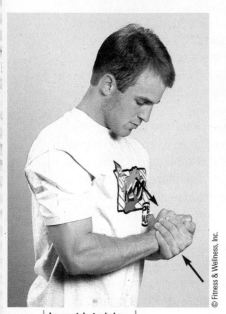
© Fitness & Wellness, Inc.

| Isometric training. |

Dynamic training is the most popular mode for strength training. Its main advantage is that strength is gained through the full range of motion. Most daily activities are dynamic in nature. We are constantly lifting, pushing, and pulling objects, and strength is needed through a complete range of motion. Another advantage is that improvements are easily measured by the amount lifted.

Dynamic training programs can be conducted without weights or with free weights (barbells and dumbbells) or on fixed resistance machines, variable resistance machines, and **isokinetic** equipment. When you perform dynamic exercises without weights (for example, pull-ups, push-ups), with free weights, or with fixed resistance machines, you move a constant resistance (weight) through a joint's full range of motion.

A limitation of dynamic training is that the greatest resistance that can be lifted equals the maximum weight that can be moved at the weakest angle of the joint. This is because of changes in muscle length and angle of pull as the joint moves through its range of motion.

Progressive overload principle Training concept stating that the demands placed on a system (for example, cardiorespiratory or muscular) must be increased systematically and progressively over time to cause physiological adaptation (development or improvement).

Specificity of training Targeting the specific body system or area the person is attempting to improve (aerobic endurance, anaerobic capacity, strength, flexibility).

Isometric Strength-training method that uses muscle contractions producing little or no movement, such as pushing or pulling against immovable objects.

Dynamic Strength-training method that uses muscle contractions with movement.

Isokinetic Strength-training method in which the speed of the muscle contraction is kept constant because the equipment (machine) provides an accommodating resistance to match the user's force through the range of motion.

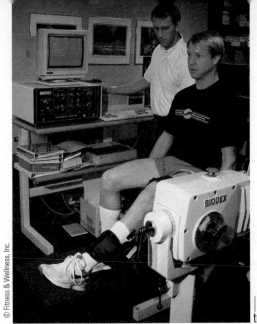
Isokinetic training.

As strength training became more popular, new strength-training machines were developed. This technology brought about isokinetic and variable resistance training. These training programs require special machines equipped with mechanical devices that provide varying amounts of resistance, with the intent of overloading the muscle group maximally through the entire range of motion.

A distinction of isokinetic training is that the speed of the muscle contraction is kept constant because the machine provides resistance to match the user's force through the range of motion. Another possible advantage of isokinetic training is that specific speeds used in various sport skills can be duplicated more closely with this type of training, which may enhance performance (specificity of training). A disadvantage is that the equipment is not readily available to many people.

The benefits of isokinetic and variable resistance training are similar to the other dynamic training methods. Theoretically, strength gains should be better because maximum resistance is applied at all angles. Research, however, has not shown this type of training to be more effective than other modes of dynamic training.

| RESISTANCE | **Resistance** in strength training is the equivalent of intensity in cardiorespiratory exercise prescription. The amount of resistance, or weight lifted, depends on whether the individual is trying to develop muscular strength or muscular endurance.

To stimulate strength development, a resistance of approximately 80 percent of the maximum capacity (1 RM) is recommended.[14] For example, a person who can press 150 pounds should work with at least 120 pounds (150 × .80). Using less than 80 percent will increase muscular endurance rather than strength. Because of the extra time needed to determine the 1 RM on each lift to ensure that the person is indeed working above 80 percent, a rule of thumb that many authors and coaches accept is that individuals should perform between 3 and 12 repetitions maximum (3 to 12 RM) for adequate strength gains.

For example, if a person is training with a resistance of 120 pounds and cannot lift it more than 12 times, the training stimulus is adequate for strength development. Once the person can lift the weight more than 12 times, the resistance should be increased by 5 to 10 pounds, and the person again should build up to 12 repetitions. If training is conducted with more than 12 repetitions, primarily muscular endurance will be developed.

Research on strength indicates that the closer a person trains to the 1 RM, the greater the strength gains. A disadvantage of constantly working at or near the 1 RM is that it increases the risk for injury.

Highly trained athletes seeking maximum strength development often use 3 to 6 repetitions maximum. Working around 10 repetitions maximum seems to produce the best results in terms of muscular hypertrophy. From a health-fitness point of view, 8 to 12 repetitions to near-fatigue are recommended for adequate development. We live in an "dynamic world" in which muscular strength and endurance both are required to lead an enjoyable life. Therefore, working near a 10-repetition threshold seems offer the most improved overall performance.

| SETS | In strength training, a **set** has been defined as the number of repetitions performed for a given exercise. For example, a person lifting 120 pounds 8 times has performed 1 set of 8 repetitions (1 × 8 × 120). The number of sets recommended for optimum development is 3 sets per exercise. You should allow between 1 and 3 minutes between sets of the same exercise.

Because of the characteristics of muscle fiber, the number of sets that can be done is limited. As the number of sets increases, so does muscle fatigue and subsequent recovery time. Therefore, if too many sets are performed, strength gains may be lessened. A recommended program for beginners in their first year of training is 3 heavy sets, up to the maximum number of repetitions, preceded by 1 or 2 light warm-up sets using about 50 percent of the 1 RM.

To make the exercise program more time-effective, two or three exercises that require different muscle groups may be alternated. In this way, an individual will not have to wait too long before proceeding to a new set on a different exercise. For example, bench press, leg extensions, and abdominal crunches may be combined so the person can go almost directly from one set to the next.

To avoid muscle soreness and stiffness, new participants ought to build up gradually to the 3 sets of maximal repetitions. This can be done by doing only 1 set of each exercise with a lighter resistance on the first day. During the second session, 2 sets of each exercise can be performed: the first light, and the second with the regular resistance. On the third session, 3 sets could be performed: 1 light and 2 heavy. After that, a person should be able to do all 3 heavy sets.

| FREQUENCY OF TRAINING | Strength training should be done either with a total-body workout two to three times per week, or more frequently if using a split-body routine (upper body one day, lower body the next). After a maximum strength workout, the muscles should be rested for about 48 hours to allow adequate recovery.

People who are not completely recovered in 2 or 3 days most likely are overtraining and, therefore, not reaping the full benefits of their program. In that case, decreasing the total number of sets or exercises performed during the previous workout is recommended.

To achieve significant strength gains, a minimum of 8 weeks of consecutive training is needed. Once an adequate level of strength is achieved, one training session per week will be sufficient to maintain the new strength level.

| Strength-Training Exercise Guidelines |

As you prepare to design your strength training program, keep the following guidelines in mind.

1. Select exercises that will involve all major muscle groups: chest, shoulders, back, legs, arms, hip, and trunk.
2. Never lift weights alone. Always have someone work out with you in case you need a spotter or help with an injury. When you use free weights, one to two spotters are recommended for certain exercises (bench press, squats, overhead press).
3. Warm up properly prior to lifting weights by performing a light-to–moderate–intensity aerobic activity for 5 to 7 minutes and some gentle stretches for a few minutes.
4. Exercise larger muscle groups first—such as those in the chest, back, and legs—before exercising smaller muscle groups (arms, abdominals, ankles, neck). The bench press exercise works the chest, shoulders, and back of the upper arms (triceps), whereas the triceps extension works the back of the upper arms only.

5. Exercise opposing muscle groups for a balanced workout. After you work the chest (bench press), work the back (rowing torso). If you work the biceps (arm curl), work the triceps (triceps extension).
6. Perform all exercises in a controlled manner. Avoid fast and jerky movements and do not throw the entire body into the lifting motion. Failure to do so increases the risk of injury and decreases the effectiveness of the exercise. Do not arch the back when lifting a weight.
7. Perform each exercise through the entire possible range of motion.
8. Breathe naturally and do not hold your breath as you lift the resistance (weight). Inhale during the eccentric phase (bringing the weight down) and exhale during the concentric phase (lifting or pushing the weight up). Practice proper breathing with lighter weights when you are learning a new exercise.
9. Avoid holding your breath while straining to lift a weight. Holding your breath greatly increases the pressure inside the chest and abdominal cavity, making it practically impossible for the blood in the veins to return to the heart. Although rare, a sudden high intrathoracic pressure may lead to dizziness, a blackout, a stroke, a heart attack, or a hernia.
10. Discontinue training if you experience unusual discomfort or pain. High tension (heavy resistance) loads used in strength training can exacerbate potential injuries. Discomfort and pain are signals to stop and determine what's wrong. Be sure to properly evaluate your condition before you continue training.
11. Stretch out for a few minutes at the end of each strength-training workout to help muscles return to their normal resting length and to minimize muscle soreness and risk of injury.

| Designing a Strength-Training Program |

Two strength-training programs are illustrated at the end of this chapter (pages 167–174). Only a minimum of equipment is required for the first program, "Strength-Training Exercises Without Weights." (Exercises 1 through 11). This program can be done within the walls of your own home. Your body weight is used as the primary resistance for most exercises. A few exercises call for a friend's help or some basic implements from around the house to provide more resistance.

Resistance Amount of weight lifted in strength training.

Set Number of repetitions in strength training (e.g., 1 set of 12 repetitions).

"Strength-Training Exercises With Weights" (Exercises 12 through 20) require machines such as those shown in the photographs. Some of these machines use fixed resistance; others use variable resistance. Many of these exercises also can be done with free weights.

Depending on the facilities available to you, you should be able to choose one of the two training programs outlined in this chapter. The resistance and the number of repetitions you use should be based on whether you want to increase your muscular strength or your muscular endurance. Do up to 10–12 repetitions maximum for strength gains and muscle hypertrophy, and more than 12 for muscular endurance.

As pointed out, three training sessions per week on nonconsecutive days is an ideal arrangement for proper development. Because both strength and endurance are required in daily activities, 3 sets of about 8 to 12 repetitions maximum for each exercise are enough. In doing this, you will obtain good strength gains and yet be close to the endurance threshold.

Perhaps the only exercises that call for more repetitions are abdominal exercises. The abdominal muscles are considered primarily antigravity or postural muscles. Hence, a little more endurance may be required. When doing abdominal work, most people do about 20 repetitions.

If time is a concern in completing a strength-training exercise program, the American College of Sports Medicine recommends as a minimum: (a) 1 set of 8 to 12 repetitions performed to near-fatigue and (b) 8 to 10 exercises involving the major muscle groups of the body, conducted twice a week[15] (see Figure 7.4). This recommendation is based on research showing that this training generates 70 to 80 percent of the improvements reported in other programs using 3 sets of about 10 RM. You are now ready to write your own strength-training prescription using Assessment 7-2.

FIGURE **7.4** STRENGTH-TRAINING GUIDELINES.

Mode:	8 to 10 dynamic strength-training exercises involving the body's major muscle groups
Resistance:	Enough to perform 8 to 12 repetitions to near-fatigue (10 to 15 repetitions for older and more frail individuals)
Sets:	A minimum of 1 set
Frequency:	At least two times per week

Based on the recommended quantity and quality of exercise for developing and maintaining cardiorespiratory and muscular fitness and flexibility in healthy adults by the American College of Sports Medicine, *Medicine and Science in Sports and Exercise*, 30 (1998): 975–991.

MUSCULAR FLEXIBILITY

Flexibility is defined as the ability of a joint to move freely through its full range of motion. Health care professionals and practitioners have generally underestimated and overlooked the contribution of good muscular flexibility to overall fitness and preventive health care.

Significance of Flexibility

We often have to make rapid or strenuous movements we are not accustomed to making, and this may cause injury. And physical therapists have indicated that improper body mechanics are often the result of poor flexibility.

A decline in flexibility can cause poor posture and subsequent aches and pains that lead to limited and painful joint movement. Inordinate tightness is uncomfortable and debilitating. Approximately 80 percent of all low back problems in the United States are attributable to improper alignment of the vertebral column and pelvic girdle, a direct result of inflexible and weak muscles. This backache syndrome costs American industry billions of dollars each year in lost productivity, health services, and worker's compensation.[16]

Participating in a regular flexibility program helps a person maintain good joint mobility, increases resistance to muscle injury and soreness, prevents low back and other spinal column problems, improves and maintains good postural alignment, promotes proper and graceful body movement, improves personal appearance and self-image, and helps to develop and maintain motor skills throughout life. In addition, flexibility exercises have been prescribed successfully to treat dysmenorrhea[17] (painful menstruation) and general neuromuscular tension (stress). Regular stretching helps decrease the aches and pains caused by psychological stress and contributes to a decrease in anxiety, blood pressure, and breathing rate.[18]

Furthermore, stretching exercises in conjunction with calisthenics are helpful in warm-up routines to prepare the human body for more vigorous aerobic or strength-training exercises, as well as in cool-down routines following exercise to help the person return to a normal resting state. Fatigued muscles tend to contract to a shorter-than-average resting length, and stretching exercises help fatigued muscles reestablish their normal resting length.

Total range of motion around a joint is highly specific and varies from one joint to the other (hip, trunk, shoulder), as well as from one individual to the next. The amount of muscular flexibility relates primarily to genetic

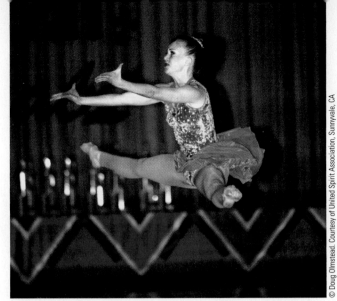

Adequate flexibility helps to develop and maintain sports skill throughout life.

factors and frequency of physical activity. Other factors that influence range of motion about a joint include joint structure, ligaments, tendons, muscles, skin, tissue injury, adipose tissue (fat), body temperature, age, and gender.

Because of the specificity of flexibility, determining an ideal level of flexibility is difficult. Nevertheless, flexibility is important to everyone's health, and even more so during the aging process.

Guidelines for Flexibility Development

Although genetics play a crucial role in body flexibility, range of joint mobility can be increased and maintained through a regular flexibility exercise program. Because range of motion is highly specific to each body part, a comprehensive stretching program, which includes all body parts and adheres to the basic guidelines for flexibility development, should be followed to obtain optimal results.

The progressive overload and specificity of training principles discussed in conjunction with strength development also apply to the development of muscular flexibility. To increase the total range of motion of a joint, the specific muscles surrounding that joint have to be stretched progressively beyond their accustomed length. Principles of mode, intensity, repetitions, and frequency of exercise also can be applied to flexibility programs.

MODE OF EXERCISE
Three modes of stretching exercises can be used to increase flexibility: (a) ballistic stretching, (b) slow-sustained stretching, and (c) proprioceptive neuromuscular facilitation stretching. Although research has indicated that all three types of stretching are effective in developing better flexibility, each technique has certain advantages.

Ballistic (or dynamic) **stretching** exercises are most often performed using jerky, rapid, and bouncy movements that provide the necessary force to lengthen the muscles. Studies have shown that this type of stretching helps to develop flexibility, but the ballistic actions may cause muscle soreness and injury because of small tears to the soft tissue.

Precautions must be taken not to overstretch ligaments, because they undergo plastic or permanent elongation. If the stretching force cannot be controlled, as in fast, jerky movements, ligaments easily can be overstretched. This, in turn, leads to excessively loose joints, which increases the risk for injuries, including joint dislocation and **subluxation**. Slow, gentle, and controlled ballistic stretching (instead of jerky, rapid, and bouncy movements), however, is quite effective in developing flexibility and can be performed safely by most individuals.

With **slow-sustained stretching** technique, muscles are lengthened gradually through a joint's complete range of motion, and the final position is held for a few seconds. Using a slow-sustained stretch causes the muscles to relax so greater length can be achieved. This type of stretch causes little pain and has a low risk for injury. Slow-sustained stretching exercises are used most frequently in and are recommended for flexibility development programs.

Proprioceptive neuromuscular facilitation (PNF) stretching has become more popular in the last few years. This technique is based on a "contract and relax" method and requires the assistance of another person. The procedure is as follows:

1. The person assisting with the exercise provides an initial force by slowly pushing in the direction of the desired stretch. The initial stretch does not cover the entire range of motion.

2. The person being stretched then applies force in the opposite direction of the stretch, against the assistant, who tries to hold the initial degree of stretch as closely as possible. This creates an isometric contraction at that angle.

3. After 4 or 5 seconds of isometric contraction, the muscle(s) being stretched

Flexibility Ability of a joint to move freely through its full range of motion.

Ballistic stretching Exercises performed using jerky, rapid, and bouncy movements.

Subluxation Partial dislocation of a joint.

Slow-sustained stretching Technique whereby the muscles are lengthened gradually through a joint's complete range of motion and the final position is held for a few seconds.

Proprioceptive neuromuscular facilitation (PNF) Stretching technique in which muscles are stretched out progressively with intermittent isometric contractions.

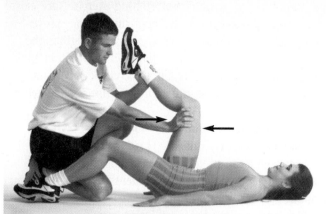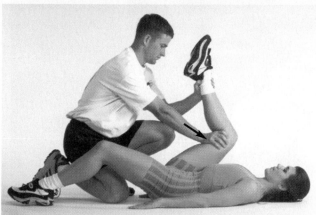

Proprioceptive neuromuscular facilitation (PNF) stretching technique.

are relaxed completely. The assistant then slowly increases the degree of stretch to a greater angle.

4. The isometric contraction is then repeated for another 4 or 5 seconds, after which the muscle is relaxed again. The assistant then can slowly increase the degree of stretch one more time. This procedure is repeated two to five times, until the exerciser feels mild discomfort. On the last trial, the final stretched position should be held for several seconds.

Theoretically, with the PNF technique, the isometric contraction helps relax the muscle(s) being stretched, which results in greater muscle length. Some fitness leaders believe that PNF is more effective than slow-sustained stretching. Another benefit of PNF is an increase in strength of the muscle(s) being stretched. Research has shown an approximate 17 percent and 35 percent increase in absolute strength and muscular endurance, respectively, in the hamstring muscle group after 12 weeks of PNF stretching.[19] The results were consistent in both men and women. These increases are attributed to the isometric contractions performed during PNF. The disadvantages are more pain with PNF, need for a second person to assist, and more time necessary to conduct each session.

| **INTENSITY OF EXERCISE** | Before you start any flexibility exercises, the muscles always should be **warmed up** using some calisthenic exercises. Failing to do a proper warm-up increases the risk for muscle pulls and tears. For this reason, a good time to do flexibility exercises is after aerobic workouts: Higher body temperature can increase joint range of motion significantly.

When you do flexibility exercises, the intensity or degree of stretch should be only to a point of mild discomfort. Pain does not have to be a part of the stretching routine.

Excessive pain is an indication that the load is too high and may lead to injury. Stretching should be done to slightly below the pain threshold. As participants reach this point, they should try to relax the muscle or muscles being stretched as much as possible. After completing the stretch, gradually bring the body part back to the starting point.

| **REPETITIONS** | In an exercise session, the time required for flexibility development is based on the number of repetitions performed and the length of time each repetition (the final stretched position) is held. The general recommendation is that each exercise be done four or five times, holding the final position each time for about 10 to 30 seconds.

As flexibility increases, the individual can gradually increase the time each repetition is held, to a maximum of a minute. Individuals who are susceptible to flexibility injuries should limit each stretch to 20 seconds.

| **FREQUENCY OF TRAINING** | Flexibility exercises should be conducted five to six times a week in the initial stages of the program. After a minimum of 6 to 8 weeks of almost daily stretching, flexibility levels can be maintained with only two to three sessions per week, using about three repetitions of 10 to 15 seconds each. Figure 7.5 provides a summary of flexibility development guidelines.

Designing a Flexibility Program

To improve body flexibility, each major muscle group should be subjected to at least one stretching exercise. A complete set of exercises for developing muscular flexibility is presented at the end of this chapter (Exercises 21 through 33). With some of the exercises, you may not be able to hold a final stretched position

FIGURE 7.5 GUIDELINES FOR DEVELOPMENT OF FLEXIBILITY.

Mode:	Static or dynamic (slow ballistic or proprioceptive neuromuscular facilitation) stretching to include every major joint of the body
Intensity:	Stretch to the point of mild discomfort
Repetitions:	Repeat each exercise at least 4 times and hold the final stretched position for 10 to 30 seconds
Frequency:	2–3 days per week

Based on the recommended quantity and quality of exercise for developing and maintaining cardiorespiratory and muscular fitness and flexibility in healthy adults by the American College of Sports Medicine, *Medicine and Science in Sports and Exercise* 30 (1998): 975–991.

(examples are lateral head tilts and arm circles), but you still should perform the exercise through the joint's full range of motion. Depending on the number and the length of the repetitions, a complete workout will last between 15 and 30 minutes. You can use Assessment 7-3 at the end of this chapter to design your own stretching program.

PREVENTING AND REHABILITATING LOW BACK PAIN

Few people make it through life without having low-back pain at some point. An estimated 75 million Americans have chronic low back pain each year. Back pain is considered chronic if it persists longer than three months. About 80 percent of the time, backache syndrome is preventable and is caused by (a) physical inactivity, (b) poor postural habits and body mechanics, or (c) excessive body weight.

People tend to think of back pain as a skeleton problem, but the spine's curvature, alignment, and movement are controlled by surrounding muscles. Lack of physical activity is the most common reason for chronic low-back pain. In particular, a major contributor to back pain is excessive sitting, which causes back muscles to shorten, stiffen, and become weaker.

Deterioration or weakening of the abdominal and gluteal muscles, along with tightening of the lower back (erector spinae) muscles, brings about an unnatural forward tilt of the pelvis. This tilt puts extra pressure on the spinal vertebrae, causing pain in the lower back. Accumulation of fat around the midsection of the body contributes to the forward tilt of the pelvis, which further aggravates the condition.

Low back pain is frequently associated with faulty posture and improper body mechanics (body positions in all of life's daily activities, including sleeping, sitting, standing, walking, driving, working, and exercising). Incorrect posture and poor mechanics, as explained in Figure 7.6, increase strain not only on the lower back but on many other bones, joints, muscles, and ligaments as well.

> Faulty posture and weak and inelastic muscles are the leading causes of chronic low back problems in the United States.

In most cases, back pain is present only with movement and physical activity. However, if the pain is severe and persists even at rest, the first step is to consult a physician, who can rule out any disc damage and may prescribe proper bed rest using several pillows under the knees for leg support (see Figure 7.6). This position helps release muscle spasms by stretching the muscles involved. In addition, a physician may prescribe a muscle relaxant or anti-inflammatory medication (or both) and some type of physical therapy. Back pain can be reduced greatly by including some specific stretching and strengthening exercises in the regular fitness program.

In most cases of low back pain, even with severe pain, people feel better within days or weeks without treatment from health care professionals.[20] To relieve symptoms, you may use over-the-counter pain relievers and hot or cold packs. You should also stay active to avoid further weakening of the back muscles. Low-impact activities like walking, swimming, water aerobics, and cycling are recommended. Once you are pain-free in the resting state, you need to start correcting the muscular imbalance by stretching the tight muscles and strengthening the weak ones. Stretching exercises always are performed first.

If there is no indication of disease or injury, such as leg numbness or pain, a herniated disk, or fractures, spinal manipulation by a chiropractor or other health care professional can provide pain relief. Spinal manipulation as a treatment modality for low back pain has been endorsed by the federal Agency for Health Care Policy and Research. The guidelines suggest that spinal manipulation may help to alleviate discomfort and pain during the first few weeks of an acute low back pain episode. Generally, benefits are seen within 10 treatments. People who have had chronic pain for over 6 months should avoid spinal manipulation until they have been thoroughly examined by a physician.

Warm-up Starting a workout slowly.

FIGURE 7.6 YOUR BACK AND HOW TO CARE FOR IT.

HOW TO STAY ON YOUR FEET WITHOUT TIRING YOUR BACK

To prevent strain and pain in everyday activities, change from one task to another before fatigue sets in: lie down between chores. Check body position frequently, drawing in the abdomen, flattening the back, bending the knees slightly.

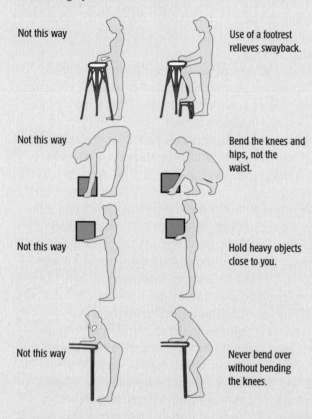

Not this way   Use of a footrest relieves swayback.

Not this way   Bend the knees and hips, not the waist.

Not this way   Hold heavy objects close to you.

Not this way   Never bend over without bending the knees.

HOW TO PUT YOUR BACK TO BED

For proper bed posture, a firm mattress is essential. Bedboards, sold commercially or devised at home, may be used with soft mattresses. Bedboards, preferably, should be made of 3/4-inch plywood. Faulty sleeping positions intensify swayback and result not only in backache but in numbness, tingling, and pain in arms and legs.

Incorrect:
Lying flat on back makes swayback worse.

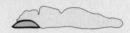

Use of high pillow strains neck, arms, shoulders.

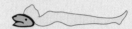

Sleeping face down exaggerates swayback, strains neck and shoulders.

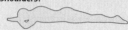

Bending one hip and knee does not relieve swayback.

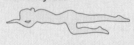

Correct:
Lying on side with knees bent effectively flattens the back. Flat pillow may be used to support neck, especially when shoulders are broad.

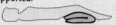

Sleeping on back is restful and correct when knees are properly supported.

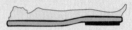

Raise the foot of the mattress 8 inches to discourage sleeping on the abdomen.

Proper arrangement of pillows for resting or reading in bed.

HOW TO SIT CORRECTLY

A back's best friend is a straight, hard chair. If you can't get the chair you prefer, learn to sit properly on whatever chair you get. **To correct sitting position from forward slump:** Throw head well back, then bend it forward to pull in the chin. This will straighten the back. Now tighten abdominal muscles to raise the chest. Check position frequently.

Relieve strain by sitting well forward, flatten back by tightening abdominal muscles, and cross knees.

Use of footrest relieves swayback. Aim is to have knees higher than hips.

Correct way to sit while driving, close to pedals. Use seat belt or hard backrest, available commercially.

TV slump leads to "dowager's hump," strains neck and shoulders.

If chair is too high, swayback is increased.

Keep neck and back in as straight a line as possible with the spine. Bend forward from hips.

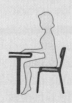

Driver's seat too far from pedals emphasizes curve in lower back.

Strained reading position. Forward thrusting strains muscles of neck and head.

Several exercises for preventing and rehabilitating the backache syndrome are given at the end of this chapter (pages 177–178). These exercises can be done twice or more daily when a person has back pain. Under normal circumstances, doing these exercises three to four times a week is enough to prevent the syndrome.

Psychological stress may also lead to back pain.[21] Excessive stress causes muscles to contract. In the case of the lower back, frequent tightening of the muscles can throw the back out of alignment and constrict blood vessels that supply oxygen and nutrients to the back. If you suffer from excessive stress and back pain at the same time, proper stress management (see Chapter 3) should be a part of your comprehensive back-care program.

MANAGEMENT OF EXERCISE-RELATED INJURIES

To enjoy and maintain physical fitness, preventing injury during a conditioning program is essential. Exercise-related injuries, nonetheless, are common in individuals who participate in exercise programs. Surveys show that more than half of all new exercise participants will incur injuries during the first 6 months of the conditioning program.

The four most common causes of injuries are (a) high-impact activities, (b) rapid conditioning programs—doing too much too quick, (c) improper shoes or training surfaces, and (d) anatomical predisposition (body propensity). High-impact activities and a substantial increase in quantity, intensity, and duration of activities are the most common causes of injuries, by far. The body requires time to adapt to more intense activities. Most of these injuries could be prevented through a more gradual and proper conditioning program.

The best treatment always has been prevention itself. If an activity is causing unusual discomfort or chronic irritation, you need to treat the cause by decreasing the intensity, switching activities, or using better equipment such as proper-fitting shoes.

In cases of acute injury, the standard treatment is rest, cold application, compression or splinting (or both), and elevation of the affected body part. This commonly is referred to as RICE:

R = Rest
I = Ice application
C = Compression, and
E = Elevation.

Providing proper rest for the injured area is critical during the recovery process. Cold should be applied three to five times a day for 15 to 20 minutes at a time during the first 24 to 36 hours by submerging the injured area in cold water, using an ice bag, or applying ice massage to the affected part. An elastic bandage or wrap can be used for compression. Elevating the body part decreases blood flow to it.

The purpose of these four types of treatment is to minimize swelling in the area, which hastens recovery time. After the first 36 to 48 hours, heat can be used if there is no further swelling or inflammation. If you have doubts regarding the nature or seriousness of the injury (such as suspected fracture), however, you should seek a medical evaluation.

Obvious deformities (such as in fractures, dislocations, or partial dislocations) call for splinting, cold application with an ice bag, and medical attention. Never try to reset any of these conditions by yourself, because muscles, ligaments, and nerves could be further damaged. Treatment of these injuries always should be in the hands of specialized medical personnel. A quick reference guide for the signs or symptoms and treatment of exercise-related problems is provided in Table 7.2.

EXERCISE INTOLERANCE

As you start your exercise program, be sure to stay within the safe limits for exercise participation. The best method to determine whether you are exercising too strenuously is to check your heart rate and make sure it does not exceed the limits of your target zone. Exercising above this target zone may not be safe for unconditioned or high-risk individuals. You do not need to exercise beyond your target zone to gain the desired benefits for the cardiorespiratory system.

In addition, several physical signs will tell you when you are exceeding functional limitations. These include a rapid or irregular heart rate, difficult breathing, nausea, vomiting, lightheadedness, headaches, dizziness, pale or flushed skin, extreme weakness, lack of energy, shakiness, sore muscles, cramps, and tightness in the chest. If you notice any of these symptoms, you should seek medical attention before continuing your exercise program. One of the most important things you need to learn when exercising is to listen to your body.

Your recovery heart rate can also be an indicator of overexertion. To a certain extent, recovery heart rate is related to fitness level. The higher your cardiorespiratory fitness level, the faster your heart rate will decrease following exercise. As a rule of thumb, heart rate should be below 120 beats per minute 5 minutes into recovery. If your heart rate is above 120, you have most likely overexerted yourself or could possibly have some other

TABLE 7.2   REFERENCE GUIDE FOR EXERCISE-RELATED PROBLEMS

Injury	Signs/Symptoms	Treatment*
Bruise (contusion)	Pain, swelling, discoloration	Cold application, compression, rest
Dislocations/Fractures	Pain, swelling, deformity	Splinting, cold application, seek medical attention
Heat cramps	Cramps, spasms, and muscle twitching in the legs, arms, and abdomen	Stop activity, get out of the heat, stretch, massage the painful area, drink plenty of fluids
Heat exhaustion	Fainting, profuse sweating, cold/clammy skin, weak/rapid pulse, weakness, headache	Stop activity, rest in a cool place, loosen clothing, rub body with cool/wet towel, drink plenty of fluids, stay out of heat for 2–3 days
Heat stroke	Hot/dry skin, no sweating, serious disorientation, rapid/full pulse, vomiting, diarrhea, unconsciousness, high body temperature	*Seek immediate medical attention*, request help and get out of the sun, bathe in cold water / spray with cold water / rub body with cold towels, drink plenty of cold fluids
Joint sprains	Pain, tenderness, swelling, loss of use, discoloration	Cold application, compression, elevation, rest, heat after 36 to 48 hours (if no further swelling)
Muscle cramps	Pain, spasm	Stretch muscle(s), use mild exercises for involved area
Muscle soreness and stiffness	Tenderness, pain	Mild stretching, low-intensity exercise, warm bath
Muscle strains	Pain, tenderness, swelling, loss of use	Cold application, compression, elevation, rest, heat after 36 to 48 hours (if no further swelling)
Shin splints	Pain, tenderness	Cold application prior to and following any physical activity, rest, heat (if no activity is carried out)
Side stitch	Pain on the side of the abdomen below the rib cage	Decrease level of physical activity or stop altogether, gradually increase level of fitness
Tendonitis	Pain, tenderness, loss of use	Rest, cold application, heat after 48 hours

* Cold should be applied 3 to 4 times a day for 15 minutes. Heat can be applied 3 times a day for 15 to 20 minutes.

cardiac abnormality. If you decrease the intensity or duration of exercise and you still have a fast heart rate 5 minutes into recovery, consult your physician.

LEISURE-TIME PHYSICAL ACTIVITY

Although individuals have notable differences, the average person in developed countries has about 3.5 hours of "free" or leisure-time daily. Unfortunately, in the current automated society, most of this time is spent in sedentary living.

Leisure-time physical activity is usually viewed as any activity undertaken during an individual's discretionary time that helps to increase resting energy or caloric expenditure. These activities are selected based on personal interests. Motivational factors for participation include health, aesthetics, weight control, competition and challenge, fun, social interaction, mental arousal, relaxation, and stress management.

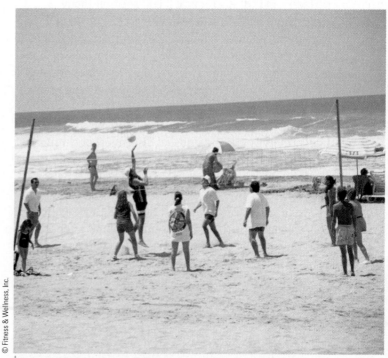

© Fitness & Wellness, Inc.

Leisure-time activities should promote energy expenditure and enhance overall health and fitness.

Frequently, leisure-time physical activity does not include exercise performed during a regular exercise program. It consists of activities such as walking, hiking, gardening, yard work, occupational work and chores, and moderate sports such as tennis, table tennis, badminton, golf, and croquet.

Every small increase in daily physical activity contributes to the development of health and wellness. Small increases in physical activity produce large decreases in early risk for disease and premature death. Therefore, health-conscious people will make a concerted effort to spend their leisure time in activities that promote energy expenditure, provide a break from daily tasks, and contribute to health-related fitness.

MOTIVATION AND BEHAVIOR MODIFICATION

Scientific evidence of the benefits derived from living a healthy lifestyle continues to mount each day. Although the data are impressive, most people still don't adhere to a healthy lifestyle. Understanding why people do not live a healthy lifestyle may help increase your readiness and motivation to do so. To answer this question, one has to examine what motivates people and what actions are required to make permanent changes in behavior (**behavior modification**).

Transtheoretical Model

For most people, changing chronic/unhealthy behaviors to stable/healthy behaviors is often a challenging process. Change usually does not occur all at once, but is rather a lengthy process that involves several stages. To aid in this process, psychologists James Prochaska, John Norcross, and Carlo DiClemente developed the transtheoretical model for behavior change.[22] This model recognizes six stages in the process of willful change. The stages of change describe underlying processes that people go through to change most problem behaviors and adopt healthy behaviors. Most frequently, the model is used to change health-related behaviors such as physical inactivity, smoking, nutrition, weight problems, stress, and alcohol abuse.

Stages of Change

The six stages of change in the transtheoretical model are precontemplation, contemplation, preparation, action, maintenance, and termination/adoption. After years of study, researchers found that applying specific behavioral-change techniques during each stage of the model increases the success rate for change. Understanding each stage of this model will help you determine where you are in relation to your personal healthy-lifestyle behaviors. It will also help you identify techniques to make successful changes.

PRECONTEMPLATION People in this stage are not considering or do not want to change a particular behavior. They typically deny having a problem and have no intent to change in the foreseeable future. These people are usually unaware or underaware of the problem. Other people around them, including family, friends, health care practitioners, and co-workers, however, identify the problem quite clearly. Precontemplators do not care about the problem behavior and may even avoid information and materials that address the issue. They tend to avoid free screenings and workshops that can help identify and change the problem, even if financial compensation is made for attendance. These people frequently have an active resistance to change and seem resigned to accept the unhealthy behavior as "their fate."

Precontemplators are the most difficult people to reach for behavioral change. They often think that change isn't even a possibility. Educating them about the problem behavior is critical to help them start the process of change. Knowledge is power, and the challenge is to find ways to help them realize that they will be ultimately responsible for the consequences of their behavior. Frequently, they may initiate change only when under pressure from others.

CONTEMPLATION In this stage, people acknowledge that they have a problem and begin to seriously think about overcoming it. Although they are not quite ready for change, they are weighing the pros and cons of change. People may remain in this stage for years, but in their minds they are planning to take some action within the next six months. Education and peer support are quite valuable during this stage.

PREPARATION In the **preparation stage**, people are seriously considering and planning to change a behavior within the next month. They are taking initial steps for change and may even try it for a short while, such as stopping smoking for a day or exercising only a few times during this

Behavior modification
A process to permanently change destructive or negative behaviors and replace them with positive behaviors.

Precontemplation stage
Stage of change in which people are unwilling to change behavior.

Contemplation stage
Stage of change in which people are considering changing behavior in the next 6 months.

Preparation stage Stage of change in which people are getting ready to make a change within the next month.

Please indicate which response most accurately describes your current _____ behavior (in the blank space identify the behavior: smoking, physical activity, stress, nutrition, weight control). Next, select the statement below (select only one) that best represents your current behavior pattern. To select the most appropriate statement, fill in the blank for one of the first three statements if your current behavior is a problem behavior. (For example, you may say, "I currently smoke and I do not intend to change in the foreseeable future," or "I currently do not exercise but I am contemplating changing in the next 6 months.") If you have already started to make changes, fill in the blank in one of the last three statements. (In this case, you may say: "I currently eat a low-fat diet but I have only done so within the last 6 months," or "I currently practice adequate stress management techniques and I have done so for over 6 months.") As you can see, you may use this form to identify your stage of change for any type of health-related behavior.

1. I currently _____ and I do not intend to change in the foreseeable future.

2. I currently _____ but I am contemplating changing in the next 6 months.

3. I currently _____ regularly but I intend to change in the next month.

4. I currently _____ but I have done so only within the last 6 months.

5. I currently _____ and I have done so for more than 6 months.

6. I currently _____ and I have done so for more than 5 years.

Stages of Change

1 =	Precontemplation	4 =	Action
2 =	Contemplation	5 =	Maintenance
3 =	Preparation	6 =	Termination/Adoption

month. During this stage, people define a general goal for behavioral change (to quit smoking by the last day of the month) and write specific objectives necessary to accomplish this goal (see Goal Setting discussion, page 162). Continued peer and environmental support are recommended during the preparation phase.

ACTION This stage requires the greatest commitment of time and energy from the individual. Here people are actively doing things to change or modify their problem behavior or to adopt a new health behavior. The **action stage** requires that the person follow the specific guidelines set forth for that particular behavior. For example, a person has actually completely stopped smoking, is exercising aerobically three times per week according to exercise prescription guidelines, or is maintaining a diet that derives less than 30 percent of its calories from fat. Relapse is common during this stage, and the individual may regress to previous stages. Once people maintain the action stage for 6 consecutive months, they move into the maintenance stage.

MAINTENANCE During the **maintenance stage**, the person continues to maintain the behavioral change for a period of up to 5 years. The maintenance phase requires continued adherence to the specific guidelines that govern the behavior (complete smoking cessation, exercising aerobically three times per week, or practicing proper stress management techniques). It is at this time that a person works to reinforce the gains made through the various stages of change and strives to prevent lapses and relapse.

TERMINATION/ADOPTION Once a behavior has been maintained for over 5 years, a person is said to be in the **termination** or **adoption phase** and exits from the cycle of change without fear of **relapse**. In the case of negative behaviors that have stopped, the stage of change is referred to as termination. If a positive behavior has been maintained for over 5 years, this stage is designated as the adoption stage. Many experts believe that after this period of time, any former addictions, problems, or lack of compliance with healthy behaviors no longer present an obstacle in the quest for wellness. The change has now become a part of one's lifestyle. This phase is the ultimate goal for all people searching for a healthier lifestyle.

You may use the form provided in Figure 7.7 to determine where you stand in respect to old behaviors that you want to change or new ones that you wish to adopt. As you use this form, you will realize that you are at different stages for different behaviors. For instance, you may be in the termination stage for aerobic exercise and smoking, in the action stage for strength training, but only in the contemplation stage for a healthy diet. Realizing where you are with respect to different behaviors will help you design a better action plan for a healthy lifestyle.

Motivation

Motivation is often set forth as an explanation for why some people succeed and others don't. Although motivation comes from within, external factors trigger the inner desire to accomplish a given task. These external factors, then, control behavior.

When studying motivation, you'll find it helpful to understand people's locus of control. People who believe they have control over events in their lives are said to have an internal locus of control. People with an external locus of control believe that what happens to them is a result of chance—the environment—and is unrelated to their behavior.

People with an internal locus of control are healthier and have an easier time initiating and adhering to a wellness program. In contrast, those who perceive that they have no control think of themselves as powerless and vulnerable. Becoming motivated is often a challenge. These people are also at greater risk for illness. When illness strikes, restoring a sense of control is vital to regain health.

Few people have either a completely external or a completely internal locus of control. They fall somewhere along a continuum, and their location along the continuum relates to their health. Also, the more external one's locus of control, the harder it is to adhere to exercise and other healthy lifestyle behaviors. Fortunately, one can develop a more internal locus of control. Understanding that most events in life are not controlled genetically or environmentally helps people pursue goals and gain control over their lives. Three impediments, however, can keep people from taking action: problems of competence, confidence, and motivation.[23]

1. Problems of competence. Lacking the skills to get a given task done leads to decreased competence. If your friends play basketball regularly, but you don't know how to play, you might not be inclined to participate. The solution to the problem of competence is to master the skills needed to participate. Most people are not born with all-inclusive natural abilities, including playing sports.

   A college professor continuously watched a group of students play an entertaining game of basketball every Friday at noon. Having no basketball skills, he was reluctant to play. The desire to join in the fun was strong enough that he enrolled in a beginning course at the college to learn to play the game. To his surprise, most students were impressed that he was willing to do this. Now, with greater competence, he is able to join Friday's "pick-up" games.

   Another alternative is to select an activity in which you are skilled. It may not be basketball, but it could well be aerobics. Don't be afraid to try new activities. Similarly, if your body weight is a problem, you could learn to cook low-fat meals. Try different recipes until you find dishes you like.

2. Problems of confidence. When the skills are there but you don't believe you can get it done, problems with confidence arise. Fear and feelings of inadequacy often interfere with the ability to perform the task.

   You never should talk yourself out of something until you have given it a fair try. If the skills are there, the sky is the limit. Initially, try to visualize yourself doing the task and getting it done. Repeat this several times, then give it a try. You will surprise yourself.

   Sometimes lack of confidence develops when the task appears insurmountable. In these situations, dividing a goal into smaller realistic objectives helps to accomplish the task. You may know how to swim, but swimming a continuous mile may take several weeks to accomplish. Set up your training program so that each day you swim a little farther until you are able to swim the entire mile. If on a given day you don't meet your objective, try it again, reevaluate, cut back a little, and, most important, don't give up.

3. Problems of motivation. In problems of motivation, both the competence and the confidence are there, but the individual is unwilling to change because the reasons for change are not important to him or her. For example, people begin contemplating a smoking cessation program only when the reasons for quitting outweigh the reasons for smoking.

   When it comes to quality of life, lack of knowledge and lack of goals are the primary causes of unwillingness to change. Knowledge often determines goals, and goals determine motivation. How badly you want it dictates how hard you'll work at it. Many people are unaware of the magnitude of the benefits of a wellness program. Unfortunately, when it comes to a healthy lifestyle, there may not be a second chance. A stroke, a heart attack, or cancer can lead to irreparable or fatal consequences. Greater understanding of what leads to disease may be all that is needed to initiate change.

Action stage Stage of change in which people are actively changing a negative behavior or adopting a new, healthy behavior.

Maintenance stage Stage of change in which people maintain behavioral change for up to 5 years.

Termination/adoption stage Stage of change in which people have eliminated an undesirable behavior or maintained a positive behavior for over 5 years.

Relapse To slip or fall back into unhealthy behavior(s) or fail to maintain healthy behaviors.

Motivation The desire and will to do something.

Also, feeling physically fit is difficult to explain unless you have experienced it yourself. Feelings of fitness, self-esteem, confidence, health, and quality of life cannot be conveyed to someone who is accustomed to sedentary living. In a way, wellness is like reaching the top of a mountain. The quietness, the clean air, the lush vegetation, the flowing water in the river, the wildlife, and the majestic valley below are difficult to explain to someone who has spent a lifetime within city limits.

| Behavior Modification |

Over the course of many years, we all develop habits that at some point in time we would like to change. Old habits die hard. Behavior modification requires continual effort. The sooner we implement a healthy lifestyle program, the greater the health benefits and quality of life that lie ahead. The following principles can be adopted to help change behavior:

1. Self-analysis. The first step in behavior modification is a decisive desire to do so. If you have no interest in changing a behavior, you won't do it. A person who has no intention of quitting smoking will not quit, regardless of what anyone may say or how strong the evidence is against it. In your self-analysis, you may want to prepare a list of reasons for continuing or discontinuing a certain behavior. When the reasons for change outweigh the reasons for not changing, you are ready for the next step.

2. Behavior analysis. Determine the frequency, circumstances, and consequences of the behavior to be altered or implemented. If the desired outcome is to decrease your consumption of fat, you first must find out what foods in your diet are high in fat, when you eat them, and when you don't eat them. Knowing when you don't eat them points to circumstances under which you exert control of your diet and will help as you set goals.

3. Goal setting. Goals motivate change in behavior. The stronger the goal (desire), the more motivated you'll be to either change unwanted behaviors or implement new healthy behaviors. The discussion on goal setting that follows will help you write goals and prepare an action plan to achieve those goals. The process will aid with behavior modification.

4. Social support. Surround yourself with people who either will work toward a common goal with you or will encourage you along the way. When attempting to quit smoking, try to do so with others who are trying to quit. You also may get help from friends who already have done so. Peer support is a strong incentive for behavioral change.

During this process, it's equally important to avoid people who will not support you. Friends who have no desire to quit smoking actually may tempt you to smoke and encourage relapse to unwanted behaviors. People who are beyond the goal you are trying to reach may not be supportive either. For instance, someone may say: "I can do 6 consecutive miles." Your response should be: "I'm proud that I can jog 3 consecutive miles."

5. Monitoring. Continuous behavior monitoring increases awareness of the desired outcome. Sometimes this principle by itself is sufficient to cause change. For example, keeping track of daily food intake reveals sources of fat in the diet. It can help you cut down gradually or completely eliminate high-fat foods before consuming them. If the goal is to increase daily fruit and vegetable intake, keeping track of the number of servings you eat each day will raise awareness and may help increase their intake.

6. Positive outlook. You should take a positive approach from the beginning and believe in yourself. Following the guidelines set out in this chapter will help you pace yourself so you can work toward change. Also look at the outcomes—how much healthier you will be, how much better you will look, or how far you will be able to jog, for instance.

7. Reinforcement. People tend to repeat behaviors that are rewarded and disregard those that are not rewarded or are punished. If you have been successful in cutting down your fat intake during the week, reward yourself by going to a show or buying a new pair of shoes. Do not reinforce yourself with destructive behaviors such as eating a high-fat dinner. If you fail to change a desired behavior (or to implement a new one), you may want to put off buying those new shoes. When a positive behavior becomes habitual, give yourself an even better reward. Treat yourself to a vacation weekend, buy a new bike, or get new clothing.

| Goal Setting |

Goals are critical to initiate change. Goals motivate behavioral change and provide a plan of action. Goals are most effective when they are

- Well planned. Only a well-conceived action plan will help you attain your goal. The items listed below will help you design your plan of action. Note that you set both general and specific objectives. The general objective is the ultimate goal you intend to achieve. The specific objectives are the steps required to reach this general objective. For example, a general objective might be to achieve recommended body weight. Several specific objectives could be to (a) lose an average of 1 pound (or 1 fat percentage point) per week (b) monitor body weight before breakfast every morning (c) assess body composition every 2 weeks (d) limit fat intake to less than 25 percent of total calories (e) eliminate all pastries from the diet during this time, and (f) exercise in the proper target zone for 45 minutes, five times per week.

- Personalized. Goals that you set for yourself are more motivational than goals someone else sets for you.
- Written. An unwritten goal is simply a wish. A written goal, in essence, becomes a contract with yourself. Show this goal to a friend or an instructor and have him or her witness, by way of a signature, the contract you made with yourself.
- Realistic. Goals should be within reach. If you have not exercised regularly, it would be unrealistic to start a daily exercise program consisting of 45 minutes of step aerobics at a vigorous intensity level. Unattainable goals lead to discouragement and loss of interest. Setting smaller, attainable goals is better.

   At times, even with realistic goals, problems arise. Try to anticipate potential difficulties as much as possible and plan for ways to deal with them. If your goal is to jog 30 minutes on 6 consecutive days, what are your alternatives if the weather turns bad? Possible solutions are to jog in the rain, find an indoor track, jog at a different time of day when the weather improves, or participate in a different aerobic activity, such as stationary cycling, swimming, or step aerobics.

- Measurable. Write your goals so they are clear, and state specifically the objective to accomplish. "I will lose weight" is not clear enough and is not measurable. A better example is "I will decrease my body fat to 17 percent."
- Time-specific. A goal always should have a specific date set for completion. This date should be realistic but not too distant in the future.
- Monitored. Monitoring your progress as you move toward a goal reinforces behavior. Keeping a physical activity log or doing a body composition assessment periodically determines where you are at any given time.
- Evaluated. Periodic reevaluations are vital for success. You may find that a given goal is unreachable. If so, reassess the goal. On the other hand, if a goal is too easy, you will lose interest and may stop working toward it. Once you achieve a goal, set a new one to improve or maintain what you have achieved. Goals keep you motivated.

BEHAVIORAL GUIDELINES TO ENHANCE EXERCISE ADHERENCE

Different things motivate different people to join and remain in a fitness program. Regardless of the initial reason for beginning a physical activity or an exercise program, you now need to plan for ways to make your workout fun. The psychology behind it is simple. If you enjoy an activity, you will continue to do it. If you don't, you will quit. Some of the following suggestions may help:

1. Start your exercise program slowly. Adhering to new behaviors takes time. Don't be discouraged if you can exercise only a few minutes or if you miss one or more exercise sessions. The key to success is perseverance.
2. Select aerobic activities you enjoy doing. Picking an activity you don't enjoy makes you less likely to keep exercising. Don't be afraid to try out a new activity, even if that means learning new skills.
3. Combine different activities. You can train by doing two or three different activities the same week. Some people find that this counteracts the monotony of repeating the same activity every day. Try **lifetime sports**. Many endurance sports such as racquetball, basketball, soccer, badminton, in-line skating, cross-country skiing, and surfing (paddling the board) provide a nice break from regular workouts.
4. Set aside a regular time for exercise. If you don't plan ahead, exercise is a lot easier to skip. Holding your exercise hour "sacred" helps you adhere to the program.
5. Obtain the proper equipment for exercise. A poor pair of shoes, for example, can increase the risk for injury, discouraging you right from the beginning.
6. Find a friend or a group of friends to exercise with. Social interaction makes exercise more fulfilling. Besides, exercise is harder to skip if someone else is waiting for you.
7. Set goals and share them with others. Quitting is tougher when someone else knows what you are trying to accomplish. When you reach a specific goal, reward yourself with a new pair of shoes or a jogging suit.
8. Don't become a chronic exerciser. Learn to listen to your body. Overexercising can lead to chronic fatigue and injuries. Exercise should be enjoyable, and in the process you will need to "stop and smell the roses."
9. Exercise in different places and facilities. This practice adds variety to your workouts.

Lifetime sports Sports that a person can do throughout the lifespan.

10. Exercise to music. People who listen to fast-tempo music tend to exercise more vigorously and longer. Using headphones when exercising outdoors, however, can be dangerous. Even indoors, it is preferable not to use headphones, so that you can still be aware of your surroundings.

11. Keep a regular record of your activities so you can monitor your progress and compare it with previous months and years.

12. Conduct periodic assessments. Improving to a higher fitness category is a reward in itself.

13. If health problems arise, see a physician. When in doubt, "better safe than sorry."

14. Exercise for a lifetime. To stay fit, you need to maintain a regular exercise program, even during vacations. If you have to interrupt your program for reasons beyond your control, do not attempt to resume your training at the same level you left off. Rather, build up gradually again.

The real challenge will come now: a lifetime commitment to physical activity and exercise. To make the commitment easier, enjoy yourself and have fun along the way. If you base your program on your interests and what you enjoy doing most, then adhering to your new active lifestyle will not be difficult.

Your activities over the next few weeks or months should help you develop positive behaviors that will carry on throughout life. If you truly commit to an active lifestyle and experience the feeling of being physically fit, there will be no looking back. If you don't get there, you won't know what it's like. Fitness and wellness is a process, and you need to put forth a constant and deliberate effort to achieve and maintain a higher quality of life. Improving the quality of your life, and most likely your longevity, is in your hands. Only you can take control of your lifestyle and thereby reap the benefits of wellness.

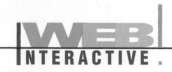

INTERACTIVE.

WEB ACTIVITIES

■ **Warm-up and Stretching Exercises to Enhance Your Performance** Learn several techniques for proper warm-ups and stretches to help you reduce your risk of injury and enhance your performance. This site lists specific types of warm-ups for basketball, baseball, running, walking, racquet sports, and golf.
http://www.vitality.com/vfm/performance.html

■ **Exercise Library** This site, from Fitness Link, features an anatomical diagram of muscles of the body. Click on one of several muscles to view exercises designed to improve the strength and tone of that muscle.
http://fitnesslink.com/mind/all-mind.shtml

■ **Training for Sport** This site, sponsored by Adidas, features the five beliefs of training for sport and a personalized training plan based on your current level of athletic ability, your sport, and your needs.
http://www.trainingforsport.com/path_home.htm

■ **The Virtual Gym** Get the most out of exercise equipment found at the gym with less risk of injury.

You can select specific muscles of the body and learn what piece of gym equipment is best to improve strength and endurance of that muscle.
http://www.fitnesslink.com/virtualgym

InfoTrac
You can find additional readings related to wellness via InfoTrac College Edition, an on-line library of more than 900 journals and publications. Follow the instructions for accessing InfoTrac that came packaged with your textbook, then search for articles using a key word search.

Suggested Reading Cedric X. Bryant and James A. Peterson, "Prescribing Exercise for Healthy Adults: An Individualized Approach" *JOPERD—The Journal of Physical Education, Recreation & Dance* 70, no. 6 (Aug, 1999): 29.

1. What are the four factors that characterize a sound exercise program?

2. Why is it important to perform both warm-up exercises prior to and cool-down exercises after a fitness routine?

3. What are the five guidelines recommended by the American College of Sports Medicine (ACSM) regarding the quantity and quality of exercise for developing and maintaining cardiorespiratory fitness and desirable body composition in a healthy adult?

4. List several types of exercises for each group of cardiorespiratory endurance activities.

Web Activity

Phys.com calculators

http://www.phys.com/c_tools/calculators3/01home/calculators.htm

Sponsor CondéNet, a division of Advance Internet Inc., is the site for the popular *Self* magazine. Consultants for this site include physicians, registered dietitians, exercise specialists, and others.

Description This site features a total of ten personal assessments in a fun interactive site. There are also quizzes, exercise slide slows with color photographs and diagrams, a search engine, and an "Ask the Professionals" section.

Available Activities Investigate the many activities at this site, including

1. Personal assessments for your body, including body fat, ideal weight, health risk, fitness, and nutrition (caloric needs, fat needs, protein needs)
2. The Ideal Sport Finder
3. Workouts
4. Motivation Quiz
5. Personal Nutritionist
6. Sports Injury Center

Web Work

1. From the home page, click on each of the links under "Your body."

2. Complete each of the following personal assessments:
   - body mass
   - body fat percentage
   - ideal weight
   - health risk
3. Next, click on the links under the "Nutrition" section and complete each of these personal assessments:
   - Caloric needs
   - Fat needs
   - Protein needs
   - Carbohydrate needs
4. Using these directions, complete the other personal assessments.

Helpful Hints

1. Completion of each of the above interactive links will provide you with a valuable self-assessment on your physical dimension of wellness.

For additional Web activities, links, and suggested readings, visit our Health, Fitness, and Wellness Resource Center at http://health.wadsworth.com.

NOTES

1. W. M. Bortz II, "Disuse and Aging," *Journal of the American Medical Association* 248 (1982): 1203–1208.

2. U. S. Department of Health and Human Services, *Physical Activity and Health: A Report of the Surgeon General* (Atlanta, GA: U.S. Department of Health and Human Services, Centers for Disease Control and Prevention, National Center for Chronic Disease Prevention and Health Promotion, 1996).

3. American College of Sports Medicine, *Guidelines for Exercise Testing and Prescription* (Baltimore: Williams & Wilkins, 2000).

4. See note 3.

5. G. Borg, "Perceived Exertion: A Note on History and Methods," *Medicine and Science in Sports and Exercise* 5 (1983): 90–93.

6. R. F. DeBusk, U. Stenestrand, M. Sheehan, and W. L. Haskell "Training Effects of Long Versus Short Bouts of Exercise in Healthy Subjects," *The American Journal of Cardiology* 65 (1990): 1010–1013.

7. American College of Sports Medicine, "Position Stand: The Recommended Quantity and Quality of Exercise for Developing and Maintaining Cardiorespiratory and Muscular Fitness, and Flexibility in Healthy Adults," *Medicine and Science in Sports and Exercise* 30 (1998): 975–991.

8. See note 2.

9. American College of Sports Medicine, "Position Stand: Exercise and Type 2 Diabetes," *Medicine and Science in Sports and Exercise* 32 (2000): 1345–1360.

10. See note 7.

11. W. Campbell, M. Crim, V. Young, and W. J. Evans, "Increased Energy Requirements and Changes in Body Composition with Resistance Training in Older Adults," *Journal of Clinical Nutrition* 60 (1994): 167–175.

12. W. W. Campbell, M. C. Crim, V. R. Young, and W. J. Evans, "Increased Energy Requirements and Changes in Body Composition with Resistance Training in Older Adults," *American Journal of Clinical Nutrition* 60 (1994): 167–175.

13. W. S. Evans, "Exercise, Nutrition and Aging," *Journal of Nutrition* 122 (1992): 796–801.

14. W. W. K. Hoeger, D. R. Hopkins, S. L. Barette, and D. F. Hale, "Relationship Between Repetitions and Selected Percentages of One Repetition Maximum: A Comparison Between Untrained and Trained Males and Females," *Journal of Applied Sport Science Research* 4, no. 2 (1990): 47–51.

15. See note 3.

16. S.A. Plowman, "Physical Fitness and Healthy Low Back Function," *President's Council on Physical Fitness and Sports: Physical Activity and Fitness Research Digest*, Series 1, no. 3 (1993): 3.

17. University of California at Berkeley, *The Wellness Guide to Lifelong Fitness* (New York: Random House, 1993): 198.

18. "Stretch Yourself Younger," *Consumer Reports on Health*, 11 (August 1999): 6–7.

19. J. Kokkonen and S. Lauritzen, "Isotonic Strength and Endurance Gains Through PNF Stretching," *Medicine and Science in Sports and Exercise* 27 (1995): S22:127.

20. R. Deyo, "Chiropractic Care for Back Pain: The Physician's Perspective," *HealthNews* 4 (September 10, 1998).

21. A. Brownstein, "Chronic Back Pain Can Be Beaten," *Bottom Line/Personal Health* 13 (October 1999): 3–4.

22. J. O. Prochaska, J. C. Norcross, and C. C. DiClemente, *Changing for Good* (New York: William Morrow and Co., 1994).

23. G. S. Howard, D. W. Nance, and P. Myers, *Adaptive Counseling and Therapy* (San Francisco: Jossey-Bass, 1987).

EXERCISE 1 — STEP-UP

ACTION

Step up and down using a box or chair approximately 12 to 15 inches high (a). Conduct one set using the same leg each time you go up, and then conduct a second set using the other leg. You also could alternate legs on each step-up cycle. You may increase the resistance by holding an object in your arms (b). Hold the object close to the body to avoid increased strain in the lower back.

MUSCLES DEVELOPED

Gluteal muscles, quadriceps, gastrocnemius, and soleus

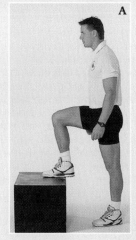
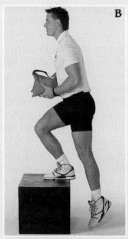

EXERCISE 2 — ROWING TORSO

ACTION

Raise your arms laterally (abduction) to a horizontal position and bend your elbows to 90°. Have a partner apply enough pressure on your elbows to gradually force your arms forward (horizontal flexion) while you try to resist the pressure. Next, reverse the action, horizontally forcing the arms backward as your partner applies sufficient forward pressure to create resistance.

MUSCLES DEVELOPED

Posterior deltoid, rhomboids, and trapezius

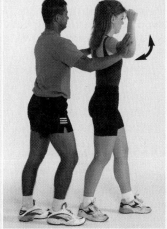

EXERCISE 3 — PUSH-UP

ACTION

Maintaining your body as straight as possible (a), flex the elbows, lowering the body until you almost touch the floor (b), then raise yourself back up to the starting position.
If you are unable to perform the push-up as indicated, decrease the resistance by supporting the lower body with the knees rather than the feet (c) or using an incline plane and supporting your hands at a higher point than the floor (d). If you wish to increase the resistance, have someone else add resistance to your shoulders as you are coming back up (e).

MUSCLES DEVELOPED

Triceps, deltoid, pectoralis major, abdominals, and erector spinae

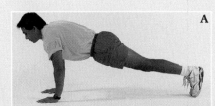
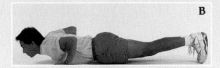
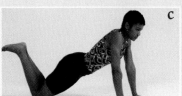
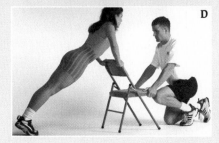
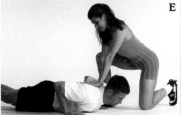

EXERCISE 4 ABDOMINAL CRUNCH AND BENT-LEG CURL-UP

ACTION

Start with your head and shoulders off the floor, arms crossed on your chest, and knees slightly bent (a). The greater the flexion of the knee, the more difficult the curl-up. Now curl up to about 30° (**abdominal crunch**—illustration b) or curl up all the way (**bent-leg curl-up**—illustration c), then return to the starting position without letting the head or shoulders touch the floor or allowing the hips to come off the floor. If you allow the hips to raise off the floor and the head and shoulders to touch the floor, you most likely will "swing up" on the next crunch or curl-up, which minimizes the work of the abdominal muscles. If you cannot curl up with the arms on the chest, place the hands by the side of the hips or even help yourself up by holding on to your thighs (illustrations d and e). Do not perform the curl-up exercise with your legs completely extended, because this will strain the lower back. For additional resistance during the abdominal crunch, have a partner add slight resistance to your shoulders as you "crunch up" (illustration f).

MUSCLES DEVELOPED

Abdominal muscles and hip flexors

NOTE:

The bent-leg curl-up exercise should be used only by individuals of at least average fitness without a history of lower back problems. New participants and those with a history of lower back problems should use the abdominal crunch exercise in its place.

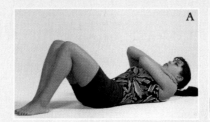
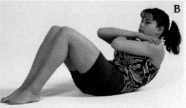
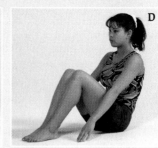
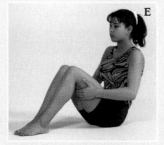
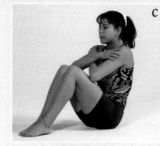
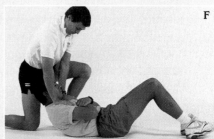

Photos © Fitness & Wellness, Inc.

EXERCISE 5 LEG CURL

ACTION

Lie on the floor face down. Cross the right ankle over the left heel (a). Apply resistance with your right foot while you bring the left foot up to 90° at the knee joint (b). Apply enough resistance so the left foot can only be brought up slowly. Repeat the exercise, crossing the left ankle over the right heel.

MUSCLES DEVELOPED

Hamstrings (and quadriceps)

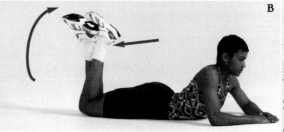
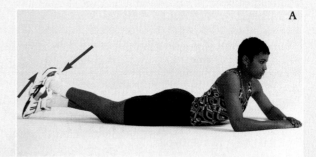

Photos © Fitness & Wellness, Inc.

EXERCISE 6   MODIFIED DIP

ACTION

Place your hands and feet on opposite chairs with knees slightly bent (make sure that the chairs are well stabilized). Dip down at least to a 90° angle at the elbow joint, then return to the initial position. To increase the resistance, have someone else hold you down by the shoulders on the way up (see illustration c). You may also perform this exercise using a gymnasium bleacher or box and with the help of a partner, as illustrated in photo d.

MUSCLES DEVELOPED

Triceps, deltoid, and pectoralis major

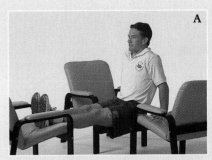

A

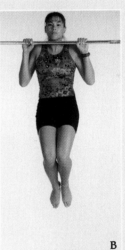

B

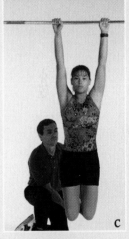

C

EXERCISE 7   PULL-UP

ACTION

Suspend yourself from a bar with a pronated (thumbs-in) grip (a). Pull your body up until your chin is above the bar (b), then lower the body slowly to the starting position. If you are unable to perform the pull-up as described, either have a partner hold your feet to push off and facilitate the movement upward (illustrations c and d) or use a lower bar and support your feet on the floor (e).

MUSCLES DEVELOPED

Biceps, brachioradialis, brachialis, trapezius, and latissimus dorsi

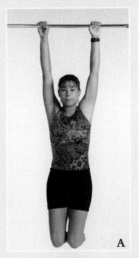

A

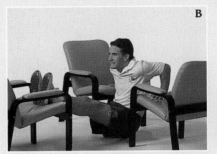

B

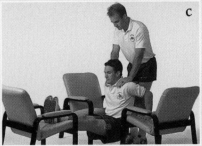

C

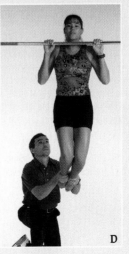

D

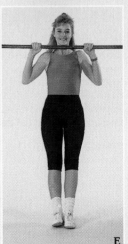

E

EXERCISE 8 ARM CURL

ACTION
Using a palms-up grip, start with the arm completely extended and, with the aid of a sandbag or bucket filled (as needed) with sand or rocks (a), curl up as far as possible (b), then return to the initial position (b). Repeat the exercise with the other arm.

MUSCLES DEVELOPED
Biceps, brachioradialis, and brachialis

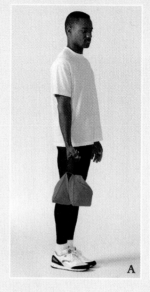
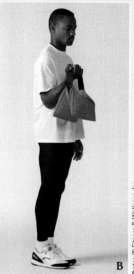

EXERCISE 9 HEEL RAISE

ACTION
From a standing position with feet flat on the floor (a), raise and lower your body weight by moving at the ankle joint only (b). For added resistance, have someone else hold your shoulders down as you perform the exercise.

MUSCLES DEVELOPED
Gastrocnemius and soleus

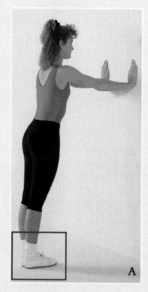
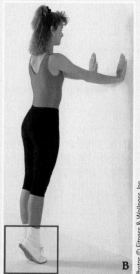

EXERCISE 10 LEG ABDUCTION AND ADDUCTION

ACTION
Both participants sit on the floor. The person on the left places the feet on the inside of the other person's feet. Simultaneously, the person on the left presses the legs laterally (to the outside—abduction), while the person on the right presses the legs medially (adduction). Hold the contraction for 5 to 10 seconds. Repeat the exercise at all three angles, and then reverse the pressing sequence. The person on the left places the feet on the outside and presses inward, while the person on the right presses outward.

MUSCLES DEVELOPED
Hip abductors (rectus femoris, sartori, gluteus medius and minimus) and adductors (pectineus, gracilis, adductor magnus, adductor longus, and adductor brevis)

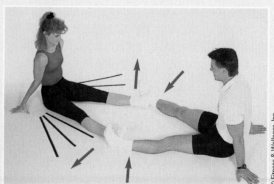

EXERCISE **11** PELVIC TILT

ACTION
Lie flat on the floor with the knees bent at about a 90°
angle (a). Tilt the pelvis by tightening the abdominal
muscles, flattening your back against the floor, and
raising the lower gluteal area ever so slightly off the
floor (b). Hold the final position for several seconds.
The exercise can also be performed against a wall (c).

AREAS STRETCHED
Low back muscles and ligaments

AREAS STRENGTHENED
Abdominal and gluteal muscles

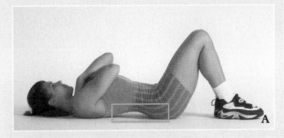
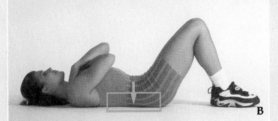
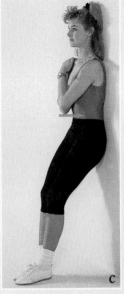

Photos © Fitness & Wellness, Inc.

|EXERCISES| STRENGTH-TRAINING WITH WEIGHTS

EXERCISE **12** ARM CURL

ACTION
Using a supinated or palms-up grip, start with the arms
almost completely extended (a). Curl up as far as
possible (b), then return to the starting position.

MUSCLES DEVELOPED
Biceps, brachioradialis, and brachialis

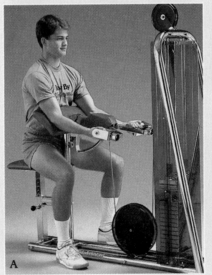
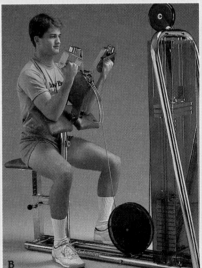

Photos © Universal Gym Equipment, Inc.

EXERCISE **13** BENCH PRESS

ACTION
Lie down on the bench with the head by the weight stack, the bench press bar above the
chest, and the knees bent so the feet rest on the far end of the bench (a). Grasp the bar
handles and press upward until the arms are completely extended (b), then return to the
original position. Do not arch the back during this exercise.

MUSCLES DEVELOPED
Pectoralis major, triceps, and deltoid

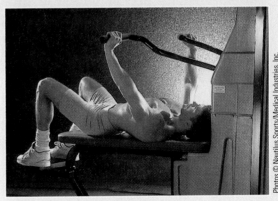

Photos © Nautilus Sports/Medical Industries, Inc.

EXERCISE 14   ABDOMINAL CRUNCH AND BENT-LEG CURL-UP

See Exercise 4 in this chapter.

EXERCISE 15   LEG EXTENSION

ACTION
Sit in an upright position with the feet under the padded bar and grasp the handles at the sides (a). Extend the legs until they are completely straight (b), then return to the starting position.

MUSCLES DEVELOPED
Quadriceps

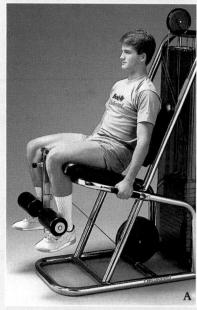
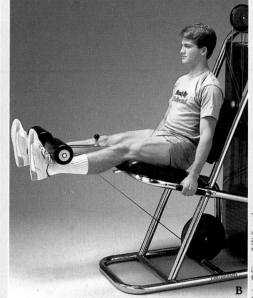

A

B

Photos © Fitness & Wellness, Inc.

EXERCISE 16   LEG CURL

ACTION
Lie with the face down on the bench, legs straight, and place the back of the feet under the padded bar (a). Curl up to at least 90° (b), and return to the original position.

MUSCLES DEVELOPED
Hamstrings

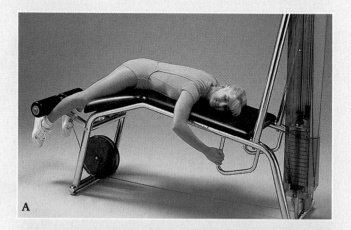

A

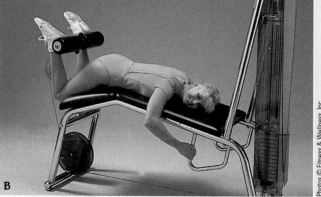

B

Photos © Fitness & Wellness, Inc.

EXERCISE 17 LAT PULL-DOWN

ACTION
Starting from a sitting position, hold the exercise bar with a wide grip (a). Pull the bar down until it touches the base of the neck (b), then return to the starting position. (If heavy resistance is used, stabilization of the body may be required either by using equipment as shown or by having someone else hold you down by the waist or shoulders.

MUSCLES DEVELOPED
Latissimus dorsi, pectoralis major, and biceps

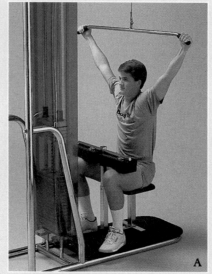
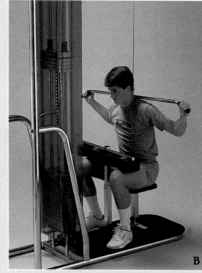

A B

EXERCISE 18 HEEL RAISE

ACTION
Start with your feet either flat on the floor or the front of the feet on an elevated block (a), then raise and lower yourself by moving at the ankle joint only (b). If additional resistance is needed, you can use a squat strength-training machine.

MUSCLES DEVELOPED
Quadriceps

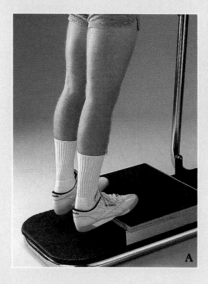
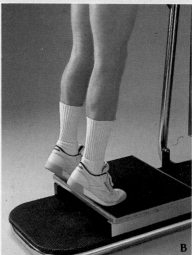

A B

EXERCISE 19 ROWING TORSO

ACTION
Sit in the machine with your arms in front of you, elbows bent and resting against the padded bars (a). Press back as far as possible, drawing the shoulder blades together (b). Return to the original position.

MUSCLES DEVELOPED
Posterior deltoid, rhomboids, and trapezius

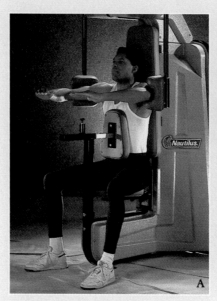
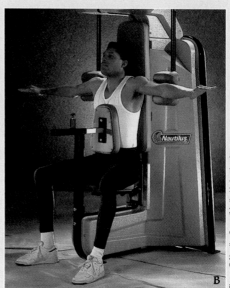

A B

EXERCISE 20 BENT-ARM PULLOVER

ACTION
Sit back into the chair and grasp the bar behind your head (a). Pull the bar over your head all the way down to your abdomen (b), and slowly return to the original position.

MUSCLES DEVELOPED
Latissimus dorsi, pectoral muscles, deltoid, and serratus anterior

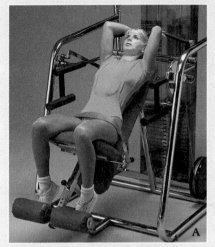
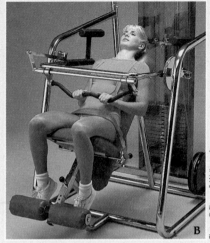

A

B

Photos © Fitness & Wellness, Inc.

|EXERCISES| FLEXIBILITY

EXERCISE 21 LATERAL HEAD TILT

ACTION
Slowly and gently tilt the head laterally. Repeat several times to each side.

AREAS STRETCHED
Neck flexors and extensors and ligaments of the cervical spine

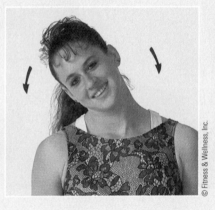

© Fitness & Wellness, Inc.

EXERCISE 22 ARM CIRCLES

ACTION
Gently circle your arms all the way around. Conduct the exercise in both directions.

AREAS STRETCHED
Shoulder muscles and ligaments

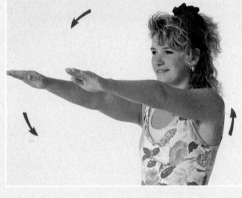

© Fitness & Wellness, Inc.

EXERCISE 23 SIDE STRETCH

ACTION
Stand straight up, feet separated to shoulder width, and place your hands on your waist. Now move the upper body to one side and hold the final stretch for a few seconds. Repeat on the other side.

AREAS STRETCHED
Muscles and ligaments in the pelvic region

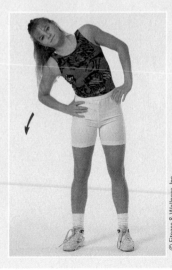

© Fitness & Wellness, Inc.

EXERCISE 24 BODY ROTATION

ACTION
Place your arms slightly away from your body, and rotate the trunk as far as possible, holding the final position for several seconds. Conduct the exercise for both the right and left sides of the body. You also can perform this exercise by standing about 2 feet away from the wall (back toward the wall) and then rotating the trunk, placing the hands against the wall.

AREAS STRETCHED
Hip, abdominal, chest, back, neck, and shoulder muscles; hip and spinal ligaments

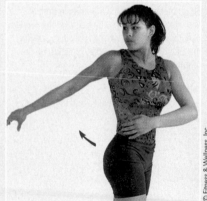

© Fitness & Wellness, Inc.

EXERCISE 25 CHEST STRETCH

ACTION
Place your hand on the shoulder of your partner who will in turn push you down by your shoulders. Hold the final position for a few seconds.

AREAS STRETCHED
Chest (pectoral) muscles and shoulder ligaments

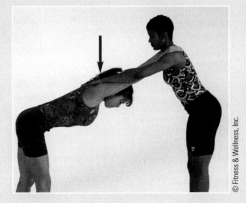

© Fitness & Wellness, Inc.

EXERCISE 26 SHOULDER HYPEREXTENSION STRETCH

ACTION
Have a partner grasp your arms from behind by the wrists and slowly push them upward. Hold the final position for a few seconds.

AREAS STRETCHED
Deltoid and pectoral muscles, and ligaments of the shoulder joint

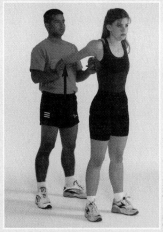

© Fitness & Wellness, Inc.

EXERCISE 27 SHOULDER ROTATION STRETCH

ACTION
With the aid of surgical tubing or an aluminum or wood stick, place the tubing or stick behind your back and grasp the two ends using a reverse (thumbs-out) grip. Slowly bring the tubing or stick over your head, keeping the elbows straight. Repeat several times (bring the hands closer together for additional stretch).

AREAS STRETCHED
Deltoid, latissimus dorsi, and pectoral muscles; shoulder ligaments

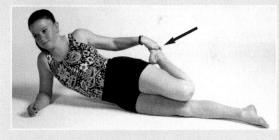

© Fitness & Wellness, Inc.

EXERCISE 28 QUAD STRETCH

ACTION
Lie on your side and move one foot back by flexing the knee. Grasp the front of the ankle and pull the ankle toward the gluteal region. Hold for several seconds. Repeat with the other leg.

AREAS STRETCHED
Quadriceps muscle, and knee and ankle ligaments

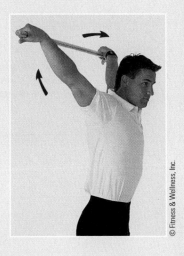

© Fitness & Wellness, Inc.

EXERCISE 29 HEEL CORD STRETCH

ACTION
Stand against the wall or at the edge of a step, and stretch the heel downward, alternating legs. Hold the stretched position for a few seconds.

AREAS STRETCHED
Heel cord (Achilles tendon), gastrocnemius and soleus muscles

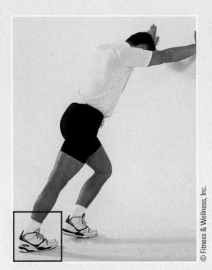

© Fitness & Wellness, Inc.

EXERCISE 30 ADDUCTOR STRETCH

ACTION
Stand with your feet about twice shoulder width and place your hands slightly above the knee. Flex one knee and slowly go down as far as possible, holding the final position for a few seconds. Repeat with the other leg.

AREAS STRETCHED
Hip adductor muscles

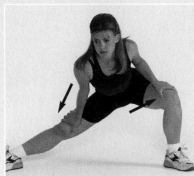

© Fitness & Wellness, Inc.

EXERCISE 31 SITTING ADDUCTOR STRETCH

ACTION
Sit on the floor and bring your feet in close to you, allowing the soles of the feet to touch each other. Now place your forearms (or elbows) on the inner part of the thigh and push the legs downward, holding the final stretch for several seconds.

AREAS STRETCHED
Hip adductor muscles

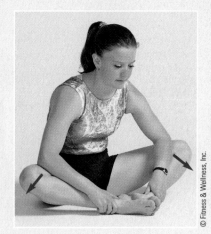

EXERCISE 32 SIT-AND-REACH STRETCH

ACTION
Sit on the floor with legs together and gradually reach forward as far as possible. Hold the final position for a few seconds. This exercise also may be performed with the legs separated, reaching to each side as well as to the middle.

AREAS STRETCHED
Hamstrings and lower back muscles, and lumbar spine ligaments

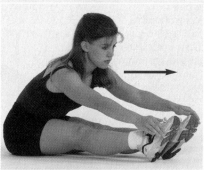

EXERCISE 33 TRICEPS STRETCH

ACTION
Place the right hand behind your neck. Grasp the right arm above the elbow with the left hand. Gently pull the elbow backward. Repeat the exercise with the opposite arm.

AREAS STRETCHED
Back of upper arm (triceps muscle) and shoulder joint

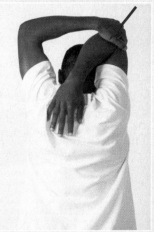

NOTE:
Exercises 34 through 41 are also flexibility exercises and can be added to your stretching program.

EXERCISES FOR THE PREVENTION AND REHABILITION OF LOW-BACK PAIN

EXERCISE 34 SINGLE-KNEE TO CHEST STRETCH

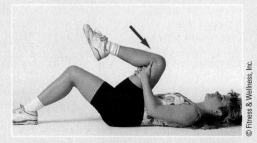

ACTION
Lie down flat on the floor. Bend one leg at approximately 100° and gradually pull the opposite leg toward your chest. Hold the final stretch for a few seconds. Switch legs and repeat the exercise.

AREAS STRETCHED
Lower back and hamstring muscles, and lumbar spine ligaments

EXERCISE 35 DOUBLE-KNEE TO CHEST STRETCH

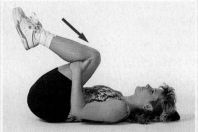

ACTION
Lie flat on the floor and then curl up slowly into a fetal position. Hold for a few seconds.

AREAS STRETCHED
Upper and lower back and hamstring muscles; spinal ligaments

EXERCISE 36 UPPER AND LOWER BACK STRETCH

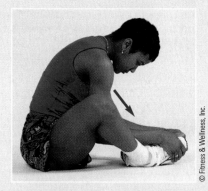

ACTION
Sit on the floor and bring your feet in close to you, allowing the soles of the feet to touch each other. Holding on to your feet, bring your head and upper chest gently toward your feet.

AREAS STRETCHED
Upper and lower back muscles and ligaments

EXERCISE 37 SIT-AND-REACH STRETCH

See Exercise 32 in this chapter.

EXERCISE 38 BACK EXTENSION STRETCH

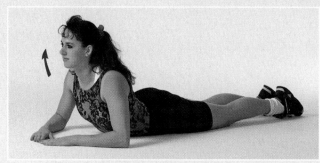

ACTION
Lie face down on the floor with the elbows by the chest, forearms on the floor, and the hands beneath the chin. Gently raise the trunk by extending the elbows until you reach an approximate 90° angle at the elbow joint. Be sure the forearms remain in contact with the floor at all times. DO NOT extend the back beyond this point. Hyperextension of the lower back may lead to or aggravate an existing back problem. Hold the stretched position for about 10 seconds.

AREAS STRETCHED
Abdominal region.

ADDITIONAL BENEFITS
Restore lower back curvature

EXERCISE 39 GLUTEAL STRETCH

ACTION

Sit on the floor, bend your right leg and place your right ankle slightly above the left knee. Grasp the left thigh with both hands and gently pull the leg toward your chest. Repeat the exercise with the opposite leg.

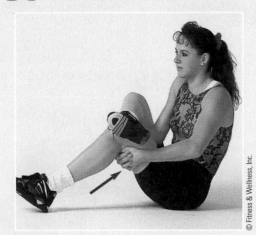

AREAS STRETCHED

Buttock area (gluteal muscles)

EXERCISE 40 TRUNK ROTATION AND LOWER BACK STRETCH

ACTION

Sit on the floor and bend the right leg, placing the right foot on the outside of the left knee. Place the left elbow on the right knee and push against it. At the same time, try to rotate the trunk to the right (clockwise). Hold the final position for a few seconds. Repeat the exercise with the other side.

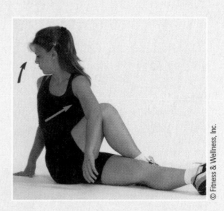

AREAS STRETCHED

Lateral side of the hip and thigh; trunk and lower back

EXERCISE 41 HIP FLEXORS STRETCH

ACTION

Kneel down on an exercise mat, a soft surface, or place a towel under your knees. Raise the left knee off the floor and place the left foot about three feet in front of you. Place your left hand over your left knee and the right hand over the back of the right hip. Keeping the lower back flat, slowly move forward and downward as you apply gentle pressure over the right hip. Repeat the exercise with the opposite leg forward

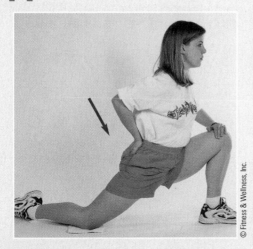

AREAS STRETCHED

Flexor muscles in front of the hip joint

EXERCISE 42 PELVIC TILT

See Exercise 11 in this chapter.

NOTE:

This is the most important exercise for use in prevention and treatment of low back pain. This exercise should be incorporated as a part of your daily physical activity and exercise program.

EXERCISE 43 ABDOMINAL CRUNCH AND ABDOMINAL CURL-UP

See Exercise 4 in this chapter.

It is important that you do not stabilize your feet when performing either of these exercises, because doing so decreases the work of the abdominal muscles. Also, remember not to "swing up" but rather to curl up as you perform these exercises.

CARDIORESPIRATORY EXERCISE PRESCRIPTION

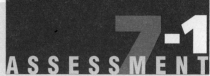

Name: _____   Date: _____   Grade: _____

Instructor: _____   Course: _____   Section: _____

Age: _____

Necessary Lab Equipment:
None required.

Objective:
To write your own cardiorespiratory endurance exercise prescription.

Intensity of exercise

1. Estimate your own maximal heart rate (MHR)

    MHR = 220 minus age (220 − age)

    MHR = 220 − _____ = _____ bpm

2. Training intensities (TI) = MHR × TI

    55% TI = _____ × .55 = _____ bpm

    65% TI = _____ × .65 = _____ bpm

    90% TI = _____ × .90 = _____ bpm

3. **Cardiorespiratory Training Zone.** The recommended cardiorespiratory training zone is found between the 55% and 90% training intensities. Individuals who have been physically inactive or are in the poor or fair cardiorespiratory fitness categories should use the 55% training intensity during the first few weeks of the exercise program.

    Recommended Cardiorespiratory Training Zone:

    Moderate Intensity = _____ bpm (55%TI) to _____ bpm (65% TI)

    High Intensity = _____ bpm (65%TI) to _____ bpm (90% TI)

    Rate of Perceived Exertion (see Figure 7.2, page 144):

    _____ to _____

Mode of Exercise

Select any activity or combination of activities that you enjoy doing. The activity has to be continuous in nature and must get your heart rate up to your recommended cardiorespiratory training zone and keep it there for as long as you exercise. Indicate your preferred mode(s) of exercise:

1. _____   2. _____   3. _____

4. _____   5. _____   6. _____

Duration and Frequency of Exercise

Please indicate how long each exercise session will last, the days of the week, and the time of day that you will exercise.

Duration: [ ] minutes

Select the days of the week and time of day that you will exercise.

☐ Monday   :   ☐ Tuesday   :   ☐ Wednesday   :   ☐ Thursday   :

☐ Friday   :   ☐ Saturday   :   ☐ Sunday   :

Exercise Site(s) and Friends

Indicate place(s) where you will exercise:

_____

_____

_____

List the friends that will exercise with you:

_____

_____

_____

Cardiorespiratory Exercise Training and Rate of Perceived Exertion

Perform an aerobic exercise workout and exercise at the perceived exertion intensities listed below. Following 5 minutes of exercise at those perceived exertion intensities, check your pulse and determine your exercise heart rate.

Physical activity performed: [ ]

Perceived Exertion	10-second pulse	Exercise Heart Rate (bpm)
Fairly light		
Somewhat hard		
Hard		

Indicate how your own perceived exertion during this activity relates to the RPE scale. Were your exercise heart rates as expected on the RPE scale? If not, what conclusion can you draw from your perceived exertion and your recommended exercise intensity computed in this assessment?

_____

_____

_____

_____

_____

_____

MUSCULAR STRENGTH/ENDURANCE PRESCRIPTION

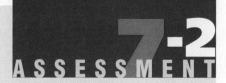

Name: _____ Date: _____ Grade: _____

Instructor: _____ Course: _____ Section: _____

Necessary Lab Equipment:

No equipment if the "Strength-Training Exercises Without Weights" program is selected. Strength-training machines or free weights if "Strength-Training Exercises With Weights" are used.

Objective:

Write a strength-training exercise program that may be carried out throughout life.

Lab Preparation:

Wear exercise clothing and prepare to participate in a sample strength-training exercise session. All of the strength-training exercises are illustrated in this chapter on pages 167–174.

Instructions:

Select one of the two strength-training exercise programs. Perform all of the recommended exercises and, with the exception of the bent-leg curl-up or abdominal crunch exercises, determine the resistance required to do approximately 10 repetitions maximum (for "Strength Training Exercises Without Weights," simply indicate the total number of repetitions performed). For the bent-leg curl-up and abdominal crunch exercises, perform or build up to about 20 repetitions.

I. Strength-Training Exercises Without Weights

Exercise	Repetitions	Sets
Step-up		
Rowing torso		
Push-up		
Abdominal crunch or Bent-leg curl-up (select one)		
Leg curl		
Modified dip		
Pull-up or Arm curl (select one)		
Heel raise		
Leg abduction and adduction		
Pelvic tilt		

II. Strength-Training Exercises With Weights*

Exercise	Repetitions	Resistance
Arm curl		
Bench press		
Abdominal crunch or Bent-leg curl-up (select one)		
Leg extension		
Leg curl		
Lab pull-down		
Heel raise		
Rowing torso		
Bent-arm pullover		

*Most of these exercises can also be performed with free weights.

III. Days of the week that you will strength train:

☐ M ☐ T ☐ W ☐ TH ☐ F ☐ S ☐ SU

IV. Muscular Strength Workout

Perform a strength-training workout according to the program you have developed. If you are not strength-training regularly, be sure to perform only one set of each exercise using light resistances only. Briefly explain your experience and indicate the exercise, resistances, repetitions, and number of sets performed. Also indicate how you felt during the workout, a few hours later, and the day thereafter.

_____

_____

_____

_____

_____

_____

_____

_____

_____

_____

_____

_____

MUSCULAR FLEXIBILITY PRESCRIPTION

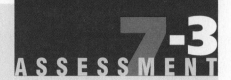

Name: _____   Date: _____   Grade: _____

Instructor: _____   Course: _____   Section: _____

Necessary Lab Equipment:
Minor implements such as a chair, a table, an elastic band (surgical tubing or a wood or aluminum stick), and a stool or steps.

Objective:
To introduce the participant to a sample stretching exercise program that may be carried out throughout life.

Instructions:
Wear exercise clothing and prepare to participate in a sample stretching exercise session. All of the flexibility exercises are illustrated in this chapter on pages 174–178).

Introduction

Perform all of the recommended flexibility exercises given in Chapter 7. Use a combination of slow-sustained and proprioceptive neuromuscular facilitation stretching techniques. Indicate the technique(s) used for each exercise, and, where applicable, the number of repetitions performed and the length of time that the final degree of stretch was held.

I.   Stretching Exercises

Exercise	Stretching Technique[1]	Repetitions	Length of Final Stretch
Lateral head tilt			NA[2]
Arm circles			NA
Side stretch			NA
Body rotation			
Chest stretch			
Shoulder hyperextension			
Shoulder rotation			NA
Quad stretch			
Heel cord stretch			
Adductor stretch			
Sitting adductor stretch			
Sit-and-reach stretch			
Triceps stretch			
Single-knee to chest stretch			

[1]SSS = Slow-sustained stretching, PNF = Proprioceptive neuromuscular facilitation
[2]Not Applicable

Double-knee to chest stretch

Upper and lower back stretch

Back extension

Gluteal stretch

Trunk rotation and lower back stretch

Hip flexors stretch

II. Days of the week that you will strength train:

M   T   W   TH   F   S   SU

IIII. Stretching Program

Using the flexibility program that you have designed, perform a stretching exercise session. Briefly explain your experience with this program and your feelings about your present flexibility level and potential implications for your future fitness and health.

8 NUTRITION AND WELLNESS

- Identify the trends and eating habits of the average American.

- Discuss reasons for food choices.

- List the six basic elements of nutrition and define their functions and sources.

- Identify the types of fat and the roles of fat in the body.

- Describe cholesterol and its functions.

- Differentiate the types of carbohydrates and the role of fiber.

- Identify the types of vitamins and their sources and functions.

- Identify the minerals the body needs, their sources, and their functions.

- List some ways to prevent food-borne diseases.

- Describe the DRI.

- Define and describe the Food Guide Pyramid and Daily Values.

- Demonstrate how to read food labels on packaged products.

- Develop personalized guidelines for a nutritional wellness plan.

185

SIX DECADES AGO, the typical American family was a classic Norman Rockwell vision: Dad in his shirt and tie sat at the head of the table while Mom, complete with ruffled apron, hurried to bring dinner to her smiling family. It was the age of two-parent, one-career families who sat down to a home-cooked meal three times a day.

As a nation, our lifestyles, and therefore, our eating habits have changed dramatically. Our lives have become more fast-paced with both parents in the work force. Dinner is more likely to be a frozen entree popped into the microwave or a hamburger and fries grabbed on the run from a fast-food drive-through. Today, fewer people sit down to breakfast or lunch at home, and as many as a fourth of all Americans eat dinner at a fast-food restaurant.

You choose to eat a meal about 1,000 times a year. Eating is so habitual that people hardly give it any thought, yet you choose when to eat, what to eat, and how much to eat about 70,000 times in a lifetime. A single day's intake of nutrients may affect body organs and their functions only slightly, but over years and decades, the effects of those intakes are cumulative. Sound **nutrition** contributes to a long and healthy life.

excessive food to the extent that a person develops obesity. Excessive intakes of vitamins and minerals are another form of overnutrition.

Some people consume too few vegetables and fruits and too much meat; other people consume inadequate servings of dairy products. Table 8.1 summarizes some USDA guidelines to promote health and prevent disease.

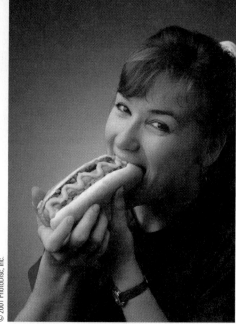

© 2001 PhotoDisc, Inc.

Fast foods should be limited in your diet.

BENEFITS OF NUTRITION

Your body renews its structures continuously: Each day it replaces some old muscle, bone, skin, and blood with new tissues. In this way some of the food you eat today becomes part of your body tomorrow. The best food for you, then, is the kind that supports today's growth and maintenance of strong muscles, sound bones, healthy skin, and produces sufficient blood to cleanse and nourish all parts of your body.

Your food choices combine with other life choices to create a pattern that raises or lowers your chances of developing diseases later. Good nutrition both promotes health and helps prevent disease.

To manage your nutrition in your own best interest, you have to learn what foods to eat, for not all are equally nutritious. You will want to avoid undernutrition, which is reducing intake of food **energy** or **nutrients** severely enough to cause disease or to make you more susceptible to disease.[1] Examples of undernutrition include iron deficiency anemia and starvation.

At the same time, overnutrition threatens people's health. Overnutrition is overconsuming food energy or nutrients sufficiently to cause disease or susceptibility to disease. Examples of overnutrition include consuming

EATING HEALTHY AT FAST-FOOD RESTAURANTS

If much of your fare comes from fast-food restaurants or cafeterias, that's okay, as long as you make food choices like these:

- Look for chains that offer healthy alternatives such as whole-grain buns, salads, or baked potatoes.
- For breakfast, choose English muffins or pancakes. Limit hash browns, bacon, sausage, croissants, butter, and Danish rolls.
- If you can, choose a salad bar; select fat-free or low-fat dressing.
- Skip the soda; drink juice, low-fat milk, or water instead.
- Baked potatoes: A good option, but get a vegetable topping (such as broccoli) if you can instead of butter or sour cream.
- Hamburgers: Get a single, plain burger; for condiments, choose mustard or catsup. Avoid or limit bacon and mayonnaise.
- Chicken: Order skinless, or take the skin off yourself. Avoid "extra crispy," because the crispness comes from added fat. Avoid chicken nuggets; they usually contain ground-up chicken skin, which is high in fat.
- Mexican: Choose chicken tacos or burritos instead of beef; order soft flour tortillas instead of fried corn tortillas; choose dishes with lots of beans and vegetables and little sour cream.
- Pizza: Choose vegetable toppings. Limit sausage, pepperoni, and hamburger.

TABLE 8.1 DIETARY GUIDELINES FOR AMERICANS/NUTRITION AND YOUR HEALTH

1. *Eat a variety of foods daily.* Include these foods everyday: fruits and vegetables; whole grain and enriched breads, cereals, and other products made from grains; milk and milk products; meats, fish poultry, and eggs; and dried peas and beans.

2. *Maintain healthy weight.* To increase calorie expenditures, increase physical activity. To decrease calorie intake, control overeating by eating slowly, taking smaller portions, and avoiding second helpings; eat fewer fatty foods and sweets and less sugar, drink fewer alcoholic beverages, and eat more foods that are low in calories and high in nutrients.

3. *Choose a diet low in fat, saturated fat, and cholesterol.* Choose low-fat protein sources such as lean meats, fish, poultry, and dry peas and beans; use eggs and organ meats in moderation; limit intake of fats on and in food; trim fats from meats; broil, bake, or boil—don't fry; limit breaded and deep-fried foods; read food labels for fat contents.

4. *Choose a diet with plenty of vegetables, fruits, and grain products.* Substitute starchy foods for foods high in fats and sugars; select whole-grain breads and cereals, fruits and vegetables, and dried beans and peas, to increase fiber and starch intake.

5. *Use sugars only in moderation.* Use less sugar, syrup, and honey; reduce intakes of concentrated sweets like candy, soft drinks, cookies, and the like; select fresh fruit or fruits canned in light syrup or their own juices; read food labels—sucrose, glucose, dextrose, maltose, lactose, fructose, syrups, and honey are all sugars; eat sugar less often to reduce dental caries.

6. *Use salt and sodium only in moderation.* Learn to enjoy the flavors of unsalted foods; flavor foods with herbs, spices, and lemon juice; reduce salt in cooking; add little or no salt at the table; limit salty foods like potato chips, pretzels, salted nuts, popcorn, condiments (soy sauce, steak sauce, and garlic salt), some cheese, pickled foods and cured meats, and some canned vegetables and soups; read food labels for sodium or salt contents, especially in processed and snack foods; use lower-sodium products when available.

7. *If you drink alcoholic beverages, do so in moderation.* For individuals who drink, limit all alcoholic beverages (including wine, beer, liquors, and so on) to one (for women) or two (for men) drinks per day. "One drink" means 12 oz of beer, 3 oz of wine, or 1½ oz of distilled spirits.[a] People who should *not* drink alcohol include pregnant women,[b] those who must drive, those taking medication, those who have trouble limiting alcohol intakes,[c] and children and adolescents.

[a]For an expanded discussion of what constitutes "a drink," see Chapter 13.
[b]For a discussion of the risks of drinking during pregnancy, see Chapter 13.
[c]For discussions of driving and alcohol, as well as of alcohol addiction, see Chapter 13.

Source: U.S. Department of Agriculture, U.S. Department of Health and Human Services, *Nutrition and Your Health: Dietary Guidelines for Americans*, 3d ed. (Washington, D.C.: Government Printing Office, 1990).

FOOD CHOICES

Because your accumulated food choices profoundly influence your health, it is worth questioning why you eat when you do, why you choose the foods you do, and, most importantly, whether they supply the nutrients you need.

To the question of what prompts you to eat, you may reply that it is hunger. Hunger is the physiological need to eat, a negative, unpleasant sensation. However, the physiological need for food is not the only stimulus that triggers eating behavior. Another cue is appetite, the psychological desire to eat. This may arise in response to the sight, smell, or thought of food even when you do not need to eat. You may have an appetite when you are not hungry—or the reverse. That is, you may be hungry but have no appetite.

As for the question of why to choose the particular foods you do, several answers come to mind:

- Personal preference (you like them).
- Habit or ethnic tradition (they are familiar; you always eat them).
- Social pressure (they are offered; you feel you can't refuse).
- Availability (they are there and ready to eat).
- Convenience (you are too rushed to prepare anything else).
- Economy (you can afford them).
- Emotional needs (some foods can make you feel better for a while).
- Values or beliefs (they fit your religious tradition or honor the environment).
- Nutritional value (you think they are good for you).

All but one of these reasons are psychological and social reasons; only the last one suggests consciousness of nutrition's importance to your wellness. But this is not to say that your other reasons for choosing foods are invalid or will necessarily damage your

Nutrition The science of foods, of the nutrients and other substances they contain, and of their actions within the body.

Energy The capacity to do work or produce heat.

Nutrients Substances obtained from food and used in the body to promote growth, maintenance, and repair. The essential nutrients are those the body cannot make for itself in sufficient quantity to meet physiological need and which, therefore, must be obtained from food.

FIGURE **8.1** FOODS AND THEIR ENERGY-YIELDING NUTRIENTS IN THEM.

Foods contain carbohydrates, protein, fat, vitamins, minerals, and water. Portion sizes shown are useful for diet planning. The meat portion is moderate (3 ounces) and the vegetable portion, ample (1 cup)—consistent with recommended guidelines.

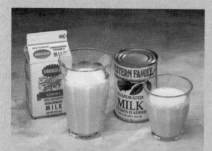

Milk = carbohydrate plus protein (plus vitamins, minerals, and water).

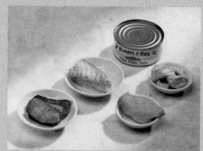

Meat = protein plus fat (plus vitamins, minerals, and water).

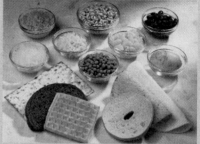

Bread (and starchy vegetables) = carbohydrate (plus protein, vitamins, and minerals).

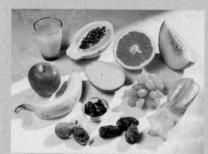

Fruit = carbohydrate (plus vitamins, minerals, and water).

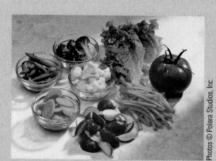

Vegetable (except starchy vegetables) = carbohydrate plus protein (plus vitamins, minerals, and water).

Photos © Polara Studios, Inc.

health. Food nourishes not only the body but also the mind and spirit. After you have learned about nutrition, you will be in a position to design a diet that meets your body's needs and honors your preferences, social values, and other individual needs.

THE SIX BASIC ELEMENTS OF NUTRITION

Foods supply nutrients, fiber, and other materials. Nutrients are substances obtained from food that promote growth, maintenance, or repair. All nutrients fall into six basic categories: proteins, fats, carbohydrates, vitamins, minerals, and water. They provide everything the body needs to continue healthy functioning, including

- growth and the formation of new tissue
- repair of damaged tissue
- production of energy

- conduction of nerve impulses
- reproduction

Three classes of nutrients provide energy the body can use: protein, fat and carbohydrate. The body uses energy from these nutrients to do its work and to generate heat. The units used to measure energy are **calories**, familiar to everyone as a reflection of how "fattening" a food is. Protein and carbohydrate each provide 4 kilocalories per gram and fat provides 9 kilocalories per gram. Figure 8.1 displays foods and the energy-yielding nutrients they contain.

One other compound people ingest provides energy: the alcohol of alcoholic beverages. Alcohol is not a nutrient, because it does not promote the body's growth, maintenance, or repair; but it is counted as an energy source because it provides 7 kilocalories per gram. Vitamins and minerals do not provide energy, but they do assist in energy-processing reactions and other metabolic functions. Water provides a medium for these reactions to occur.

| Protein |

Protein is an energy-yielding nutrient providing 4 calories per gram. Protein can be used as an energy source, but it is best utilized as the major structural and working material of cells; it provides the basic materials for cell growth and repair. Proteins are made of **amino acids**, each of which is composed of carbon, oxygen, hydrogen, and nitrogen. Protein helps build skin, blood, muscles, and bone; aids in the formation of hormones; regulates the body's chemical processes; forms enzymes; carries nutrients to all body cells; and is a major constituent of the immune system.

Most Americans rely heavily on animal sources of protein, including milk, milk products, eggs, meat, poultry, and fish. Good plant sources of protein are

- Legumes, such as dried beans, dried peas, dried lentils, peanuts, soybeans, and soy products.
- Grains, such as oats, rice, barley, cornmeal, and whole-grain breads and pastas.
- Nuts and seeds, such as walnuts, cashews, pecans, sunflower seeds, and sesame seeds.
- Vegetables, such as broccoli and dark leafy green vegetables.

Proteins, whether derived from plant or animal sources, are made up of about 20 amino acids. From these 20 building blocks, our bodies create various proteins to build and repair tissue, regulate the formation of hormones and enzymes, and maintain the body's chemical balance. Of the 20 amino acids, the body can manufacture 11. The other 9, called "**essential amino acids**," must be obtained from the foods we eat.

Complete proteins (such as chicken) contain all of the essential amino acids. **Incomplete proteins** (such as pinto beans and brown rice) may contain only some of the essential amino acids or may contain all of them but in insufficient amounts to allow humans to synthesize protein. However, an incomplete protein source can be combined with another food that supplies the missing essential amino acids. One good combination is peanut butter on whole-grain bread; another is black beans and rice.

Only about 15 percent of the total calories should come from protein. Most Americans eat more than twice the amount of protein they need. An American woman, for example, needs only about 46 to 48 grams of protein a day, the equivalent of a cup of low-fat yogurt, a cup of low-fat milk, and 4 ounces of chicken. Protein is essential for the body's growth and repair, but too much can be harmful. Contrary to popular belief, excess protein consumed beyond energy and physiological needs is not stored as muscle, but is stored as fat.

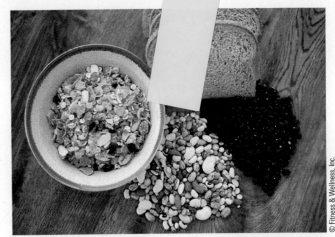

Legumes, grains, and nuts also provide protein.

Excessive protein causes the body to excrete calcium (needed for strengthening bones and teeth). If a person eats too much protein, the extra nitrogen is excreted in urine, which can strain the kidneys. Nutritionist and author Jane Brody said, "Americans excrete the most expensive urine in the world. If it were economical to collect and dry it, tons of nitrogen could be harvested from the nation's toilet bowls each day."[2]

People who are **vegetarians** avoid some or all foods of animal origin. People who eat animal products sparingly usually realize several health benefits, including reduced risk of heart disease, lower levels of cholesterol and other fats in the blood, lower blood pressure, and lower weight.

The wide array of available foods allows most vegetarians to get the proper balance of necessary nutrients. Strict vegetarians do need to make extra effort to get essential amino acids, certain necessary minerals (especially calcium, iron, and zinc), and certain vitamins (such as vitamin B_{12} and vitamin D), because the

Calories Units used to measure energy; determined from the heat food releases when burned. Calories reflect the extent to which a food's energy can be stored in body fat.

Protein Compounds composed of amino acids necessary for growth or tissue repair; protein also functions as enzymes, hormones, regulators of fluid and electrolyte balance, acid-base regulators, transporters, and antibodies.

Amino acids Building blocks of protein; "amino" means "containing nitrogen."

Essential amino acids Amino acids that cannot be produced by the body at all or are produced in the body in insufficient amounts to meet its needs; they must be provided by the diet.

Complete proteins A dietary protein containing all nine essential amino acids in the same relative amounts that human beings require.

Incomplete proteins Dietary proteins that do not contain all the essential amino acids in sufficient quantities for human protein synthesis.

Vegetarians People who omit meat, fish, and poultry from their diets. Lacto-ovo-vegetarians use milk and milk products and eggs as well as plant foods; strict vegetarians eat only plant foods.

FIGURE 8.2 VEGETARIAN PROTEIN CHOICES.

Choose from two or more of these columns to obtain balanced assortments of amino acids for the human body's use.

Grains	Legumes	Seeds and Nuts	Vegetables
Barley	Dried beans	Cashews	Broccoli
Bulgur	Dried lentils	Nut butters	Leafy greens
Cornmeal	Dried peas	Other nuts	Others
Oats	Peanuts	Sesame seeds	
Pasta	Soy products	Sunflower seeds	
Rice		Walnuts	
Whole-grain breads			

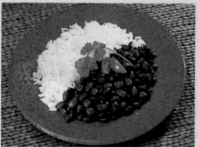
Beans and rice.

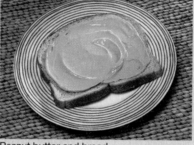
Peanut butter and bread.

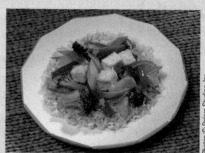
Soybean curd (tofu) and rice.

Photos © Polara Studios, Inc.

best sources of these are milk, eggs, and meat. Good non-animal sources of these nutrients include fortified cereals and soy products, tofu, legumes, almonds, asparagus, dark green vegetables, and whole-grain breads.

If you are a vegetarian, consider these suggestions to help avoid nutritional deficiencies:

- Combine complementary proteins to make sure you get complete proteins. In essence, combine vegetables or legumes with grains—beans and corn (staples in Mexican cuisine), beans and rice, tofu and rice, black bean and rice soup.
- Eat at least one cup of dark green vegetables a day to boost your iron intake. Combine foods rich in vitamin C with foods rich in iron; the vitamin C helps the body absorb iron.
- If you don't drink milk, eat at least two cups of legumes (dried beans and peas) or calcium-fortified tofu a day to provide you with adequate calcium.
- Eat a wide range of foods to better your chances of getting balanced nutrients.

Depending on how strict your diet is, you may need to use a nutritional supplement. Check with a nutrition expert, a registered dietitian, for advice. Figure 8.2 displays healthy vegetarian protein choices.

Fat

Fat is another energy-yielding nutrient. The most concentrated form of food energy, fat provides 9 kilocalories per gram, more than twice the calories in a gram of carbohydrate or protein. Fats provide valuable services: They transport fat-soluble vitamins in the body, insulate and protect body organs, regulate hormones, contribute to growth, provide a concentrated source of energy, and are essential for healthy skin. Fats give foods their flavor, texture, and palatability. Fats also provide foods with aromas that encourage people to eat them. Fat provides satiety, a feeling of fullness.

Although the right amount of fat is essential to growth and functioning of the body, too much fat is harmful. Excess dietary fat can lead to high blood

CALORIE VALUE OF NUTRIENTS

1 gram of carbohydrate	4 calories
1 gram of protein	4 calories
1 gram of fat	9 calories

FIGURE **8.3** FAT AND CALORIES.

Fat hides calories in food. When you trim fat, you trim calories.

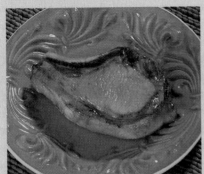

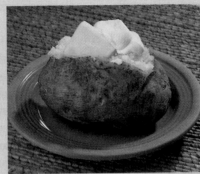

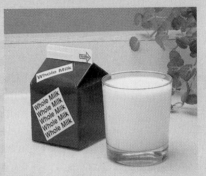

Small pork chop with ½ inch border of fat (25 grams fat) = 275 cal.

Large potato with 1 tbsp butter and 1 tbsp sour cream (14 grams fat) = 350 cal.

Whole milk, 1 c (8 grams fat) = 150 cal.

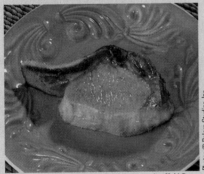

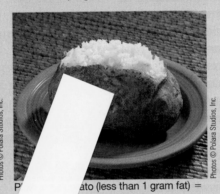

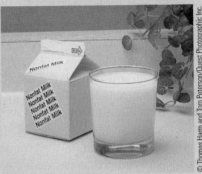

Small pork chop with fat trimmed off (13 grams fat) = 165 cal.

P_____ ato (less than 1 gram fat) = ____

Nonfat milk, 1 c (less than 1 gram fat) = 90 cal.

pressure, stroke, heart disease, diabetes, and other diseases. Excessive body fat is a leading factor in heart disease (see Chapter 11). It also has been linked to cancers of the colon, breast, uterus, and prostate.

The average American eats much more fat than is recommended or healthy. Experts recommend that no more than 30 percent of the total calories in the diet should come from fat. On a 30 percent fat diet, if you eat 1,600 calories a day, you should have no more than 53 grams of fat; for 2,000 calories a day, no more than 67 grams of fat.

To figure out the fat content of individual foods, multiply the grams of fat by 9 and divide this by the total calories in that food. You then multiply that number by 100 to get the percentage. For example, if a food label lists a total of 100 calories and 7 grams of fat, the fat content is 63 percent of total calories. This simple guideline can help you quickly assess the fat in your diet, and you can use this information to select foods that are lower in fat.

Reducing fat intake offers a fringe benefit to people who wish to cut calories. A spoonful of fat contains more than twice as many calories as a spoonful of sugar or pure protein. By removing the fat from a food, you can drastically reduce the calorie count. Figure 8.3 shows that the single most effective step you can take to reduce the energy value of a food is to eat it with less fat.

TYPES OF FATS Fats can be categorized as saturated, monounsaturated, or polyunsaturated based on their chemical structure. Each has health implications. **Saturated fats** are solid at room temperature and most come from animal sources. The only exceptions are coconut oil, palm oil, and palm kernel oil (the "tropical oils"), which are highly saturated but still liquid at room temperature. Saturated fats raise the level of low-density lipoproteins (the most harmful kind of cholesterol) in the bloodstream and have been linked to heart disease (see Chapter 11) and other

Fat Lipids in food or in the body that provide the body with a continuous fuel supply, protect it from mechanical shock, and carry fat-soluble vitamins.

Saturated fats Fats carrying the maximum possible numbers of hydrogen atoms; usually found in animal products such as butter and lard.

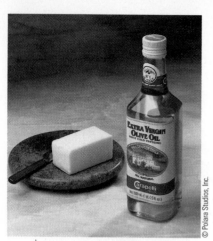

At room temperature unsaturated fats (such as those found in oil) are usually liquid, whereas saturated fats (such as those found in butter) are solid.

degenerative diseases. Examples of foods high in saturated fats are butter, cream, lard, bacon, beef, veal, lamb, poultry skin, and many processed food items.

Monounsaturated fats are liquid at room temperature. They are found in peanuts, cashews, olives, and avocados, as well as olive oil, peanut oil, cottonseed oil, and canola oil.

Polyunsaturated fats are found in most vegetable oils and, with a few exceptions, are liquid at room temperature. Foods containing polyunsaturated fats include fish, margarine, walnuts, almonds, pecans, corn oil, safflower oil, sunflower oil, sesame oil, and soybean oil.

Registered dietitians advise that people consume monounsaturated and polyunsaturated fats more often than saturated fats because of the negative effects of saturated fats on blood lipids. However, an even greater concern is total dietary fat. The most important dietary steps you can take to prevent disease are to control total dietary fat and to control your body weight.

Some mono-unsaturated and poly-unsaturated fats are **hydrogenated** during manufacturing. During this process, hydrogen is added to the fat to increase shelf life and to make the product harder or more spreadable. Hydrogenated fats are found in shortening, margarine, some crackers, and some nut butters. Eating a vegetable oil that has been hydrogenated may carry as many health risks as eating saturated fat.

> The most important dietary steps you can take to prevent disease are to control total dietary fat and to control your body weight.

CHOLESTEROL | **Cholesterol** is another type of fat. Despite its negative publicity, cholesterol does play beneficial roles in the body. It aids in digestion, is a major component of the membranes that protect nerve fibers, aids in production of vitamin D, and helps the body produce sex hormones. Too much cholesterol in the bloodstream, however, places a person at significantly higher risk for developing heart disease. Cholesterol forms a major part of the deposits that accumulate along arteries and increase the risk of heart attacks and strokes.

Blood levels of cholesterol are affected by being overweight and consuming a high-fat diet. Cholesterol blood level is not affected as much by cholesterol intake as by total fat intake. To test your knowledge about fat, see Assessment 8-1.

> One of the best ways to reduce the production of cholesterol in the body is to reduce the intake of saturated fat.

Carbohydrate

The third energy-yielding nutrient is carbohydrate. **Carbohydrates** provide 4 kilocalories per gram. Carbohydrates supply the body with the energy needed for daily activities. Because they are digested more easily and metabolized more efficiently and quickly than proteins, they are a preferred source of energy. The two different kinds of carbohydrates are **simple carbohydrates** (sugars) and **complex carbohydrates** (starches).

The terms "complex carbohydrate" and "simple carbohydrate" refer to an important distinction among carbohydrates—simply stated, the distinction between starch and fiber versus sugars. Another important distinction among the simple carbohydrates (sugars) is that they come in both natural (dilute) and processed (concentrated) form—simply stated, fruit versus candy.

> An 8-ounce can of Coke has approximately 10 teaspoons of sugar.

The simple carbohydrates are the sugars. All sugars are chemically similar to glucose and can be converted to glucose in the body. All of their names end in "-ose," which makes them easy to recognize as carbohydrates. The four sugars most important in human nutrition are glucose (the body's fuel), fructose (the sweet sugar of fruits, honey, and maple syrup), sucrose (table sugar), and lactose (milk sugar). Simple carbohydrates come mostly from fruits and milk or in concentrated forms such as sugar, honey, and other sweets.

Registered dietitians recommend that you consume abundant quantities of

> In terms of nutrition, there is no significant difference between honey and sugar.

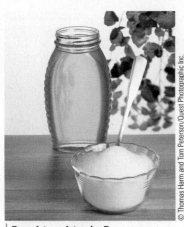

| Pure fat = fat only. Pure sugar equals carbohydrate only. |

fruits and vegetables that contain sugars, but they urge you in the same breath to "avoid consuming too much sugar." What's the difference?

Part of the answer lies in the phrase "empty calories." When you eat an apple, you receive about 100 calories from the sugars in it, together with a little vitamin A, a bit of thiamine, some vitamin C, a moderate dose of fiber, a healthy bit of potassium, and several dozen other nutrients. By contrast, a 12-ounce cola beverage gives you about 150 calories from sugar without any other nutrients. In fact, it creates a sort of debt, because to avoid overconsuming calories, you now have to derive all the nutrients you need in a day from food containing 150 fewer calories.

The same criticism applies to both honey and sugar. Some people believe that honey is an ideal substitute for sugar because they say it offers nutrients along with sugar. However, honey only contains a minute trace of some nutrients, so relative to a person's daily need, these tiny amounts don't add up to much. Honey is almost identical to sugar chemically. In terms of nutrition, there's no significant difference between honey and sugar.

HONEY VERSUS SUGAR

Some people believe honey to be the ideal substitute for sugar because, they say, it offers nutrients with its sweetness, rather than just empty calories. True, honey does contain traces of a few vitamins and minerals, but relative to a person's daily need, these nutrients don't add up to much. A tablespoon of honey (65 calories) offers one-tenth of a milligram of iron, for example, but an adult's daily need for iron can be as high as 15 milligrams or more. Consequently, to meet the need for iron, an adult would need 150 tablespoons in a day—almost 10,000 calories of honey! (Most people can eat only 2,000 to 3,000 calories a day without getting fat.) The nutrients in honey just do not add up as fast as the calories do, so honey, like sugar, is a relatively empty-calorie food. Honey is almost identical to sugar chemically, too. And spoon for spoon, sugar contains fewer calories than honey, because the sugar crystals take up more space.

The word "sugar" does not always appear on food labels. Instead, manufacturers may list the various kinds of sweeteners separately. The label may have a long list of ingredients including corn syrup, corn starch, sucrose, and honey. These hidden sugars can be deceptive.

SUGAR SUBSTITUTES People dream of calorie-less doughnuts, calorie-free candy, and ice cream with the calories of skim milk. At the same time, consumers insist that no risks to health must accompany calorie savings. The desire of most people to control body weight yet experience the taste of sugar has lead to the introduction of sugar substitutes.

People can choose from two sets of substitutes: One is the sugar alcohols, which are energy-yielding sweeteners (sometimes referred to as "nutritive sweeteners"); the other is the artificial sweeteners, which provide virtually no energy or calories.

The sugar alcohols are familiar to people who use special dietary products. Among them are maltitol, mannitol, sorbitol, and xylitol. A benefit of sugar alcohols is that ordinary mouth bacteria cannot metabolize them as rapidly as they metabolize sugar, so sugar alcohols do not contribute to tooth decay.

The person who wishes to reduce energy intake should be aware that the sugar alcohols do provide as much energy (that is, calories) as sucrose, even though these products may be labeled "sugar-free." For this person, artificial sweeteners may offer a preferable alternative.

Artificial sweeteners also make foods taste sweet without promoting tooth decay. Unlike sugar alcohols, they have the added advantages of being calorie-free. The most commonly used synthetic sweeteners are saccharin and aspartame.

Monounsaturated fats Fatty acids that lack two hydrogen atoms and have one double bond between carbons; found in olive oil, canola oil, and peanut oil.

Polyunsaturated fats Fatty acids that lack four hydrogen atoms and have two or more double bonds between carbons; found in safflower, sunflower, corn, soybean, and cottonseed oils.

Hydrogenation A chemical process by which hydrogens are added to monounsaturated or polyunsaturated fats to reduce the number of double bonds and make the product more saturated (solid) and more resistant to spoilage.

Cholesterol A type of fat called a "sterol"; necessary for synthesis of sex hormones, adrenal hormones, and vitamin D; cholesterol is obtained from the diet and made in the body.

Carbohydrates Compounds composed of carbon, oxygen, and hydrogen atoms. Carbohydrates provide about half of all energy needed by muscles and other tissues and is the preferred fuel for the brain and nervous system.

Simple carbohydrates Sugars in the form of fruits and milk or honey, sucrose, corn syrup, and fructose.

Complex carbohydrates Polysaccharides composed of straight or branched chains of monosaccharides.

Saccharin is used primarily in soft drinks and as a table sweetener. Due to questions about its safety, these products must carry warnings. Saccharin has another disadvantage: It does not taste exactly like sugar.

Aspartame received FDA approval and has been added to a variety of foods, including diet drinks, gum, cereals, gelatins, and puddings. The popularity of this product is due to its taste, which is almost like sugar. People seem to prefer aspartame also because of its reported safety. Aspartame appears to be safe for use by all people except those with a rare inherited disorder known as phenylketonuria.

As a sweet-toothed species, many people perceive sugar substitutes as the only way to cheat the scales. Evidence seems to suggest that artificial sweeteners, used in moderation as part of a well-balanced diet, pose no health risks.

| **COMPLEX CARBOHYDRATES** | The complex carbohydrates are composed of long chains of glucose units. Starch, the principle complex carbohydrate in grains and vegetables, is the chief energy source for human beings throughout the world and is highly desirable in the diet. Starch provides the body with the glucose it needs in the form it uses best. And if the starchy foods you eat are wholesome—such as whole-grain breads (not refined white bread), potatoes (not potato chips), or whole-grain cereals (not the sugary kind)—then your body obtains many of the other nutrients it needs, along with a steady supply of glucose. Most people would do well to boost their intakes of such starch foods.

Diets high in complex carbohydrates help to keep the blood sugar at a constant level and reduce the risks of heart disease, cancer, and other degenerative diseases. The best sources of complex carbohydrates are grains, such as wheat, rice, oats, corn, rye, barley, and millet; potatoes, sweet potatoes, and yams; fruits; vegetables; and legumes, such as soybeans, garbanzo beans, black-eyed peas, kidney beans, butter beans, and peanuts.

Because they are nutritionally dense, most complex carbohydrate foods are rich in vitamins and minerals. Many contain a significant amount of protein. Complex carbohydrates provide a steady source of energy, making them an excellent choice for physically active people (especially endurance athletes). Complex carbohydrates also are stored in the muscles and the liver as **glycogen**, which fuels the body when it needs sudden bursts of energy. For most people, nearly half of daily calories come from carbohydrates, at least 80 percent of which are complex carbohydrates.

Fiber, another complex carbohydrate in food, is mostly indigestible by human beings and therefore yields no calories. Fiber holds water and so provide the bulk

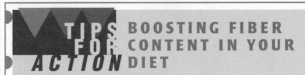

inside the intestines that enables the muscle of the digestive tract walls to push their contents along. Foods high in fiber also make softer stools. The subject may be unglamorous, but it intensely interests anyone who suffers from the consequences of a lack of fiber: constipation (hard, sluggish stools), hemorrhoids (swollen, painful rectal veins that bulge out from straining to pass hard stools), or a host of other intestinal ills.

Because fiber keeps the intestinal contents moving, it helps to prevent infection of the appendix (appendicitis). Additionally, fiber helps to control blood cholesterol levels, a risk factor for heart disease. (Certain fibers bind cholesterol and keep it from being absorbed in the body; it is excreted with the feces instead.) Fiber also helps control the blood glucose concentration and so helps to prevent diabetes. Some fibers bind cancer-causing agents in the digestive tract and keep them from being absorbed by or from touching the intestinal walls.

Fiber may also help prevent obesity. The person who eats fiber-rich foods chews longer and fills up sooner on fewer calories. Consistently, foods that are high in fiber are often low in calories and vice versa, so it is hard to eat a diet high in fiber and also gain weight.

Plant foods, especially those with their skins intact, are high in fiber. Fiber breaks down when foods are refined or cooked. Apples have more fiber than applesauce; apple juice has none. If you want to eat a diet high in fiber, choose whole grains, whole fruits, and whole vegetables most of the time. Most Americans eat about 15 grams of fiber a day. The National Cancer Institute recommends doubling that amount, to about 30 grams of fiber a day. The fiber content of selected foods can be

TABLE 8.2 FIBER CONTENT OF SELECTED FOODS

	Serving Size	Grams of Dietary Fiber
Grains		
Bread, white	1 slice	0.6
Bread, whole wheat	1 slice	1.5
Oat bran, dry	⅓ cup	4.0
Oatmeal, dry	⅓ cup	2.7
Rice, brown, cooked	½ cup	2.4
Rice, white, cooked	½ cup	0.8
Fruits		
Apple, with skin	1 small	2.8
Apricots, with skin	4 fruit	3.5
Banana	1 small	2.2
Blueberries	¾ cup	1.4
Figs, dried	3 fruit	4.6
Grapefruit	½ fruit	1.6
Pear, with skin	1 large	5.8
Prunes, dried	3 medium	1.7
Vegetables		
Asparagus, cooked	½ cup	1.8
Broccoli, cooked	½ cup	2.4
Carrots, cooked, sliced	½ cup	2.0
Peas, green, frozen, cooked	½ cup	4.3
Tomatoes, raw	1 medium	1.0
Legumes		
Kidney beans, cooked	½ cup	6.9
Lima beans, canned	½ cup	4.3
Pinto beans, cooked	½ cup	5.9
Beans, white, cooked	½ cup	5.0
Lentils, cooked	½ cup	5.2
Peas, black-eyed, canned	½ cup	4.7

From James W. Anderson, *Plant Fiber in Foods*, 2d Edition, University of Kentucky, College of Medicine, HCF Nutrition Foundation, P.O. Box 22124, Lexington, KY 40522.

found in Table 8.2. Assessment 8-2 includes questions related to your fiber intake.

| Vitamins and Minerals |

Vitamins and **minerals** occur in foods in much smaller quantities than do the energy-yielding nutrients, and they make no contribution of energy themselves. Nor do they contribute building material, except for the minerals of bone. Instead they are mostly helpers, or facilitators, of body processes. They are, nonetheless, a powerful group of substances, as their absence attests. Vitamin A deficiency can cause blindness; a lack of niacin causes mental illness; a lack of iron causes anemia. The consequences of deficiencies are so dire and the effects of restoring the needed nutrients so dramatic that they make wonderful stories for faddists to tell: Are you bald? Impotent? Do you have pimples? Are you nearsighted? The right vitamin will cure whatever ails you, they say.

Actually, a vitamin or mineral can cure only the disease caused by a deficiency of that vitamin or mineral. Also, an overdose of any vitamin or mineral can make people as sick as a deficiency can, and it can even cause death. For most healthy people, a balanced diet of ordinary foods supplies enough, but not too much, of each of the vitamins and minerals. The vitamins are listed along with some of their more important roles in Table 8.3. The vitamins fall into two categories.

1. Fat-soluble vitamins, including vitamins A, D, E, and K, are stored in the body's fat cells. They are not excreted in the urine and are accumulated in the fat tissues of the body. If you consume too many, they can be toxic.
2. Water-soluble vitamins, including vitamin C and the B-complex vitamins, dissolve readily in water and are excreted in the urine. Megadoses of these vitamins can also be toxic.

Vitamins C and E (and **beta-carotene**, a vitamin A precursor) function as **antioxidants**, preventing oxygen from combining with other substances that it may damage. During normal **metabolism**, oxygen changes carbohydrates and fats into energy. In this process, oxygen is transformed into stable forms of water and carbon dioxide. A small amount of oxygen, however, ends up in an unstable form, referred to as oxygen-free radicals—which can damage healthy tissue. The presence of antioxidants protects cell membranes and DNA from this damage, which is believed to assist in

Glycogen A storage form of carbohydrate in the liver and muscle.

Dietary fiber The part of the plant that is not digested in the small intestine and that provides the bulk needed to keep the digestive system running smoothly; found in vegetables, fruits, grains, and legumes.

Vitamins Organic, essential nutrients required in small amounts to perform specific functions that promote growth, maintenance, or repair; vitamins do not provide energy, but are necessary in energy-yielding reactions.

Minerals Inorganic elements; some minerals are required in small amounts and are therefore essential.

Beta-carotene An orange pigment with antioxidant activity; a vitamin A precursor made by plants.

Antioxidants A compound that protects other compounds from oxidation by being oxidized itself. This process protects valuable cellular substances from being altered or destroyed; in the body it helps prevent damage to cells and body fluids.

Metabolism All of the chemical reactions that occur within living cells; energy metabolism includes the reactions by which the body obtains and spends the energy from food.

TABLE 8.3   MAJOR FUNCTIONS OF VITAMINS

Nutrient	Good Sources	Major Functions	Deficiency Symptoms
Vitamin A	Milk, cheese, eggs, liver, yellow and dark green fruits and vegetables	Required for healthy bones, teeth, skin, gums, and hair; maintenance of inner mucous membranes, thus increasing resistance to infection; adequate vision in dim light.	Night blindness; decreased growth; decreased resistance to infection; rough, dry skin
Vitamin D	Fortified milk, cod liver oil, salmon, tuna, egg yolk	Necessary for bones and teeth; needed for calcium and phosphorus absorption.	Rickets (bone softening), fractures, muscle spasms
Vitamin E	Vegetable oils, yellow and green leafy vegetables, margarine, wheat germ, whole grain breads and cereals	Related to oxidation and normal muscle and red blood cell chemistry.	Leg cramps, red blood cell breakdown
Vitamin K	Green leafy vegetables, cauliflower, cabbage, eggs, peas, potatoes	Essential for normal blood clotting.	Hemorrhaging
Vitamin B_1 (Thiamin)	Whole grain or enriched bread, lean meats and poultry, fish, liver, pork, poultry, organ meats, legumes, nuts, dried yeast	Assists in proper use of carbohydrates; normal functioning of nervous system; maintenance of good appetite.	Loss of appetite, nausea, confusion, cardiac abnormalities, muscle spasms
Vitamin B_2 (Riboflavin)	Eggs, milk, leafy green vegetables, whole grains, lean meats, dried beans and peas	Contributes to energy release from carbohydrates, fats, and proteins; needed for normal growth and development, good vision, and healthy skin.	Cracking of the corners of the mouth, inflammation of the skin, impaired vision.
Vitamin B_6 (Pyridoxine)	Vegetables, meats, whole grain cereals, soybeans, peanuts, potatoes	Necessary for protein and fatty acids metabolism and for normal red blood cell formation.	Depression, irritability, muscle spasms, nausea
Vitamin B_{12}	Meat, poultry, fish, liver, organ meats, eggs, shellfish, milk, cheese	Required for normal growth, red blood cell formation, nervous system and digestive tract functioning.	Impaired balance, weakness, drop in red blood cell count
Niacin	Liver and organ meats, meat, fish, poultry, whole grains, enriched breads, nuts, green leafy vegetables, and dried beans and peas	Contributes to energy release from carbohydrates, fats, and proteins; normal growth and development; and formation of hormones and nerve-regulating substances.	Confusion, depression, weakness, weight loss
Biotin	Liver, kidney, eggs, yeast, legumes, milk, nuts, dark green vegetables	Essential for carbohydrate metabolism and fatty acid synthesis.	Inflamed skin, muscle pain, depression, weight loss
Folate	Leafy green vegetables, organ meats, whole grains and cereals, dried beans	Needed for cell growth and reproduction and for red blood cell formation.	Decreased resistance to infection
Pantothenic Acid	All natural foods, especially liver, kidney, eggs, nuts, yeast, milk, dried peas and beans, green leafy vegetables	Related to carbohydrate and fat metabolism.	Depression, low blood sugar, leg cramps, nausea, headaches
Vitamin C (Ascorbic acid)	Fruits, vegetables	Helps protect against infection; required for formation of collagenous tissue, normal blood vessels, teeth, and bones.	Slow-healing wounds, loose teeth, hemorrhaging, rough scaly skin, irritability

preventing the development of heart disease, cancer, and even emphysema.

| MINERALS | Minerals are the inorganic elements; some minerals are required in small amounts and therefore are essential. Minerals are classified as **major minerals** and **trace minerals**. Major minerals are essential nutrients found in the human body in amounts larger than 5 grams, and trace minerals are found in the body in amounts less than 5 grams. Because they are needed in such small amounts, minerals can be extremely toxic if consumed in excess.

Table 8.4 lists selected minerals of both types, along with their sources and functions. Many people suffer from

TABLE **8.4** MAJOR FUNCTIONS OF MINERALS

Nutrient	Good Sources	Major Functions	Deficiency Symptoms
Calcium	Milk, yogurt, cheese, green leafy vegetables, dried beans, sardines and salmon with edible bones	Required for strong teeth and bone formation; maintenance of good muscle tone, heartbeat, and nerve function.	Bone pain and fractures, periodontal disease, muscle cramps
Copper	Seafood, meats, beans, nuts, whole grains	Helps with iron absorption and hemoglobin formation; required to synthesize the enzyme cytochrome oxidase.	Anemia (although deficiency is rare in humans)
Iron	Organ meats, lean meats, seafoods, eggs, dried peas and beans, nuts, whole and enriched grains, green leafy vegetables	Major component of hemoglobin; aids in energy utilization.	Nutritional anemia, overall weakness
Phosphorus	Meats, fish, milk, eggs, dried beans and peas, whole grains, processed foods	Required for bone and teeth formation; energy release regulation.	Bone pain and fracture, weight loss, weakness
Zinc	Milk, meat, seafood, whole grains, nuts, eggs, dried beans	Essential component of hormones, insulin, and enzymes; used in normal growth and development.	Loss of appetite, slow-healing wounds, skin problems
Magnesium	Green leafy vegetables, whole grains, nuts, soybeans, seafood, legumes	Needed for bone growth and maintenance; carbohydrate and protein utilization; nerve function; temperature regulation.	Irregular heartbeat, weakness, muscle spasms, sleeplessness
Sodium	Table salt, processed foods, meat	Needed for body fluid regulation; transmission of nerve impulses; heart action.	Rarely seen
Potassium	Legumes, whole grains, bananas, orange juice, dried fruits, potatoes	Required for heart action; bone formation and maintenance; regulation of energy release; acid-base regulation.	Irregular heartbeat, nausea, weakness
Selenium	Seafood, meat, whole grains	Component of enzymes; functions in close association with vitamin E.	Muscle pain, possible heart muscle deterioration, possible hair and nail loss

FOR OPTIMAL BONE HEALTH:

- Drink plenty of milk. Most adults get about half their calcium from milk. One cup of milk—whether whole milk, 2%, 1%, or skim milk—provides 300 milligrams of calcium.
- Eat foods rich in vitamin D; they help your body absorb calcium. Primary sources are milk and dairy products.
- Avoid too much meat and other protein-rich foods, because they make your body excrete calcium.
- Cut down on alcohol, caffeine, and phosphates (found in soda) because they take the place of calcium-rich beverages in your diet.
- Be involved in weight-bearing physical activities.
- Maintain a healthy body weight; avoid being too thin. The bones need the stimulation to grow dense by supporting a healthy body.
- If you smoke, stop.

deficiencies of two important minerals—calcium and iron.

Calcium Calcium helps regulate the heart, maintain proper fluid balance in the cells, transmit nerve impulses, and clot the blood. Among its other functions, calcium aids in the formation of bones, which is important to people of all ages. A low calcium intake during childhood and adolescence limits the bone's ability to achieve an optimal peak mass and density. Bone tissue is active, bone cells are replaced throughout adulthood, therefore you need plenty of calcium to help your bones maintain strength and density. Women have smaller, less-dense bones than men and

Major minerals Essential mineral nutrients found in the human body in amounts larger than 5 grams; sometimes called "macrominerals."

Trace minerals Essential mineral nutrients found in the human body in amounts less than 5 grams; sometimes called "microminerals."

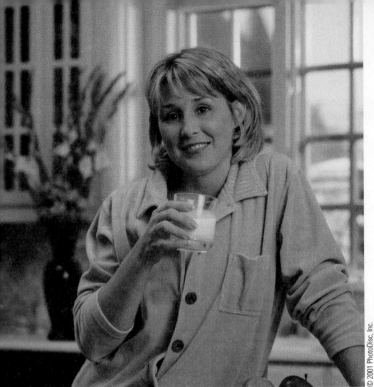

Consuming dairy foods today will help reduce your risk of osteoporosis tomorrow.

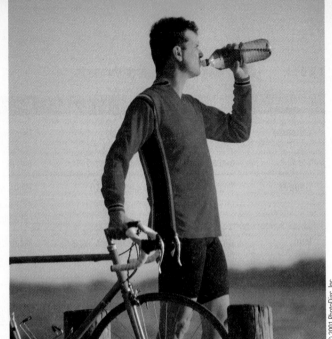

Water is the most vital nutrient.

are about eight times more likely to develop osteoporosis, a disease characterized by weak and porous bones that are likely to fracture.

Unlike many diseases that make themselves known through symptoms such as pain, osteoporosis is silent. The body sends no signals saying bone loss is occurring. This disease is called "the silent thief" for this reason. People need to take action they are young to protect their bones and reduce osteoporosis. Assessment 8-3 can help you determine risk for osteoporosis.

Bones respond to physical activity by becoming denser and stronger. If you for example, your leg bones will respond by more mass. If you use your arms regularly to li or swing a tennis racket, the bones in your arms stronger.

Iron A deficiency of iron in means too few red blood cells in the bloodstream cause a condition called iron deficiency an , characterized by weakness, pallor, shortness of breath, susceptibility to infection, shortened attention span, impaired learning abilities, loss of vision, and other serious physical problems. Women who are menstruating run a particular risk of iron deficiency. As many as 15 percent of American women of childbearing age may have an iron deficiency because of blood lost during menstruation.

On the other hand, too much iron can cause infections, tissue damage, and severe liver damage, and it may also increase the risk for heart disease. Because the proper balance is so important, you should consult with your doctor before taking any iron supplement.

Water

Next to air, water is the element most necessary for human survival. You could survive much longer without food than you could without water. Water is the major component of blood, which carries oxygen and nutrients to all cells in the body. It helps your body use the other nutrients in your diet, aids your body in getting rid of wastes, helps you digest foods, maintains the proper electrolyte balance in the body, lubricates joints, and regulates body temperature—to name just a few functions.

Approximately 60 percent of your body is made of water. You get some water from the foods you eat. Fruits, for example, are as much as 80 percent water. Especially good choices are melons and apples. Even foods you don't typically think of as containing much water, such as bread and meat, can be anywhere from 33 to 50 percent water. In addition to the foods you eat, you should drink eight to ten 8-ounce glasses of water a day—more if you are large, physically active, live in a hot climate, or perspire excessively.

You cannot always rely on thirst to indicate a water deficit. A rough indicator is the color of your urine. If it is dark amber color or has a strong odor, you are not drinking enough water. Passing a full bladder of colorless or pale yellow urine at least four times a day means you are getting enough water. The following—in addition to drinking plenty of water—will help you maintain proper intake:

- Avoid caffeine. It increases the body's need for water while it increases the amount of water the body puts out.
- Avoid alcohol. You need 8 ounces of water to metabolize a single ounce of alcohol.

TABLE 8.5 1989 RECOMMENDED DIETARY ALLOWANCES (RDA)

	Energy (Kcal)	Protein (g)	Vitamin A (μg RE)	Vitamin E (mg TE)	Vitamin K (μg)	Vitamin C (mg)	Iron (mg)	Zinc (mg)	Iodine (μg)	Selenium (μg)
Infants										
0.0–0.5	650	13	375	3	5	30	6	5	40	10
0.5–1.0	850	14	375	4	10	35	10	5	50	15
Children										
1–3	1300	16	400	6	15	40	10	10	70	20
4–6	1800	24	500	7	20	45	10	10	90	20
7–10	2000	28	700	7	30	45	10	10	120	30
Males										
11–14	2500	45	1000	10	45	50	12	15	150	40
15–18	3000	59	1000	10	65	60	12	15	150	50
19–24	2900	58	1000	10	70	60	10	15	150	70
25–50	2900	63	1000	10	80	60	10	15	150	70
51+	2300	63	1000	10	80	60	10	15	150	70
Females										
11–14	2200	46	800	8	45	50	15	12	150	45
15–18	2200	44	800	8	55	60	15	12	150	50
19–24	2200	46	800	8	60	60	15	12	150	55
25–50	2200	50	800	8	65	60	15	12	150	55
51+	1900	50	800	8	65	60	10	12	150	55
Pregnancy	+300	60	800	10	65	70	30	15	175	65
Lactation										
1st 6 mo.	+500	65	1300	12	65	95	15	19	200	75
2nd 6 mo.	+500	62	1200	11	65	90	15	16	200	75

- Cut back on protein to a healthy level. The wastes produced from proteins build up in the kidneys, and you need extra water to flush them out.
- Drink a steady amount of water throughout the day to keep your body well supplied.

DEFINING NUTRIENT NEEDS: DIETARY REFERENCE INTAKES

Defining the amounts of energy, nutrients, and other dietary components that best support health is a huge task. For more than 50 years, nutrition experts produced a set of energy and nutrient standards known as the Recommended Dietary Allowances (RDA) for healthy people in the United States. Over the years, these standards were revised periodically as new evidence became available.

A major revision of nutrient recommendations occurred in 1997.[3] The revised recommendations are called **Dietary Reference Intakes (DRI)**. The revised recommendations include key nutrients crucial to health.[4]

The DRI include four sets of values:

Estimated Average Requirement. Nutrition experts review hundreds of research studies to determine how much of a nutrient is needed in the diet to maintain a specific function, such as the amount of calcium needed to minimize bone loss in later life.[5] A population-wide average is selected, an **Estimated Average Requirement,** an amount that appears sufficient to maintain a specific body function.

Recommended Dietary Allowance. The intake to recommend for most healthy people, a **Recommended Dietary Allowance**. This value is considered generous, to meet the needs of most people. To ensure that vitamin and mineral RDAs meet the needs of as many people as possible, they are set high. Table 8.5 displays the RDAs.

Adequate Intake. For nutrients that lack enough scientific evidence to determine an Estimated Average Requirement (which is needed

Dietary Reference Intakes (DRI) A set of nutrient values for the dietary nutrient intakes of healthy people; these values are used for planning and assessing diets and include Estimated Average Requirements, Recommended Dietary Allowances, Adequate Intakes, and Tolerable Upper Intake Levels.

Estimated Average Requirement (EAR) The amount of a nutrient that will maintain a specific biochemical or physiological function in half of the population.

Recommended Dietary Allowances (RDA) The average daily amount of a nutrient considered adequate to meet the known nutrient needs of most healthy people; a goal for dietary intakes by individuals.

Age (yr)	Thiamin RDA (mg/day)	Riboflavin RDA (mg/day)	Niacin RDA (mg/day)[a]	Biotin AI (µg/day)	Pantothenic acid AI (mg/day)	Vitamin B₆ RDA (mg/day)	Folate RDA (µg/day)[b]	Vitamin B₁₂ RDA (µg/day)	Choline AI (mg/day)	Vitamin C RDA (mg/day)	Vitamin A RDA (µg/day)[c]	Vitamin D AI (µg/day)[d]
Infants[f]												
0.0–0.5	0.2	0.3	2	5	1.7	0.1	65	0.4	125	40	400	5
0.5–1.0	0.3	0.4	4	6	1.8	0.3	80	0.5	150	50	500	5
Children												
1–3	0.5	0.5	6	8	2	0.5	150	0.9	200	15	300	5
4–8	0.6	0.6	8	12	3	0.6	200	1.2	250	25	400	5
Males												
9–13	0.9	0.9	12	20	4	1.0	300	1.9	375	45	600	5
14–18	1.2	1.3	16	25	5	1.3	400	2.4	550	75	900	5
19–30	1.2	1.3	16	30	5	1.3	400	2.4	550	90	900	5
31–50	1.2	1.3	16	30	5	1.3	400	2.4	550	90	900	5
51–70	1.2	1.3	16	30	5	1.7	400	2.4	550	90	900	10
>70	1.2	1.3	16	30	5	1.7	400	2.4	550	90	900	15
Females												
9–13	0.9	0.9	12	20	4	1.0	300	1.8	375	45	600	5
14–18	1.0	1.0	14	25	5	1.2	400	2.4	400	65	700	5
19–30	1.1	1.1	14	30	5	1.3	400	2.4	425	75	700	5
31–50	1.1	1.1	14	30	5	1.3	400	2.4	425	75	700	5
51–70	1.1	1.1	14	30	5	1.5	400	2.4	425	75	700	10
>70	1.1	1.1	14	30	5	1.5	400	2.4	425	75	700	15
Pregnancy												
≤18	1.4	1.4	18	30	6	1.9	600	2.6	450	80	750	5
19–30	1.4	1.4	18	30	6	1.9	600	2.6	450	85	770	5
31–50	1.4	1.4	18	30	6	1.9	600	2.6	450	85	770	5
Lactation												
≤18	1.4	1.6	17	35	7	2.0	500	2.8	550	115	1200	5
19–30	1.4	1.6	17	35	7	2.0	500	2.8	550	120	1300	5
31–50	1.4	1.6	17	35	7	2.0	500	2.8	550	120	1300	5

[a] Niacin recommendations are expressed as niacin equivalents (NE), except for recommendations for infants younger than 6 months, which are expressed as preformed niacin.
[b] Folate recommendations are expressed as dietary folate equivalents (DFE).
[c] Vitamin A recommendations are expressed as retinol activity equivalents (RAE).

[d] Vitamin D recommendations are expressed as cholecalciferol and assume an absence of adequate exposure to sunlight.
[e] Vitamin E recommendations are expressed as α-tocopherol.
[f] For all nutrients, values for infants are AI.

to set an RDA), an **Adequate Intake (AI)** is established instead of an RDA. An AI reflects the average amount of a nutrient that a group of healthy people consumes. (Table 8.6 displays the 1997–2001 Dietary Reference Intakes, which consist of two values: the RDA and the AI.)

Tolerable Upper Intake Level. This is the level at which a nutrient is likely to become toxic. The recommended intakes for nutrients are generous, and although they do not necessarily cover every person for every

nutrient, they probably should not be exceeded by much. People's tolerances for high doses of nutrients vary, and somewhere above the recommended intake is the **Tolerable Upper Intake Level**.[6] Nutrient recommendations fall within a range, with marginal and danger zones both below and above it. Upper levels are useful in guarding against the overconsumption of nutrients, which is most likely to occur when people use supplements or fortified foods regularly. (Table 8.7 displays the Tolerable Upper Intake Levels.)

| Vitamins | | Minerals | | | | | | | | | | | |
Vitamin E RDA (mg/day)[a]	Vitamin K AI (µg/day)	Calcium AI (mg/day)	Phosphorus RDA (mg/day)	Magnesium RDA (mg/day)	Iron RDA (mg/day)	Zinc RDA (mg/day)	Iodine RDA (µg/day)	Selenium RDA (µg/day)	Copper RDA (µg/day)	Manganese AI (mg/day)	Fluoride AI (mg/day)	Chromium AI (µg/day)	Molybdenum RDA (µg/day)
4	2.0	210	100	30	0.27	2	110	15	200	0.003	0.01	0.2	2
5	2.5	270	275	75	11	3	130	20	220	0.6	0.5	5.5	3
6	30	500	460	80	7	3	90	20	340	1.2	0.7	11	17
7	55	800	500	130	10	5	90	30	440	1.5	1.0	15	22
11	60	1300	1250	240	8	8	120	40	700	1.9	2	25	34
15	75	1300	1250	410	11	11	150	55	890	2.2	3	35	43
15	120	1000	700	400	8	11	150	55	900	2.3	4	35	45
15	120	1000	700	420	8	11	150	55	900	2.3	4	35	45
15	120	1200	700	420	8	11	150	55	900	2.3	4	30	45
15	120	1200	700	420	8	11	150	55	900	2.3	4	30	45
11	60	1300	1250	240	8	8	120	40	700	1.6	2	21	34
15	75	1300	1250	360	15	9	150	55	890	1.6	3	24	43
15	90	1000	700	310	18	8	150	55	900	1.8	3	25	45
15	90	1000	700	320	18	8	150	55	900	1.8	3	25	45
15	90	1200	700	320	8	8	150	55	900	1.8	3	20	45
15	90	1200	700	320	8	8	150	55	900	1.8	3	20	45
15	75	1300	1250	400	27	13	220	60	1000	2.0	3	29	50
15	90	1000	700	350	27	11	220	60	1000	2.0	3	30	50
15	90	1000	700	360	27	11	220	60	1000	2.0	3	30	50
19	75	1300	1250	360	10	14	290	70	1300	2.6	3	44	50
19	90	1000	700	310	9	12	290	70	1300	2.6	3	45	50
19	90	1000	700	320	9	12	290	70	1300	2.6	3	45	50

Source: Adapted with permission from the *Dietary Reference Intakes* series, National Academy Press, Copyright 1997, 1998, 2000, 2001, by the National Academy of Sciences. Courtesy of the National Academy Press, Washington, D.C.

DAILY VALUES AND FOOD LABELS

The Food and Drug Administration developed a system for food labeling, referred to as "**Daily Values**," based on a 2,000 calorie diet. Each nutrient contained in a serving of the product is expressed as a percent of that nutrient's daily recommended intake. This means that, assuming a person consumes a 2,000 calorie diet, they will obtain that percent of the daily value from

Adequate Intakes (AI) The average amount of a nutrient that appears sufficient to maintain a specific criteria; a value used as a guide for nutrient intake when a RDA cannot be determined.

Tolerable Upper Intake Level (TUIL) The maximum amount of a nutrient that appears safe for most healthy people and beyond which there is an increased risk of adverse effects.

Daily Values Reference Values of daily requirements developed by the Food and Drug Administration (FDA) specifically for use on food labels.

TABLE 8.7 TOLERABLE UPPER INTAKE LEVELS

Age (yr)	Vitamins								Minerals		
	Niacin (mg/day)ᵃ	Vitamin B₆ (mg/day)	Folate (µg/day)ᵇ	Choline (mg/day)	Vitamin C (mg/day)	Vitamin A (µg/day)ᶜ	Vitamin D (µg/day)ᵈ	Vitamin E (mg/day)ᵉ	Calcium (mg/day)	Phosphorus (mg/day)	Magnesium (mg/day)
Infants											
0.0–0.5	—	—	—	—	—	600	25	—	—	—	—
0.5–1.0	—	—	—	—	—	600	25	—	—	—	—
Children											
1–3	10	30	300	1000	400	600	50	200	2500	3000	65
4–8	15	40	400	1000	650	900	50	300	2500	3000	110
9–13	20	60	600	2000	1200	1700	50	600	2500	4000	350
Adolescents											
14–18	30	80	800	3000	1800	2800	50	800	2500	4000	350
Adults											
19–70	35	100	1000	3500	2000	3000	50	1000	2500	4000	350
>70	35	100	1000	3500	2000	3000	50	1000	2500	3000	350
Pregnancy											
≤18	30	80	800	3000	1800	2800	50	800	2500	3500	350
19–50	35	100	1000	3500	2000	3000	50	1000	2500	3500	350
Lactation											
≤18	30	80	800	3000	1800	2800	50	800	2500	4000	350
19–50	35	100	1000	3500	2000	3000	50	1000	2500	4000	350

a The UL for niacin and folate apply to synthetic forms obtained from supplements, fortified foods, or a combination of the two.
b The UL for vitamin A applies to the preformed vitamin only.
c The UL for vitamin E applies to any form of supplemental α-tocopherol, fortified foods, or a combination of the two.
d The UL for magnesium applies to synthetic forms obtained from supplements or drugs only.

a serving of the product. These percentages require adjustments by the individual depending on daily caloric needs.

Both the RDA and the Daily Values apply only to healthy people. They are not intended for people who are ill and who may require additional nutrients.

Reading the food label (Figure 8.4) can help you make wise food choices. By law, the FDA requires that all the nutrients in a food must be listed on the label in language the consumer can understand. By law, every food label also must include the following:

- The common name of the product
- The name and address of the manufacturer, distributor, or packer
- The net contents of the package (count, measure, or weight)
- The ingredients listed in descending order, with the most plentiful ingredient listed first

If the product makes any nutritional claims, the law requires that the following nutritional information be listed on the label under the heading "Nutritional Information":

- Serving or portion size
- Servings per container
- Calories per serving
- Carbohydrates (in grams) per serving
- Fats (in grams) per serving
- Vitamins, minerals, and proteins (as percentages of the RDA) per serving
- The amount of eight "indicator nutrients"—protein, vitamin A, niacin, thiamine, riboflavin, vitamin C, calcium, and iron

CONSUMER CONCERNS ABOUT FOODS

From time to time people raise concerns regarding food safety issues, including additives, **irradiation**, and food-borne illness.

Food additives are chemical agents added to processed foods to help preserve them or to change their appearance or enhance their flavor. Food additives fall into the general categories of antioxidants, emulsifiers, flavorings, preservatives, and sweeteners.

Antioxidants, such as BA and BHT, are synthetic chemicals used to keep oils and fats from becoming rancid. Emulsifiers suspend the flavor oils throughout the product, improving both flavor and appearance. A

					Minerals					
Iron (mg/day)	Zinc (mg/day)	Iodine (µg/day)	Selenium (µg/day)	Copper (µg/day)	Manganese (mg/day)	Fluoride (mg/day)	Molybdenum (µg/day)	Boron (mg/day)	Nickel (mg/day)	Vanadium (mg/day)
40	4	—	45	—	—	0.7	—	—	—	—
40	5	—	60	—	—	0.9	—	—	—	—
40	7	200	90	1000	2	1.3	300	3	0.2	—
40	12	300	150	3000	3	2.2	600	6	0.3	—
40	23	600	280	5000	6	10	1100	11	0.6	—
45	34	900	400	8000	9	10	1700	17	1.0	—
45	40	1100	400	10,000	11	10	2000	20	1.0	1.8
45	40	1100	400	10,000	11	10	2000	20	1.0	1.8
45	34	900	400	8000	9	10	1700	17	1.0	—
45	40	1100	400	10,000	11	10	2000	20	1.0	—
45	34	900	400	8000	9	10	1700	17	1.0	—
45	40	1100	400	10,000	11	10	2000	20	1.0	—

Note: An Upper Limit was not established for vitamins and minerals not listed and for those age groups listed with a dash (—) because of a lack of data, not because these nutrients are safe to consume at any level of intake. All nutrients can have adverse effects when intakes are excessive.

Source: Adapted with permission from the *Dietary Reference Intakes* series, National Academy Press. Copyright 1997, 1998, 2000, 2001, by the National Academy of Sciences. Courtesy of the National Academy Press, Washington, DC.

number of artificial agents are used in processed foods to enhance flavor. Some—such as sodium nitrate, used in corned beef and bacon as well as other red meats—are also used as coloring agents or preservatives. Preservatives inhibit bacterial growth, giving processed foods a longer shelf life.

In an attempt to improve the quality of food, some manufacturers use radiation to treat both fresh and processed foods. Essentially, foods are exposed to gamma radiation, which lengthens the shelf life of the product and destroys any microorganisms that might have contaminated the food. The process of irradiation does not make food radioactive. The FDA has approved irradiation to enhance food safety.

Food contaminated with bacteria or parasites can cause food-borne illness, characterized by nausea, vomiting, abdominal pain, bloating, gas, and diarrhea. The symptoms of food-borne illness most often begin within 5 to 8 hours of eating the contaminated food. Symptoms, however, depend on the type of organism that causes the illness; they may begin as soon as 30 minutes after eating the food or may not develop for as long as several weeks afterward. When symptoms do not develop for days or weeks, the problem often is misdiagnosed because it cannot be related readily to a specific food.

Although many cases of food-borne illness can be traced to food served at restaurants, approximately one-third can be traced to careless or unsafe handling and preparation of food in the home. To protect yourself from food-borne illness at home, do the following:

- When you shop, put meat, poultry, and fish in separate plastic bags so their drippings don't contaminate your other groceries.
- Check the expiration date on all meat, poultry, and fish before you buy it. When possible, get meat that was put in the cooler that day. Buy only what you can use within the next few days unless you are planning to freeze it. Keep meat, poultry, and fish in the refrigerator (that is, unfrozen) no longer than 3 days.
- Never buy meat, poultry, fish, or fresh produce from counters that are not clean.
- Refrigerate perishable foods (including fresh produce) as soon as you get home from the store. Make sure your refrigerator keeps foods at 40°F or cooler; bacteria thrive at temperatures as low as 45°F.
- Never thaw foods on the counter. Foods should be thawed in the refrigerator,

Irradiation Sterilizing a food by exposure to energy waves; this process kills microorganisms and insects.

FIGURE 8.4 INFORMATION ON NEW FOOD LABEL.

Nutrition Facts Title

The new title "Nutrition Facts" signals the new label.

Serving Size

Similar food products now have similar serving sizes. This makes it easier to compare foods. Serving sizes are based on amounts people actually eat.

New Label Information

Some label information may be new to you. The new nutrient list covers those most important to your health. You may have seen this information on some old labels, but it is now required.

Vitamins and Minerals

Only two vitamins, A and C, and two minerals, calcium and iron, are required on the food label. A food company can voluntarily list other vitamins and minerals in the food.

Label Numbers

Numbers on the nutrition label may be rounded for labeling.

NUTRITION FACTS

Serving Size 1 cup (228g)
Servings Per Container 2

Amount Per Serving

Calories 90	Calories from Fat 30

	% Daily Value*
Total Fat 3g	**5%**
Saturated Fat 0g	**0%**
Cholesterol 0mg	**0%**
Sodium 300mg	**13%**
Total Carbohydrate 13g	**4%**
Dietary Fiber 3g	**12%**
Sugars 3g	
Protein 3g	

Vitamin A	80%	•	Vitamin C	60%
Calcium	4%	•	Iron	4%

*% Daily Values are based on a 2000 calorie diet. Your daily values may be higher or lower depending on your calorie needs:

	Calories	2000	2500
Total Fat	Less than	65g	80g
Sat Fat	Less than	20g	25g
Cholesterol	Less than	300mg	300mg
Sodium	Less than	2400mg	2400mg
Total Carbohydrate		300g	375g
Dietary Fiber		25g	30g

Calories per gram:
Fat 9 • Carbohydrates 4 • Protein 4

Foods that have only a few of the nutrients required on the standard label can use a short label format. What's on the label depends on what's in the food. Small- and medium-sized packages with very little label space also can use a short label.

% Daily Value

% Daily Value shows how a food fits into a 2,000-calorie reference diet.

You can use % Daily Value to compare foods and see how the amount of a nutrient in a serving of food fits in a 2,000-calorie reference diet.

Daily Values Footnote

Daily Values are the new label reference numbers. These numbers are set by the government and are based on current nutrition recommendations.

Some labels list the daily values for a daily diet of 2,000 and 2,500 calories. Your own nutrient needs may be less than or more than the Daily Values on the label.

Calories Per Gram Footnote

Some labels tell the approximate number of calories in a gram of fat, carbohydrate, and protein.

Some food packages make claims such as "light," "low-fat," and "cholesterol-free." These claims can be used only if a food meets strict government definitions. Here are some of the meanings:

Label claim	Definition*
Calorie-Free	Less than 5 calories
Light or Lite	1/3 fewer calories or 50% less fat; if more than half the calories are from fat, fat content must be reduced by 50% or more
Light in Sodium	50% less sodium
Fat-Free	Less than 1/2 gram fat
Low-Fat	3 grams or less fat**
Cholesterol-Free	Less than 2 milligrams cholesterol and 2 grams or less saturated fat**
Low Cholesterol	20 milligrams or less cholesterol and 2 grams or less saturated fat**
Sodium-Free	Less than 5 milligrams sodium**
Very Low Sodium	35 milligrams or less sodium**
Low-Sodium	140 milligrams or less sodium**
High Fiber	5 grams or more fiber

*Per Reference Amount (standard serving size). Some claims have higher nutrient levels for main dish products and meal products, such as frozen entrees and dinners.
**Also per 50 g for products with small serving sizes (reference amount is 30 g or less or 2 tbsp or less).

Some food packages may now carry health claims. A health claim is a label statement that describes the relationship between a nutrient and a disease or health-related condition. A food must meet certain nutrient levels to make a health claim. Seven types of health claims are allowed. These nutrient-disease relationships include

A diet:	And:
High in calcium	Osteoporosis (brittle bone disease)
High in fiber-containing grain products, fruits, and vegetables	Cancer
High in fruits or vegetables (high in dietary fiber or vitamins A or C)	Cancer
High in fiber from fruits, vegetables, and grain products	Heart disease
Low in fat	Cancer
Low in saturated fat and cholesterol	Heart disease
Low in sodium	High blood pressure

in the microwave, or submerged in cold water. Cook food as soon as it is defrosted.

- Wash your hands thoroughly with soap and running hot water before handling any food, after you've touched any raw meat (including poultry and fish), and before you eat.
- Use paper towels to wipe up meat juices, then discard the paper towels. Wash sponges in the dishwasher at least every other day. Wash dishcloths and kitchen towels in hot water and machine dry. Hang kitchen towels promptly after each use to air-dry and discourage growth of bacteria.
- Wash utensils and cutting boards thoroughly with hot, soapy water after preparing raw meat, poultry, or fish and before using them to prepare other uncooked foods, such as salad ingredients. When possible, use separate cutting boards.
- If you use a wood cutting board for meat or poultry, never use it to prepare other foods, regardless of how well you wash it. Wood can absorb bacteria, and it is difficult to clean thoroughly.
- Wash cutting boards with soap and hot water after each use and allow them to air-dry. Wash glass, solid wood, and plastic cutting boards in the dishwasher. Discard a plastic cutting board when it gets excessively cut up.
- Sanitize cutting boards at least once a week with a solution of 2 teaspoons of chlorine (household) bleach in 1 quart of water. Leave the bleach solution standing on the surface of the cutting board for 5 minutes, rinse well, and allow to air-dry.
- Avoid eating raw eggs (common in homemade ice cream, homemade mayonnaise, Caesar salad, hollandaise sauce, and homemade "energy" drinks). Cook eggs until both the yolks and whites are set (not runny).
- Cook all meat, poultry, and fish thoroughly. An estimated 5 percent of all meat is contaminated with *E. coli* bacteria, and these bacteria are not destroyed by refrigeration or freezing. Approximately 25 percent of all chicken marketed in the United States is contaminated with salmonella bacteria. The only way to destroy any bacteria in meat is to cook it thoroughly. The juices of pork and chicken should run clear, with no trace of pink in the meat. Cook beef until it is at least medium rare; the more rare the beef, the greater the risk for food-borne illness. Cook fish until the thickest part is opaque and flakes easily with a fork. Ground meat and poultry pose the greatest risk for contamination, because bacteria on the surface can be mixed into the meat during grinding. Make sure all ground meat is cooked thoroughly, with no traces of pink.

- Never place cooked meat on the same plate that held the raw meat.
- Do not leave cooked foods standing at room temperature for longer than 2 hours; refrigerate leftovers immediately.

Finally, if you have any question regarding the safety of a food item, it is best to not eat it. The rule of thumb is "When in doubt, throw it out."

HOW TO CHOOSE NUTRITIOUS FOODS

Altogether, people need about 40 vitamins and minerals. How can they meet their needs for all these nutrients? Eating wisely usually does not mean making drastic changes, more often it just means fine-tuning your current diet a little. Eat this food more often, and eat that food a little less often. For many people, a helpful way to plan adequate, balanced diets is the Food Guide Pyramid.

Food Guide Pyramid

The **Food Guide Pyramid**, shown in Figure 8.5, can help a diet planner design an adequate and balanced diet. The pyramid conveys three essential elements of a healthy diet:

- Proportion. Eat different amounts every day from the basic food groups. The shape of the pyramid tells you at a glance that grains, vegetables, and fruits should make up the bulk of your diet.
- Moderation. Use fats and sugars sparingly.
- Variety. Choose different foods from each major food group every day.

The widest level of the pyramid, or the base, indicates the foods you should eat in greater amounts. The top level, indicates the foods you should eat in smaller amounts.

LEVEL 1: BREADS AND GRAINS At the base of the pyramid are grains, cereals, pastas, and breads. It is recommended that 6 to 11 servings a day come from foods in this group. These foods supply complex carbohydrate, riboflavin, thiamin, niacin, iron, and other nutrients. Within this group, you should focus on whole-grain foods that are lowest in fat and eat refined foods from this group (white bread, white rice, refined cereals) in moderation.

Food Guide Pyramid A food group plan that assigns foods to five major food groups; developed by the U.S. Department of Agriculture.

FIGURE **8.5** FOOD GUIDE PYRAMID.

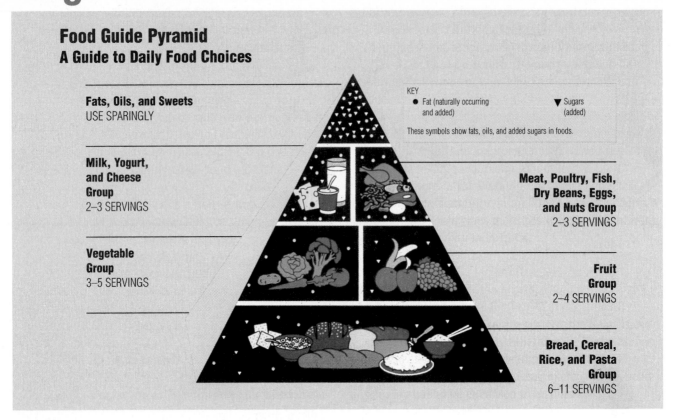

Food Guide Pyramid
A Guide to Daily Food Choices

Fats, Oils, and Sweets
USE SPARINGLY

Milk, Yogurt,
and Cheese
Group
2–3 SERVINGS

Vegetable
Group
3–5 SERVINGS

Meat, Poultry, Fish,
Dry Beans, Eggs,
and Nuts Group
2–3 SERVINGS

Fruit
Group
2–4 SERVINGS

Bread, Cereal,
Rice, and Pasta
Group
6–11 SERVINGS

KEY
● Fat (naturally occurring and added)   ▼ Sugars (added)
These symbols show fats, oils, and added sugars in foods.

Trying to get as many as 11 servings a day of complex carbohydrates may seem overwhelming until you figure out what a serving is. Some examples of a single serving from the grains, cereals, pastas, and breads group are

- ½ cup of cooked rice
- ½ cup of cooked cereal, or 1 ounce of dry cereal (about one-fourth of a bowl)
- 1 pancake
- 3 pretzels or 6 snack crackers
- 1 tortilla
- ½ of a hamburger bun

LEVEL 2: VEGETABLES AND FRUITS | Most vegetables and fruits are naturally low in calories and rich in nutrients. You should eat 3 to 5 servings of vegetables a day. Vegetables supply carbohydrate, Vitamin A, folate, and other nutrients. A serving of vegetables is considered to be ½ cup of chopped fresh, frozen, or canned vegetables; ¼ cup of dried vegetables; 1 cup of raw leafy vegetables; or ¾ cup of vegetable juice (fresh, frozen, or canned). To save the nutrients in vegetables, they should not be cooked in water or overcooked. Baking, steaming, and microwaving vegetables best preserves the nutrients.

Eating them raw, when possible, is also beneficial. Eating well-scrubbed skins (of apples or potatoes, for instance) boosts fiber in the diet, as does eating the edible seeds of fruits (such as the seeds in strawberries, raspberries, and pomegranates).

The USDA recommends at least two to four servings of fresh fruits or fruit juices each day. Fruits supply carbohydrate, Vitamins A and C, potassium, and other nutrients. A serving is considered to be 1 whole fresh fruit (such as a medium banana or medium apple); ½ cup of raw, cooked, or canned fruit; ¼ cup of dried fruit; or ¾ cup of fruit juice (fresh, frozen, or canned).

LEVEL 3: MEATS AND DAIRY | You need fewer servings of meats and dairy, so they fall nearer the top of the pyramid. The USDA recommends 2 to 3 servings a day of meats or meat alternatives. These foods supply protein, iron, niacin, folate, zinc, and other nutrients. The best sources are low in fat: fish, skinless poultry, lean cuts of meat, dried beans, and peas, for example.

Skim milk and whole milk have equal amounts of calcium.

The key with meats is to serve smaller portions than you probably are accustomed to. A single serving of cooked protein is only 2 to 3 ounces, or about the size of a deck of playing cards. The following non-meat proteins can substitute for 1 ounce of meat:

- 3 ounces of tofu
- 1 egg
- 2 tablespoons of peanut butter
- ½ cup of dried beans or peas, cooked
- ¼ cup nuts

Adults need 2 to 3 servings of dairy products daily. Dairy products provide carbohydrate, calcium, riboflavin, protein, Vitamin D, and other nutrients. Teenagers and pregnant or breast-feeding women need 3 to 4 servings. Pregnant or breast-feeding teens need 4 servings. Again, the best of these are low in fat, such as low-fat or skim milk, 1% cottage cheese, and part-skim cheeses (such as ricotta and mozzarella).

A single serving of dairy food consists of 1 cup of milk, 1 cup of yogurt, 2 ounces of processed cheese, 1½ ounces of natural cheese, ½ cup of cottage cheese, or 1½ cups of ice cream or frozen yogurt.

LEVEL 4: FATS AND SUGARS

The foods at the tip of the pyramid—fats, oils, and sweets—should be eaten sparingly. No recommended servings are given. A diet with too much saturated fat can increase the risk of heart disease. Sugars are high in calories but have no nutritional value. Excessive sugar contributes to tooth decay. Eating too many sweets fills you up without providing the nutrients you need for a balanced diet.

The beauty of the Food Guide Pyramid lies in its simplicity and ease of learning. It is not rigid; it can be used with great flexibility. For example, cheese can be substituted for milk because both supply the same nutrients (calcium, protein, and riboflavin) in about the same amounts.

When you plan your meals, remember that your own body is unique. It responds to food in its own characteristic ways according to its genetic inheritance and current needs. For example, a sedentary young woman who tends to gain weight may need to take steps to reduce her intake of fat, but an active young man who tends to stay thin might need to consume more calorie-dense foods. She needs to avoid storing excess calories from fat; he needs them to add body weight. The point here is to think carefully about your own body and its needs before taking any dietary actions. Assessment 8-4 can help you evaluate the quality of your diet. If you have special concerns, see a nutrition expert—a registered dietitian.

STRATEGIES: SELECTING NUTRITIOUS FOODS

To select nutritious foods:

1. Given the choice between whole foods and refined, processed foods, choose the former (apples rather than apple pie; potatoes rather than potato chips). Fewer nutrients have been refined out of the whole foods; less fat, salt, and sugar have been added.
2. When choosing meats, choose the lean ones. Select fish or poultry often, beef seldom. Ask for broiled, not fried, to control your fat intake.
3. Use both raw and cooked vegetables and fruits. Raw foods offer more fiber and vitamins, such as folate and thiamin that are destroyed by cooking. Cooking foods frees other vitamins and minerals for absorption.
4. Include milk, milk products, or other calcium sources for the calcium you need. Use low-fat or nonfat items to reduce fat and calories.
5. Learn to use margarine, butter, and oils sparingly; only a little gives flavor; a lot overloads you with fat and calories.
6. Vary your choices. Eat broccoli today, carrots tomorrow, and corn the next day. Eat Chinese today, Italian tomorrow, and hot dogs and beans on Saturday.
7. Load your plate with vegetables and unrefined starchy foods. A small portion of meat or cheese is all you need for protein.
8. When choosing breads and cereals, choose the whole-grain varieties.

To select nutritious fast foods:

9. Choose the broiled sandwich with lettuce, tomatoes, and other goodies—and hold the mayo—rather than the fish or chicken patties coated with breadcrumbs and cooked in fat.
10. Select a salad—and use more plain vegetables than those mixed with oily or mayonnaise-based dressings.
11. Order chili with more beans than meat. Choose a soft bean burrito over tacos with fried shells.
12. Drink low-fat milk rather than a cola beverage.

When choosing from a vending machine:

13. Choose cracker sandwiches over chips and pork rinds (virtually pure fat). Choose peanuts, pretzels, and popcorn over cookies and candy.
14. Choose milk and juices over cola beverages.

NUTRIENT SUPPLEMENTS

Billions of dollars are spent on vitamin pills—actually, vitamin-mineral supplements—each year. Some people who haven't learned enough about nutrition think they need supplements as insurance against their own poor food choices. Indeed, their food choices may be poor, but taking supplements is no guarantee that they will obtain the particular nutrients they need. It is just as likely that they will duplicate the nutrients their food supply provides and still lack the ones they need. The only way to be sure to get the needed assortment of nutrients is to construct a balanced diet from a variety of foods. Besides, no supplement can give you all the nutrients you get from food.

No one supplement can match a balanced diet, and no combination of supplements can, either. No one knows enough yet to construct a synthetic substitute for food. Even in hospitals where the most advanced technology is available and advanced formulas are supplied for patients who cannot eat, these formulas only enable patients to survive. The patients do not thrive until they are consuming food again.

Nutrient supplements are useful at times. A person may need a specific nutrient to counteract a specific deficiency—iron for iron-deficiency anemia, for example. But it takes medical training and tests to make a correct diagnosis; people cannot diagnose their own deficiencies.

Other times that you may consider taking a supplement: (1) If your energy intake is below 1,500 calories per day, because you will have difficulty consuming enough food to meet your vitamin and mineral needs; and (2) if you know that, for whatever reason, you will be eating irregularly for a limited time.

Whenever a health care provider has recommended a supplement, carefully follow directions as to the type and dose to take. A single, balanced, vitamin-mineral supplement should suffice. Look for one in which the nutrient levels are at or slightly below the RDA and avoid preparations that have high levels of nutrients to avoid toxicities.

Remember, you will still be getting some nutrients from food.

High doses of vitamins and minerals should be avoided. Excessive intakes can cause as many health problems as deficient intakes. Table 8.7 lists tolerable upper intake levels or levels that are likely to cause toxicity. Be sure to keep your intake at a safe level, not too low and not too high.

Iron supplementation frequently is recommended for women who have heavy menstrual flow. Some pregnant and lactating women also may require supplements. In specific instances, supplements should be selected with the advice of a registered dietitian.

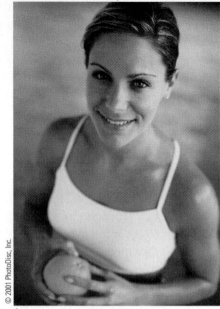

Once you are achieving the dietary behaviors you seek, congratulate yourself.

For healthy people with a balanced diet, most supplements do not seem to provide additional benefits. They do not help people run faster, jump higher, relieve stress, improve sexual prowess, cure a common cold, or boost energy levels.

If your diet does not follow the recommended guidelines, it is best to make changes in your diet rather than rely on a pill for nutrient needs. Outline the changes you need to make, then design a plan that helps you accomplish those changes. Little by little, start to substitute nutritious foods for some empty-calorie foods. Once you are achieving the dietary behaviors you desire, congratulate yourself. You'll begin to feel better and your body will appreciate it!

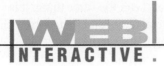

WEB ACTIVITIES

■ **American Dietetic Association** This comprehensive site features daily food tips, frequently asked questions, nutrition resources, and links to other reliable Web sites on nutrition.
http://www.eatright.org

■ **Dietary Guidelines** from the Food and Nutrition Information Center. This site not only features the 2000 American Dietary guidelines, but also has links to historical dietary guidelines (since 1894) and dietary guidelines from 20 countries.
http://www.nal.usda.gov/fnic/dga/index.html

■ **CyberDiet's Eating Out Guidelines** This site features information on healthy food selections from the following cuisines: USA, France, India, Mexico, Italy, Thailand, Japan, China, and Greece.
http://www.CyberDiet.com/foodfact/eatguide.html

■ **The Cyberkitchen** This very interactive site, sponsored by Shape Up America, will show you how to balance your dietary intake with your physical activity to maintain healthy weight. You provide personal information regarding your age, gender, height, weight, and activity level, and the Cyberkitchen provides you with a healthy diet plan to meet your goals (weight loss or weight gain). It's fun and educational.
http://www.shapeup.org/kitchen/frameset1.htm

■ **The Diet Analysis Web Site** This interactive site allows you to enter a variety of foods to receive a complete nutritional review of your diet based on the Recommended Dietary Allowances for your age and gender.
http://dawp.anet.com/cgi-bin/w3-msql/dawp.html

■ **The Interactive Food Guide Pyramid** Click on the different components of the Food Guide Pyramid to learn how to incorporate the proper nutrients into your daily diet.
http://www.nal.usda.gov:8001/py/pmap.htm

InfoTrac

You can find additional readings related to wellness via InfoTrac College Edition, an on-line library of more than 900 journals and publications. Follow the instructions for accessing InfoTrac that came packaged with your textbook, then search for articles using a key word search.

Suggested Reading Marisa Fox, "Brave New Foods," *Women's Sports and Fitness* 3, no. 6 (June 2000): 104.

1. What is the name of a plant chemical found in tomatoes, red grapefruit, and other fruits and vegetables that is linked to lower rates of cancer and heart disease?
2. What are some of the benefits of eating eggs? What are some of the drawbacks?
3. What are the common types of phytochemicals found in soy? What are some of the health benefits of soy products?

Web Activity
Nutrition Analysis Tool
http://www.ag.uiuc.edu/~food-lab/nat

Sponsor University of Illinois—Urbana/Champaign Council on Food and Agricultural Research.

Description This site features a personalized nutrition assessment tool that allows you to analyze the foods you eat for a variety of nutrients.

Available Activities

1. This site consists of an interactive personalized diet analysis tool that will provide you with nutrient content of foods that you select from a comprehensive database.

   • Nutrition Analysis
   • Energy Calculator
   • Soy Food Finder

Web Work

1. Click on the "Step by Step" button.
2. Enter your age and gender. Click the "Step 2" button.
3. Select the nutrient or nutrients that you would like to include in your analysis.
4. Go back to the home page and select the "Direct to NAT" link. Add the first food to your personal diet list by clicking in the white box above this list and typing the name of the food you wish to add. Then press Enter or click on "Add Food."
5. The Nutrient Analysis Tool now searches its extensive database. NAT will return a list of all the food items that match the word or words you typed in. The personal diet list keeps track of all the foods you add, the serving size and number of servings for each food, and the total gram weight of each food you add.
6. Scroll down the list of foods from the database that match your typed food and click on the radio button that best corresponds to it. Then, click on the "Add Selected Food" button below this list.

7. Type the number of servings in the appropriate box and use the scroll-down menu to select your serving size. Click on the "Add this Amount" button.

8. This takes you back to the "Add New Food" page. Type in the name of the second food product that you would like analyzed and follow the instructions above. Repeat steps #4–8 for each new food you desire to add to your personal diet list.

9. Finally, click on the "Analyze Food" button to receive your results for the selected nutrients.

Helpful Hints

1. The database has almost every type of food, but some foods may be listed under a different name. http://www.eatright.org

2. If you have trouble finding a particular food, try using other words that mean the same thing. It is best to start with general terms and then narrow the choices down by using more specific terms that describe the food, its contents, or even how it is prepared.

For additional Web activities, links, and suggested readings, visit our Health, Fitness, and Wellness Resource Center at http://health.wadsworth.com.

NOTES

1. E. Whitney et al., Understanding Nutrition, 8th Edition (St. Paul: West Publishing, 1999).

2. J. Brody, *Jane Brody's Nutrition Book* (NY: Bantam Books, 1987).

3. Committee on Dietary Reference Intakes, Dietary Reference Intakes for Calcium, Phosphorus, Magnesium, Vitamin D, and Fluoride (Washington, DC:, National Academy Press, 1997).

4. Committee on Dietary Reference Intakes, Dietary Reference Intakes for Thiamin, Riboflavin, Niacin, Vitamin B$_6$, Folate, Vitamin B$_{12}$, Pantothenic acid, Biotin, and Choline (Washington, DC:, National Academy Press, 1998).

5. J. King, "The Need to Consider Functional Endpoints in Defining Nutrient Requirements," *American Journal of Clinical Nutrition* 63 (1996): 983S.

6. W. Mertz, "Risk Assessment of Essential Trace Elements: New Approaches to Setting Recommended Dietary Allowances and Safety Limits," *Nutrition Reviews* 53 (1995): 179–185.

TEST FOR FATS

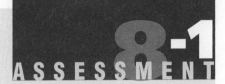

Name: _____   Date: _____   Grade: _____

Instructor: _____   Course: _____   Section: _____

True/False

1. Egg yolks contain the "bad" cholesterol called LDL.

2. Mayonnaise made from canola oil has less fat than regular mayonnaise, which is generally made from soybean oil.

3. The more unsaturated fat a food has, the more it will raise blood-cholesterol levels.

4. Polyunsaturated fats are converted to saturated fats when heated, such as in deep-fat frying.

5. A jar of peanut butter labeled "cholesterol free" is better than regular brands.

6. A label that reads "95% fat free" means the food derives only 5 percent of its calories from fat.

7. The best way to decrease blood-cholesterol levels is to eat less cholesterol.

8. A third of the average U.S. woman's fat intake comes from salad dressing, margarine, cheese, and beef.

9. A label that reads "low cholesterol" means the food has fewer calories than regular brands and no saturated fat.

10. Veggie burgers are always a low-fat alternative to hamburgers.

Multiple Choice

Select the best answer to the following questions.

11. A product's label says it contains only vegetable oils. It would be
    a. high in only saturated fat.
    b. high in only unsaturated fat.
    c. high in either saturated fat or unsaturated fat.
    d. high in unsaturated fat and might contain some cholesterol.

12. A woman has a total blood-cholesterol level of 220 mg/dl and an HDL level of 60 mg/dl. What is this person's ratio of total cholesterol to HDL cholesterol? Is she at high or low risk for heart disease?
    a. 3:7 ratio and low risk
    b. 2:7 ratio and low risk
    c. 7:2 ratio and low risk
    d. 4:5 ratio and high risk

13. A 5-ounce serving of ground beef has how much more fat than the same size serving of skinless chicken breast?
    a. 50 percent   c. 75 percent
    b. 65 percent   d. 95 percent

14. There are 30 grams of fat and 309 calories in an avocado. What is the percentage of fat calories?
    a. 42 percent   c. 87 percent
    b. 62 percent   d. 97 percent

15. A food is considered low-fat if it has how many grams of fat per 100 calories?
    a. 3   c. 10
    b. 5   d. 30

16. According to the American Heart Association, people ideally should adopt a low-fat diet that contains no more than 30 percent fat calories
    a. starting at birth.
    b. at 2 years of age.
    c. at puberty.
    d. in early adulthood.

17. An olive-oil label states that the product is "extra light." This means
    a. it has a lighter color and taste than other olive oils.
    b. it weighs less.
    c. it has fewer calories.
    d. it is lower in saturated fats.

18. Whole milk gets 48 percent of its calories from fat. What percentage of calories come from fat in 2% low-fat milk?
    a. 2 percent   c. 25 percent
    b. 15 percent   d. 30 percent

19. Experts recommend limiting your saturated-fat intake to no more than 10 percent of total calorie intake. If you eat 2,000 calories per day, your saturated-fat allowance would be
    a. 10 grams   c. 27 grams
    b. 22 grams   d. 36 grams

20. A Taco Bell taco salad contains how many teaspoons of fat?
    a. 9   c. 15
    b. 12   d. 25

From Elizabeth Somer, "Facing Fats," *SHAPE* (January, 1994). Reprinted with permission.

Answers:

1. **False.** LDL is a carrier of cholesterol in the blood. It is not found in food.

2. **False.** They contain similar amounts of fat and calories.

3. **False.** The more *saturated* fat in your diet, the more your blood-cholesterol level will be raised.

4. **False.** However, frying does expose these fats to oxygen, and once oxidized, they can increase heart-disease risk.

5. **False.** Cholesterol is found only in animal products.

6. **False.** The label refers only to fat content by weight. The percentage of calories from fat would be much higher. For instance, a 95% fat-free Janet Lee Chopped Ham contains 60% fat calories (2 grams of fat per 30-calorie slice).

7. **False.** Reducing your saturated fat intake is the most important dietary factor for lowering blood cholesterol.

8. **True.** The average woman in the United States gets 9 percent of her fat from salad dressing, 8 percent from margarine, 8 percent from cheese and 7 percent from beef, for a total of one-third.

9. **False.** A food can be cholesterol-free and still be high in calories and/or saturated fat.

10. **False.** Commercial veggie burgers get anywhere from 6 to 66 percent of their calories from fat.

11. **c.** Most vegetable oils are high in unsaturated fats. However, manufacturers also use tropical oils, such as palm or coconut oils, which are as saturated as lard.

12. **a.**

13. **d.**

14. **c.**

15. **a.** There are 9 calories per gram of fat, so a food that has 3 grams of fat per 100 calories is 27% fat; a food that is less than 30% fat is considered low fat.

16. **b.**

17. **a.**

18. **d.**

19. **b.**

20. **c.**

To find your score, total your correct answers.

18 or more: All of that label reading has paid off! You are a bona fide fat sleuth.

15 to 17: You put the average American to shame. If you practice what you know, your diet is probably within the low-fat zone.

12 to 14: You keep company with the majority of Americans and may be confused when it comes to fat. Review the answers and see if you can improve your score.

Less than 12: Oops. It's time to take the fat issue more seriously.

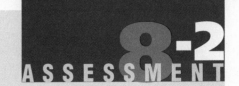

Name: _____

Date: _____   Grade: _____

Instructor: _____

Course: _____   Section: _____

Are You Meeting Your Fiber Quota?

To find out how close you come to meeting your daily fiber quota, keep track of everything you eat for 3 days. Then, take the quiz below and add up your points. This quiz was developed with assistance from nutrition lecturer Liz Applegate and nutrition professor Judith Stern, both at the University of California, Davis.

1. What type of bread (including rolls and muffins) did you usually eat?

   a. whole-wheat or whole-grain   +4
   b. white or partial whole-wheat   +2

2. How many servings of oat products did you average daily? (1 serving = 1 cup cooked oatmeal or oat bran.)

   a. 2 or more   +4
   b. 1   +3
   c. 1/2   +2
   d. none   0

3. How many times during the last 3 days did you eat beans (legumes), such as kidney beans, pintos, garbanzos, soybeans, lentils, and split peas?

   a. 3 or more   +4
   b. 2   +3
   c. 1   +2
   d. none   0

4. How many times during the 3-day period did you eat high-fiber breakfast cereals?

   a. 3 or more   +4
   b. 2   +3
   c. 1   +2
   d. none   0

5. How many times during the 3-day period did you eat cooked whole-grain side dishes, such as brown rice or barley?

   a. 3 or more   +4
   b. 2   +3
   c. 1   +2
   d. none   0

6. Approximately how many servings of canned or fresh fruits and vegetables did you eat daily? (Use an average from the previous 3 days. 1 serving = 1/2 cup cooked or 1 cup or 1 piece raw.)

   a. 7 or more   +5
   b. 5–6   +4
   c. 3–4   +2
   d. 1–2   +1
   e. none   −2

Scoring: If your overall score is over 20, your fiber intake is probably adequate. If it is lower, try to increase your fiber intake using the foods mentioned above. Be sure to increase your water intake when you eat more fiber.

Check Your Calcium Intake

If you are not a fan of dairy products, you may be coming up far short of your calcium needs. But even if you are a milk lover, how much calcium your body actually absorbs depends upon your genetic makeup and other factors. And how much you retain depends upon your intake of salt and protein. This duo may increase the elimination of calcium, causing your body to steal calcium it needs from your bones.

The following quiz was developed with the assistance of Robert P. Heaney, professor of medicine at Creighton University School of Medicine, Omaha, Nebraska. It can tell you how close your diet comes to providing the appropriate amount of bone food. Just check the answer that applies to you.

1. I eat a serving of yogurt (8 ounces), milk (1 cup), or cheese (1 ounce) at least once a day.

   ____ True   +3
   ____ False   −1

2. Dairy products give me gas and bloating, so I avoid them.

   ____ True   −1
   ____ False   +1

3. I make sure I eat one or more of the following nondairy sources of calcium at least 3 times a week: leafy green vegetables (kale or broccoli), shellfish (oysters or clams), or canned fish with edible bones (salmon or sardines).

   ____ True   +1
   ____ False   0

4. I make an effort to slip dairy foods into my diet whenever I can (grating cheese over salads, for example).

____ True   +1
____ False   0

5. I eat calcium-enriched forms of products (such as breakfast cereal or fruit juice) whenever possible.

____ True   +1
____ False   −1

6. When given a choice, I drink carbonated soft drinks over low-fat dairy drinks or water.

____ True   −1
____ False   0

7. I tend to get my protein from meats.

____ True   −1
____ False   +1

8. I usually salt food automatically without tasting it.

____ True   −1
____ False   +1

Scoring: If you scored between 7 and 9, you are laying the dietary foundation for a rock-solid skeleton. (Remember, though, that even if you scored a perfect 9, you may still have a bone deficit if you are inactive, underweight or post-menopausal, have a family history of osteoporosis, or take aluminum-based antacids or other calcium-robbing drugs.) If you scored between 4 and 6, try to include more low-fat dairy products and go easy on the calcium bandits. If you scored below 4, your skeleton may be becoming perilously porous. Learn to love low-fat yogurt and make friends with skim milk. Ask your doctor about taking a calcium supplement.

Can You Find the Hidden Salt?

If you've already banned the saltshaker from the table and sworn off salty snacks—good for you! But to keep your intake at the recommended one-teaspoon-a-day limit takes a bit more vigilance. Three-fourths of your dietary sodium is hidden in already-prepared foods, experts say. And many salt-laced foods, such as cereal, diet soda, and instant pudding don't taste a bit salty.

Just how good are you at avoiding this hidden salt? If you're eating more potassium-rich fresh fruits and vegetables than packaged convenience foods, for example, you're probably doing great.

Take this quiz to find out where you stand on the hidden salt scale.

1. When barbecuing meat or fish, I'm more likely to brush on herbs or homemade marinara sauce than commercial ketchup, barbecue sauce, or soy sauce.

____ True   +1
____ False   −1

2. The fresh or frozen fruits and vegetables and lean meats in my grocery cart usually crowd out the canned, and processed foods.

____ True   +1
____ False   −1

3. I buy only the low-salt type of margarine.

____ True   +1
____ False   −1

4. I usually have dehydrated, instant versions of soups, sauces, salad dressings, oatmeal, or other foods on hand.

____ True   −1
____ False   +1

5. I steam, microwave, broil, or stir-fry vegetables rather than boil them.

____ True   +1
____ False   −1

6. Processed cheese never passes my lips.

____ True   +1
____ False   −1

7. I rinse canned foods such as tuna, ham, and beans before preparing them.

____ True   +1
____ False   −1

8. I'm a sucker for deli food—cold cuts, prepared salads, pastrami, ham, smoked fish, and so on.

____ True   −1
____ False   +1

9. I usually order my hamburger with the works—pickles, ketchup, mustard and special sauce.

____ True   −1
____ False   +1

10. When dining out, I usually order oil and vinegar dressing for my salad and ask for gravies and sauces on the side.

____ True   +1
____ False   −1

Scoring: 8–10: You're a top-notch salt sleuth. 5–7: There's room for improvement. Scan food labels closely for the key phrases "sodium-free" or "very low sodium." Below 5: You're probably relying on too many prepared condiments and packaged convenience foods. Try to cut down on these.

IS OSTEOPOROSIS IN YOUR FUTURE?

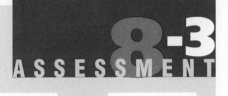

Name: _____ Date: _____ Grade: _____

Instructor: _____ Course: _____ Section: _____

Risk factors you CANNOT control:

		YES	NO
1.	Are you female?	☐	☐
2.	Do you have a family history of osteoporosis?	☐	☐
3.	Are your ancestors from the British Isles, northern Europe, China, or Japan?	☐	☐
4.	Are you very fair-skinned?	☐	☐
5.	Are you small-boned?	☐	☐
6.	Are you over age 35?	☐	☐
7.	Have you had your ovaries removed, or did you have an early menopause?	☐	☐
8.	Are you allergic to milk and milk products?	☐	☐
9.	Have you never been pregnant?	☐	☐
10.	Do you have cancer or kidney disease?	☐	☐
11.	Do you have to take chemotherapy, steroids, anticonvulsants, or anticoagulants?	☐	☐

Risk factors you CAN control:

		YES	NO
12.	Do you smoke?	☐	☐
13.	Do you drink alcohol?	☐	☐
14.	Do you avoid milk and cheese in your diet?	☐	☐
15.	Do you get very little exercise?	☐	☐
16.	Do you drink a lot of soft drinks?	☐	☐
17.	Is your diet high in protein?	☐	☐
18.	Do you consume a lot of caffeine (five or more cups of coffee per day or equivalent)?	☐	☐
19.	Are you amenorrheic (without a monthly period)?	☐	☐
20.	Do you get less than 1,000 mg of calcium a day?	☐	☐
21.	Is your body weight very low?	☐	☐
22.	Do you go on extreme or crash diets?	☐	☐
23.	Do you have a high sodium (salt) intake?	☐	☐

If you answered "yes" to three (3) of the above questions, you are at risk for osteoporosis and may want to ask your doctor to give you a bone density screening test. The more questions you answered "yes" to, the higher your risk of developing osteoporosis in the future.

Many clinical studies suggest that osteoporosis is a preventable disease. As you can see from the quiz, you can do several things right now to help prevent osteoporosis in your future.

Adapted from *Marion Laboratories, Inc.*

RATE YOUR DIET

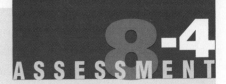
Name: _____ Date: _____ Grade: _____

Instructor: _____ Course: _____ Section: _____

These 39 questions will give you a rough sketch of your typical eating habits. the (+) or (–) number for each answer instantly pats you on the back for good eating habits or alerts you to problems you didn't even know you had. The quiz focuses on fat, saturated fat, cholesterol, sodium, sugar, fiber, and fruits and vegetables. It doesn't attempt to cover everything in your diet. Also, it doesn't try to measure precisely how much of the key nutrients you eat.

Instructions

Next to each answer is a number with a + or − sign in front of it. *Circle the number that corresponds to the answer you choose.* That's your score for the question. If two or more answers apply, circle each one. Then average them to get your score for the question.

How to average. In answering question 19, for example, if your sandwich-eating is equally divided among tuna salad (−2), roast beef (+1) and turkey breast (+3), add the three scores (which gives you +2) and then divide by three. That gives you a score of +²/₃ for the question. Round it to +1.

Pay attention to serving sizes, which we give when needed. For example, a serving of vegetables is ¹/₂ cup. If you usually eat one cup of vegetables at a time, count it as two servings.

Fruits, Vegetables, Grains & Beans

1. How many servings of fruit or 100% fruit juice do you eat per day? *(OMIT fruit snacks like Fruit Roll-Ups and fruit-on-the-bottom yogurt. One serving = one piece or ¹/₂ cup of fruit or 6 oz. of fruit juice.)*
   - (a) 0 . . . . –3
   - (b) less than 1 . . . . . . –2
   - (c) 1 0
   - (d) 2 . . . . +1
   - (e) 3 . . . . +2
   - (f) 4 or more . . . . +3

2. How many servings of non-fried vegetables do you eat per day? *(One serving = ¹/₂ cup. INCLUDE potatoes.)*
   - (a) 0 . . . . –3
   - (b) less than 1 . . . . . . –2
   - (c) 1 0
   - (d) 2 . . . . +1
   - (e) 3 . . . . +2
   - (f) 4 or more . . . . +3

3. How many servings of vitamin-rich vegetables do you eat per week? *(One serving = ¹/₂ cup, ONLY count broccoli, Brussels sprouts, carrots, collards, kale, red pepper, spinach, sweet potatoes, or winter squash.)*
   - (a) 0 . . . . –3
   - (b) 1 to 3 . . . .+1
   - (c) 4 to 6 . . . . +2
   - (d) 7 or more . . . . +3

4. How many servings of leafy green vegetables do you eat per week? *(One serving = ¹/₂ cup cooked or 1 cup raw. ONLY count collards, kale, mustard greens, romaine lettuce, spinach, or Swiss chard.)*
   - (a) 0 . . . . –3
   - (b) less than 1 . . . . . . –2
   - (c) 1 to 2 . . . .+1
   - (d) 3 to 4 . . . . +2
   - (e) 5 or more . . . . +3

5. How many times per week does your lunch or dinner contain grains, vegetables, or beans, but little or no meat, poultry, fish, or eggs?
   - (a) 0 . . . . –1
   - (b) 1 to 2 . . . .+1
   - (c) 3 to 4 . . . . +2
   - (d) 5 or more . . . . +3

6. How many times per week do you eat dried beans, split peas, or lentils? *(OMIT green beans.)*
   - (a) 0 . . . . –3
   - (b) less than 1 . . . . . . –1
   - (c) 1 0
   - (d) 2 . . . . +1
   - (e) 3 . . . . +2
   - (f) 4 or more . . . . +3

7. How many servings of grains do you eat per day? *(One serving = 1 slice of bread, 1 oz. of crackers, 1 large pancake, 1 cup pasta or cold cereal, or ¹/₂ cup granola, cooked cereal, rice or bulgar. OMIT heavily sweetened cold cereals.)*
   - (a) 0 . . . . –3
   - (b) 1 to 2 0
   - (c) 3 to 4 . . . .+1
   - (d) 5 to 7 . . . . +2
   - (e) 8 or more . . . . +3

Source: From *Nutrition Action Healthletter*, May 1996. Reprinted with permission.

8. What type of bread, rolls, etc., do you eat?

   (a) 100% whole wheat as the only flour .... +3

   (b) whole wheat flour as the 1st or 2nd flour .... +2

   (c) rye, pumpernickel, or oatmeal .... +1

   (d) white, French, or Italian 0

9. What kind of breakfast cereal do you eat?

   (a) whole-grain (like oatmeal or Wheaties) .... +3

   (b) low-fiber (like Cream of Wheat or Corn Flakes) 0

   (c) sugary low-fiber (like Frosted Flakes) or
       low-fat granola .... −1

   (d) regular granola .... −2

10. How many times per week do you eat high-fat red meats
    *(hamburgers, pork chops, ribs, hot dogs, pot roast, sausage,
    bologna, steaks other than round steak, etc.)*?

    (a) 0 .... +3   (d) 2 .... −2

    (b) less than 1 ...... +2   (e) 3 .... −3

    (c) 1 .... −1   (f) 4 or more .... −4

11. How many times per week do you eat lean red meats *(hot
    dogs or luncheon meats with no more than 2 grams of fat per
    serving, round steak, or pork tenderloin)*?

    (a) 0 .... +3   (d) 2–3 .... −1

    (b) less than 1 ...... +1   (e) 4–5 .... −2

    (c) 1 0   (f) 6 or more .... −3

12. After cooking, how large is the serving of read meat you eat?
    *(To convert from raw to cooked, reduce by 25 percent. For
    example, 4 oz. of raw meat shrinks to 3 oz. after cooking.
    There are 16 oz. in a pound.)*

    (a) 6 oz. or more ....−3   (c) 3 oz. or less 0

    (b) 4 to 5 oz. ....−2   (d) don't eat red meat .... +3

13. If you eat red meat, do you trim the visible fat when you cook
    or eat it?

    (a) yes .... +1   (b) no .... −3

14. What kind of ground meat or poultry do you eat?

    (a) regular ground beef .... −4

    (b) ground beef that's 11% to 25% fat .... −3

    (c) ground chicken or 10% fat ground beef .... −2

    (d) ground turkey .... −1

    (e) ground turkey breast .... +3

    (f) don't eat ground meat or poultry .... +3

15. What chicken parts do you eat?

    (a) breast .... +3   (d) wing .... −2

    (b) drumstick .... +1   (e) don't eat poultry ..... +3

    (c) thigh .... −1

16. If you eat poultry, do you remove the skin before eating?

    (a) yes .... +2   (b) no .... −3

17. If you eat seafood, how many times per week? *(Omit deep-
    fried foods, tuna packed in oil, and mayonnaise-laden tuna
    salad—low-fat mayo is okay.)*

    (a) less than 1 0   (c) 2 .... +2

    (b) 1 .... +1   (d) 3 or more .... +3

Mixed Foods

18. What is your most typical breakfast? *(SUBTRACT an extra 3
    points if you also eat sausage.)*

    (a) biscuit sandwich or croissant sandwich .... −4

    (b) croissant, danish, or doughnut .... −3

    (c) don't eat breakfast .... −3

    (d) pancakes, French toast, or waffles .... −1

    (e) cereal, toast, or bagel .... +3

    (f) low-fat yogurt or low-fat cottage cheese .... +3

19. What sandwich fillings do you eat?

    (a) regular luncheon meat, or bologna .... −3

    (b) tuna, egg, or chicken salad or ham .... −2

    (c) peanut butter .... +1

    (d) roast beef .... +1

    (e) low-fat luncheon meat .... +1

    (f) tuna or chicken salad made with fat-free mayo ...... +3

    (g) turkey breast or hummus .... +3

20. What do you order on your pizza?

    (a) at least one vegetable topping .... +3

    (b) one lean meat topping 0

    (c) one high-fat meat topping (sausage, pepperoni) ..... −2

    (d) more than 1 high-fat meat topping .... −3

21. What do you put on your pasta?

    (a) sautéed vegetables .... +3

    (b) tomato sauce or red clam sauce .... +2

    (c) meat sauce or meat balls .... −1

    (d) pesto or another oily sauce .... −2

    (e) Alfredo or another creamy sauce .... −4

22. How many times per week do you eat deep-fried foods *(fish,
    chicken, french fries, potato chips, etc.*?

    (a) 0 .... +3   (d) 3 .... −2

    (b) 1 0   (e) 4 or more .... −3

    (c) 2 .... −1

23. At a salad bar, what do you choose?
    (a) no dressing, lemon, or vinegar . . . . +3
    (b) fat-free dressing . . . . +2
    (c) low- or reduced-calorie dressing. . . . . +1
    (d) oil and vinegar . . . . −1
    (e) regular dressing . . . . −2
    (f) cole slaw, pasta salad, or potato salad. . . . . −2

24. How many servings of low-fat calcium-rich foods do you eat
    per day? *(One serving = ⅔ cup low-fat or non-fat milk or
    yogurt, 1 oz. low-fat cheese, 1½ oz. sardines, 3½ oz. canned
    salmon with bones, 1 oz. tofu enriched with calcium, 1 cup
    collards or kale, or 200 mg of a calcium supplement.)*
    (a) 0 . . . . −3   (d) 2. . . . . +2
    (b) less than 1 . . . . . . −1   (e) 3 or more . . . . +3
    (c) 1 . . . . +1

Fats and Oils

25. What do you put on your bread, toast, bagel, or English
    muffin?
    (a) stick butter or cream cheese . . . . −4
    (b) stick margarine or whipped butter . . . . −3
    (c) regular tub margarine . . . . −2
    (d) light tub margarine or whipped light butter . . . . −1
    (e) jam, fat-free margarine, or fat-free cream cheese 0
    (f) nothing . . . . +3

26. What do you spread on your sandwiches?
    (a) mayonnaise. . . . . −2
    (b) light mayonnaise. . . . . −1
    (c) catsup, mustard, or fat-free mayonnaise . . . . +1
    (d) nothing. . . . . +2

27. With what do you make tuna salad, pasta salad, chicken salad,
    etc.?
    (a) mayonnaise. . . . . . −2   (c) fat-free mayonnaise. . . 0
    (b) light mayonnaise. . −1   (d) low-fat yogurt . . . . +2

28. What do you use to sauté vegetables or other foods?
    *(Vegetable oil includes safflower, corn, sunflower, and
    soybean.)*
    (a) butter or lard . . . . . −3   (d) olive or canola oil. . . . . +1
    (b) margarine . . . . −2   (e) broth . . . . +2
    (c) vegetable oil or   (f) cooking spray. . . . . . . +3
        light margarine . . . −1

Beverages

29. What do you drink on a typical day?
    (a) water, or low-fat or skim milk . . . . +3
    (b) caffeine-free coffee or tea 0
    (c) diet soda . . . . −1
    (d) coffee or tea (up to 4 a day) . . . . −1
    (e) regular soda (up to 2 a day) . . . . −2
    (f) regular soda (3 or more a day) . . . . −3
    (g) coffee or tea (5 or more a day) . . . . −3

30. What kind of "fruit" beverage do you drink?
    (a) orange, grapefruit, prune, or pineapple juice . . . . +3
    (b) apple, grape, or pear juice. . . . . +1
    (c) cranberry juice blend or cocktail 0
    (d) fruit "drink," "ade," or "punch" . . . . −3

31. What kind of milk do you drink?
    (a) whole . . . . −3   (c) 1% low-fat. . . . . +2
    (b) 2% fat 0   (d) skim. . . . . +3

Desserts and Snacks

32. What do you eat as a snack?
    (a) fruits or vegetables . . +3   (d) cookies or fried chips . . −2
    (b) low-fat yogurt . . . . . +2   (e) nuts or granola bar. . . . −2
    (c) low-fat crackers . . . . +1   (f) candy bar or pastry . . . −3

33. Which of the following "salty" snacks do you eat? *(AVERAGE
    two or more scores if necessary.)*
    (a) potato chips, corn chips, or popcorn . . . . −3
    (b) tortilla chips . . . . −2
    (c) salted pretzels or light microwave popcorn . . . . −1
    (d) unsalted pretzels. . . . . +2
    (e) baked tortilla or potato chips or homemade
        air-popped popcorn. . . . . +3
    (f) don't eat salty snacks . . . . +3

34. What kind of cookies do you usually eat?
    (a) fat-free cookies. . . . . +2
    (b) graham crackers or reduced-fat cookies . . . . +1
    (c) oatmeal cookies. . . . . −1
    (d) sandwich cookies (like Oreos) . . . . −2
    (e) chocolate coated, chocolate chip, or peanut butter . . . . −3
    (f) don't eat cookies. . . . . +3

35. What kind of cake or pastry do you eat?

    (a) cheesecake . . . . –4

    (b) pie or doughnuts . . . . –3

    (c) cake with frosting . . . . –2

    (d) cake without frosting . . . . –1

    (e) muffins 0

    (f) angel food, fat-free cake, or fat-free pastry . . . . +1

    (g) don't eat cakes or pastries . . . . +3

36. What kind of frozen dessert do you usually eat? *(SUBTRACT 1 point for each of the following toppings: hot fudge, nuts, or chocolate candy bars or pieces.)*

    (a) gourmet ice cream . . . . –3

    (b) regular ice cream . . . . –2

    (c) frozen yogurt or light ice cream 0

    (d) sorbet, sherbet, or ices 0

    (e) non-fat frozen yogurt or fat-free ice cream . . . . +3

SCORING YOUR DIET

Add up your score for each question.

Score

Score		
0 or below	Oops!	There is much room for improvement. Work on one positive change at a time.
1 to 29	Hmmm.	Don't be discouraged. This eating business is tough.
30 to 59	Yesss!	Congratulations. You can invite us over to eat any day.
60 or above	C-o-o-o-l.	Our photographer should be at your door any second.

9 BODY COMPOSITION ASSESSMENT

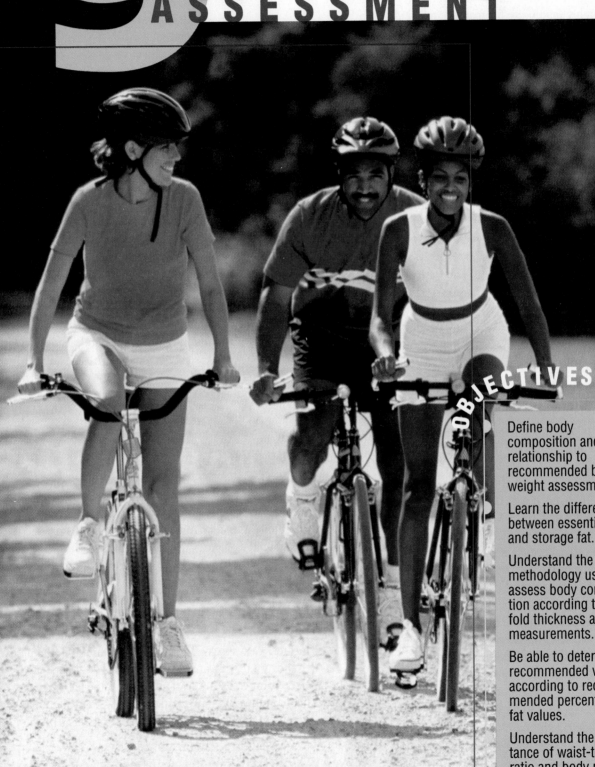

OBJECTIVES

Define body composition and its relationship to recommended body weight assessment.

Learn the difference between essential fat and storage fat.

Understand the methodology used to assess body composition according to skinfold thickness and girth measurements.

Be able to determine recommended weight according to recommended percent body fat values.

Understand the importance of waist-to-hip ratio and body mass index.

221

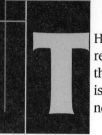

THE TERM **BODY COMPOSITION** is used in reference to the fat and nonfat components of the human body. The fat component usually is called fat mass or **percent body fat**. The nonfat component is termed **lean body mass**.

For many years, people relied on height/weight charts to determine **recommended body weight**. We now know, however, that these tables can be highly inaccurate for many people and fail to identify critical fat values associated with higher risk for disease. The proper way to determine recommended weight is through body composition by finding out what percent of total body weight is fat and what amount is lean tissue.

Once the fat percentage is known, recommended body weight can be calculated from recommended body fat. Recommended body weight, also called "healthy weight," is defined as the body weight at which there seems to be no harm to human health. This includes the absence of any medical condition that would improve with weight loss and a fat distribution pattern that is not associated with increased risk for illness.

> To determine whether people are truly overweight or falsely at recommended body weight, body composition should be established.

Although various techniques for determining percent body fat were developed several years ago, many people still are unaware of these procedures and continue to depend on height/weight charts to find out their recommended body weight. The standard height/weight tables were first published in 1912. They were based on average weights (including shoes and clothing) for men and women who obtained life insurance policies between 1888 and 1905. The recommended body weight on these tables is categorized according to gender, height, and frame size. Because no scientific guidelines are given to determine frame size, most people choose their frame size based on the column in which the weight comes closest to their own!

To determine whether people are **overweight** or falsely at recommended body weight, body composition must be established. **Obesity** means an excess of body fat. If body weight is the only criterion, an individual easily can be overweight according to height/weight charts, yet not have any excess body fat. Football players, body builders, weight lifters, and other athletes with large muscle size are typical examples. Some of these athletes who appear to be 20 or 30 pounds overweight really have little body fat.

TOO FAT?

The inaccuracy of height/weight charts was illustrated clearly when a young man who weighed about 225 pounds applied to join a city police force but was turned down without an interview. The reason? He was "too fat," according to the height/weight charts. When this young man's body composition later was assessed at a preventive medicine clinic, he was shocked to find out that only 5 percent of his total body weight was in the form of fat—considerably lower than the recommended standard. In the words of the technical director of the clinic, "The only way this fellow could come down to the chart's target weight would have been through surgical removal of a large amount of his muscle tissue."

At the other end of the spectrum, some people who weigh very little and are viewed by many as skinny or underweight can actually be classified as obese because of their high body fat content. People who weigh as little as 100 pounds but are more than 30 percent fat (about one-third of their total body weight) are not uncommon. These cases are found more often in sedentary people and those who are always dieting. Physical inactivity and constant negative caloric balance both lead to a loss in lean body mass (see Chapter 10). These examples clearly illustrate that body weight alone does not always tell the true story.

ESSENTIAL AND STORAGE FAT

Total fat in the human body is classified into two types: essential fat and storage fat. **Essential fat** is needed for normal physiological function. Without it, human health deteriorates. This type of fat is found in tissues such as muscles, nerve cells, bone marrow, intestines, heart, liver, and lungs. This essential fat constitutes about 3 percent of the total weight in men and 12 percent in women (see Figure 9.1). The percentage is higher in women because it includes sex-specific fat, such as that found in the breast tissue, the uterus, and other sex-related fat deposits.

Storage fat is the fat stored in adipose tissue, mostly beneath the skin (subcutaneous fat) and around major organs in the body. This fat serves three basic functions:

1. As an insulator to retain body heat
2. As energy substrate for metabolism
3. As padding against physical trauma to the body

FIGURE 9.1 TYPICAL BODY COMPOSITION OF AN ADULT MAN AND WOMAN.

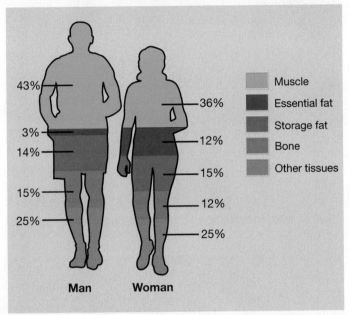

- 43%
- 3%
- 14%
- 15%
- 25%

- 36%
- 12%
- 15%
- 12%
- 25%

- Muscle
- Essential fat
- Storage fat
- Bone
- Other tissues

Man   **Woman**

The amount of storage fat does not differ between men and women except that men tend to store fat around the waist; women, around the hips and thighs.

TECHNIQUES FOR ASSESSING BODY COMPOSITION

Body composition can be assessed through several procedures. The most common techniques are (a) hydrostatic or underwater weighing, (b) skinfold thickness, (c) girth measurements, (d) bioelectrical impedance, and (e) air displacement. Because these procedures yield estimates of body fat, each technique may yield slightly different values. Therefore, when you assess your body composition, the same technique should be used for pre- and post-test comparisons.

Sophisticated techniques to assess body composition are presently available, but the equipment is costly and not readily accessible to the general population. These procedures are used primarily in research and medical facilities. In addition to measuring lean tissue and body fat, some of these newer methods also provide information on total body water and bone mass. Among these techniques are magnetic resonance imaging (MRI), dual energy X-ray absorptiometry (DEXA), computed tomography (CT), and total body electrical conductivity (TOBEC). However, in terms of predicting percent body fat, none appears to be more accurate than hydrostatic weighing.

Hydrostatic Weighing

Hydrostatic weighing is the standard of body composition assessment. Almost all other techniques to determine body composition are validated against hydrostatic weighing. It is the most accurate technique available if it is administered properly and if the individual is able to perform the test adequately. The psychological factor of being weighed while submerged in water makes hydrostatic weighing difficult to administer to the **aquaphobic**.

In this procedure, the subject is submerged in a tank of water and weighed after exhaling all air from the lungs. The resulting figures determine the percentages of lean tissue and fat in the body. The person's residual lung volume (the amount of air left in the lungs following complete forceful exhalation) must be measured to accurately determine percent body fat. If the residual volume cannot be measured, as is the case in many health/fitness centers, the volume is estimated using predicting equations, which may sacrifice the accuracy of the assessment.

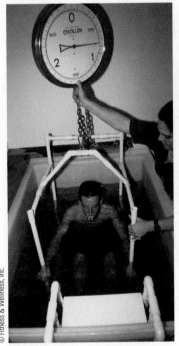

© Fitness & Wellness, Inc.

| Hydrostatic weighing technique used for body composition assessment. |

Body composition The fat and nonfat components of the human body; important in assessing recommended body weight.

Percent body fat Proportional amount of fat in the body based on the person's total weight; includes both essential and storage fat.

Lean body mass Body weight without body fat.

Recommended body weight Body weight at which there seems to be no harm to human health; healthy weight.

Overweight An excess amount of weight against a given standard, such as height or recommended percent body fat.

Obesity An excessive accumulation of body fat, usually at least 30 percent above recommended body weight.

Essential fat Minimal amount of body fat needed for normal physiological functions; constitutes about 3 percent of total weight in men and 12 percent in women.

Storage fat Body fat in excess of essential fat; stored in adipose tissue.

Hydrostatic weighing Underwater weighing technique to assess body composition; considered one of the most accurate techniques for body composition assessment.

Aquaphobic Having a fear of water.

Because of the cost, time, and complexity of hydrostatic weighing, most health and fitness programs prefer **anthropometric measurement techniques**, which correlate quite well with hydrostatic weighing. These techniques, primarily skinfold thickness and girth measurements, allow a quick, simple, and inexpensive estimate of body composition.

| Skinfold Thickness |

Assessing body composition using **skinfold thickness** is based on the principle that approximately half of the body's fatty tissue is directly beneath the skin. Valid and reliable estimates of this tissue give a good indication of percent body fat.

The skinfold test is done with the aid of pressure calipers. Several sites must be measured to reflect the total percentage of fat: triceps, suprailium, and thigh skinfolds for women; and chest, abdomen, and thigh for men (Figure 9.2). All measurements should be taken on the right side of the body.

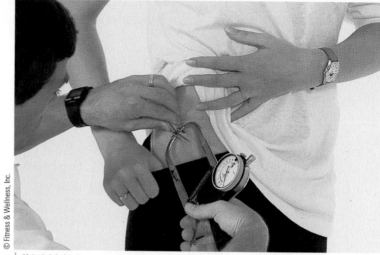

© Fitness & Wellness, Inc.

| Skinfold thickness technique used for the assessment of body composition. |

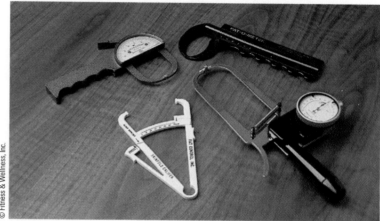

© Fitness & Wellness, Inc.

| Various types of skinfold calipers can be used to assess skinfold thickness. |

FIGURE 9.2 ANATOMICAL LANDMARKS FOR SKINFOLD MEASUREMENTS.

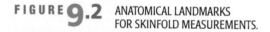

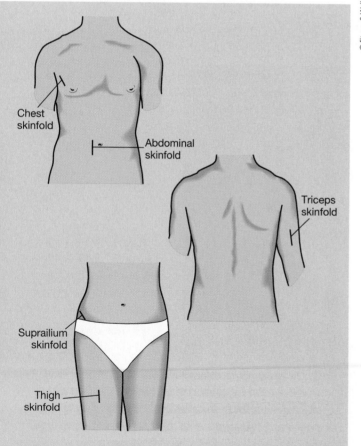

Chest skinfold

Abdominal skinfold

Triceps skinfold

Suprailium skinfold

Thigh skinfold

Even the skinfold technique requires some training to obtain accurate measurements. Also, different technicians may produce slightly different measurements from the same person. Therefore, the same technician should take pre- and post-measurements.

Measurements should be done at the same time of the day, preferably in the morning, because changes in water hydration from activity and exercise can increase skinfold girth. The procedure for assessing percent body fat using skinfold thickness is given in Figure 9.3. If skinfold calipers* are available to you, you may assess your percent body fat with the help of your instructor or an experienced technician. Use the appropriate Table 9.1, 9.2, or 9.3 to estimate body composition from your measurements.

---

*This instrument is available at most colleges and universities. If unavailable, you can purchase an inexpensive yet reliable skinfold caliper from: Fat Control Inc., P.O. Box 10117, Towson, MD 21204, Phone 301/296-1993.

FIGURE 9.3 — PROCEDURE FOR BODY FAT ASSESSMENT ACCORDING TO SKINFOLD THICKNESS TECHNIQUE.

1. Select the proper anatomical sites. For men, chest, abdomen, and thigh skinfolds are used. For women, use triceps, suprailium, and thigh skinfolds (*see* Figure 9.2). Take all measurements on the right side of the body with the person standing. The correct anatomical landmarks for skinfolds are:

   Chest: a diagonal fold halfway between the shoulder crease and the nipple.

   Abdomen: a vertical fold taken about one inch to the right of the umbilicus.

   Triceps: a vertical fold on the back of the upper arm, halfway between the shoulder and the elbow.

   Thigh: a vertical fold on the front of the thigh, midway between the knee and hip.

   Suprailium: a diagonal fold above the crest of the ilium (on the side of the hip).

2. Measure each site by grasping a double thickness of skin firmly with the thumb and forefinger, pulling the fold slightly away from the muscular tissue. The calipers are held perpendicular to the fold, and the measurement is taken ½ inch below the finger hold. Each site is measured three times, and the values are read to the nearest .1 to .5 mm. The average of the two closest readings is recorded as the final value. The readings should be taken without delay to avoid excessive compression of the skinfold. Releasing and refolding the skinfold is required between readings.

3. In pre- and post-assessments, the measurement should be conducted at the same time of day. The best time is early in the morning to avoid water hydration changes resulting from activity or exercise.

4. Percent fat is obtained by adding the three skinfold measurements and looking up the respective values on Table 9.1 for women, Table 9.2 for men under age 40, and Table 9.3 for men over age 40.

For example, if the skinfold measurements for an 18-year-old female are: (a) triceps = 16, (b) suprailium = 4, and (c) thigh = 30 (total = 50), the percent body fat is 20.6%

Anthropometric measurement techniques Measurement of body girths at different sites.

Skinfold thickness Technique to assess body composition by measuring a double thickness of skin at specific body sites.

TABLE 9.1 — PERCENT FAT ESTIMATES FOR WOMEN CALCULATED FROM TRICEPS, SUPRAILIUM, AND THIGH SKINFOLD THICKNESS

Sum of 3 Skinfolds	22 or Under	23 to 27	28 to 32	33 to 37	38 to 42	43 to 47	48 to 52	53 to 57	58 and Over
23– 25	9.7	9.9	10.2	10.4	10.7	10.9	11.2	11.4	11.7
26– 28	11.0	11.2	11.5	11.7	12.0	12.3	12.5	12.7	13.0
29– 31	12.3	12.5	12.8	13.0	13.3	13.5	13.8	14.0	14.3
32– 34	13.6	13.8	14.0	14.3	14.5	14.8	15.0	15.3	15.5
35– 37	14.8	15.0	15.3	15.5	15.8	16.0	16.3	16.5	16.8
38– 40	16.0	16.3	16.5	16.7	17.0	17.2	17.5	17.7	18.0
41– 43	17.2	17.4	17.7	17.9	18.2	18.4	18.7	18.9	19.2
44– 46	18.3	18.6	18.8	19.1	19.3	19.6	19.8	20.1	20.3
47– 49	19.5	19.7	20.0	20.2	20.5	20.7	21.0	21.2	21.5
50– 52	20.6	20.8	21.1	21.3	21.6	21.8	22.1	22.3	22.6
53– 55	21.7	21.9	22.1	22.4	22.6	22.9	23.1	23.4	23.6
56– 58	22.7	23.0	23.2	23.4	23.7	23.9	24.2	24.4	24.7
59– 61	23.7	24.0	24.2	24.5	24.7	25.0	25.2	25.5	25.7
62– 64	24.7	25.0	25.2	25.5	25.7	26.0	26.2	26.4	26.7
65– 67	25.7	25.9	26.2	26.4	26.7	26.9	27.2	27.4	27.7
68– 70	26.6	26.9	27.1	27.4	27.6	27.9	28.1	28.4	28.6
71– 73	27.5	27.8	28.0	28.3	28.5	28.8	29.0	29.3	29.5
74– 76	28.4	28.7	28.9	29.2	29.4	29.7	29.9	30.2	30.4
77– 79	29.3	29.5	29.8	30.0	30.3	30.5	30.8	31.0	31.3
80– 82	30.1	30.4	30.6	30.9	31.1	31.4	31.6	31.9	32.1
83– 85	30.9	31.2	31.4	31.7	31.9	32.2	32.4	32.7	32.9
86– 88	31.7	32.0	32.2	32.5	32.7	32.9	33.2	33.4	33.7
89– 91	32.5	32.7	33.0	33.2	33.5	33.7	33.9	34.2	34.4
92– 94	33.2	33.4	33.7	33.9	34.2	34.4	34.7	34.9	35.2
95– 97	33.9	34.1	34.4	34.6	34.9	35.1	35.4	35.6	35.9
98–100	34.6	34.8	35.1	35.3	35.5	35.8	36.0	36.3	36.5
101–103	35.2	35.4	35.7	35.9	36.2	36.4	36.7	36.9	37.2
104–106	35.8	36.1	36.3	36.6	36.8	37.1	37.3	37.5	37.8
107–109	36.4	36.7	36.9	37.1	37.4	37.6	37.9	38.1	38.4
110–112	37.0	37.2	37.5	37.7	38.0	38.2	38.5	38.7	38.9
113–115	37.5	37.8	38.0	38.2	38.5	38.7	39.0	39.2	39.5
116–118	38.0	38.3	38.5	38.8	39.0	39.3	39.5	39.7	40.0
119–121	38.5	38.7	39.0	39.2	39.5	39.7	40.0	40.2	40.5
122–124	39.0	39.2	39.4	39.7	39.9	40.2	40.4	40.7	40.9
125–127	39.4	39.6	39.9	40.1	40.4	40.6	40.9	41.1	41.4
128–130	39.8	40.0	40.3	40.5	40.8	41.0	41.3	41.5	41.8

Body density is calculated based on the "Generalized equation for predicting body density of women" developed by A. S. Jackson, M. L. Pollock, and A. Ward, *Medicine and Science in Sports and Exercise* 12 (1980): 175–182. Percent body fat is determined from the calculated body density using the Siri formula.

TABLE 9.2 — PERCENT FAT ESTIMATES FOR MEN 40 AND UNDER CALCULATED FROM CHEST, ABDOMEN, AND THIGH SKINFOLD THICKNESS

Sum of 3 Skinfolds	Under 19	20 to 22	24 to 25	26 to 28	29 to 31	32 to 34	35 to 37	38 to 40
8– 10	.9	1.3	1.6	2.0	2.3	2.7	3.0	3.3
11– 13	1.9	2.3	2.6	3.0	3.3	3.7	4.0	4.3
14– 16	2.9	3.3	3.6	3.9	4.3	4.6	5.0	5.3
17– 19	3.9	4.2	4.6	4.9	5.3	5.6	6.0	6.3
20– 22	4.8	5.2	5.5	5.9	6.2	6.6	6.9	7.3
23– 25	5.8	6.2	6.5	6.8	7.2	7.5	7.9	8.2
26– 28	6.8	7.1	7.5	7.8	8.1	8.5	8.8	9.2
29– 31	7.7	8.0	8.4	8.7	9.1	9.4	9.8	10.1
32– 34	8.6	9.0	9.3	9.7	10.0	10.4	10.7	11.1
35– 37	9.5	9.9	10.2	10.6	10.9	11.3	11.6	12.0
38– 40	10.5	10.8	11.2	11.5	11.8	12.2	12.5	12.9
41– 43	11.4	11.7	12.1	12.4	12.7	13.1	13.4	13.8
44– 46	12.2	12.6	12.9	13.3	13.6	14.0	14.3	14.7
47– 49	13.1	13.5	13.8	14.2	14.5	14.9	15.2	15.5
50– 52	14.0	14.3	14.7	15.0	15.4	15.7	16.1	16.4
53– 55	14.8	15.2	15.5	15.9	16.2	16.6	16.9	17.3
56– 58	15.7	16.0	16.4	16.7	17.1	17.4	17.8	18.1
59– 61	16.5	16.9	17.2	17.6	17.9	18.3	18.6	19.0
62– 64	17.4	17.7	18.1	18.4	18.8	19.1	19.4	19.8
65– 67	18.2	18.5	18.9	19.2	19.6	19.9	20.3	20.6
68– 70	19.0	19.3	19.7	20.0	20.4	20.7	21.1	21.4
71– 73	19.8	20.1	20.5	20.8	21.2	21.5	21.9	22.2
74– 76	20.6	20.9	21.3	21.6	22.0	22.2	22.7	23.0
77– 79	21.4	21.7	22.1	22.4	22.8	23.1	23.4	23.8
80– 82	22.1	22.5	22.8	23.2	23.5	23.9	24.2	24.6
83– 85	22.9	23.2	23.6	23.9	24.3	24.6	25.0	25.3
86– 88	23.6	24.0	24.3	24.7	25.0	25.4	25.7	26.1
89– 91	24.4	24.7	25.1	25.4	25.8	26.1	26.5	26.8
92– 94	25.1	25.5	25.8	26.2	26.5	26.9	27.2	27.5
95– 97	25.8	26.2	26.5	26.9	27.2	27.6	27.9	28.3
98–100	26.6	26.9	27.3	27.6	27.9	28.3	28.6	29.0
101–103	27.3	27.6	28.0	28.3	28.6	29.0	29.3	29.7
104–106	27.9	28.3	28.6	29.0	29.3	29.7	30.0	30.4
107–109	28.6	29.0	29.3	29.7	30.0	30.4	30.7	31.1
110–112	29.3	29.6	30.0	30.3	30.7	31.0	31.4	31.7
113–115	30.0	30.3	30.7	31.0	31.3	31.7	32.0	32.4
116–118	30.6	31.0	31.3	31.6	32.0	32.3	32.7	33.0
119–121	31.3	31.6	32.0	32.3	32.6	33.0	33.3	33.7
122–124	31.9	32.2	32.6	32.9	33.3	33.6	34.0	34.3
125–127	32.5	32.9	33.2	33.5	33.9	34.2	34.6	34.9
128–130	33.1	33.5	33.8	34.2	34.5	34.9	35.2	35.5

Body density is calculated based on the "Generalized equation for predicting body density of men" developed by A. S. Jackson and M. L. Pollock, *British Journal of Nutrition* 40 (1978): 497–504. Percent body fat is determined from the calculated body density using the Siri formula.

TABLE 9.3 — PERCENT FAT ESTIMATES FOR MEN OVER 40 CALCULATED FROM CHEST, ABDOMEN, AND THIGH SKINFOLD THICKNESS

Sum of 3 Skinfolds	41 to 43	44 to 46	47 to 49	50 to 52	53 to 55	56 to 58	59 to 61	62 and Over
8– 10	3.7	4.0	4.4	4.7	5.1	5.4	5.8	6.1
11– 13	4.7	5.0	5.4	5.7	6.1	6.4	6.8	7.1
14– 16	5.7	6.0	6.4	6.7	7.1	7.4	7.8	8.1
17– 19	6.7	7.0	7.4	7.7	8.1	8.4	8.7	9.1
20– 22	7.6	8.0	8.3	8.7	9.0	9.4	9.7	10.1
23– 25	8.6	8.9	9.3	9.6	10.0	10.3	10.7	11.0
26– 28	9.5	9.9	10.2	10.6	10.9	11.3	11.6	12.0
29– 31	10.5	10.8	11.2	11.5	11.9	12.2	12.6	12.9
32– 34	11.4	11.8	12.1	12.4	12.8	13.1	13.5	13.8
35– 37	12.3	12.7	13.0	13.4	13.7	14.1	14.4	14.8
38– 40	13.2	13.6	13.9	14.3	14.6	15.0	15.3	15.7
41– 43	14.1	14.5	14.8	15.2	15.5	15.9	16.2	16.6
44– 46	15.0	15.4	15.7	16.1	16.4	16.8	17.1	17.5
47– 49	15.9	16.2	16.6	16.9	17.3	17.6	18.0	18.3
50– 52	16.8	17.1	17.5	17.8	18.2	18.5	18.8	19.2
53– 55	17.6	18.0	18.3	18.7	19.0	19.4	19.7	20.1
56– 58	18.5	18.8	19.2	19.5	19.9	20.2	20.6	20.9
59– 61	19.3	19.7	20.0	20.4	20.7	21.0	21.4	21.7
62– 64	20.1	20.5	20.8	21.2	21.5	21.9	22.2	22.6
65– 67	21.0	21.3	21.7	22.0	22.4	22.7	23.0	23.4
68– 70	21.8	22.1	22.5	22.8	23.2	23.5	23.9	24.2
71– 73	22.6	22.9	23.3	23.6	24.0	24.3	24.7	25.0
74– 76	23.4	23.7	24.1	24.4	24.8	25.1	25.4	25.8
77– 79	24.1	24.5	24.8	25.2	25.5	25.9	26.2	26.6
80– 82	24.9	25.3	25.6	26.0	26.3	26.6	27.0	27.3
83– 85	25.7	26.0	26.4	26.7	27.1	27.4	27.8	28.1
86– 88	26.4	26.8	27.1	27.5	27.8	28.2	28.5	28.9
89– 91	27.2	27.5	27.9	28.2	28.6	28.9	29.2	29.6
92– 94	27.9	28.2	28.6	28.9	29.3	29.6	30.0	30.3
95– 97	28.6	29.0	29.3	29.7	30.0	30.4	30.7	31.1
98–100	29.3	29.7	30.0	30.4	30.7	31.1	31.4	31.8
101–103	30.0	30.4	30.7	31.1	31.4	31.8	32.1	32.5
104–106	30.7	31.1	31.4	31.8	32.1	32.5	32.8	33.2
107–109	31.4	31.8	32.1	32.4	32.8	33.1	33.5	33.8
110–112	32.1	32.4	32.8	33.1	33.5	33.8	34.2	34.5
113–115	32.7	33.1	33.4	33.8	34.1	34.5	34.8	35.2
116–118	33.4	33.7	34.1	34.4	34.8	35.1	35.5	35.8
119–121	34.0	34.4	34.7	35.1	35.4	35.8	36.1	36.5
122–124	34.7	35.0	35.4	35.7	36.1	36.4	36.7	37.1
125–127	35.3	35.6	36.0	36.3	36.7	37.0	37.4	37.7
128–130	35.9	36.2	36.6	36.9	37.3	37.6	38.0	38.5

Body density is calculated based on the "Generalized equation for predicting body density of men" developed by A. S. Jackson and M. L. Pollock, *British Journal of Nutrition* 40 (1978): 497–504. Percent body fat is determined from the calculated body density using the Siri formula.

Girth Measurements

A simpler method to determine body fat is by measuring circumferences at various body sites. All this technique requires is a standard measuring tape, and good accuracy can be achieved with little practice. The limitation is that it may not be valid for athletic individuals (men or women) who participate actively in strenuous physical activity or people who can be classified visually as thin or obese.

The required procedure for **girth measurements** is given in Figure 9.4. Measurements for women include the upper arm, hip, and wrist; for men, the waist and wrist. Tables 9.4 and 9.5 translate these measurements into body density and percent fat estimates for women and men, respectively.

> **Girth measurements**
> Technique to assess body composition by measuring circumferences at specific body sites.

FIGURE 9.4 PROCEDURE FOR BODY FAT ASSESSMENT ACCORDING TO GIRTH MEASUREMENTS.

Girth Measurements for Women*

1. Using a regular tape measure, determine the following girth measurements in centimeters (cm):

   Upper Arm: Measure halfway between the shoulder and the elbow.

   Hip: Measure at the point of largest circumference.

   Wrist: Take the girth in front of the bones where the wrist bends.

2. Obtain the person's age.

3. Using Table 9.4, find the girth measurement for each site and age in the lefthand columns. Look up the constant values in the righthand columns. These values will allow you to derive body density (BD) by substituting the constants in the following formula:

   BD = A − B − C + D

4. Using the derived body density, calculate percent body fat (%F) according to the following equation:

   %F = (495 ÷ BD) − 450**

   Example: Jane is 20 years old, and the following girth measurements were taken: biceps = 27 cm, hip = 99.5 cm, wrist = 15.4 cm.

Data	Constant		
Upper Arm = 27 cm	A	=	1.0813
Age = 20	B	=	.0102
Hip = 99.5 cm	C	=	.1206
Wrist = 15.4 cm	D	=	.0971

   BD = A − B − C + D
   BD = 1.0813 − .0102 − .1206 + .0971 = 1.0476

   %F = (495 ÷ BD) − 450
   %F = (495 ÷ 1.0476) − 450 = 22.5

Girth Measurements for Men***

1. Using a regular tape measure, determine the following girth measurements in inches (the men's measurements are taken in inches as contrasted with centimeters for women):

   Waist: Measure at the umbilicus (belly button)

   Wrist: Measure in front of the bones where the wrist bends.

2. Subtract the wrist from the waist measurement.

3. Obtain the person's weight in pounds.

4. Look up the percent body fat (%F) in Table 9.5 by using the difference obtained in Step 2 above and the person's body weight.

Example: John weighs 160 pounds, and his waist and wrist girth measurements are 36.5 and 7.5 inches, respectively.

   Waist girth = 36.5 inches
   Wrist girth = 7.5 inches
   Difference = 29.0 inches
   Body weight = 160.0 lbs.
   %F = 22

---

* Reproduced by permission from R. B. Lambson, "Generalized Body Density Prediction Equations for Women Using Simple Anthropometric Measurements." (Ph.D. diss. Brigham Young University, August 1987).

** From W. E. Siri, *Body Composition From Fluid Spaces and Density*, (Berkeley: University of California, Donner Laboratory of Medical Physics, 1956).

*** Table 3.5 reproduced by permission from A. G. Fisher, and P. E. Allsen, *Jogging* (Dubuque, IA: Wm. C. Brown, 1987). This table was developed according to the generalized body composition equation for men using simple measurement techniques by K. W. Penrouse, A. G Nelson, and A G. Fisher, *Medicine and Science in Sports and Exercise* 17, no. 2 (1985): 189. © American College of Sports Medicine 1985.

TABLE 9.4 CONVERSION CONSTANTS FROM GIRTH MEASUREMENTS TO CALCULATE BODY DENSITY FOR WOMEN

Upper Arm (cm)	Constant A	Age	Constant B	Hip (cm)	Constant C	Hip (cm)	Constant C	Wrist (cm)	Constant D
20.5	1.0966	17	.0086	79	.0957	114.5	.1388	13.0	.0819
21	1.0954	18	.0091	79.5	.0963	115	.1394	13.2	.0832
21.5	1.0942	19	.0096	80	.0970	115.5	.1400	13.4	.0845
22	1.0930	20	.0102	80.5	.0976	116	.1406	13.6	.0857
22.5	1.0919	21	.0107	81	.0982	116.5	.1412	13.8	.0870
23	1.0907	22	.0112	81.5	.0988	117	.1418	14.0	.0882
23.5	1.0895	23	.0117	82	.0994	117.5	.1424	14.2	.0895
24	1.0883	24	.0122	82.5	.1000	118	.1430	14.4	.0908
24.5	1.0871	25	.0127	83	.1006	118.5	.1436	14.6	.0920
25	1.0860	26	.0132	83.5	.1012	119	.1442	14.8	.0933
25.5	1.0848	27	.0137	84	.1018	119.5	.1448	15.0	.0946
26	1.0836	28	.0142	84.5	.1024	120	.1454	15.2	.0958
26.5	1.0824	29	.0147	85	.1030	120.5	.1460	15.4	.0971
27	1.0813	30	.0152	85.5	.1036	121	.1466	15.6	.0983
27.5	1.0801	31	.0157	86	.1042	121.5	.1472	15.8	.0996
28	1.0789	32	.0162	86.5	.1048	122	.1479	16.0	.1009
28.5	1.0777	33	.0168	87	.1054	122.5	.1485	16.2	.1021
29	1.0775	34	.0173	87.5	.1060	123	.1491	16.4	.1034
29.5	1.0754	35	.0178	88	.1066	123.5	.1497	16.6	.1046
30	1.0742	36	.0183	88.5	.1072	124	.1503	16.8	.1059
30.5	1.0730	37	.0188	89	.1079	124.5	.1509	17.0	.1072
31	1.0718	38	.0193	89.5	.1085	125	.1515	17.2	.1084
31.5	1.0707	39	.0198	90	.1091	125.5	.1521	17.4	.1097
32	1.0695	40	.0203	90.5	.1097	126	.1527	17.6	.1109
32.5	1.0683	41	.0208	91	.1103	126.5	.1533	17.8	.1122
33	1.0671	42	.0213	91.5	.1109	127	.1539	18.0	.1135
33.5	1.0666	43	.0218	92	.1115	127.5	.1545	18.2	.1147
34	1.0648	44	.0223	92.5	.1121	128	.1551	18.4	.1160
34.5	1.0636	45	.0228	93	.1127	128.5	.1558	18.6	.1172
35	1.0624	46	.0234	93.5	.1133	129	.1563		
35.5	1.0612	47	.0239	94	.1139	129.5	.1569		
36	1.0601	48	.0244	94.5	.1145	130	.1575		
36.5	1.0589	49	.0249	95	.1151	130.5	.1581		
37	1.0577	50	.0254	95.5	.1157	131	.1587		
37.5	1.0565	51	.0259	96	.1163	131.5	.1593		
38	1.0554	52	.0264	96.5	.1169	132	.1600		
38.5	1.0542	53	.0269	97	.1176	132.5	.1606		
39	1.0530	54	.0274	97.5	.1182	133	.1612		
39.5	1.0518	55	.0279	98	.1188	133.5	.1618		
40	1.0506	56	.0284	98.5	.1194	134	.1624		
40.5	1.0495	57	.0289	99	.1200	134.5	.1630		
41	1.0483	58	.0294	99.5	.1206	135	.1636		
41.5	1.0471	59	.0300	100	.1212	135.5	.1642		
42	1.0459	60	.0305	100.5	.1218	136	.1648		
42.5	1.0448	61	.0310	101	.1224	136.5	.1654		
43	1.0434	62	.0315	101.5	.1230	137	.1660		
43.5	1.0424	63	.0320	102	.1236	137.5	.1666		
44	1.0412	64	.0325	102.5	.1242	138	.1672		
		65	.0330	103	.1248	138.5	.1678		

(Continued)

WELLNESS: GUIDELINES FOR A HEALTHY LIFESTYLE

Upper Arm (cm)	Constant A	Age	Constant B	Hip (cm)	Constant C	Hip (cm)	Constant C	Wrist (cm)	Constant D
		66	.0335	103.5	.1254	139	.1685		
		67	.0340	104	.1260	139.5	.1691		
		68	.0345	104.5	.1266	140	.1697		
		69	.0350	105	.1272	140.5	.1703		
		70	.0355	105.5	.1278	141	.1709		
		71	.0360	106	.1285	141.5	.1715		
		72	.0366	106.5	.1291	142	.1721		
		73	.0371	107	.1297	142.5	.1728		
		74	.0376	107.5	.1303	143	.1733		
		75	.0381	108	.1309	143.5	.1739		
				108.5	.1315	144	.1745		
				109	.1321	144.5	.1751		
				109.5	.1327	145	.1757		
				110	.1333	145.5	.1763		
				110.5	.1339	146	.1769		
				111	.1345	146.5	.1775		
				111.5	.1351	147	.1781		
				112	.1357	147.5	.1787		
				112.5	.1363	148	.1794		
				113	.1369	148.5	.1800		
				113.5	.1375	149	.1806		
				114	.1382	149.5	.1812		
						150	.1818		

Bioelectrical Impedance

The **bioelectrical impedance** technique is much simpler to administer, but it does require costly equipment. In this technique, the individual is hooked up to a machine that runs a weak (totally painless) electrical current through the body to analyze body composition (body fat, lean body mass, and body water). The technique is based on the principle that lean tissue is a better conductor of electricity than fat tissue is. The easier the conductance, the leaner the individual.

The accuracy of current equations used to estimate percent body fat with this technique is still questionable. More research is required before the equations approach the accuracy of hydrostatic weighing, skinfolds, or girth measurements.

An advantage of bioelectrical impedance is that results are highly reproducible. Unlike other techniques, in which experienced technicians are necessary to obtain valid results, almost anyone can administer bioelectrical impedance. And, although the test results may not be completely accurate, this instrument is valuable in assessing body composition changes over time.

If this instrument or some other type of equipment for body composition assessment is available to you, you can use it to determine your percent body fat. You may want to compare the results with other techniques. Following all manufacturer's instructions will ensure the best possible result.

Air Displacement

Air displacement is a relatively new technique that holds considerable promise as a valid method for the assessment of body composition. With this technique, an individual sits inside a small chamber (commercially known as the **Bod Pod**). Body volume is determined by subtracting the air volume with the person inside the chamber from the volume of the empty chamber.

Bioelectrical impedance Technique to assess body composition by running a weak electrical current through the body.

Air displacement Technique to assess body composition by calculating the body volume from the air displaced by an individual sitting inside a small chamber.

Bod Pod Commercial name of the equipment used for the air displacement technique.

TABLE 9.5 ESTIMATED PERCENT BODY FAT FOR MEN OBTAINED FROM WAIST MINUS WRIST GIRTH MEASUREMENTS (IN INCHES) AND BODY WEIGHT (IN POUNDS)

Waist Minus Wrist Girth Measurement

Body Weight	22	22.5	23	23.5	24	24.5	25	25.5	26	26.5	27	27.5	28	28.5	29	29.5	30	30.5	31	31.5	32	32.5	33	33.5	34	34.5	35	35.5	36	36.5	37	37.5	38	38.5	39	39.5	40	40.5	41	41.5	42	42.5	43	43.5	44	44.5	45	45.5	46	46.5	47	47.5	48	48.5	49	49.5	50
120	4	6	8	10	12	14	16	18	20	21	23	25	27	29	31	33	35	37	39	41	43	45	47	49	50	52	54	56	58																												
125	4	6	7	9	11	13	15	16	18	20	22	23	25	27	29	31	33	35	37	39	41	43	45	46	48	50	52	54	56	58																											
130	3	5	7	9	11	12	14	16	18	19	21	23	24	26	28	30	32	33	35	37	39	41	43	44	46	48	50	52	53	55	57																									
135	3	5	7	9	10	12	14	15	17	19	20	22	24	25	27	29	31	33	34	36	38	40	42	43	45	47	49	50	52	54	55	56																							
140	3	5	7	8	10	12	13	15	17	18	20	22	23	25	27	28	30	32	33	35	37	39	40	42	44	46	47	49	51	52	54	55	56																					
145	3	5	6	8	10	11	13	15	16	18	19	21	23	24	26	28	29	31	33	34	36	38	39	41	43	44	46	48	49	51	53	54	55	55																			
150	2	4	6	7	9	11	12	14	15	17	19	20	22	23	25	27	28	30	32	33	35	36	38	40	41	43	45	46	48	50	51	53	54	55	55																		
155	2	4	6	7	9	10	12	13	15	17	18	20	21	23	24	26	28	29	31	32	34	36	37	39	41	42	44	45	47	48	50	52	53	54	55	55																
160	2	4	5	7	9	10	11	13	15	16	18	19	21	22	24	26	27	29	30	32	34	35	37	38	40	41	43	45	46	48	49	51	52	53	54	54	54															
165	2	4	5	6	8	10	11	12	14	15	17	18	20	21	23	24	26	28	29	31	32	34	35	37	39	40	42	43	45	47	48	50	51	52	54	54	54	54														
170	2	3	5	6	8	9	11	12	13	15	16	18	19	21	22	24	25	27	28	30	31	33	35	36	38	39	41	42	44	45	47	49	50	52	53	54	54	54	54													
175	2	3	4	6	7	9	10	12	13	14	16	17	19	20	22	23	25	26	28	29	31	32	34	35	37	39	40	42	43	45	46	48	49	51	52	53	53	53	53	53												
180	2	3	4	5	7	8	10	11	12	14	15	17	18	19	21	22	24	25	27	28	29	31	32	34	35	37	38	40	41	43	44	46	47	48	50	51	52	53	53	53	53											
185	2	3	4	5	6	8	9	10	12	13	15	16	17	19	20	22	23	24	26	27	29	30	32	33	35	36	38	39	40	42	43	45	46	48	49	50	51	52	53	53	53	53										
190	2	2	4	5	6	7	9	10	11	13	14	15	17	18	20	21	22	24	25	27	28	29	31	32	34	35	37	38	39	41	42	44	45	46	48	49	50	51	52	52	52	52	52								
195	2	2	4	5	6	7	8	10	11	12	14	15	16	18	19	20	22	23	25	26	27	29	30	32	33	34	36	37	39	40	41	43	44	45	47	48	49	50	51	52	52	52	52	52							
200	2	2	3	4	6	7	8	9	11	12	13	15	16	17	19	20	21	23	24	25	27	28	30	31	32	34	35	36	38	39	41	42	43	45	46	47	49	50	51	52	52	52	52	52	52						
205	2	2	3	4	5	6	8	9	10	11	13	14	15	17	18	19	21	22	23	25	26	27	29	30	31	33	34	35	37	38	40	41	42	44	45	46	48	49	50	51	52	52	52	52	52	52					
210	2	2	3	4	5	6	7	9	10	11	12	14	15	16	18	19	20	21	23	24	25	27	28	29	31	32	33	35	36	37	39	40	41	43	44	45	47	48	49	51	51	51	51	51	51	51	51				
215	2	2	3	4	5	6	7	8	10	11	12	13	15	16	17	19	20	21	22	24	25	26	28	29	30	32	33	34	36	37	38	40	41	42	44	45	46	48	49	50	51	51	51	51	51	51	51	51			
220	2	2	3	4	5	6	7	8	9	11	12	13	14	16	17	18	20	21	22	23	25	26	27	29	30	31	33	34	35	37	38	39	40	42	43	44	46	47	48	49	51	51	51	51	51	51	51	51	51		
225	2	2	3	4	5	5	6	8	9	10	11	13	14	15	16	18	19	20	22	23	24	25	27	28	29	31	32	33	34	36	37	38	40	41	42	43	45	46	47	49	50	51	51	51	51	51	51	51	51	51	
230	2	2	3	4	4	5	6	7	8	10	11	12	13	15	16	17	18	20	21	22	23	25	26	27	28	30	31	32	34	35	36	37	39	40	41	42	44	45	46	47	49	50	51	51	51	51	51	51	51	51	51
235	2	2	3	3	4	5	6	7	8	9	11	12	13	14	15	17	18	19	20	22	23	24	25	27	28	29	30	32	33	34	35	37	38	39	40	42	43	44	45	47	48	49	50	51	51	51	51	51	51	51	51
240	2	2	3	3	4	5	6	7	8	9	10	12	13	14	15	16	18	19	20	21	23	24	25	26	28	29	30	31	33	34	35	36	37	39	40	41	42	44	45	46	47	49	50	50	50	50	50	50	50	50	50
245	2	2	3	3	4	5	6	6	7	9	10	11	12	13	15	16	17	18	19	21	22	23	24	26	27	28	29	30	32	33	34	35	37	38	39	40	41	43	44	45	46	48	49	50	50	50	50	50	50	50	50
250	2	2	3	3	4	4	5	6	7	8	9	11	12	13	14	15	16	18	19	20	21	22	24	25	26	27	28	30	31	32	33	34	36	37	38	39	40	42	43	44	45	46	48	49	50	50	50	50	50	50	50
255	2	2	3	3	4	4	5	6	7	8	9	10	11	13	14	15	16	17	18	20	21	22	23	24	26	27	28	29	30	32	33	34	35	36	38	39	40	41	42	44	45	46	47	48	50	50	50	50	50	50	50
260	2	2	3	3	4	4	5	6	7	8	9	10	11	12	13	15	16	17	18	19	20	22	23	24	25	26	27	29	30	31	32	33	34	36	37	38	39	40	41	43	44	45	46	47	48	50	50	50	50	50	50
265	2	2	3	3	4	4	5	5	6	7	8	9	10	12	13	14	15	16	17	18	19	21	22	23	24	25	26	28	29	30	31	32	33	35	36	37	38	39	40	42	43	44	45	46	47	48	49	49	49	49	49
270	2	2	3	3	3	4	5	5	6	7	8	9	10	11	12	13	14	16	17	18	19	20	21	22	24	25	26	27	28	29	31	32	33	34	35	36	37	38	40	41	42	43	44	45	46	47	48	49	48	48	48
275	2	2	3	3	3	4	5	5	6	7	8	9	10	11	12	13	14	15	16	17	18	19	20	21	23	24	25	26	27	28	29	30	31	32	34	35	36	37	38	39	40	41	42	43	45	46	47	48	47	47	47
280	2	2	3	3	3	4	4	5	6	7	8	8	9	11	12	13	14	15	16	17	18	19	20	21	22	23	24	25	26	27	28	30	31	32	33	34	35	36	37	38	39	40	42	43	44	45	46	47	46	46	46
285	2	2	3	3	3	4	4	5	6	6	7	8	9	10	11	12	13	14	15	16	17	18	20	20	21	22	23	24	26	27	28	29	30	31	32	33	34	35	36	38	39	40	41	42	43	44	45	46	45	45	45
290	2	2	3	3	3	4	4	5	6	6	7	8	9	10	11	11	12	13	14	15	16	17	19	19	20	21	22	23	24	25	26	27	28	30	31	32	33	34	35	36	37	38	39	40	41	42	43	44	43	44	44
295	2	2	3	3	3	4	4	5	5	6	7	8	9	10	10	11	12	13	14	15	16	17	18	18	19	20	21	22	23	24	25	26	28	29	30	31	32	33	34	35	36	37	38	39	40	41	42	43	42	43	43
300	2	2	3	4	4	5	5	5	6	7	8	8	9	10	11	12	12	13	14	15	16	16	17	18	19	20	20	21	22	23	24	24	25	26	27	28	28	29	30	31	32	33	34	35	36	37	37	38	39	42	43

The amount of air in the person's lungs is also taken into consideration when determining the actual body volume. Body density and percent body fat are then calculated from the obtained body volume.

Initial research has shown that this technique compares very favorably with hydrostatic weighing and it is less cumbersome to administer. The procedure takes only about 5 minutes to perform. Additional research is needed, however, to determine its accuracy among different age groups, ethnic backgrounds, and athletic populations. Although body composition assessment through air displacement is a relatively easy procedure, the Bod Pod is not readily available in fitness centers and exercise laboratories because of its high cost.

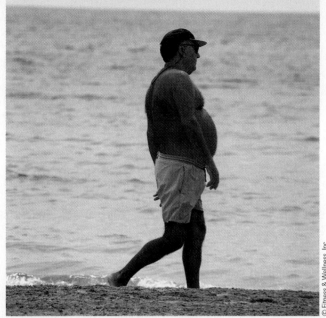

Individuals who accumulate body fat around the midsection of the body are at greater risk for disease than those who accumulate body fat in other areas of the body.

© Fitness & Wellness, Inc.

WAIST-TO-HIP RATIO

Scientific evidence suggests that the way people store fat affects their risk for disease. Some individuals tend to store fat in the abdominal area (called the "apple" shape). Others store it primarily around the hips and thighs (in gluteal femoral fat, which produces the "pear" shape).

Obese individuals with a lot of abdominal fat are clearly at higher risk for coronary heart disease, congestive heart failure, hypertension, adult-onset diabetes (Type II), and strokes than are obese people with similar amounts of total body fat that is stored primarily in the hips and thighs. Relatively new evidence also indicates that, among individuals with high abdominal fat, those whose fat deposits are around internal organs (visceral fat) are at even greater risk for disease than those whose abdominal fat is primarily beneath the skin (subcutaneous fat).[1]

Because of the higher risk for disease in individuals who tend to store a lot of fat in the abdominal area, instead of the hips and thighs, a **waist-to-hip ratio** test was designed to estimate the risk. The waist measurement is taken at the point of smallest circumference, and the hip measurement is taken at the point of greatest circumference.

The waist-to-hip ratio differentiates the "apples" from the "pears." Men tend to be apples, and women tend to be pears. The panel recommends that men need to lose weight if the waist-to-hip ratio is 1.0 or higher. Women need to lose weight if the ratio is .85 or higher (see Table 9.6). More conservative estimates indicate that the risk starts to increase when the ratio exceeds .95 and .80 for men and women, respectively. For example, the waist-to-hip ratio for a man with a 40-inch waist and a 38-inch hip would be 1.05 (40 ÷ 38). This ratio may indicate higher risk for disease.

TABLE 9.6 — DISEASE RISK ACCORDING TO WAIST-TO-HIP RATIO

Waist-to-Hip Ratio		
Men	Women	Disease Risk
≤0.95	≤0.80	Very Low
0.96–0.99	0.81–0.84	Low
≥1.00	≥0.85	High

BODY MASS INDEX

Another technique scientists use to determine thinness and excessive fatness is the **body mass index (BMI)**. This index incorporates height and weight to estimate critical fat values at which the risk for disease increases.

BMI is calculated by dividing the weight in kilograms by the square of the height in meters or multiplying body weight in pounds by 705, and dividing this figure by the square of the height in inches. For example, the BMI for an individual who weighs 172 pounds (78 kg) and is 67 inches (1.7 m) tall would be 27 $[78 ÷ (1.7)^2]$ or $[172 × 705 ÷ (67)^2]$. You can also look up your BMI in Table 9.7 according to your height and weight.

Waist-to-hip ratio A measurement to assess potential risk for disease based on distribution of body fat.

Body mass index (BMI) Ratio of weight to height, used to determine thinness and fatness.

TABLE 9.7 BODY MASS INDEX

Determine your BMI by looking up the number where your weight and height intersect on the table. According to your results, look up your disease risk in Table 9.8.

Height	Weight																												
	110	115	120	125	130	135	140	145	150	155	160	165	170	175	180	185	190	195	200	205	210	215	220	225	230	235	240	245	250
5'0"	21	22	23	24	25	26	27	28	29	30	31	32	33	34	35	36	37	38	39	40	41	42	43	44	45	46	47	48	49
5'1"	21	22	23	24	25	26	26	27	28	29	30	31	32	33	34	35	36	37	38	39	40	41	42	43	43	44	45	46	47
5'2"	20	21	22	23	24	25	26	27	27	28	29	30	31	32	33	34	35	36	37	37	38	39	40	41	42	43	44	45	46
5'3"	19	20	21	22	23	24	25	26	27	27	28	29	30	31	32	33	34	35	35	36	37	38	39	40	41	42	43	43	44
5'4"	19	20	21	21	22	23	24	25	26	27	27	28	29	30	31	32	33	33	34	35	36	37	38	39	39	40	41	42	43
5'5"	18	19	20	21	22	22	23	24	25	26	27	27	28	29	30	31	32	32	33	34	35	36	37	37	38	39	40	41	42
5'6"	18	19	19	20	21	22	23	23	24	25	26	27	27	28	29	30	31	31	32	33	34	35	36	36	37	38	39	40	40
5'7"	17	18	19	20	20	21	22	23	23	24	25	26	27	27	28	29	30	31	31	32	33	34	34	35	36	37	38	38	39
5'8"	17	17	18	19	20	21	21	22	23	24	24	25	26	27	27	28	29	30	30	31	32	33	33	34	35	36	36	37	38
5'9"	16	17	18	18	19	20	21	21	22	23	24	24	25	26	27	27	28	29	30	30	31	32	32	33	34	35	35	36	37
5'10"	16	17	17	18	19	19	20	21	22	22	23	24	24	25	26	27	27	28	29	29	30	31	32	32	33	34	34	35	36
5'11"	15	16	17	17	18	19	20	20	21	22	22	23	24	24	25	26	26	27	28	29	29	30	31	31	32	33	33	34	35
6'0"	15	16	16	17	18	18	19	20	20	21	22	22	23	24	24	25	26	26	27	28	28	29	30	31	31	32	33	33	34
6'1"	15	15	16	16	17	18	18	19	20	20	21	22	22	23	24	24	25	26	26	27	28	28	29	30	30	31	32	32	33
6'2"	14	15	15	16	17	17	18	19	19	20	21	21	22	22	23	24	24	25	26	26	27	28	28	29	30	30	31	31	32
6'3"	14	14	15	16	16	17	17	18	19	19	20	21	21	22	22	23	24	24	25	26	26	27	27	28	29	29	30	31	31
6'4"	13	14	15	15	16	16	17	18	18	19	19	20	21	21	22	23	23	24	24	25	26	26	27	27	28	29	29	30	30

According to BMI, the lowest risk for chronic disease is in the 22 to 25 range[2] (see Table 9.8). Individuals are classified as overweight between 25 and 30. BMIs above 30 are defined as obese and below 20 as **underweight**. As compared with individuals with a BMI below 25, mortality rates are up to 25 percent higher for people with a BMI between 25 and 30, and 50 to 100 percent higher for those with a BMI above 30.[3] Approximately 20 percent of U. S. adults have a body BMI of 30 or more.

BMI is a useful tool to screen the general population, but one weakness, similar to height/weight charts, is that it fails to differentiate fat from lean body mass or take into account where most of the fat is located (waist-to-hip ratio). Using BMI, athletes (such as body builders and football players) with a large amount of muscle mass easily can fall in the moderate- or even high-risk categories. Therefore, body composition and waist-to-hip ratios are better procedures to determine recommended body weight and health risk.

TABLE 9.8 DISEASE RISK ACCORDING TO BODY MASS INDEX (BMI)

BMI	Disease Risk
<20.00	Moderate to Very High
20.00 to 21.99	Low
22.00 to 24.99	Very Low
25.00 to 29.99	Low
30.00 to 34.99	Moderate
35.00 to 39.99	High
≥40.00	Very High

DETERMINING RECOMMENDED BODY WEIGHT

After finding out your percent body fat, you can determine your current body composition classification according to Table 9.9. In this table, you will find the health fitness and the high physical fitness percent fat standards.

For example, the recommended health fitness fat percentage for a 20-year-old female is 28 percent or less.

TABLE 9.9 BODY COMPOSITION CLASSIFICATION ACCORDING TO PERCENT BODY FAT

			MEN		
Age	Excellent	Good	Moderate	Overweight	Significantly Overweight
≤19	12.0	12.1–17.0	17.1–22.0	22.1–27.0	≥27.1
20–29	13.0	13.1–18.0	18.1–23.0	23.1–28.0	≥28.1
30–39	14.0	14.1–19.0	19.1–24.0	24.1–29.0	≥29.1
40–49	15.0	15.1–20.0	20.1–25.0	25.1–30.0	≥30.1
≥50	16.0	16.1–21.0	21.1–26.0	26.1–31.0	≥31.1
			WOMEN		
Age	Excellent	Good	Moderate	Overweight	Significantly Overweight
≤19	17.0	17.1–22.0	22.1–27.0	27.1–32.0	≥32.1
20–29	18.0	18.1–23.0	23.1–28.0	28.1–33.0	≥33.1
30–39	19.0	19.1–24.0	24.1–29.0	29.1–34.0	≥34.1
40–49	20.0	20.1–25.0	25.1–30.0	30.1–35.0	≥35.1
≥50	21.0	21.1–26.0	26.1–31.0	31.1–36.0	≥36.1

High physical fitness standard

Health fitness standard

The health fitness standard is established at the point at which there seems to be no harm to health in terms of percent body fat. A high physical fitness range for this same woman would be between 18 and 23 percent.

It's even possible to fall below the high physical fitness standard numbers. Many highly trained male athletes are as low as 3 percent, and some female distance runners have been measured at 6 percent body fat (which may not be healthy).

Although people generally agree that the mortality rate is greater for obese people, some evidence indicates that the same is true for underweight people. "Underweight" and "thin" do not necessarily mean the same thing. A healthy thin person has total body fat around the high fitness percentage, whereas an underweight person has extremely low body fat, even to the point of compromising the essential fat.

The 3 percent essential fat for men and 12 percent for women seem to be the lower limits for people to maintain good health. Below these percentages, normal physiologic functions can be seriously impaired.

Some experts point out that a little storage fat (in addition to the essential fat) is better than none at all. As a result, the health and high fitness standards for percent fat in Table 9.9 are set higher than the minimum essential fat requirements, at a point beneficial to optimal health and well-being. Finally, because lean tissue decreases with age, one extra percentage point is allowed for every additional decade of life.

Your recommended body weight is computed based on the selected health or high fitness fat percentage for your age and gender. Your decision to select a "desired" fat percentage should be based on your current percent body fat and your personal health/fitness objectives. To compute your own recommended body weight:

1. Determine the pounds of body weight in fat (FW). Multiply body weight (BW) by the current percent fat (%F) expressed in decimal form (FW = BW × %F).
2. Determine lean body mass (LBM) by subtracting the weight in fat from the total body weight (LBM = BW − FW). (Anything that is not fat is part of the lean component.)
3. Select a desired body fat percentage (DFP) based on the health or high fitness standards given in Table 9.9.
4. Compute recommended body weight (RBW) according to the formula: RBW = LBM ÷ (1.0 − DFP).

As an example of these computations, a 19-year-old female who weighs 160 pounds and is 30 percent fat would like to know what her recommended body weight would be at 22 percent:

Gender: female
Age: 19
BW: 160 lbs.
%F: 30% (.30 in decimal form)

1. FW = BW × %F
   FW = 160 × .30 = 48 lbs.
2. LBM = BW − FW
   LBM = 160 − 48 = 112 lbs.
3. DFP: 22% (.22 in decimal form)
4. RBW = LBM ÷ (1.0 − DFP)
   RBW = 112 ÷ (1.0 − .22)
   RBW = 112 ÷ .78 = 143.6 lbs.

In Assessments 9-1 and 9-2, you will have the opportunity to determine your own body composition, recommended body weight, and disease risk according to waist-to-hip ratio and BMI.

Other than hydrostatic weighing, skinfold thickness seems to be the most practical and valid technique to estimate body fat. If skinfold calipers are available, use this technique to assess percent body fat. If calipers are unavailable, you can estimate your percent fat according to the girth measurements technique or another technique available to you. (You may wish to use several techniques and compare the results.)

Underweight Extremely low body weight.

IMPORTANCE OF REGULAR BODY COMPOSITION ASSESSMENTS

Children do not start life with a weight problem. Although a small group struggles with weight throughout life, most are not overweight when they reach age 20 or so.

Current trends indicate that starting at age 25, the average man and woman in the United States gains 1 pound of weight per year. Thus, by age 65, the average American will have gained 40 pounds of weight. Because of the typical reduction in physical activity in our society, however, the average person also loses a half a pound of lean tissue each year. Therefore, over this span of 40 years, there has been an actual fat gain of 60 pounds accompanied by a 20-pound loss of lean body mass[4] (see Figure 9.5). These changes cannot be detected unless body composition is assessed periodically.

If you are on a diet/exercise program, you should repeat the computations about once a month to monitor changes in body composition. This is important because lean body mass is affected by weight reduction programs and amount of physical activity. As lean body mass changes, so will your recommended body weight. To make valid comparisons, the same technique should be used for pre- and post-assessments.

Changes in body composition resulting from a weight control/exercise program were illustrated in a co-ed aerobics course taught during a 6-week summer term. Students participated in aerobic dance routines four times a week, 60 minutes each time. On the first and last days of class, several physiological parameters, including body composition, were assessed. Students also were given information on diet and nutrition, and they followed their own weight control program.

At the end of the 6 weeks, the average weight loss for the entire class was 3 pounds (see Figure 9.6). Because body composition was assessed, however, class members were surprised to find that the average fat loss was actually 6 pounds, accompanied by a 3-pound increase in lean body mass.

> Starting at age 25, the average adult in the United States gains 1.5 pounds of body fat per year.

When you diet, your body composition should be reassessed periodically because of the effects of negative caloric balance on lean body mass. As is discussed in Chapter 10, dieting alone does decrease lean body mass. This lean body mass loss can be reduced or eliminated by combining a sensible diet with physical exercise.

FIGURE 9.5 TYPICAL BODY COMPOSITION CHANGES FOR ADULTS IN THE UNITED STATES.

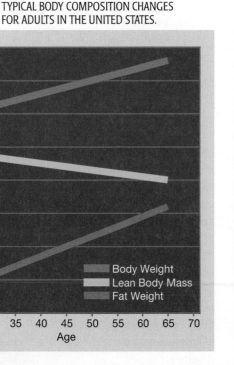

FIGURE 9.6 EFFECTS OF A 6-WEEK AEROBICS PROGRAM ON BODY COMPOSITION.

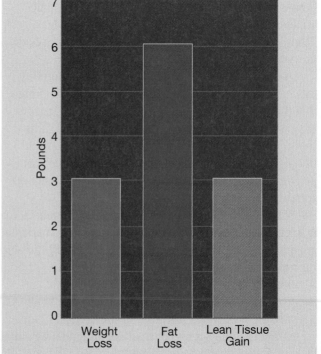

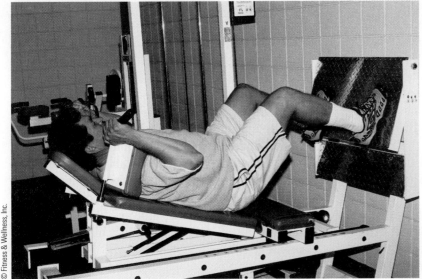

| A person can lose fat and gain lean body mass while body weight may remain unchanged or even increase slightly during the early stages of an exercise program. |

© Fitness & Wellness, Inc.

WEB INTERACTIVE.

WEB ACTIVITIES

■ **Body Mass Index** A comprehensive site from Shape Up, America describing body mass measurements, including a chart.
http://www.shapeup.org/bmi/index.html

■ **Body Composition and Somatype** This site features a table listing male and female percent body fat ranges, body fat myths and truths, and specific activities to help achieve proper body composition.
http://www.worldguide.com/Fitness/med.html

■ **Skinfold Caliper Measurements** This site describes how and where to take these measurements, as well as the equations used to determine body fat.
http://www.solid.net/lowcarb/lylemcd/skinfold.htm

■ **Calculate Your BMI**, using your height and weight. BMI stands for body mass index, a ratio between weight and height. It is a mathematical formula that correlates body fat with lean tissue. BMI is a better predictor of disease risk than body weight alone. This site also features tools to calculate your ideal weight and your target heart rate.
http://www.drkoop.com/wellness/weight_loss/#

InfoTrac

You can find additional readings related to wellness via InfoTrac College Edition, an on-line library of more than 900 journals and publications. Follow the instructions for accessing InfoTrac that came packaged with your textbook, then search for articles using a key word search.

Suggested Reading "Body Fat," *Harvard Women's Health Watch* 6, no. 10 (June 1999): Item 99172002.

1. Physiologically, what accounts for gender differences in body composition and distribution of fat?
2. What role does ethnicity play in body composition?
3. What physiological activities take place in the body in response to dieting and when caloric intake subsequently increases?

Web Activity
CyberDiet Tools
http://www.cyberdiet.com

Sponsor The co-founders, Cynthia Fink and Timi Gustafson, R.D., created CyberDiet in 1995. The information on CyberDiet is peer-reviewed by licensed registered dietitians as well as other health care providers.

Description Dedicated to the belief that healthy weight management and lifestyle change must come from a combination of balanced nutrition, regular exercise, and behavioral modification, CyberDiet provides a wealth of fun and well-presented nutritional information. Cyberdiet.com is a comprehensive resource for those seeking a change to a healthier lifestyle. Through articles, meal plans, recipes, interactive tools, nutritional programs, and much more, Cyberdiet.com provides the latest and one of the most comprehensive nutritional and weight management information sites available on the Internet.

Available Activities

1. The "Nutritional Profile" gives specific recommendations for calorie levels and nutritional needs, geared to your specific weight management goals.
2. "Body Mass Index" is a risk predictor that can help determine whether you will be negatively affected by your current weight and/or be at risk for obesity-related diseases, such as heart attacks, strokes, and so on.
3. The "Waist/Hip Ratio calculator" can pinpoint signs that your weight and weight distribution are becoming health risks.
4. The "CyberDiet Activity and Target Heart Rate calculators" provide basic information for safe and healthy exercise.
5. Through partnership with Wellmed, CyberDiet provides a complete and confidential health risk assessment.

Web Work

1. From the Cyberdiet.com home page, go to the "Self-Assessment" box and click on the "Nutrition Profile" link.
2. Enter your name, age, gender, height, and weight. Use the pull-down menu to select your preferred units for weight (pounds or kilograms) and height (feet or centimeters).
3. Use the pull-down menu to select your frame size (small, medium, or large) and your activity level (from sedentary to extremely active).
4. Then, click on the "Complete Profile" button at the bottom of the page.
5. You will then receive your calculated BMI reading and helpful tips regarding weight management. You will also be given the opportunity to select your desired weight goals (lose, maintain, or gain) and select a rate of desired weight change (from ½ pound per week to 2 pounds per week). When completed, click on the "Complete Your Profile" button.
6. You will then receive a series of tables describing the appropriate number of calories as well as amounts of a variety of nutrients (fat, protein, carbohydrates, vitamins, minerals, cholesterol, and fiber) that you should consume daily to help you achieve your weight goal.

Helpful Hints

1. It is most useful to complete all of the assessments because the results of one often are important in the evaluation of another.
2. To obtain the most from your interactive experience at CyberDiet.com, return to the home page and select one of a variety of links including a daily food planner, eating right, fast food facts, dining out, diet detective, and smart chef.

For additional Web activities, links, and suggested readings, visit our Health, Fitness, and Wellness Resource Center at http://health.wadsworth.com.

NOTES

1. C. Bouchard, G. A. Bray, and V. S. Hubbard, "Basic and Clinical Aspects of Regional Fat Distribution," *American Journal of Clinical Nutrition* 52 (1990): 946–950.
2. E. E. Calle, M. J. Thun, J. M. Petrelli, C. Rodriguez, and C. W. Heath, "Body-Mass Index and Mortality in a Prospective Cohort of U.S. Adults," *The New England Journal of Medicine* 341 (1999): 1097–1105.
3. K. M. Flegal, M. D. Carrol, R. J. Kuczmarski, and C. L. Johnson, "Overweight and Obesity in the United States: Prevalence and Trends, 1960–1994," *International Journal of Obesity and Related Metabolic Disorders* 22 (1998): 39–47.
4. J. H. Wilmore, "Exercise and Weight Control: Myths, Misconceptions, and Quackery," (lecture given at annual meeting of American College of Sports Medicine, Indianapolis, June 1994).

BODY COMPOSITION ASSESSMENT AND RECOMMENDED BODY WEIGHT DETERMINATION

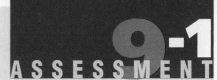

ASSESSMENT 9-1

Name: _____   Date: _____   Grade: _____

Instructor: _____   Course: _____   Section: _____

Necessary Lab Equipment:
Skinfold calipers and standard measuring tapes.

Objective:
To assess percent body fat using skinfold thickness and/or girth measurements and to determine recommended body weight based on percent body fat.

Instructions:
If skinfold calipers are available, use the skinfold thickness technique to assess your percent body fat (see Figures 9.2 and 9.3, pages 224–225). If calipers are unavailable, estimate the percent fat according to the girth measurements technique. You may wish to use both techniques and compare the results. Compute your recommended body weight according to your current and recommended percent body fat guidelines provided in Table 9.9, page 233).

I. Percent Body Fat According to Skinfold Thickness

Men

Chest (mm): _____

Abdomen (mm): _____

Thigh (mm): _____

Total (mm): _____

Percent Fat: _____

Women

Triceps (mm): _____

Suprailium (mm): _____

Thigh (mm): _____

Total (mm): _____

Percent Fat: _____

II. Percent Fat According to Girth Measurements

Men

Waist (inches): _____

Wrist (inches): _____

Difference: _____

Body Weight: _____

Percent Fat: _____

Women

Upper Arm (cm): _____   Constant A = _____

Age: _____   Constant B = _____

Hip (cm): _____   Constant C = _____

Wrist (cm): _____   Constant D = _____

BD* = A − B − C + D

BD = _____ − _____ − _____ + _____ = _____

Percent Fat = (495 ÷ BD) − 450 = (495 ÷ _____) − 450 = _____

*Body density

Interpretation of Body Composition Results

Briefly indicate your feelings about the results of your body composition analysis. If more than one technique was performed, how well do the results correlate with each other?

_____

_____

_____

_____

_____

_____

_____

State your body composition goal, why you desire to attain that goal, and indicate how important is the attainment of this goal to you. Also indicate changes that you feel you will need to make in your daily activity and diet habits to achieve this goal.

_____

_____

_____

_____

_____

_____

_____

_____

_____

_____

_____

_____

_____

_____

_____

_____

_____

III. Recommended Body Weight Determination

A. Body Weight (BW): _____

B. Current Percent Fat (%F)**: _____

C. Fat Weight (FW) = BW × %F

FW = _____ × _____ = _____

D. Lean Body Mass (LBM) = BW − FW = _____ − _____ = _____

E. Age: _____

F. Desired Fat Percent (DFP – *see* Table 9.9): _____

G. Recommended Body Weight (RBW) = LBM ÷ (1.0 − DFP**)

RBW = _____ ÷ (1.0 − _____) = _____

**Express percentages in decimal form (e.g., 25% = .25)

IV. Disease Risk and Recommended Body Weight Analysis

Briefly address how the results of your waist-to-hip ratio and body mass index tests relate to your potential risk for disease.

_____

_____

_____

_____

_____

_____

_____

_____

Based on your recommended body weight computation, indicate how you feel about this target weight and whether this weight is a realistic goal for you to attain.

_____

_____

_____

_____

_____

_____

_____

_____

WEIGHT AND HEALTH: DISEASE RISK ASSESSMENT

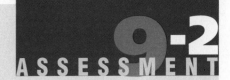

Name: _____   Date: _____   Grade: _____

Instructor: _____   Course: _____   Section: _____

Necessary Lab Equipment:
Scale and standard measuring tapes.

Objective:
Determine disease risk based on the waist-to-hip ratio and the body mass index (BMI).

Instructions:
Determine your height, waist, and hip measurements in inches. Record your body weight in pounds. Compute your waist-to-hip ratio and BMI as indicated below.

I. Waist-to-Hip Ratio

Waist (inches): _____

Hip (inches): _____

Ratio (waist ÷ hip): _____   Disease risk: _____

Recommended Standards

Waist-to-Hip Ratio

Men	Women	Disease Risk
<.95	<.80	Very Low
.96–.99	.81–.84	Low
>1.0	>.85	High

II. Body Mass Index

Weight (pounds): _____

Height (inches): _____

BMI = Weight × 705 ÷ (Height × Height)

BMI = _____ × 705 ÷ (_____ × _____)

BMI = _____   Disease risk: _____

Recommended Standards

BMI	Disease Risk
< 20.00	Moderate to Very High
20.00 to 21.99	Low
22.00 to 24.99	Very Low
25.00 to 29.99	Low
30.00 to 34.99	Moderate
35.00 to 39.99	High
≥ 40.00	Very High

10

WEIGHT MANAGEMENT, EATING DISORDERS, AND WELLNESS

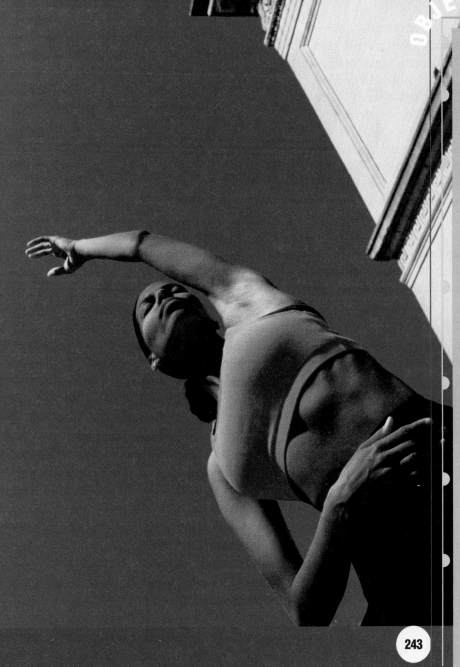

OBJECTIVES

Understand the health consequences of obesity.

Learn about fad diets and other myths and fallacies regarding weight control.

Become familiar with eating disorders and their associated medical problems and behavior patterns; understand the need for professional help to treat these conditions.

Become familiar with the physiology of weight loss, including setpoint theory and the effects of diet on basal metabolic rate.

Recognize the role of a lifetime exercise program as the key to a successful weight loss and maintenance program.

Learn how to implement a physiologically sound weight reduction and weight maintenance program.

Learn behavior modification techniques that help a person adhere to a lifetime weight maintenance program.

243

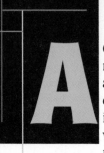

ACHIEVING AND MAINTAINING recommended body weight is a major objective of a physical fitness program. Next to poor cardiorespiratory fitness, excessive body fat is the most common problem in fitness and wellness assessments. (The assessment of recommended weight was discussed in Chapter 9.)

Two terms commonly used with reference to people who weigh more than recommended are "overweight" and "obesity." Obesity is the point at which excess body fat can lead to serious health problems. Obesity is a health hazard of epidemic proportions in most developed countries around the world. According to the World Health Organization, an estimated 35 percent of the adult population in industrialized nations is obese. Obesity has been established at a body mass index (BMI) of 30 or higher.

In the United States, 63 percent of men and 55 percent of women are overweight (with a BMI greater than 25) and 21 percent of men and 27 percent of women are obese (see Figure 10.1).[1] An estimated 97 million people are overweight and 30 million are obese.[2] Between 1960 and 1994, the overall (men and women combined) prevalence of adult obesity increased from about 13 percent to 22.5 percent. Most of this increase occurred in the 1990s.[3] In the last decade alone, the average weight of American adults increased by about 15 pounds. The prevalence of obesity is even higher in some ethnic groups, especially African Americans and Hispanic Americans.

About 44 percent of all women and 29 percent of all men are on a diet at any given moment.[4] People spend about $40 billion yearly attempting to lose weight. More

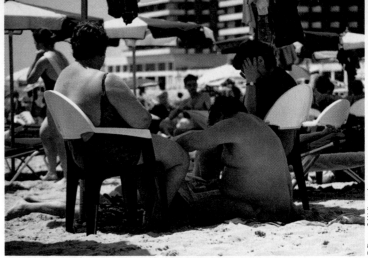

Obesity is a health hazard of epidemic proportions in developed countries.

than $10 billion goes to memberships in weight reduction centers, and another $30 billion to diet food sales. Furthermore, according to the National Institutes of Health, the total cost attributable to obesity-related disease is approximately $100 billion per year.

As the second leading cause of preventable death in the United States, overweight and obesity have been associated with several serious health problems and account for 15 to 20 percent of the annual mortality rate. About 300,000 deaths each year are caused by excessive body weight. In 1998, the American Heart Association identified obesity as one of the six major risk factors for coronary heart disease. Obesity also is a risk factor for hypertension; congestive heart failure; high blood lipids; atherosclerosis; stroke; thromboembolitic disease; varicose veins; Type II diabetes; osteoarthritis; gallbladder disease; sleep apnea; respiratory problems; ruptured intervertebral discs; and endometrial, breast, prostate, and colon cancers. Furthermore, it is implicated in psychological maladjustment and a higher accidental death rate.

> The lack of exercise, not the weight problem itself, possibly is the cause of many of the health risks associated with obesity.

OVERWEIGHT VERSUS OBESITY

Overweight and **obesity** are not the same thing. Many overweight people (carrying an excess of 10 to 20 pounds) are not obese. Although research findings from studies are inconsistent, the health consequences of a few extra pounds of body fat might be exaggerated and may apply primarily to severely overweight individuals.

FIGURE 10.1 PERCENTAGE OF THE ADULT POPULATION THAT IS OBESE AND OVERWEIGHT IN THE UNITED STATES.

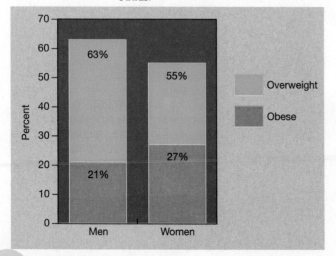

Data from the Aerobics Research Institute in Dallas confirm that, as body fat increases, so do blood cholesterol and triglycerides. The study also showed that the higher the fitness level, the lower the mortality rate, regardless of body weight.[5] This finding is significant because obese men who were fit had a lower risk of death than unfit men of average weight and the same risk as fit men of average weight. Thus, at least partially, lack of physical activity and not the weight problem itself may be the cause of premature death in some obese people.

Although the premature mortality of obese men in the study who become active decreased regardless of whether they lost weight, few obese men in the study were fit. This pattern holds true in life. Most obese people either don't exercise or are unable to do so because of functional limitations when they attempt to participate in traditional fitness activities such as jogging, walking, and cycling. Those who do exercise tend to lose weight.

A few pounds of excess weight may not be harmful to most people, but this is not always the case. People with excessive body fat who have diabetes and other cardiovascular risk factors (elevated blood lipids, high blood pressure, physical inactivity, and poor eating habits) benefit from weight loss. Even a modest reduction of 5 to 10 percent can reduce high blood pressure and total cholesterol levels. People who have a few extra pounds of weight but who otherwise are healthy and physically active, exercise regularly, and eat a healthy diet may not be at greater risk for early death.

Nonetheless, recommended body composition is a primary objective of overall physical fitness and enhanced quality of life. Individuals at recommended body weight are able to participate in a wide variety of moderate-to-vigorous activities without functional limitations. These people have the freedom to enjoy most of life's recreational activities to their fullest potential. Excessive body weight does not afford an individual the fitness level to enjoy vigorous lifetime activities such as basketball, soccer, racquetball, surfing, mountain cycling, and mountain climbing. Maintaining high fitness and recommended body weight gives a person a degree of independence throughout life that most people in developed nations no longer enjoy.

| Tolerable Weight |

Many people want to lose weight so they will look better. That's a noteworthy goal. The problem, however, is that they have a distorted image of what they would really look like if they were to reduce to what they think is their ideal weight. Hereditary factors play a big role, and only a small fraction of the population has the genes for a "perfect body."

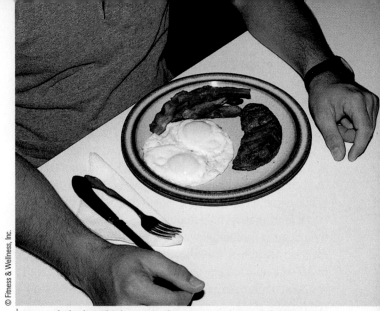

© Fitness & Wellness, Inc.

Low-carbohydrate/high-protein diets create nutritional deficiencies and can contribute to the development of cardiovascular disease, cancer, and osteoporosis.

When people set their own target weight, they should be realistic. Attaining the "excellent" levels of percent body fat (shown in Table 9.9, page 233) is extremely difficult for some. It is even more difficult to maintain, unless the person makes a commitment to a vigorous lifetime exercise program and permanent dietary changes. Few people are willing to do that. The "moderate" percent body fat category may be more realistic for many people.

A question you should ask yourself is "Am I happy with my weight?" Part of enjoying a higher quality of life is being happy with yourself. If you are not, you either need to do something about it or learn to live with it.

If you are above the moderate percent body fat category, you should try to come down and stay in this category, for health reasons. Being in the moderate category seems to pose no detriment to health.

If you are in the moderate category but would like to be lower, you need to ask yourself two more questions "How badly do I want it? Do I want it badly enough to implement lifetime exercise and dietary changes?" If you are not willing to change, you should stop worrying about your weight and deem the moderate category "tolerable" for you.

| The Weight Loss Dilemma |

For most people, **yo-yo dieting** carries as great a health risk as being overweight and remaining overweight in the first place. Epidemiological data show that frequent fluctuations in weight (up or down)

Overweight Excess weight according to a given standard, such as height or recommended percent body fat; less than obese.

Obesity A chronic disease characterized by excessive body fat in relation to lean body mass.

Yo-yo dieting Constantly losing and gaining weight.

markedly increase the risk of dying of cardiovascular disease.

Based on the findings that constant losses and regains can be hazardous to health, quick-fix diets should be replaced by a slow but permanent weight loss program (as described under "Exercise: The Key to Weight Loss and Weight Maintenance" on page 253). Individuals reap the benefits of recommended body weight when they achieve that weight and stay there throughout life.

Unfortunately, only about 10 percent of all people who begin a traditional weight loss program without exercise are able to lose the desired weight. Worse, only 5 in 100 are able to keep the weight off. The body is highly resistant to permanent weight changes through caloric restrictions alone.

Traditional diets have failed because few of them incorporate lifetime changes in food selection and exercise as fundamental to successful weight loss. When the diet stops, weight gain begins. The $40 billion diet industry tries to capitalize on the idea that weight can be lost quickly without taking into consideration the consequences of fast weight loss or the importance of lifetime behavioral changes to ensure proper weight loss and maintenance.

In addition, various studies indicate that most people, especially obese people, underestimate their energy intake. Those who try to lose weight but fail to do so are often described as "diet-resistant." One study found that, while on a "diet," a group of obese individuals with a self-reported history of diet resistance underreported their average daily caloric intake by almost 50 percent (1,028 self-reported calories versus 2,081 actual—see Figure 10.2).[6] These individuals also overestimated their amount of daily physical activity by about 25 percent (1,022 calories self-reported versus 771 actual). These differences represent an additional 1,304 calories of energy unaccounted for by the subjects in the study. The findings indicate that failing to lose weight often is related to misreports of actual food intake and level of physical activity.

| The Diet Craze |

Because we continue to hope that the latest diet to hit the market will really work this time, fad diets continue to appeal to people of all shapes and sizes. These diets may work for while, but most of the time the success is short-lived. These diets deceive people and claim the person will lose weight by following all instructions. Most fad diets are very low in calories and deprive the body of certain nutrients, generating a metabolic imbalance. Under these conditions, a lot of the weight lost is in the form of water and protein, and not fat.

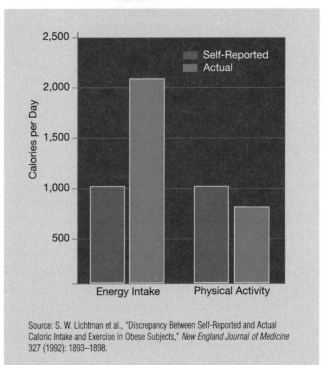

FIGURE 10.2 DIFFERENCES BETWEEN SELF-REPORTED AND ACTUAL DAILY CALORIC INTAKE AND EXERCISE IN OBESE INDIVIDUALS ATTEMPTING TO LOSE WEIGHT.

Source: S. W. Lichtman et al., "Discrepancy Between Self-Reported and Actual Caloric Intake and Exercise in Obese Subjects," *New England Journal of Medicine* 327 (1992): 1893–1898.

Close to half the weight lost on a crash diet consists of lean (protein) tissue. When the body uses protein instead of a combination of fats and carbohydrates as a source of energy, weight is lost as much as 10 times faster. A gram of protein produces half the amount of energy that fat does. Muscle protein is made up of one-fifth of protein and four-fifths water. Therefore, each pound of muscle yields only one-tenth the energy of a pound of fat. As a result, most of the weight lost is in the form of water, which on the scale, of course, looks good.

The largest diet craze in the market today are the low-carbohydrate diet plans. Although small variations exist between them, in general, "low-carb" diets limit the intake of carbohydrate-rich foods like bread, potatoes, rice, pasta, cereals, crackers, juices, sodas, sweets (candy, cake, cookies), and even fruits and vegetables. Dieters are allowed to eat all the protein-rich foods they desire, including steak, ham, chicken, fish,

> When I get calls about the latest diet fad, I imagine a trick birthday cake candle that keeps lighting up and we have to keep blowing it out.
>
> —Dr. Kelly Brownell, Yale University.

bacon, eggs, nuts, cheese, tofu, high-fat salad dressings, butter, and small amounts of a few fruits and vegetables. Examples of these diets are the Atkins Diet, The Zone, Protein Power, the Scarsdale Diet, the Carbohydrate Addict's diet, and Sugar Busters.

Consumption of carbohydrates causes a rise in blood sugar (glucose). During the process of digestion, carbohydrates are converted into glucose, a basic fuel used by every cell in the body. As blood glucose rises, insulin is released from the pancreas. Insulin is a hormone that facilitates the entry of glucose into the cells, thus lowering the glucose level in the bloodstream.

Not all carbohydrates cause a similar rise in blood glucose. The rise in glucose is based on the speed of digestion, which depends on a number of factors, including the size of the food particles. Small-particle carbohydrates breakdown rapidly and cause a quick, sharp rise in blood glucose. Thus, to gauge a food's effect on blood glucose, carbohydrates are classified by the **glycemic index**.

A high glycemic index signifies a quick rise in blood glucose. At the top of the 100-point scale is glucose itself. This index is not directly related to simple and complex carbohydrates, and index numbers are not always what one might expect. Rather, it is based on the actual laboratory-measured speed of absorption. Processed foods generally have a high glycemic index, whereas high-fiber foods tend to have a lower index (see Table 10.1).

The body functions best when blood sugar remains at a constant level. This is best accomplished with low–glycemic index foods (foods with a high glycemic index are useful to replenish depleted glycogen stores following prolonged or exhaustive exercise). Elimination of all high–glycemic index foods from the diet is not necessary. Combining them with low–glycemic index items or with some fat and protein brings the average index down. Regular consumption of high glycemic foods, nonetheless, can increase the risk of cardiovascular disease, especially in people at risk for diabetes.

Proponents of low-carb diets indicate that, if a person eats less carbohydrate and more protein, the pancreas will produce less insulin—and as insulin drops, the body turns to its own fat deposits for energy. There is no scientific proof, however, that high levels of insulin lead to weight gain. None of the authors of these diets have published any studies that validate these claims. Yet, these authors base their diets on the faulty premise that high insulin leads to overweight. In fact, we know the opposite to be true—excessive body fat causes insulin levels to rise.

Low-carb diets are contrary to the nutrition advice of most national leading health organizations, who recommend a diet low in animal fat and saturated fat and high in complex carbohydrates. Without fruits, vegetables, and grains, high-protein diets lack many vitamins, minerals, and fiber—all dietary factors that protect against an array of ailments and diseases. The major risk associated with low-carb diets is an increased risk of heart disease because high-protein foods are also high in fat content. Because of the low carbohydrate intake, the body also loses vitamin B, calcium, and potassium. Potential bone loss can further accentuate the risk for osteoporosis. Weakness, nausea, bad breath, constipation, irritability, lightheadedness, and fatigue are side effects commonly associated with these diets. Long-term adherence to a high-protein diet can also increase the risk of certain types of cancer.

In addition to the low-carb diets, "combo diets" such as the Schwarzbein and Suzanne Somers diets are also popular as of late. The Schwarzbein diet claims that eating proteins and nonstarchy carbohydrates together will keep the food from being stored as fat. The Suzanne Somers diet doesn't allow you to eat proteins within 3 hours of carbohydrates, and if fruits are eaten, the dieter must wait at least 20 minutes before eating other carbohydrate foods. Both of these diets allow consumption of high-protein/high-fat food items, which increases risk for heart disease.

Other diets allow only certain specialized foods. Most of these diets create a nutritional deficiency, which at times is even fatal. If people realized that no magic foods will provide all of the necessary nutrients and that a person has to eat a variety of foods to be well-nourished, the diet industry would not be as successful.

The reason many of these diets succeed is because a large number of foods are restricted on the diet, thus people tend to eat less food.

TABLE 10.1 GLYCEMIC INDEX OF SELECTED FOODS

Food Item	Index	Food Item	Index
Glucose	100	Muesli	56
Carrots	92	Peas	51
Honey	87	White pasta	50
Baked potatoes	85	Oatmeal	59
White rice	72	Whole wheat pasta	42
White bread	69	Oranges	40
Whole wheat bread	69	Apples	39
Bananas	62	Low-fat yogurt	33
Boiled potatoes	62	Fructose	20
Corn	59	Peanuts	13

Glycemic index A scale of 1 to 100 that rates the body's speed of absorption of various carbohydrates; 100 is the fastest. Formulated by rating the plasma glucose response of carbohydrate-containing foods with the response produced by the same amount of carbohydrate from a standard source, usually glucose or white bread.

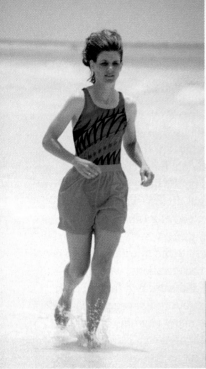

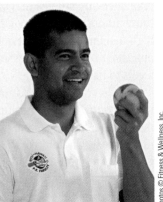

| Achieving and maintaining a high physical fitness percent body fat standard requires a lifetime commitment to regular physical activity and proper nutrition. |

Photos © Fitness & Wellness, Inc.

With the extraordinary variety of foods available in our midst, it is unrealistic to think that people will adhere to these diets for very long. People eventually get tired of eating the same thing day in and day out and start eating less, thus leading to weight loss. If they happen to achieve the lower weight but do not make permanent dietary changes, they regain the weight quickly once they go back to their previous eating habits.

A few diets recommend exercise along with caloric restrictions—the best method for weight reduction, of course. People who adhere to these diets will succeed, so the diet has achieved its purpose. Unfortunately, if the people do not change their food selection and activity level permanently, they gain back the weight once they discontinue dieting and exercise.

Also, let's not forget that we eat for reasons other than to lose weight—we eat for pleasure and for health. Healthy eating along with regular physical activity are two of the most essential components of a wellness lifestyle, and they provide the best weight management program available today.

EATING DISORDERS

Anorexia nervosa and bulimia nervosa are physical and emotional conditions thought to stem from some combination of individual, family, and social pressures. These disorders are characterized by an intense fear of becoming fat that does not disappear even when the dieter has lost extreme amounts of weight. Anorexia nervosa and bulimia nervosa are increasing steadily in most industrialized nations where society encourages low-calorie diets and thinness.

| Anorexia Nervosa |

Approximately 19 of every 20 individuals with **anorexia nervosa** are young women. An estimated 1 percent of the female population in the United States is anorexic. Anorexic individuals seem to fear weight gain more than death from starvation. Furthermore, they have a distorted image of their body and think of themselves as being fat even when they are emaciated.

Although a genetic predisposition may contribute, the anorexic person often comes from a mother-dominated home, with possible drug addictions in the family. The syndrome may emerge following a stressful life event and uncertainty about one's ability to cope efficiently.

Because the female role in society is changing rapidly, young women seem to be especially susceptible. Life experiences such as gaining weight, starting the menstrual period, beginning college, losing a boyfriend, having poor self-esteem, being socially rejected, starting a professional career, or becoming a wife or a mother can trigger the syndrome.

These individuals typically begin a diet and at first feel in control and happy about their weight loss, even if they are not overweight. To speed the weight loss, they frequently combine extreme dieting with exhaustive exercise and overuse of laxatives and diuretics.

SYMPTOMS OF ANOREXIA NERVOSA

Diagnostic criteria for anorexia nervosa are

- Refusal to maintain body weight over a minimal normal weight for age and height (including weight loss leading to maintenance of body weight less than 85 percent of that expected or failure to make expected weight gain during periods of growth, leading to body weight less than 85 percent of that expected).
- Intense fear of gaining weight or becoming fat, even though underweight.
- Disturbance in the way in which one's body weight, size, or shape is perceived; undue influence of body weight or shape on self-evaluation; or denial of the seriousness of the current low body weight.
- In postmenarcheal females, amenorrhea (absence of at least three consecutive menstrual cycles). (A woman is considered to have amenorrhea if her periods occur only following estrogen therapy.)

Source: Reprinted with permission from the **Diagnostic and Statistical Manual of Mental Disorders**, Fourth Edition, Text Revision. Copyright 2000 American Psychiatric Association.

> **Anorexics strongly deny their condition. They are able to hide it and deceive friends and relatives quite effectively.**

Anorexics commonly develop obsessive and compulsive behaviors and emphatically deny their condition. They are pre-occupied with food, meal planning, and grocery shopping, and they have unusual eating habits. As they lose weight and their health begins to deteriorate, anorexics feel weak and tired. They might realize they have a problem, but they will not stop the starvation and will refuse to consider the behavior abnormal.

Once they have lost a lot of weight and malnutrition sets in, physical changes become more visible. Typical changes are amenorrhea (stopping menstruation), digestive problems, extreme sensitivity to cold, hair and skin problems, fluid and electrolyte abnormalities (which may lead to an irregular heartbeat and sudden stopping of the heart), injuries to nerves and tendons, abnormalities of immune function, anemia, growth of fine body hair, mental confusion, inability to concentrate, lethargy, depression, dry skin, lower skin and body temperature, and osteoporosis.

Many of the changes of anorexia nervosa can be reversed, but treatment almost always requires professional help. The sooner it is started, the better the chances for reversibility and cure. Therapy consists of a combination of medical and psychological techniques to restore proper nutrition, prevent medical complications, and modify the environment or events that triggered the syndrome.

Unfortunately, anorexics strongly deny their condition. They are able to hide it and deceive friends and relatives quite effectively. Based on their behavior, many of them meet all of the characteristics of anorexia nervosa, but it goes undetected because both thinness and dieting are socially acceptable. Only a well-trained clinician is able to make a positive diagnosis.

Bulimia Nervosa

Bulimia nervosa is more prevalent than anorexia nervosa. For many years it was thought to be a variant of anorexia nervosa, but now it is identified as a separate condition. It afflicts mainly young people. As many as one in every five women on college campuses may be bulimic, according to some estimates. Bulimia nervosa also is more prevalent than anorexia nervosa in males, although bulimia is still much more prevalent in females.

Bulimics usually are healthy-looking people, well-educated, and near recommended body weight. They

---

SYMPTOMS OF BULIMIA NERVOSA

The diagnostic criteria for bulimia nervosa are

- Recurrent episodes of binge eating. An episode of binge eating is characterized by both of the following:
  1. Eating in a discrete period of time (for example, within any 2-hour period) an amount of food that is definitely more than most people would eat during a similar period and under similar circumstances.
  2. A sense of lack of control over eating during the episode (a feeling that one cannot stop eating or control what or how much one is eating).
- Recurring inappropriate compensatory behaviors to prevent weight gain, such as self-induced vomiting; misuse of laxatives, diuretics, enemas, or other medications; fasting; or excessive exercise.
- The binge eating and inappropriate compensatory behaviors both occur, on average, at least twice a week for 3 months.
- Self-evaluation is unduly influenced by body shape and weight.
- The disturbance does not occur exclusively during episodes of anorexia nervosa.

Source: Reprinted with permission from the **Diagnostic and Statistical Manual of Mental Disorders,** Fourth Edition, Text Revision. Copyright 2000 American Psychiatric Association.

---

seem to enjoy food and often socialize around it. In actuality, they are emotionally insecure, rely on others, and lack self-confidence and self-esteem. Recommended weight and food are important to them.

The binge-purge cycle usually occurs in stages. As a result of stressful life events or the simple compulsion to eat, bulimics engage periodically in binge eating that may last an hour or longer. With some apprehension, bulimics anticipate and plan the cycle. Next they feel an urgency to begin, followed by large and uncontrollable food consumption during which they may eat several thousand calories (up to 10,000 calories in extreme cases). After a short period of relief and satisfaction, feelings of deep guilt, shame, and intense fear of gaining weight ensue. Purging seems to be an easy answer, so the bingeing cycle can continue without fear of gaining weight.

The most typical form of purging is self-induced

> **Anorexia nervosa** An eating disorder characterized by self-imposed starvation to lose and maintain very low body weight.
>
> **Bulimia nervosa** An eating disorder characterized by a pattern of binge eating and purging in an attempt to lose and maintain low body weight.

vomiting. Bulimics also frequently ingest strong laxatives and emetics. Near-fasting diets and strenuous bouts of exercise are common. Medical problems associated with bulimia nervosa include cardiac arrhythmias, amenorrhea, kidney and bladder damage, ulcers, colitis, tearing of the esophagus or stomach, tooth erosion, gum damage, and general muscular weakness.

Unlike anorexics, bulimics realize their behavior is abnormal and feel great shame about it. Fearing social rejection, they pursue the binge-purge cycle in secrecy and at unusual hours of the day.

Bulimia nervosa can be treated successfully when the person realizes that this destructive behavior is not the solution to life's problems. A change in attitude can prevent permanent damage or death.

Treatment for anorexia nervosa and bulimia nervosa is available on most school campuses through the school's counseling center or the health center. Local hospitals also offer treatment for these conditions. Many communities have support groups, frequently led by professional personnel and usually free of charge.

PHYSIOLOGY OF WEIGHT LOSS

Only a few years ago the principles governing a weight loss and maintenance program seemed to be clear, but now we know the final answers are not in yet. Traditional concepts related to weight control have centered on three assumptions: (a) that balancing food intake against output allows a person to achieve recommended weight, (b) that all fat people just eat too much, and (c) that the human body doesn't care how much (or little) fat it stores. Although these statements contain some truth, they still are open to much debate and research. We now know that the causes of obesity are complex, including a combination of genetics, behavior, and lifestyle factors.

Energy-Balancing Equation

The principle embodied in the **energy-balancing equation** is simple: If daily energy requirements could be determined accurately, caloric intake could be balanced against output. This is not always the case, though, because genetic and lifestyle-related individual differences determine the number of calories required to maintain or lose body weight.

Table 10.2 (on page 257) offers some general guidelines for estimating daily caloric intake requirements according to lifestyle patterns. This is only an estimated figure and, as discussed later in the chapter, it serves only as a starting point from which individual adjustments have to be made.

One pound of fat represents 3,500 calories. Assuming that a person's basic daily caloric expenditure is 2,500 calories, if this person were to decrease intake by 500 calories per day, it should result in a loss of one pound of fat in 7 days ($500 \times 7 = 3,500$). But research has shown—and many dieters have experienced—that even when they carefully balance caloric input against caloric output, weight loss does not always happen as predicted. Furthermore, two people with similar measured caloric intake and output seldom lose weight at the same rate.

The most common explanation regarding individual differences in weight loss and weight gain has been the variation in human metabolism from one person to another. We are all familiar with people who "can eat all day long" and not gain an ounce of weight, whereas others "cannot even dream about food" without gaining weight. Because experts did not believe that human metabolism alone could account for such extreme differences, they developed several theories that might better explain them. Setpoint theory is one of the most widely accepted results of this development.

Setpoint Theory

Results of several research studies point toward a **weight-regulating mechanism (WRM)** that has a **setpoint** for controlling both appetite and the amount of fat stored. Setpoint is hypothesized to work like a thermostat for body fat, maintaining fairly constant body weight, because the mechanism "knows" at all times the exact amount of adipose tissue stored in the fat cells. Some people have high settings; others have low settings.

If body weight decreases (as in dieting), the setpoint senses this change and triggers the WRM to increase the person's appetite or make the body conserve energy to maintain the "set" weight. The opposite also may be true. Some people have a hard time gaining weight. In this case, the WRM decreases appetite or causes the body to waste energy to maintain the lower weight.

SETPOINT AND CALORIC INTAKE | Every person has his or her own certain body fat percentage (as established by the setpoint) that the body attempts to maintain. The genetic instinct to survive tells the body that fat storage is vital, and therefore it sets an acceptable fat level. This level remains somewhat constant or may climb gradually because of poor lifestyle habits.

For instance, under strict calorie reduction, the body may make extreme metabolic adjustments in an effort to maintain its setpoint for fat. The **basal metabolic rate**, the lowest level of caloric intake necessary to sustain life, may drop dramatically when confronted with a consistent negative caloric balance, and a person's weight may plateau for days or even weeks. A low metabolic rate compounds a person's problems in maintaining recommended body weight.

These findings were substantiated by research conducted at Rockefeller University in New York.[7] The authors showed that the body resists maintaining altered weight. Obese and lifetime nonobese individuals were used in the investigation. Following a 10 percent weight loss, in an attempt to regain the lost weight, the subjects' bodies compensated by burning up to 15 percent fewer calories than expected for the new reduced weight (after accounting for the 10 percent loss). The effects were similar in the obese and nonobese participants. These results imply that, after a 10 percent weight loss, a person would have to eat less or exercise more to account for the estimated deficit of about 200 to 300 calories.

In this same study, when the participants were allowed to increase their weight to 10 percent above their "normal" body weight (pre-weight loss), their bodies burned 10 to 15 percent more calories than expected in an attempt to waste energy and return to the pre-set weight. This is another indication that the body is highly resistant to weight changes unless additional lifestyle changes are incorporated to ensure successful weight management. These changes will be discussed later in this chapter.

Dietary restriction alone will not lower the setpoint, even though the person may lose weight and fat. When the dieter goes back to the normal or even below-normal caloric intake (at which the weight may have been stable for a long time), he or she quickly regains the fat lost as the body strives to regain a comfortable fat store.

> Weight loss should be gradual, not abrupt.

Let's use a practical illustration. A person would like to lose some body fat and assumes that a stable body weight has been reached at an average daily caloric intake of 1,800 calories (no weight gain or loss occurs at this daily intake). In an attempt to lose weight rapidly, this person now goes on a strict low-calorie diet, or even worse, a near-fasting diet. Immediately the body activates its survival mechanism and readjusts its metabolism to a lower caloric balance. After a few weeks of dieting at fewer than 400 to 600 calories per day, the body can now maintain its normal functions at 1,000 calories per day.

Having lost the desired weight, the person terminates the diet but realizes that the original intake of 1,800 calories per day will have to be lowered to maintain the new lower weight. To adjust to the new lower body weight, the intake is restricted to about 1,500 calories per day. The individual is surprised to find that, even at this lower daily intake (300 fewer calories), weight comes back at a rate of 1 pound every 1 to 2 weeks. Even after the diet has ended, this new lowered metabolic rate may take several months to kick back up to its normal level.

Given this survival mechanism, individuals clearly should not go on very low-calorie diets. Not only will this slow down resting metabolic rate, but it also will deprive the body of basic daily nutrients required for normal function.

Daily intakes of 1,200 to 1,500 calories provide the necessary nutrients if those calories are distributed properly over the five basic food groups (meeting the daily required servings from each group). Of course, the individual will have to learn which foods meet the requirements and yet are low in fat and sugar.

Under no circumstances should a person go on a diet that calls for below 1,200 calories for women and 1,500 calories for men. Weight (fat) is gained over months and years, not overnight. Likewise, weight loss should be gradual, not abrupt.

LOWERING THE SETPOINT A second way in which the setpoint may work is by keeping track of the nutrients and calories consumed daily. It is thought that the body, like a cash register, records the daily food intake and the brain will not feel satisfied until the calories and nutrients have been "registered."

This setpoint for calories and nutrients seems to operate even when people participate in moderately intense exercise. Some evidence suggests that people do not become hungrier with moderate physical activity. Therefore, people can choose to lose weight either by going hungry or by stepping up their daily physical activity. Calories burned through physical activity helps to lower body fat.

The most common question regarding the setpoint is how it can be lowered so the body will feel comfortable at a lesser fat percentage. These factors seem to affect the setpoint directly by lowering the fat thermostat:

1. Aerobic exercise.
2. A diet high in complex carbohydrates.
3. Nicotine.
4. Amphetamines.

The last two are more destructive than the overweight, so they are not reasonable alternatives (as far as the extra

Energy-balancing equation A principle holding that as long as caloric input equals caloric output, the person will not gain or lose weight. If caloric intake exceeds output, the person gains weight; when output exceeds input, the person loses weight.

Weight-regulating mechanism (WRM) A feature of the hypothalamus (an area of the brain) that controls how much the body should weigh.

Setpoint Weight control theory proposing that the body has an established weight and strongly attempts to maintain that weight.

Basal metabolic rate (BMR) The lowest level of oxygen consumption necessary to sustain life.

> The only practical and sensible way to lower the setpoint is a combination of aerobic exercise and a diet high in complex carbohydrates and low in fat.

strain on the heart is concerned, smoking one pack of cigarettes per day is said to be the equivalent of carrying 50 to 75 pounds of excess body fat).

On the other hand, diets high in fats and refined carbohydrates, near-fasting diets, and perhaps even artificial sweeteners seem to raise the setpoint. Therefore, the only practical and sensible way to lower the setpoint and lose fat weight is a combination of aerobic exercise and a diet high in complex carbohydrates and low in fat.

Because of the effects of proper food management on the body's setpoint, many nutritionists believe the total *number* of calories should not be the main concern in a weight control program. Rather, it should be the *source* of those calories. In this regard, most of the weight loss effort is better spent retraining eating habits, increasing the intake of complex carbohydrates and high-fiber foods, and decreasing the consumption of refined carbohydrates (sugars) and fats. In most cases, this change in eating habits will bring about a decrease in total daily caloric intake. Because 1 gram of carbohydrates provides only 4 calories, as opposed to 9 calories per gram of fat, you could eat twice the volume of food (by weight) when you substitute carbohydrates for fat.

A NEW APPROACH

A "diet" is no longer viewed as a temporary tool to aid in weight loss but, instead, as a permanent change in eating behaviors to ensure weight management and better health. The role of increased physical activity also must be considered, because achieving weight loss, maintenance, and recommended body composition are seldom attained without a moderate reduction in caloric intake combined with a regular exercise program.

Fat can be lost by selecting the proper foods, exercising, or restricting calories. When a person tries to lose weight by dietary restrictions alone, lean body mass (muscle protein, along with vital organ protein) always decreases. The amount of lean body mass lost depends entirely on caloric limitation.

When people go on a near-fasting diet, up to half of the weight loss is lean body mass and the other half is actual fat loss (see Figure 10.3).[8] When diet is combined with exercise, close to 100 percent of the weight loss is

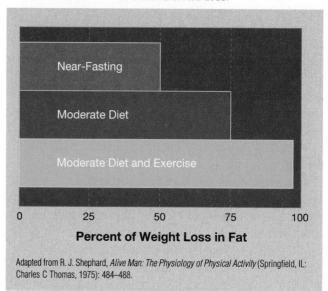

FIGURE **10.3** EFFECTS OF THREE FORMS OF DIETING ON FAT LOSS.

Near-Fasting

Moderate Diet

Moderate Diet and Exercise

0   25   50   75   100

Percent of Weight Loss in Fat

Adapted from R. J. Shephard, *Alive Man: The Physiology of Physical Activity* (Springfield, IL: Charles C Thomas, 1975): 484–488.

in the form of fat, and lean tissue actually may increase. Loss of lean body mass is never good, because it weakens the organs and muscles and slows down metabolism. Large losses of lean tissue can disturb heart function and damage other organs. Equally important is not to over-indulge (binge) following a very-low-calorie diet. This may cause changes in metabolic rate and electrolyte balance, which could trigger fatal cardiac arrhythmias.

Contrary to some beliefs, aging is not the main reason for the lower metabolic rate. It is not so much that metabolism slows down but that people slow down. As people age, they tend to rely more on the amenities of life (remote controls, cellular telephones, intercoms, single-level homes, riding lawnmowers) that lull a person into sedentary living.

Basal metabolism is directly related to lean body weight. The more lean tissue, the higher the metabolic rate. As a consequence of sedentary living and less physical activity, the lean component decreases and fat tissue increases. The human body requires a certain amount of oxygen per pound of lean body mass. Because fat is considered metabolically inert from the point of view of caloric use (that is, the body burns few calories to sustain fat), the lean tissue uses most of the oxygen, even at rest. As muscle and organ mass (lean body mass) decreases, so do the energy requirements at rest.

Reductions in lean body mass are common in aging people (primarily because of physical inactivity) and those on severely restricted diets. The loss of lean body mass also may account for a lower metabolic rate (described earlier) and the longer time it takes to kick back up.

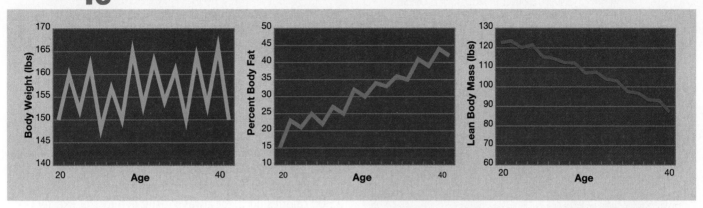

Diets with caloric intakes below 1,200 to 1,500 calories cannot guarantee the retention of lean body mass. Even at this intake level, some loss is inevitable unless the diet is combined with exercise. Despite the claims of many diets that they do not alter the lean component, the simple truth is that, regardless of what nutrients may be added to the diet, severe caloric restrictions always prompt the loss of lean tissue. Too many people go on low-calorie diets constantly. Every time they do, the metabolic rate slows down as more lean tissue is lost.

Many people in their 40s and older who weigh the same as they did when they were 20 tend to think they are at recommended body weight. During this span of 20 years or more, they may have dieted many times without participating in an exercise program. They regain the weight shortly after they terminate each diet, and most of that gain is in fat. Maybe at age 20 they weighed 150 pounds, of which only 15 percent was fat. Now at age 40, even though they still weigh 150 pounds, they might be 30 percent fat (see Figure 10.4). At recommended body weight, they wonder why they are eating very little and still having trouble staying at that weight.

EXERCISE: THE KEY TO WEIGHT LOSS AND WEIGHT MAINTENANCE

A more effective way to tilt the energy-balancing equation in your favor is by burning calories through physical activity. Exercise also seems to exert control over how much a person weighs.

Starting at age 25, the typical American gains 1 pound of weight per year. This weight gain represents a simple energy surplus of under 10 calories per day. In most cases, the additional weight accumulated in middle age comes from people becoming less physically active

and not as a result of increases in caloric intake. Dr. Jack Wilmore, a leading exercise physiologist and expert weight management researcher, stated:

> Physical inactivity is certainly a major, if not the primary, cause of obesity in the United States today. A certain minimal level of activity might be necessary for us to accurately balance our caloric intake to our caloric expenditure. With too little activity, we appear to lose the fine control we normally have to maintain this incredible balance. This fine balance amounts to less than 10 calories per day, or the equivalent of one potato chip.[9]

Exercise is crucial to losing weight and maintaining weight. Not only will exercise maintain lean tissue, but advocates of the setpoint theory say that exercise resets the fat thermostat to a new, lower level. This change may be rapid, or it may take time. A few overweight individuals have exercised faithfully almost daily, 60 minutes at a time, for a whole year before seeing significant weight change. People with a "sticky" setpoint have to be patient and persistent.

If a person is trying to lose weight, a combination of aerobic and strength-training exercises works best. Aerobic exercise is the best to offset the setpoint, and the continuity and duration of these types of activities cause many calories to be burned in the process. The role of aerobic exercise in successful lifetime weight management cannot be overestimated.

> Physical inactivity is certainly a major, if not the primary, cause of obesity in the United States today.
> —Dr. Jack Wilmore

As illustrated in Figure 10.5, greater weight loss is achieved by combining a diet with an aerobic exercise program.[10] Of even greater significance, only the individuals who participated in an 18-month post-diet

FIGURE 10.5 AEROBIC EXERCISE AND WEIGHT LOSS AND MAINTENANCE IN MODERATELY OBESE INDIVIDUALS.

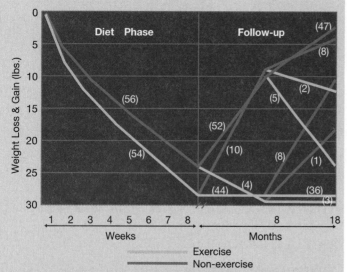

Note: Numbers in parentheses indicate number of participants.

Source: K. N., Pavlou, S. Krey, and W. P. Steffe, "Exercise as an Adjunct to Weight Loss and Maintenance in Moderately Obese Subjects," *American Journal of Clinical Nutrition* 49 (1989): 1115–1123.

Although inches and percent body fat decrease when sedentary individuals begin an exercise program, body weight often remains the same or may even increase during the first few weeks of the program. Exercise helps to increase muscle tissue, connective tissue, blood volume (as much as 500 ml, or the equivalent of 1 pound, following the first week of aerobic exercise), enzymes and other structures within the cell, and glycogen (which binds water). All of these changes lead to a higher functional capacity of the human body. With exercise, most of the weight loss becomes apparent after a few weeks of training, after the lean component has stabilized.

Although we know that a negative caloric balance of 3,500 calories does not always result in a loss of exactly 1 pound of fat, the role of exercise in achieving a negative balance by burning additional calories is significant in weight reduction and maintenance programs. Sadly, some individuals claim that the number of calories burned during exercise is hardly worth the effort. They think that cutting their daily intake by some 300 calories is easier than participating in some sort of exercise that would burn the same amount of calories. The problem is that the willpower to cut those 300 calories lasts only a few weeks, and then the person goes right back to the old eating patterns.

If a person gets into the habit of exercising regularly, say three times a week, jogging 3 miles per exercise session (about 300 calories burned), this represents 900 calories in one week, about 3,600 calories in one month, or 46,800 calories per year. This minimal amount of exercise could mean as many as 13.5 extra pounds of fat in one year, 27 in two, and so on.

aerobic exercise program were able to keep the weight off. Those who discontinued exercise gained weight. Furthermore, of those who initiated or resumed exercise during the 18-month follow-up, all were able to lose weight again. Individuals who only dieted and did not exercise regained 60 percent and 92 percent of their weight loss at the 6- and 18-month follow-ups, respectively.

Weight loss might be more rapid when aerobic exercise is combined with a strength-training program. Each additional pound of muscle tissue can raise the basal metabolic rate by about 35 calories per day.[11] Thus, an individual who adds 5 pounds of muscle tissue as a result of strength training increases the basal metabolic rate by 175 calories per day (35×5), which equals 63,875 calories per year (175×365) or the equivalent of 18.25 pounds of fat ($63,875 \div 3,500$).

Strength training is suggested especially for people who think they are at their recommended body weight, yet their body fat percentage is higher than recommended. The number of calories burned during a typical hour-long strength-training session is much less than during an hour of aerobic exercise. Because of the high intensity of strength training, the person needs frequent rest intervals to recover from each set of exercise. The average person actually lifts weights only 10 to 12 minutes during each hour of exercise. In the long run, however, the person enjoys the benefits of gains in lean tissue. (Guidelines for developing aerobic and strength-training programs are given in Chapter 7.)

CALORIC EXPENDITURE

Activity	Calories Burned Per Hour
Sitting	80–100
Standing	95–120
Light activity Cleaning house, office work, golf	240–300
Moderate activity Walking briskly (3.5 mph), gardening, cycling (5.5 mph), dancing	370–460
Strenuous activity Jogging (9 min./mile), swimming	580–730
Very strenuous Running (7 min./mile), racquetball, cross-country skiing	740–920

We tend to forget that our weight creeps up gradually over the years, not just overnight. Hardly worth the effort? And we have not even taken into consideration the increase in lean tissue, possible resetting of the setpoint, benefits to the cardiovascular system, and, most important, the improved quality of life. The fundamental reasons for overfatness and obesity, few could argue, are sedentary living and lack of physical activity.

> Regular activity seems to be the strongest predictor of success in long-term weight management.

Many of the health and disease-prevention benefits that people try to achieve by losing weight are reaped through exercise alone, even without weight loss. Exercise offers protection against premature morbidity and mortality for everyone, including people who already have risk factors for cardiovascular disease (see Chapter 11). The lack of exercise, not the weight problem itself, may cause many of the health risks associated with obesity.

Low-Intensity Versus High-Intensity Exercise for Weight Loss

Some individuals promote low-intensity exercise over high-intensity for weight loss purposes. As compared with high intensity, low-intensity exercise burns a greater proportion of calories derived from fat. The lower the intensity of exercise, the higher the percentage of fat utilization as an energy source. In theory, if you are trying to lose fat, this principle makes sense, but in reality it is misleading. The bottom line when you are trying to lose weight is to burn more calories. When your daily caloric expenditure exceeds your intake, weight is lost. The more calories you burn, the more fat you lose.

During low-intensity exercise, up to 50 percent of the calories burned may be derived from fat (the other 50 percent from glucose [carbohydrates]). With intense exercise, only 30 to 40 percent of the caloric expenditure comes from fat. Overall, however, you can burn twice as many (or more) calories during high-intensity exercise, and, subsequently more fat as well. Let's look at a practical illustration. If you exercise for 30 minutes at a moderate intensity and burn 200 calories, about 100 of those calories (50 percent) would come from fat. If you exercise at high intensity during those same 30 minutes, you may burn 400 calories, with 120 to 160 of the calories (30 to 40 percent) coming from fat. Thus, if you exercised at a low intensity, you would have to do so twice as long to burn the same number of calories. Another benefit is that the metabolic rate remains at a higher level after high-intensity exercise, so you continue to burn more calories following exercise.

Moreover, high-intensity exercise by itself appears to trigger greater fat loss than low-intensity exercise. Research conducted at Laval University in Quebec, Canada, showed that subjects who performed a high-intensity intermittent training program lost more body fat than a low- to moderate-intensity continuous aerobic endurance group.[12] Even more surprisingly, this finding occurred despite the fact that the high-intensity group burned fewer total calories per exercise session. The results support the notion that vigorous exercise is more conducive to weight loss than low- to moderate-intensity exercise.

Before you start high-intensity exercise sessions, a word of caution is in order. Be sure that it is medically safe for you to participate in such activities and that you build up gradually to that level. If you are cleared to participate in high-intensity exercise, do not attempt to do too much too quickly, because you may suffer injuries and discouragement. You must allow your body a proper conditioning period of 8 to 12 weeks, or even longer for people with a moderate-to-serious weight problem. High intensity also does not mean high impact. High-impact activities are the most common cause of exercise related injuries. Additional information on these topics is presented in Chapter 7.

The previous discussion on high- versus low-intensity exercise does not mean that low intensity is not effective. Low-intensity exercise provides substantial health benefits, and people who initiate exercise programs are more willing to participate and stay with low-intensity programs. Low-intensity exercise does promote weight loss, but it is not as effective. You will need to exercise longer to obtain the same results.

WEIGHT LOSS MYTHS

Cellulite and **spot reducing** are mythical concepts. **Cellulite** is nothing but enlarged fat cells that bulge out from accumulated body fat.

Doing several sets of daily sit-ups will not get rid of fat in the midsection of the body. When fat comes off, it does so throughout the entire body, not just the exercised area. The greatest proportion of fat may come off the biggest fat deposits, but the caloric output of a few sets of sit-ups has practically no effect on

Spot reducing Fallacious theory claiming that exercising a specific body part will result in significant fat reduction in that area.

Cellulite Term frequently used in reference to fat deposits that "bulge out"; these deposits are enlarged fat cells from excessive accumulation of body fat.

> You can't "spot reduce." When you lose fat, you lose it from all the areas in your body where it is stored.

reducing total body fat. A person has to exercise much longer to really see results.

Other touted means toward quick weight loss—rubberized sweatsuits, steam baths, mechanical vibrators— are misleading. When a person wears a sweatsuit or steps into a sauna, the weight lost is not fat but merely a significant amount of water. Sure, it looks nice when you step on the scale immediately afterward, but this represents a false loss of weight. As soon as you replace body fluids, you gain back the weight quickly.

Wearing rubberized sweatsuits not only hastens the rate of body fluid loss—fluid that is vital during prolonged exercise—but it also raises core temperature at the same time. This combination puts a person in danger of dehydration, which impairs cellular function and in extreme cases can even cause death.

Similarly, mechanical vibrators are worthless in a weight-control program. Vibrating belts and turning rollers may feel good, but they require no effort whatsoever. Fat cannot be shaken off. It is lost primarily by burning it in muscle tissue.

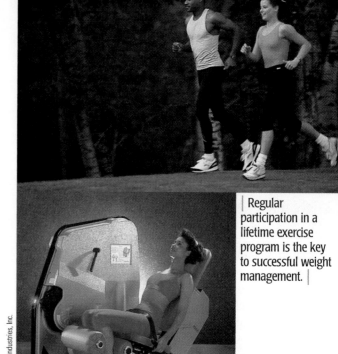

Regular participation in a lifetime exercise program is the key to successful weight management.

IMPLEMENTING A SOUND AND SENSIBLE WEIGHT LOSS PROGRAM

Dieting never has been fun and never will be. People who are overweight and are serious about losing weight, however, have to include regular exercise in their life along with proper food management and a sensible reduction in caloric intake.

Some precautions are in order, because excessive body fat is a risk factor for cardiovascular disease. Depending on the extent of the weight problem, a medical examination and possibly a stress ECG (see discussion on stress electrocardiogram in Chapter 11, page 294) may be a good idea before undertaking the exercise program. A physician should be consulted in this regard.

Significantly overweight individuals may also have to choose activities in which they will not have to support their own body weight but that still will be effective in burning calories. Injuries to joints and muscles are common in overweight individuals who participate in weight-bearing exercises such as walking, jogging, and aerobics.

Swimming may not be a good weight-loss exercise either. More body fat makes a person more buoyant and

most people are not at the skill level to swim fast enough to get the best training effect. They tend to just float along, limiting the number of calories burned as well as the benefits to the cardiorespiratory system.

Some better alternatives are riding a bicycle (either road or stationary), walking in a shallow pool, doing water aerobics, or running in place in deep water (treading water). The water exercises are gaining popularity and have proven to be effective in reducing weight without the pain and risk of injuries. Through the caloric expenditure of selected physical activities given in Table 10.3, you will be able to determine your own daily caloric requirement using Assessment 10-1.

How long should each exercise session last? To develop and maintain cardiorespiratory fitness, 20 to 30 minutes of exercise at the recommended target rate, three to five times per week, is suggested (see Chapter 7). For weight-loss purposes, many experts recommend exercising at least 45 minutes at a time, five to six times a week.

A person should not try to do too much too fast. Unconditioned beginners should start with about 15 minutes of aerobic exercise three times a week, gradually increasing the duration by approximately 5 minutes per week and the frequency by 1 day per week during the next 3 to 4 weeks.

One final benefit of exercise for weight control is that it allows fat to be burned more efficiently. Carbohydrates and fats are both sources of energy. When the glucose levels begin to drop during prolonged exercise, more fat is used as energy substrate.

Equally important is that fat-burning enzymes increase with aerobic training. Fat is lost primarily by burning it in muscle. Therefore, as the concentration of the enzymes increases, so does the ability to burn fat.

In addition to exercise and adequate food management, sensible adjustments in caloric intake are recommended. Most research finds that a negative caloric balance is required to lose weight. Perhaps the only exception is with people who are eating too few calories. A nutrient analysis often reveals that faithful dieters are not consuming enough calories. These people actually need to increase their daily caloric intake (combined with an exercise program) to get their metabolism to kick back up to a normal level.

The reasons for prescribing a lower caloric figure to lose weight are as follows.

1. Most people underestimate their caloric intake and are eating more than they should be eating.
2. Developing new behaviors takes time, and some people have trouble adjusting to new eating habits.
3. Many individuals are in such poor physical condition that they take a long time to increase their activity level enough to offset the setpoint and burn enough calories to aid in loss of body fat.
4. Some dieters have difficulty succeeding unless they can count calories.
5. A few people simply will not alter their food selection. For those who will not (who will maintain their risk for chronic diseases), a large increase in physical activity, a negative caloric balance, or a combination of the two is the only way to lose weight successfully.

You can estimate your daily caloric requirement by consulting Tables 10.2 and 10.3 and Assessment 10-1. Because this is only an estimated value, individual adjustments related to many of the factors discussed in this chapter may be necessary to establish a more precise value. Nevertheless, the estimated value does offer a beginning guideline for weight control or reduction. Assessments 10-2 and 10-3 can also be used to establish your eating patterns and sources of calories and fat in your diet.

The average daily caloric requirement without exercise is based on typical lifestyle patterns, total body weight, and gender. Individuals who hold jobs that require heavy manual labor burn more calories during the day than those who have sedentary jobs (such as working behind a desk). To find your activity level, refer to Table 10.2 and rate yourself accordingly. The number

TABLE 10.2 AVERAGE CALORIC REQUIREMENT PER POUND OF BODY WEIGHT BASED ON LIFESTYLE PATTERNS AND GENDER

	Calories Per Pound	
	Men	Women*
Sedentary—limited physical activity	13.0	12.0
Moderate physical activity	15.0	13.5
Hard Labor—strenuous physical effort	17.0	15.0

*Pregnant or lactating women add 3 calories to these values.

TABLE 10.3 ESTIMATED CALORIC EXPENDITURE BASED ON PERCEIVED EXERTION OF PHYSICAL ACTIVITY

Perceived Exertion		Caloric Expenditure (Cal/lb/min)
Very, very light	(7)*	0.030
Very light	(9)	0.040
Fairly light	(11)	0.050
Somewhat hard	(13)	0.070
Hard	(15)	0.090
Very hard	(17)	0.100
Very, very hard	(19)	0.110

* Numbers in parentheses indicate the rate of perceived exertion (RPE), see Figure 7.2, Chapter 7.

Adapted from W. W. K. Hoeger and S. A. Hoeger, "Caloric Expenditure of Selected Physical Activities," *Principles & Labs for Fitness and Wellness* (Wadsworth/Thomson Learning, 2002): 126.

given in Table 10.2 is per pound of body weight, so you multiply your current weight by that number. For example, the typical caloric requirement to maintain body weight for a moderately active male who weighs 160 pounds is 2,400 calories (160 lbs × 15 cal/lb).

To determine the average number of calories you burn daily as a result of exercise, figure out the total number of minutes you exercise weekly, then figure the daily average exercise time. For instance, a person exercising "somewhat hard" five times a week, 30 minutes each time, exercises 150 minutes per week (5 × 30). The average daily exercise time is 21 minutes (150 ÷ 7, rounded off to the lowest unit).

Next, from Table 10.3, find the energy requirement for the activity (or activities) based on its perceived exertion. In the case of "somewhat hard," the requirement is .070 calories per pound of body weight per minute of activity (cal/lb/min). With a body weight of 160 pounds, this man would burn 11.2 calories each minute (body weight × .070, or 160 × .070). In 21 minutes he burns almost 235 calories (21 × 11.2).

Now you can obtain the estimated total caloric requirement, with exercise, needed to maintain body weight. To do this, add the typical daily requirement (without exercise) and the average calories burned through exercise. In our example, it is 2,635 calories (2,400 + 235).

If a negative caloric balance is recommended to lose weight, this person has to consume fewer than 2,635 calories daily to achieve the objective. Because of the many factors that play a role in weight control, the 2,635 calories is only an estimated daily requirement. Furthermore, we cannot predict that you will lose exactly 1 pound of fat in 1 week if you cut your daily intake by 500 calories (500 × 7 = 3,500 calories, or the equivalent of 1 pound of fat).

The estimated daily caloric figure is only a target guideline for weight control. Periodic readjustments are necessary because individuals differ, and the estimated daily cost changes as you lose weight and modify your exercise habits.

To determine the target caloric intake to lose weight, multiply your current weight by 5 and subtract this amount from the total caloric requirement with exercise, as determined previously (you can figure out your own requirement using Assessment 10-1). This final caloric intake to lose weight should never be below 1,200 calories for women and 1,500 for men. If distributed properly over the various food groups, these figures are the lowest caloric intakes that provide the necessary nutrients the body needs. In terms of percentages of total calories, the daily distribution should be approximately 60 percent carbohydrates (mostly complex carbohydrates), less than 30 percent fat, and about 12 percent protein.

Many experts believe a person can take off weight more efficiently by reducing the amount of daily fat intake to 10–20 percent of the total daily caloric intake. Because 1 gram of fat supplies more than twice the amount of calories that

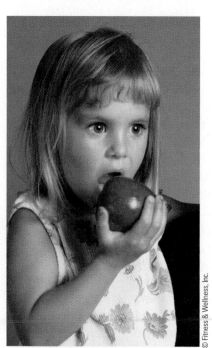
The establishment of healthy eating patterns starts at a young age.

SUBSTITUTION CHART	
Butter	Powdered butter flavoring, reduced-calorie margarine
Cooking oil	Vegetable cooking spray, broth, wine
Mayonnaise	Low-calorie salad dressing; reduced-calorie, low-fat mayonnaise
Eggs	Egg substitute or egg whites
Salad dressing	Oil-free or reduced-calorie dressing; flavored vinegars
Sour cream	Plain low-fat or nonfat yogurt, low-fat or nonfat sour cream
Cream cheese	Low-fat cream cheese, Neufchâtel cheese
Whole milk	Skim milk or 1%
Evaporated milk	Evaporated skim milk
Microwave popcorn (pre-bagged)	Air-popped or microwave-popped without fats
Ground beef	Ground chicken or turkey
Bacon and ham	Turkey ham

carbohydrates and protein do, the general tendency is not to overeat.

Further, it takes only 3 to 5 percent of ingested calories to store fat as fat, whereas it takes approximately 25 percent of ingested calories to convert carbohydrates to fat. Other research indicates that if people eat the same number of calories as carbohydrate or fat, those on the fat diet will store more fat. Successful weight-loss programs allow only small amounts of fat in the diet.

Many people have trouble adhering to a 10 percent to 20 percent fat–calorie diet. During weight loss periods, however, you are strongly encouraged to do so. Start with a 20 percent fat–calorie diet. Refer to Table 10.4 to determine the grams of fat at 10 percent, 20 percent, and 30 percent of the total calories

> Successful weight management is accomplished by making a lifetime commitment to physical activity and proper food selection.

Caloric Intake	Grams of Fat		
	10%	20%	30%
1,200	13	27	40
1,300	14	29	43
1,400	16	31	47
1,500	17	33	50
1,600	18	36	53
1,700	19	38	57
1,800	20	40	60
1,900	21	42	63
2,000	22	44	67
2,100	23	47	70
2,200	24	49	73
2,300	26	51	77
2,400	27	53	80
2,500	28	56	83
2,600	29	58	87
2,700	30	60	90
2,800	31	62	93
2,900	32	64	97
3,000	33	67	100

for selected energy intakes. Also, use the form provided in Assessment 10-2 to monitor your daily fat intake.

MONITORING YOUR DIET WITH DAILY FOOD LOGS

To help you monitor and adhere to your diet plan, you may use the daily food logs provided in Assessments 10-4 to 10-7. Before using any of these forms, make a master copy for your files so you can make future copies as needed. Guidelines are provided for 1,200-, 1,500-, 1,800-, and 2,000-calorie diet plans. These plans have been developed based on the Food Guide Pyramid and the Dietary Guidelines for Americans to meet the Recommended Dietary Allowances.[13] The objective is to meet (not exceed) the number of servings allowed for each diet plan. Each time you eat a serving of a certain food, record it in the appropriate box.

To lose weight, you should use the diet plan that most closely approximates your target caloric intake. Emphasizing low-fat/lean foods, the plan is based on the following caloric allowances for each food group:

- Bread, cereal, rice, and pasta group: 80 calories per serving.

- Fruit group: 60 calories per serving.
- Vegetable group: 25 calories per serving.
- Milk, yogurt, and cheese group (use low-fat products): 120 calories per serving.
- Meat, poultry, fish, dry beans, eggs, and nuts group: Use 300-calorie low-fat frozen entrees per serving or an equivalent amount if you prepare your own main dish (see discussion below).

As you start your diet plan, pay particular attention to food serving sizes. To find out what counts as one serving, refer to the Food Guide Pyramid (see Figure 8.5 in Chapter 8). Take care with cup and glass sizes. A standard cup is 8 ounces, but most glasses nowadays contain between 12 and 16 ounces. If you drink 12 ounces of fruit juice, in essence you are getting two servings of fruit, because a standard serving is 3/4 cup of juice.

Read food labels carefully to compare the caloric value of the serving listed on the label with the caloric guidelines provided above. Here are some examples:

- One slice of standard white bread has about 80 calories. A plain bagel may have 200 to 350 calories. Although it is low in fat, a 350-calorie bagel is equivalent to almost 4½ servings in the bread, cereal, rice, and pasta group.
- The standard serving size listed on the food label for most cereals is 1 cup. As you read the nutrition information, however, you find that for the same cup of cereal, one type of cereal has 120 calories whereas another cereal has 200 calories. Because a standard serving in the bread, cereal, rice, and pasta group is 80 calories, the first cereal would be 1½ servings and the second one 2½ servings.
- A medium-size fruit usually is considered to be 1 serving. Large fruits could provide as many as 3 servings.
- In the milk, yogurt, and cheese groups, 1 serving represents 120 calories. A cup of whole milk has about 160 calories, whereas a cup of skim milk contains 88 calories. A cup of whole milk, therefore, would provide 1⅓ servings in this food group.

To be more accurate with caloric intake and to simplify meal preparation, use commercially prepared low-fat frozen entrees as the main dish for lunch and dinner meals (only one entree for the 1,200-calorie diet plan—see Assessment 10-4). Look for entrees that provide about 300 calories and no more than 6 grams of fat per entree. These two entrees can be used as selections for the meat, poultry, fish, dry beans, eggs, and nuts group and will provide most of the daily protein requirement for the body. Along with each entree, supplement the meal with some of your servings from the other food groups. This diet plan has been used successfully in weight-loss research programs.[14] If you choose not to use these low-fat entrees, prepare a similar meal using 3 ounces (cooked) of lean meat, poultry, or fish with additional vegetables, rice, or pasta that will provide 300 calories with fewer than 6 grams of fat per dish.

In your daily logs, be sure to record the precise amount in each serving. If you choose to do so, you can run a computerized nutrient analysis to verify your caloric intake and food distribution pattern (percent of total calories from carbohydrate, fat, and protein).

BEHAVIOR MODIFICATION AND ADHERENCE TO A WEIGHT MANAGEMENT PROGRAM

Achieving and maintaining recommended body composition is by no means impossible, but this does require desire and commitment. If weight management is to become a priority in life, people must realize that they have to retrain their behavior to some extent.

Modifying old habits and developing new, positive behaviors take time. Individuals have applied the following management techniques to change detrimental behavior successfully and adhere to a positive lifetime weight control program. In developing a retraining program, people are not expected to incorporate all of the strategies listed but should note the ones that apply to them.

- Make a commitment to change. The first necessary ingredient is the desire to modify your behavior. You need to stop precontemplating and contemplating change and get going! The reasons for change must be more compelling than those for continuing your present lifestyle patterns. You must accept that you have a problem and decide by yourself whether you really want to change. If you are sincerely committed, the chances for success are enhanced already.

> The desire to lose weight must become more important than the desire to overeat or not exercise.

- Set realistic goals. Most people with a weight problem would like the pounds to melt away without realizing that the weight problem developed over several years. A sound weight reduction and maintenance program can be accomplished only by establishing new life-time eating and exercise habits, both of which take time to develop. In setting a realistic long-term goal, short-term objectives also should be planned. The long-term goal may be to decrease body fat to 20 percent of total body weight. The short-term objective may be a 1 percent decrease in body fat each month. Objectives like these allow for regular evaluation and help maintain motivation and renewed commitment to attain the long-term goal.
- Incorporate exercise into the program. Choosing enjoyable activities, places, times, equipment, and people to work with helps a person adhere to an exercise program. (Details on developing a complete exercise program are given in Chapter 7.)
- Differentiate hunger and appetite. Hunger is the actual physical need for food. Appetite is a desire for food, usually triggered by factors such as stress, habit, boredom, depression, availability of food, or just the thought of food itself. People should eat only when they have a physical need. In this regard, developing and sticking to a regular meal pattern helps control hunger.
- Eat less fat. Each gram of fat provides 9 calories, whereas protein and carbohydrates provide only 4. In essence, you can eat more food on a low-fat diet because you consume fewer calories with each serving.
- Pay attention to calories. Some people think that because a certain food is low in fat, they can eat as much as they want. Entire boxes of fat-free cookies and bags of pretzels have been consumed under this pretense. A homemade chocolate-chip cookie may have 100 calories, whereas a low-fat one may have 50. Simple math will tell you that eating one homemade

cookie is better than eating a half-dozen low-fat ones. When reading food labels, don't just look at the fat content, but pay attention to calories as well.

- Cut unnecessary items from your diet. Many people regularly drink a 140-calorie can of soda (or more) each day. Substituting a glass of water would cut 51,100 (140 × 365) calories yearly from the diet—the equivalent of 14.6 (51,000 ÷ 3,500) pounds of fat.

- Add foods to your diet that reduce cravings.[15] Many people have a biological imbalance of insulin. Insulin helps the body use and conserve energy. Some people produce so much insulin that their bodies can't use it all. This imbalance leads to an overpowering craving for carbohydrates. As they eat more carbohydrates, even more insulin is released. Foods that reduce cravings include eggs, red meat, fish, poultry, cheese, tofu, oils, fats, and nonstarchy vegetables such as lettuce, green beans, peppers, asparagus, broccoli, mushrooms, and Brussels sprouts. If you watch your portion sizes, eating foods that reduce cravings at regular meals and for snacks helps to decrease the intense desire for carbohydrates, prevent overeating, and aid weight loss.

- Avoid automatic eating. Many people associate certain daily activities with eating. For example, people may eat while cooking, watching television, or reading. Most of the time the foods consumed in these situations lack nutritional value or are high in sugar and fat.

- Stay busy. People tend to eat more when they sit around and do nothing. Occupying the mind and body with activities not associated with eating helps take away the desire to eat. Some options are walking, cycling, playing sports, gardening, sewing, visiting a library, a museum, a park. To break the routine of life, you might develop other skills and interests or try something new and exciting.

- Plan meals ahead of time. Sensible shopping is necessary to accomplish this objective. (Always shop on a full stomach, because hungry shoppers tend to buy unhealthy foods impulsively—and then snack on the way home). The shopping list should include whole-grain breads and cereals, fruits and vegetables, low-fat milk and dairy products, lean meats, fish, and poultry.

- Cook wisely.
  - Use less fat and refined foods in food preparation.
  - Trim all visible fat from meats and remove skin from poultry before cooking.
  - Skim the fat off gravies and soups.
  - Bake, broil, boil, and steam instead of frying.
  - Sparingly use butter, cream, mayonnaise, and salad dressings.

- Avoid coconut oil, palm oil, and cocoa butter.
- Prepare plenty of foods that contain fiber.
- Include whole-grain breads and cereals, vegetables, and legumes in most meals.
- Eat fruits for dessert.
- Stay away from soda, fruit juices, and fruit-flavored drinks.
- In addition to sugar, cut down on other refined carbohydrates, such as corn syrup, malt sugar, dextrose, and fructose.
- Drink plenty of water—at least six glasses a day.

- Do not serve more food than you should eat. Measure the food in portions and keep serving dishes away from the table. In this way you will eat less, have a harder time getting seconds, and have less appetite because the food is not visible. People should not be forced to eat when they are satisfied (including children after they already have had a healthy, nutritious serving).

- Try "junior size" instead of "super size." Use smaller plates, bowls, cups, and glasses. Try eating half as much food as you commonly eat. Over the years the sizes of dishes and glasses have gotten bigger. Consequently, people serve and eat a lot more food than they need. If you use a smaller plate, it will look like more food and you'll tend to eat less. Watch for portion sizes at restaurants as well. Plates and portion sizes at restaurants now are so large that people overeat and still end up with leftovers to take home. Similarly, the original bottle of Coca-Cola contained 6.5 ounces. Machines now routinely dispense 20-ounce bottles, and convenience stores sell 64-ounce "buckets" of soda (about 750 calories).

> Supersized foods create supersized people.

- Eat out infrequently. Research indicates that the more often people of all ages eat out, the more body fat they have. People who eat out six or more times per week consume an average of about 300 extra calories per day and 30 percent more fat than those who don't eat out as often.

- Eat slowly and at the table only. Eating is one of the pleasures of life, and we need to take time to enjoy it. Eating on the run is not good because the body doesn't have enough time to "register" nutritive and caloric consumption, and people overeat before the body perceives the fullness signal. Eating at the table also forces people to take time out to eat, and it deters snacking between meals, primarily because of the extra time and effort required to sit down and eat. When people are done eating, they should not sit

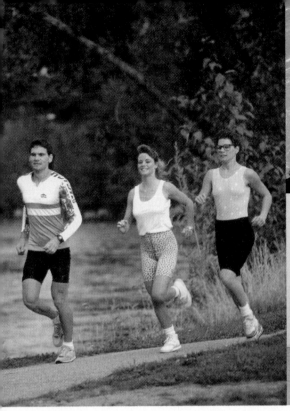
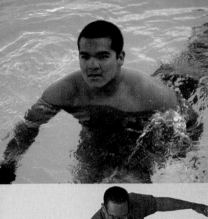
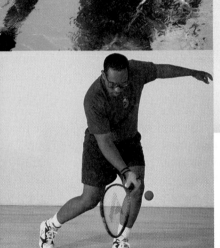
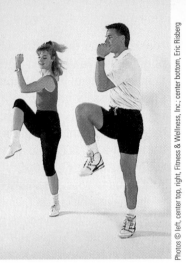

Exercising with other people and in different places helps maintain exercise adherence.

around the table but, rather, clean up and put away the food to keep from unnecessary snacking.

- Avoid social binges. Social gatherings tend to entice self-defeating behavior. Visual imagery might help before attending social gatherings. Plan ahead and visualize yourself there. Do not feel pressured to eat or drink and don't rationalize in these situations. Choose low-calorie foods and entertain yourself with other activities such as dancing and talking.

- Do not raid the refrigerator or the cookie jar. In these tempting situations, take control. Stop and think. Do not bring high-calorie, high-sugar, or high-fat foods into the house. If they are there already, store them where they are hard to get to or see. If they are out of sight or not readily available, the temptation is less. Keeping food in places such as the garage and basement discourages people from taking the time and effort to get them. By no means should you have to eliminate treats entirely, but all things should be done in moderation.

- Avoid evening food raids. Most people with weight problems do really well during the day but then "lose it" at nighttime. Excessive snacking following the evening meal is a common pitfall. Stay busy after your evening meal. Go for a short walk and get to bed earlier. In most cases the intense desire for food that you get during the evening hours disappears following a good night's rest.

- Practice stress-management techniques (discussed in Chapter 3). Many people snack and increase food consumption in stressful situations. Eating is not a stress-releasing activity and, instead, can aggravate the problem if weight control is an issue.

- Get support. People who receive support from friends, relatives, and formal support groups are much more likely to lose and maintain weight loss than those without such support. The more support you receive, the better off you will be.

- Monitor changes and reward accomplishments. Feedback on fat loss and lean tissue gain is a reward in itself. Awareness of changes in body composition also helps reinforce new behaviors. Being able to exercise without interruption for 15, 20, 30, or 60 minutes; swimming a certain distance; running a mile—all these accomplishments deserve recognition. Meeting objectives calls for rewards that are not related to eating: new clothing, a tennis racquet, a bicycle, exercise shoes, or something else that is special and you would not have acquired otherwise.

- Prepare for slips. Most people will slip and occasionally splurge. If that happens, do not despair and give up. Reevaluate and continue with your efforts. An occasional slip will not make much difference in the long run.

- Think positive. Avoid negative thoughts about how difficult changing past behaviors might be. Instead, think of the benefits you will reap, such as feeling, looking, and functioning better, plus enjoying better health and improving the quality of life. Avoid negative environments and people who will not be supportive.

IN CONCLUSION

There is no simple and quick way to take off excessive body fat and keep it off for good. Weight management is accomplished by making a lifetime commitment to physical activity and proper food selection. When taking part in a weight (fat) reduction program, people also have to decrease their caloric intake moderately and implement strategies to modify unhealthy eating behaviors.

During the process, relapses into past negative behaviors are almost inevitable. The three most common reasons for relapse are

1. Stress-related factors (such as major life changes, depression, job changes, illness).

2. Social reasons (entertaining, eating out, business travel).

3. Self-enticing behaviors (placing yourself in a situation to see how much you can get away with ("One small taste won't hurt," leading to "I'll eat just one slice," and finally, "I haven't done well, so I might as well eat some more").

Making mistakes is human and does not necessarily mean failure. Failure comes to those who give up and do not use previous experiences to build upon and, in turn, develop skills that will prevent self-defeating behaviors in the future. Where there's a will, there's a way, and those who persist will reap the rewards.

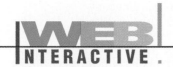

WEB ACTIVITIES

■ **Weight Management** This site describes how to select a safe weight loss plan combining exercise and healthy diet, including the FDA diet plan.
http://www.wellweb.com/nutri/weight_management.htm

■ **Nutrition Analysis Tool** This program was developed at the University of Illinois—Urbana/Champaign and consists of a free Web-based program that allows you to analyze the foods you eat for a variety of nutrients.
http://www.ag.uiuc.edu/~food-lab/nat

■ **Count Your Calories Because Your Calories Count** This interactive site, sponsored by Wake Forest University Baptist Medical Center, features a four-step assessment of your diet, including "How's Your Diet?" "Fit or Not Quiz," Calorie Counter," and "Drive Through Diet." There is also an "Eating Disorders" quiz.
http://www.bgsm.edu/nutrition/in.html

■ **Shape-Up America's Eating Smart Menu** This site describes how to establish your dietary goals and plan for success, including tips on how to incorporate physical fitness with your dietary guidelines.
http://www.shapeup.org/publications/eating.smart/textmenu.htm

■ **Eating Disorders: Don't Let Time Run Out Before You Get Help** This visually appealing site, from the

American Family Physician journal, describes the signs and symptoms of anorexia and bulimia, discusses body image and improving self-esteem, treatment for anorexia and bulimia, and how to help a friend who has an eating disorder.
http://health4teens.org/eating

InfoTrac

You can find additional readings related to wellness via InfoTrac College Edition, an on-line library of more than 900 journals and publications. Follow the instructions for accessing InfoTrac that came packaged with your textbook, then search for articles using a key word search.

Suggested Reading Tanya R. Berry and Bruce L. Howe, "Risk Factors for Disordered Eating in Female University Athletes," *Journal of Sport Behavior* 23, no. 3 (Sept. 2000): 207.

1. What are some of the variables that may contribute to patterns of disordered eating among university athletes and nonathletes? Why are student athletes at higher risk than nonathletes?

2. Athletes participating in specifically what types of university sports are most likely to suffer from patterns of disordered eating?

3. What are some of the psychosocial variables that contribute to disordered eating? Based on this study, name two significant predictors of restrained eating.

Web Activity
Eating Disorders Self-Test: Are You in Danger?
http://www.anred.com

Sponsor Anorexia and Related Eating Disorders, Inc., a nonprofit organization that provides information about various food and weight disorders, including warning signs, recovery, and prevention.

Description This excellent Web site features very comprehensive descriptions of all types of eating disorders, including anorexia, bulimia, binge eating disorder, anorexia athletica (compulsive exercising), body dysmorphic disorder (bigorexia), and many less-common eating disorders. The site features an overview, definitions and descriptions of each disorder, statistics, warning signs (food behaviors, body image behaviors, social behaviors, and feelings), medical problems, causes, treatment and recovery, and information on how to help someone who has an eating disorder, including tips for parents, partners, and other family members.

Available Activities
1. The Self-Test entitled "Are You in Danger?" consists of 33 Yes/No questions to help you ascertain if you are at risk for developing an eating disorder.

Web Work
1. From the home page, click on "site index."
2. Scroll down the comprehensive table of contents to the "Are You in Danger? A Self-Test" link.
3. Click on this link and print out the list of 33 questions.
4. Circle the number(s) corresponding to the statements that describe you and your eating behaviors.
5. After answering the questions, read the last paragraph on the page to find whether you need to seek medical and/or psychological assistance.

Helpful Hints
1. It is easiest to print out the page and simply circle each statement that applies to you.
2. The self-assessment is not a substitute for appropriate medical and psychological care by qualified licensed professionals. You should show your results of this self-assessment test to your health professional.

For additional Web activities, links, and suggested readings, visit our Health, Fitness, and Wellness Resource Center at http://health.wadsworth.com.

NOTES

1. A. Must et al., "The Disease Burden Associated with Overweight and Obesity," *Journal of the American Medical Association* 282 (1999): 1523–1529.
2. National Institutes of Health, "Clinical Guidelines on the Identification, Evaluation, and Treatment of Overweight and Obesity in Adults," NIH Publication No. 98-4083 (Washington, DC: NIH, 1998).
3. K. M. Flegal, M. D. Carrol, R. J. Kuczmarski, and C. L. Johnson, "Overweight and Obesity in the United states: Prevalence and Trends, 1960–1994," *International Journal of Obesity and Related Metabolic Disorders* 22 (1998): 39–47.
4. M. K. Serdula et al., "Prevalence of Attempting Weight Loss and Strategies for Controlling Weight," *Journal of the American Medical Association* 282 (1999): 1353–1358.
5. C. E. Barlow, H. W. Kohl III, L. W. Gibbons, and S. N. Blair, "Physical Fitness, Mortality, and Obesity," *International Journal of Obesity* 19 (1996): S41–44.
6. S. W. Lichtman et al., "Discrepancy Between Self-Reported and Actual Caloric Intake and Exercise in Obese Subjects," *New England Journal of Medicine* 327 (1992), 1893–1898.
7. R. L. Leibel, M. Rosenbaum, and J. Hirsh, "Changes in Energy Expenditure Resulting from Altered Body Weight," *New England Journal of Medicine* 332 (1995): 621–628.
8. R. J. Shepard, *Alive Man: The Physiology of Physical Activity* (Springfield, IL: Charles C Thomas, 1975): 484–488.
9. J. H. Wilmore, "Exercise, Obesity, and Weight Control," *Physical Activity and Fitness Research Digest* (Washington DC: President's Council on Physical Fitness & Sports, 1994).
10. K. N. Pavlou, S. Krey, and W. P. Steffe, "Exercise as an Adjunct to Weight Loss and Maintenance in Moderately Obese Subjects," *American Journal of Clinical Nutrition* 49 (1989), 1115–1123.
11. W. W. Campbell, M. C. Crim, V. R. Young, and W. J. Evans, "Increased Energy Requirements and Changes in Body Composition with Resistance Training in Older Adults," *American Journal of Clinical Nutrition* 60 (1994): 167–175.
12. A. Tremblay, J. A. Simoneau, and C. Bouchard. "Impact of Exercise Intensity on Body Fatness and Skeletal Muscle Metabolism," *Metabolism* 43 (1994): 814–818.
13. U.S. Department of Health and Human Services: Department of Agriculture, "Nutrition and Your Health: Dietary Guidelines for Americans." *Home and Garden Bulletin* 232, 2000;

    U.S. Department of Agriculture, Human Nutrition Information Service, "The Food Guide Pyramid," *Home and Garden Bulletin* 252 (Dec. 1992);

    National Academy Press, Food and Nutrition Board, *Recommended Dietary Allowances* (Washington DC: National Academy Press, 1989).
14. W. W. K. Hoeger, C. Harris, E. M. Long, and D. R. Hopkins, "Four-Week Supplementation With a Natural Dietary Compound Produces Favorable Changes in Body Composition," *Advances in Therapy* 15, no. 5 (1998): 305–313;

    W. W. K. Hoeger, C. Harris, E. M. Long, R. L. Kjorstad, M. Welch, T. L. Hafner, and D. R. Hopkins, "Dietary Supplementation with Chromium Picolinate/L-Carnitine Complex in Combination with Diet and Exercise Enhances Body Composition," *Journal of the American Nutraceutical Association* 2, no. 2 (1999): 40–45.
15. R. Heller and R. Heller, "How The Weight-Loss Scientists Lost Their Weight: You Can, Too," *Bottom Line/Personal Health* 18, no. 11 (1997): 9–10.

ESTIMATION OF DAILY CALORIC REQUIREMENT

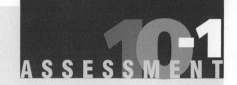

Name: Date: Grade:

Instructor: Course: Section:

Necessary Lab Equipment

Tables 10.2 (page 257) and 10.3 (page 257).

Objective

To determine your estimated daily caloric requirement with exercise for weight maintenance and/or reduction.

I. Computation Form for Daily Caloric Requirement

A. Current body weight in pounds . . . .

B. Caloric requirement per pound of body weight (use Table 10.2) . . . .

C. Typical daily caloric requirement without exercise to maintain body weight (A × B) . . . .

D. Selected physical activity (e.g., jogging)[a] . . . .

E. Number of exercise sessions per week . . . .

F. Duration of exercise session (in minutes) . . . .

G. Total weekly exercise time in minutes (E × F) . . . .

H. Average daily exercise time in minutes (G ÷ 7) . . . .

I. Caloric expenditure per pound per minute (cal/lb/min) based on perceived exertion of physical activity (use Table 10.3) . .

J. Total calories burned per minute of physical activity (A × I) . . . .

K. Average daily calories burned as a result of the exercise program (H × J) . . . .

L. Total daily caloric requirement with exercise to maintain body weight (C + K) . . . .

M. Number of calories to subtract from daily requirement to achieve a negative caloric balance
(multiply current body weight by 5) . . . .

N. Target caloric intake to lose weight (L − M)[b] . . . .

---

[a] If more than one physical activity is selected, you will need to estimate the average daily calories burned as a result of each additional activity (steps D through K) and add all of these figures to L above.

[b] This figure should never be below 1,200 calories for women or 1,500 calories for men. See Assessments 10–4 through 10–7 for the 1,200-, 1,500-, 1,800-, and 2,000-calorie-diet plans.

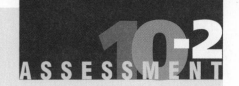
Name: _____ Date: _____ Grade: _____

Instructor: _____ Course: _____ Section: _____

Age _____ Weight _____ Number of days to be Analyzed _____

Sex ____ Male ____ Female (pregnant –P, Lactating–L, Neither–N)

Activity Rating: Sedentary (limited physical activity)   = 1
                  Moderate physical activity   = 2
                  Hard labor (strenuous physical activity)   = 3

Assignment:

This laboratory experience should be carried out as home-work assignment to be completed over the next seven days.

Lab Resources:

Food Guide Pyramid (Figure 8.5, page 206) and list of "Nutritive Value of Selected Foods" (Appendix).

Objective:

To meet the minimum daily required servings of the basic food groups and monitor total daily fat intake.

Instructions:

Keep a 7-day record of your food consumption using the Food Guide Pyramid and the form provided on the next page. Make additional copies of this form as needed (at least 3 days are recommended). Whenever you have something to eat, record the food code from the Nutritive Value of Selected Foods list contained in the Appendix, the number of calories, grams of fat, and the servings in the corresponding spaces provided for each food group. If a food item is not listed in the Nutritive Value of Selected Foods list, the information can be obtained from the food container itself or from some of the references given at the end of the list of foods in the Appendix.

Record all information immediately after each meal, because it will be easier to keep track of foods and the amounts eaten. If twice the amount of a particular serving is eaten, the calories and grams of fat must be doubled and two servings should be recorded under the respective food group.

At the end of the day, evaluate your diet by checking whether the minimum required servings for each food group were met and by calculating the total amount of fat consumed. If you have met the required servings, you are well on your way to achieving a well-balanced diet. Additionally, fat intake should not exceed 30 percent of the total daily caloric consumption. If you are on a diet, you may want to reduce fat intake to less than 20 percent of total daily calories (see Table 10.4, page 259).

Name

No.	Food	Amount	Calories	Fat (gm)	Food Groups (servings)				
					Bread, Cereal, Rice & Pasta	Vegetable	Fruit	Milk, Yogurt & Cheese	Meat, Poultry, Fish, Dry Beans, Eggs, & Nuts
1									
2									
3									
4									
5									
6									
7									
8									
9									
10									
11									
12									
13									
14									
15									
16									
17									
18									
19									
20									
21									
22									
23									
24									
25									
26									
27									
28									
29									
30									
Totals									
Recommended Amount			*	**	6–11	3–5	2–4	2–3	2–3
Deficiencies									

*Compute using Table 10.2, page 257.

**Multiply the recommended amount of calories by .30 (30%) and divide by 9 to obtain the recommended amount of grams of fat (if on a diet, multiply by .20 or .10 — see Table 10.4, page 259).

ARE YOU A PSYCHOLOGICAL OVEREATER?

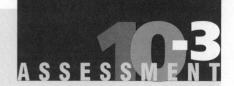

Name: _____   Date: _____   Grade: _____

Instructor: _____   Course: _____   Section: _____

NECESSARY LAB EQUIPMENT:
None required.

OBJECTIVE:
To determine if you are a psychological overeater.

INSTRUCTIONS:
Psychological overeaters generally fall into several distinct categories. Finding yourself in one of these categories is no cause for panic. Becoming aware of when, why, and where you overeat can help you avoid the triggers that lead to nonstop nibbling. To find out where you fit in, answer the questions below as follows:

0 = never	1 = once in a while
2 = fairly often	3 = regularly

The category with the highest score gives you your basic overeating style.

Nervous Night Eater

- [ ] I often skimp on meals until nightfall, then I stuff my face nonstop.
- [ ] I crave sweet, salty, or high-fat snacks.
- [ ] I often munch in front of the TV starting with the evening news on through the late show.
- [ ] I often conduct midnight raids on the refrigerator.
- [ ] I have trouble getting to sleep or staying asleep.
- [ ] I drink more than three cups of coffee a day.
- [ ] On a scale of 1 to 10, I'd say my stress level rates a 9 or 10.
- [ ] I've been called a worrywart.

Compulsive Eater

- [ ] I often skip sit-down meals and usually eat on the run.
- [ ] I'm rarely without some type of food in my mouth.
- [ ] I'd rather eat food—even when I'm not hungry—than waste it.
- [ ] I crave foods that are sweet, starchy, and soft (but I'll eat anything).
- [ ] I usually sneak food when no one is around to see me eat it.
- [ ] My favorite beverage is diet soda—lots of it.
- [ ] I'm cheery on the outside, but inside I feel lonely and blue.
- [ ] My love life is either stressful or nonexistent.

Closet Binge Eater

- [ ] About three times a month, I suddenly pig out uncontrollably.
- [ ] When I binge, I gobble food fast and steadily, easily polishing off an entire bag of cookies.
- [ ] I binge in private and usually at night.
- [ ] My binges usually are triggered when I'm upset or stressed out.
- [ ] Immediately after bingeing I feel calm, but later ashamed and furious at myself.
- [ ] After a binge, I often fast or crash-diet.
- [ ] Often after bingeing, my stomach aches or I have trouble sleeping.
- [ ] I often feel angry and depressed but don't know why.

Hand-Me-Down Eater

- [ ] My family devours king-size portions of rich food at every meal.
- [ ] My parents and siblings are overweight.
- [ ] My family frequently snacks together in front of the TV.
- [ ] The most exercise my family gets is reaching for seconds on pie.
- [ ] Both my mother and I love to cook.
- [ ] Having a well-stocked pantry makes me feel secure and loved.

Adapted from John Feltman and the editors of *Prevention Magazine,* "Improving Your Eating Style," *Food and Nutrition* (Emmaus, PA: Rodale Press, 1993). Used by permission.

- [ ] My mother always serves an extravagant dinner with rich desserts.
- [ ] My family celebrates even minor occasions with lavish feasts.

Thin/Fat

- [ ] I was overweight as a teenager and now am deathly afraid of gaining weight.
- [ ] It's a never-ending battle to stay thin.
- [ ] I eat nothing but low-calorie meals.
- [ ] I nag those close to me if they gain even a pound or two, because I detest fat people.
- [ ] My life would be ruined if I were to gain weight.
- [ ] I can tell you the fat and calorie count of nearly every food.
- [ ] Fat people are weak and have no will power.
- [ ] Bingeing is the farthest thing from my mind.

Chronic Dieter

- [ ] I've tried all the latest diets and read all the diet books, but none of them are any good.
- [ ] Within a few months of losing weight, I'm back to my former fat self.
- [ ] I often crash-diet before a party or important social event.
- [ ] I know more than most people about diets, nutrition, and psychological causes for weight gain.
- [ ] I can tell you exactly how and why I lost and regained every pound.
- [ ] I've memorized the calorie count for foods from A to Z.
- [ ] Weight-loss groups and doctors have all failed me.
- [ ] I'm into quick and easy weight loss.

Environmental Eater

- [ ] I can't resist the aromas emanating from a bakery.
- [ ] Just reading about luscious dessert recipes makes me drool.
- [ ] TV food commercials send me to the refrigerator.
- [ ] Eating food goes along with the territory of my job —power lunches, social dinners, and so on.
- [ ] I eat more than most people at meals.
- [ ] When dining out, I rarely pass up the dessert cart.
- [ ] I've begun to develop love handles on my waist and batwings under my arms.
- [ ] I rarely turn down an extra helping or a meal, even if I'm not hungry—if it's there, I'll eat it.

Couch Potato

- [ ] I prefer curling up with a bag of chips to physical activity.
- [ ] The most exercise I get these days is lifting a fork to my mouth.
- [ ] It takes fewer and fewer calories to maintain the same weight.
- [ ] I wouldn't be caught dead in workout gear.
- [ ] Walking to stores at the mall is an effort.
- [ ] I'm stressed and anxious most of the time.
- [ ] I sit behind a desk all day.
- [ ] Once I could have danced all night, but since I've gained weight, I can barely shuffle to the TV.

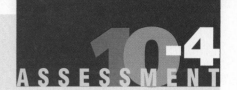
Name: Date: Grade:

Instructor: Course: Section:

Instructions:

The objective of the diet plan is to meet (not exceed) the number of servings allowed for the food groups listed. Each time you eat a food, record it in the space provided for that group, along with the appropriate serving size. Refer to the Food Guide Pyramid to find out what counts as one serving for each group listed (see Figure 8.5, page 206). Instead of the meat, poultry, fish, dry beans, eggs, and nuts group, you are allowed to have a commercially available low-fat frozen entree for your main meal (this entree should provide no more than 300 calories and less than 6 grams of fat). You can make additional copies of this form as needed.

Bread, Cereal, Rice, Pasta Group (80 calories/serving): 6 servings

1.
2.
3.
4.
5.
6.

Vegetable Group (25 calories/serving): 3 servings

1.
2.
3.

Fruit Group (60 calories/serving): 2 servings

1.
2.

Milk Group (120 calories/serving, use low-fat milk and low-fat milk products): 2 servings

1.
2.

Low-fat Frozen Entree (300 calories and less than 6 grams of fat): 1 serving

1.

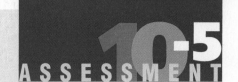

DAILY FOOD INTAKE RECORD:
1,500-CALORIE DIET PLAN

Name: _____ Date: _____ Grade: _____

Instructor: _____ Course: _____ Section: _____

Instructions:

The objective of the diet plan is to meet (not exceed) the number of servings allowed for the food groups listed. Each time you eat a food, record it in the space provided for that group, along with the appropriate serving size. Refer to the Food Guide Pyramid to find out what counts as one serving for each group listed (see Figure 8.5, page 206). Instead of the meat, poultry, fish, dry beans, eggs, and nuts group, you are allowed to have two commercially available low-fat frozen entrees for two of your main meals (these entrees should provide no more than 300 calories and less than 6 grams of fat). You can make additional copies of this form as needed.

Bread, Cereal, Rice, Pasta Group (80 calories/serving): 6 servings

1 _____

2 _____

3 _____

4 _____

5 _____

6 _____

Vegetable Group (25 calories/serving): 3 servings

1 _____

2 _____

3 _____

Fruit Group (60 calories/serving): 2 servings

1 _____

2 _____

Milk Group (120 calories/serving, use low-fat milk and low-fat milk products): 2 servings

1 _____

2 _____

Two Low-fat Frozen Entrees (300 calories and less than 6 grams of fat): 2 servings

1 _____

2 _____

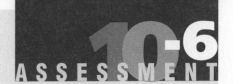
DAILY FOOD INTAKE RECORD:
1,800-CALORIE DIET PLAN

Name: _____   Date: _____   Grade: _____

Instructor: _____   Course: _____   Section: _____

Instructions:

The objective of the diet plan is to meet (not exceed) the number of servings allowed for the food groups listed. Each time you eat a food, record it in the space provided for that group, along with the appropriate serving size. Refer to the Food Guide Pyramid to find out what counts as one serving for each group listed (see Figure 8.5, page 206). Instead of the meat, poultry, fish, dry beans, eggs, and nuts group, you are allowed to have two commercially available low-fat frozen entrees for two of your main meals (these entrees should provide no more than 300 calories and less than 6 grams of fat). You can make additional copies of this form as needed.

Bread, Cereal, Rice, Pasta Group (80 calories/serving): 8 servings

1 _____   5 _____

2 _____   6 _____

3 _____   7 _____

4 _____   8 _____

Vegetable Group (25 calories/serving): 5 servings

1 _____

2 _____

3 _____

4 _____

5 _____

Fruit Group (60 calories/serving): 3 servings

1 _____

2 _____

3 _____

Milk Group (120 calories/serving, use low-fat milk and low-fat milk products): 2 servings

1 _____

2 _____

Two Low-fat Frozen Entrees (300 calories and less than 6 grams of fat): 2 servings

1 _____

2 _____

DAILY FOOD INTAKE RECORD:
2,000-CALORIE DIET PLAN

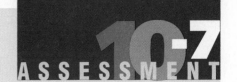

Name: _____ Date: _____ Grade: _____

Instructor: _____ Course: _____ Section: _____

Instructions:

The objective of the diet plan is to meet (not exceed) the number of servings allowed for the food groups listed. Each time you eat a food, record it in the space provided for that group, along with the appropriate serving size. Refer to the Food Guide Pyramid to find out what counts as one serving for each group listed (see Figure 8.5, page 206). Instead of

the meat, poultry, fish, dry beans, eggs, and nuts group, you are allowed to have two commercially available low-fat frozen entrees for two of your main meals (these entrees should provide no more than 300 calories and less than 6 grams of fat). You can make additional copies of this form as needed.

Bread, Cereal, Rice, Pasta Group (80 calories/serving): 10 servings

1	_____	6	_____
2	_____	7	_____
3	_____	8	_____
4	_____	9	_____
5	_____	10	_____

Vegetable Group (25 calories/serving): 5 servings

1 _____
2 _____
3 _____
4 _____
5 _____

Fruit Group (60 calories/serving): 4 servings

1 _____
2 _____
3 _____
4 _____

Milk Group (120 calories/serving, use low-fat milk and low-fat milk products): 2 servings

1 _____
2 _____

Two Low-fat Frozen Entrees (300 calories and less than 6 grams of fat): 2 servings

1 _____
2 _____

CARDIOVASCULAR WELLNESS

- Define cardiovascular disease and coronary heart disease.

- Become familiar with the incidence of cardiovascular diseases.

- Estimate your own risk of developing coronary heart disease.

- Teach the importance of a healthy lifestyle in the prevention of cardiovascular disease.

- Discuss the major risk factors that lead to the development of coronary heart disease.

- Present guidelines for cardiovascular disease prevention.

279

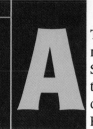

A T THE BEGINNING of the 20th century, the most common health problems in the United States were infectious diseases such as tuberculosis, diphtheria, influenza, kidney disease, polio, and other diseases of infancy. Progress in the field of medicine largely eliminated these diseases. Nevertheless, as the American people started to enjoy the "good life" (sedentary living, alcohol, fatty foods, excessive sweets, tobacco, and drugs), a parallel increase was seen in chronic diseases such as cancer, diabetes, emphysema, cirrhosis of the liver, and, in particular, diseases of the cardiovascular system.

As the incidence of chronic diseases grew, it became clear that prevention was the best medicine. Consequently, a fitness and wellness trend gradually developed over the last three decades. People began to realize that good health is largely self-controlled and that the leading causes of premature death and illness in the United States could be prevented by adhering to positive lifestyle habits.

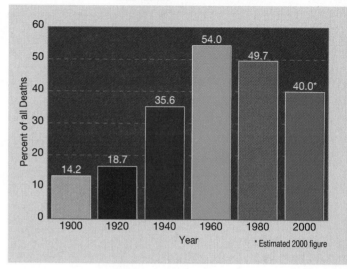

FIGURE 11.1 INCIDENCE OF CARDIOVASCULAR DISEASE IN UNITED STATES FOR SELECTED YEAR: 1900–2000.

INCIDENCE OF CARDIOVASCULAR DISEASE

As we begin the 21st century, **cardiovascular diseases** continue to be the leading cause of death in the United States. About 20 percent of the population has some form of cardiovascular disease. One in three men and one in ten women will develop a major cardiovascular problem before age 60.[1] Based on 1998 statistics, 40 percent of all deaths in the United States were attributable to heart and blood vessel disease.[2]

Cardiovascular diseases encompass all pathological conditions that affect the heart and the circulatory system (blood vessels). Some examples of cardiovascular diseases are **coronary heart disease**, peripheral vascular disease, congenital heart disease, rheumatic heart disease, atherosclerosis, strokes, high blood pressure, and congestive heart failure. According to estimates, if all deaths from the major cardiovascular diseases were eliminated, life expectancy in the United States would increase by about 10 years.[3]

Although heart and blood vessel disease is still the number-one health problem in the United States, the incidence declined by 26 percent between 1960 and 2000 (see Figure 11.1). The main reasons for this dramatic decrease are health education and better treatment modalities. More people now are aware of the risk factors for cardiovascular disease and are changing their lifestyles to lower their own potential risk for this disease. Further work remains to be done, however, because studies show that the risk of death from cardiovascular

disease is greater for the least-educated compared with the most-educated people.

According to the American Heart Association, 58.8 million people in the United States were afflicted with diseases of the cardiovascular system in 1999, including 50 million with hypertension (high blood pressure) and 12 million with coronary heart disease. Many of these people have more than one type of cardiovascular disease. The estimated cost of heart and blood vessel disease in 2000 exceeded $326 billion.[4] Heart attacks alone cost American industry approximately 132 million workdays annually, including $22 billion in lost productivity because of physical and emotional disability.

CORONARY HEART DISEASE

The major form of cardiovascular disease is coronary heart disease (CHD), a condition in which the arteries that supply the heart muscle with oxygen and nutrients are narrowed by fatty deposits such as cholesterol and triglycerides. Narrowing of the coronary arteries diminishes the blood supply to the heart muscle, which can precipitate a heart attack (see Figure 11.2).

CHD is the single leading cause of death in the United States, accounting for approximately 20 percent of all deaths and about half of all cardiovascular deaths.[5] More than half of the people who died suddenly from CHD had no previous symptoms of the disease. Further, approximately 80 percent of deaths from CHD in people under age 65 occur during the first heart attack.[6] Almost all of the risk factors for CHD are preventable and reversible, and individuals can reduce their risk. A risk

FIGURE 11.2 MYOCARDIAL INFARCTION (HEART ATTACK) AS A RESULT OF ACUTE REDUCTION IN BLOOD FLOW THROUGH ANTERIOR DESCENDING CORONARY ARTERY.

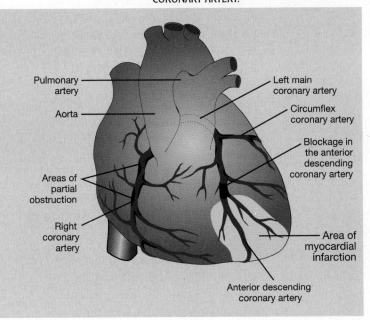

- Pulmonary artery
- Aorta
- Areas of partial obstruction
- Right coronary artery
- Left main coronary artery
- Circumflex coronary artery
- Blockage in the anterior descending coronary artery
- Area of myocardial infarction
- Anterior descending coronary artery

factor analysis to evaluate your personal risk of coronary heart disease is provided in Assessment 11-1 (page 299).

Approximately 1.1 million people have heart attacks each year, and more than 350,000 of them die as a result. More than half the time, the first symptom of coronary heart disease is the heart attack itself, and 40 percent of the people who have a first heart attack die within the first 24 hours.

Although genetic inheritance plays a role in CHD, the most important determinant is personal lifestyle. The leading risk factors contributing to CHD are the following:

- Physical inactivity
- Low HDL cholesterol
- Elevated LDL cholesterol
- Smoking
- High blood pressure
- Diabetes
- Excessive body fat
- Elevated homocysteine
- Abnormal electrocardiogram (either stress or resting ECG)
- Family history of heart disease
- Personal history of heart disease
- Elevated triglycerides
- Tension and stress
- Age

With the exception of age, family history of heart disease, and certain electrocardiogram (ECG) abnormalities, the risk factors are preventable and reversible. The leading risk factors for CHD are discussed next, along with general recommendations for risk reduction.

Studies have documented further that multiple interrelations usually exist between risk factors. Physical inactivity, for instance, often contributes to an increase in (a) body weight (fat), (b) higher cholesterol, (c) triglycerides, (d) tension and stress, (e) blood pressure, and (f) risk for diabetes. The interrelationships among leading cardiovascular risk factors are depicted in Figure 11.3.

PHYSICAL INACTIVITY

Physical inactivity is responsible for low levels of cardiorespiratory endurance, previously defined as the

Cardiovascular diseases The array of conditions that affect the heart and the blood vessels.

Coronary heart disease (CHD) Condition in which the arteries that supply the heart muscle with oxygen and nutrients are narrowed by fatty deposits, such as cholesterol and triglycerides.

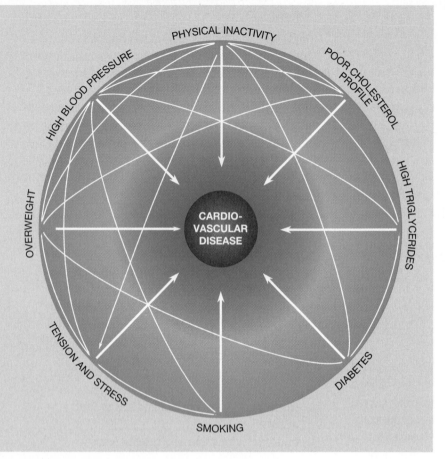

The significance of physical inactivity in contributing to cardio-vascular risk was clearly shown in 1992, when the American Heart Association named physical inactivity one of the six major risk factors for cardiovascular disease. (The other five factors are smoking, a poor cholesterol profile, high blood pressure, diabetes, and obesity.) Based on the overwhelming amount of scientific data in this area, evidence of the benefits of aerobic exercise in reducing heart disease is far too impressive to be ignored.

Research at the Institute for Aerobics Research in Dallas, Texas, clearly shows the tie between cardiorespiratory fitness and mortality, regardless of age and other risk factors[7] (see Figure 11.4). A higher level of physical fitness benefits even those who have other risk factors, such as high blood pressure and serum cholesterol, cigarette smoking, and a family history of heart disease. In most cases, unfit people in the study (group 1) without these risk factors had higher death rates than fit people (groups 4 and 5) with these same risk factors.

Although the findings show that the higher the level of cardiorespiratory fitness, the longer the life, the largest drop in premature death is seen be-tween the unfit and the moderately fit groups. Even small improvements in cardiorespiratory endurance greatly decrease the risk for cardiovascular mortality. Most adults who become physically active and engage in moderate-intensity activities can attain these fitness levels easily.

Subsequent research published in 1993 in the *New England Journal of Medicine* substantiated the importance of exercise in preventing CHD.[8] The research indicated that the benefits (to previously inactive adults) of starting a moderate-to-vigorous physical activity program were as important as quitting smoking, managing blood pressure, or controlling cholesterol. The increase in physical activity led to the same decrease as giving up cigarette smoking in relative risk for death from CHD.

ability of the lungs, heart, and blood vessels to deliver enough oxygen to the cells to meet the demands of prolonged physical activity. Improving cardiorespiratory endurance through aerobic exercise may have the greatest impact in reducing overall risk for heart disease. Although specific recommendations can be followed to improve each risk factor, a regular aerobic exercise program helps control most of the major risk factors that lead to heart disease.

Physical activity and aerobic exercise will do the following:

- Increase cardiorespiratory endurance
- Decrease and control blood pressure
- Reduce body fat
- Lower blood lipids (cholesterol and triglycerides)
- Improve HDL cholesterol
- Help control diabetes
- Increase and maintain good heart function, sometimes improving certain ECG abnormalities
- Motivate toward smoking cessation
- Alleviate tension and stress
- Counteract a personal history of heart disease

Regular physical activity seems to be the single most important factor in the prevention of coronary heart disease.

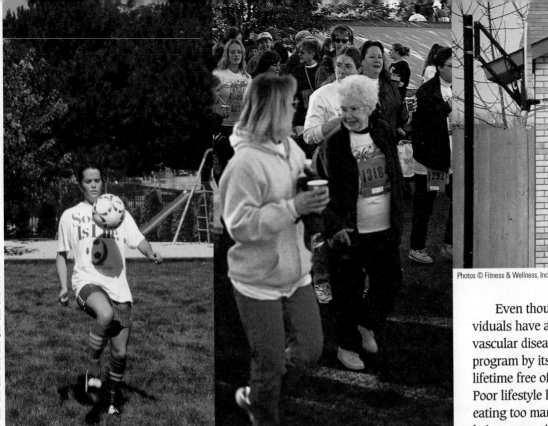

Lifetime participation in aerobic activities is one of the most important factors in prevention of cardiovascular disease.

Photos © Fitness & Wellness, Inc.

Even though physically active individuals have a lower incidence of cardiovascular disease, a regular aerobic exercise program by itself does not guarantee a lifetime free of cardiovascular problems. Poor lifestyle habits—such as smoking, eating too many fatty/salty/sweet foods, being overweight, and having high stress levels—increase cardiovascular risk and will not be eliminated completely through aerobic exercise.

Overall risk factor management is the best guideline to lower the risk for cardiovascular disease. Still, aerobic exercise is one of the most important activities in preventing and reducing cardiovascular problems.

FIGURE 11.4 AGE-ADJUSTED CARDIOVASCULAR DEATH RATES BY PHYSICAL FITNESS GROUPS.

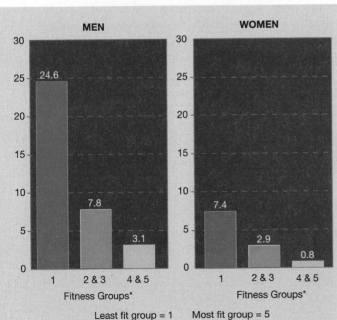

MEN

WOMEN

Fitness Groups*

Least fit group = 1   Most fit group = 5

*Death rates per 10,000 person-years of follow-up. One person-year indicates one person that was followed up one year later.

From S. N. Blair, H. W. Kohl III, R. S. Paffenbarger Jr., D. G. Clark, K. H. Cooper, and L. W. Gibbons, "Physical Fitness and All-Cause Mortality: A Prospective Study of Healthy Men and Women," *Journal of the American Medical Association* 262 (1989): 2395–2401.

ABNORMAL CHOLESTEROL PROFILE

Cholesterol is a waxy substance, technically a steroid alcohol, found only in animal fats and oils. This fatty substance is essential for specific metabolic functions in the body, but an abnormal cholesterol profile contributes to atherosclerotic plaque, a buildup of fatty tissue in the walls of the arteries. As the plaque builds up, it blocks the blood vessels that supply the heart muscle (myocardium) with oxygen and nutrients, and these obstructions can trigger a myocardial infarction or heart attack (see Figures 11.2 and 11.5).

Cholesterol is carried in the bloodstream by molecules of protein known as high-density lipoproteins (HDLs), low-density lipoproteins (LDLs), and very low-density lipoproteins (VLDLs). Subcategories of these lipoproteins have been

Cholesterol A waxy substance, technically a steroid alcohol, found only in animal fats and oil; used in making cell membranes, as a building block for some hormones, in the fatty sheath around nerve fibers, and in other necessary substances.

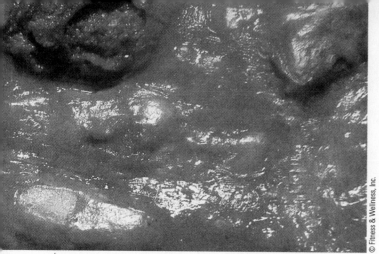

Build-up of fatty plaque on the inner lining of an artery because of atherosclerosis.

© Fitness & Wellness, Inc.

identified recently, but the discussion here focuses only on these major categories.

Cholesterol receives much attention because direct relationships have been established between cholesterol levels (high total cholesterol, high **LDL cholesterol**, and low HDL cholesterol) and the rate of CHD in both men and women. Unfortunately, the heart disguises its problems quite well and typical symptoms of heart disease, such as angina pectoris or chest pain, do not start until the arteries are about 75 percent blocked. In many cases, the first symptom is sudden death.

The general recommendation by the National Cholesterol Education Program (NCEP) is to keep total cholesterol levels below 200 mg/dl. Other health professionals recommend that total cholesterol in individuals age 30 and younger should not be higher than 180 mg/dl, and for children the level should be below 170 mg/dl. Cholesterol levels between 200 and 239 mg/dl are borderline high, and levels of 240 mg/dl and above indicate high risk for disease (see Table 11.1).

Cholesterol is transported primarily in the form of LDL and HDL. The low-density molecules tend to release cholesterol, which then may penetrate the lining or inner membrane of the arteries and speed up the process of atherosclerosis. NCEP guidelines state that an LDL value below 130 mg/dl is desirable, between 130 and 159 mg/dl is borderline high, and 160 mg/dl and above carries high risk for cardiovascular disease.

HDL cholesterol, on the other hand, tends to attract cholesterol, which is then carried to the liver to be metabolized and excreted. In a process known as **reverse cholesterol transport**, HDLs act as "scavengers," removing cholesterol from the body and preventing plaque from forming in the arteries.

The strength of HDL is in the protein molecules found in their coatings. When HDL comes in contact with cholesterol-filled cells, these protein molecules attach to the cells and take their cholesterol. The more HDL cholesterol, the better. HDL cholesterol is the "good cholesterol" and offers some protection against heart disease.

Substantial research suggests that a low level of HDL cholesterol has the strongest relationship to CHD at all levels of total cholesterol, including levels below 200 mg/dl.[9] The recommended HDL cholesterol value to minimize the risk for CHD is 45 mg/dl or higher. Guidelines for the various types of cholesterol are given in Table 11.1.

For the most part, HDL cholesterol is determined genetically. Generally, women have higher values than men. This is one of the reasons heart disease is less common in women. African-American children and adult African-American men have higher values than Caucasians. HDL cholesterol also decreases with age.

Increasing HDL cholesterol improves the cholesterol profile and decreases the risk for CHD. Habitual aerobic

F I G U R E 11.5 THE ATHEROSCLEROTIC PROCESS.

THE ATHEROSCLEROTIC PROCESS

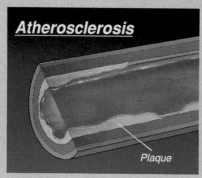
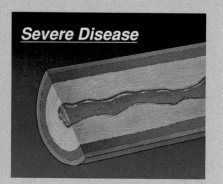

Healthy Artery   **Atherosclerosis**   **Severe Disease**

Plaque

From *Heart of a Healthy Life*. Courtesy of the American Heart Association, © 1992.

TABLE **11.1** CHOLESTEROL GUIDELINES

	Amount	Rating
Total Cholesterol	<200 mg/dl	Desirable
	200–239 mg/dl	Borderline high
	≥240 mg/dl	High risk
LDL-Cholesterol	<130 mg/dl	Desirable
	130–159 mg/dl	Borderline high
	≥160 mg/dl	High risk
HDL-Cholesterol	≥45 mg/dl	Desirable
	36–44 mg/dl	Moderate risk
	≤35 mg/dl	High risk

exercise, weight loss, and quitting smoking all have been shown to raise HDL cholesterol.[10] Beta-carotene intake promotes an increase in HDL cholesterol in some individuals.[11] Drug therapy can also lead to higher HDL cholesterol levels.

Increased HDL cholesterol and a regular aerobic (high-intensity or above 6 METs, for at least 20 minutes three times per week—see Chapter 7) exercise program are clearly related. Individual responses to aerobic exercise differ, but, generally, the more the exercise, the higher is the HDL cholesterol level.

Even when more LDL cholesterol is present than the cells can use, cholesterol seems not to cause a problem until it is oxidized by free radicals. Data suggests that a single unstable **oxygen free radical** (an oxygen compound produced during metabolism) can damage LDL particles. When oxidation occurs, white blood cells invade the arterial wall, take up the cholesterol, and clog the arteries.

The antioxidant effect of vitamins C and E and beta-carotene can also reduce the risk for CHD.[12] Vitamin C seems to inactivate free radicals, and vitamin E protects LDL from oxidation. Beta-carotene not only absorbs free radicals, keeping them from causing damage, but it also may help increase HDL levels. One to two medium-size raw carrots per day provide the recommended daily amount of beta-carotene antioxidant nutrients.

Certain cholesterol-lowering drugs may also help raise HDL levels. These agents include colestipol, niacin, cholestyramine, and gemfibrozil.[13] Some experts believe that HDL levels below 40 mg/dl in combination with triglycerides above 150 mg/dl should be treated with medication.

Many authorities also believe the ratio of LDL cholesterol to HDL cholesterol is a strong indicator of potential risk for cardiovascular disease. An LDL cholesterol to HDL cholesterol ratio of 3.5 or lower is excellent for men, and 3.0 or lower is best for women. For instance, the combination of 50 mg/dl of HDL cholesterol and 150 mg/dl of LDL cholesterol translates to a ratio of 3.0 (150 ÷ 50 = 3.0).

The average adult in the United States consumes between 400 and 600 mg of dietary cholesterol daily. However, consumption of saturated fats raises cholesterol levels more than anything else in the diet. Saturated fats produce approximately 1,000 mg of cholesterol per day.[14] Because of individual differences, some people can have a higher-than-normal intake of saturated fats and still maintain normal cholesterol levels. Others who have a lower intake can have abnormally high levels.

Saturated fats are found mostly in meats and dairy products and seldom in foods of plant origin. Poultry and fish contain less saturated fat than beef does, but should still be eaten in moderation (about 3 to 6 ounces per day). Unsaturated fats are mainly of plant origin and cannot be converted to cholesterol.

If LDL cholesterol is higher than ideal, it can be lowered by losing body fat, manipulating the diet, taking medication, and participating in a regular aerobic exercise program. Cholesterol-lowering drugs, most notably the statins group, can lower cholesterol by 25 to 50 percent in 2 to 3 months. These medications decrease absorption in the intestines or block cholesterol formation by the cells. It is better to lower LDL cholesterol without medication, because these drugs can cause muscle and joint pain and alter liver enzyme levels. People with heart disease must often take cholesterol-lowering medication, but it is best if medication is combined with lifestyle changes to augment the cholesterol-lowering effect.

To decrease LDL cholesterol, a diet low in fat, saturated fat, and cholesterol and high in fiber is recommended. Saturated fat should be replaced with monounsaturated and polyunsaturated fats because the latter tend to decrease LDL cholesterol. Exercise is important, because dietary manipulation by itself is not as effective in lowering LDL cholesterol as a combination of diet plus aerobic exercise.[15]

Fiber

To significantly lower LDL cholesterol, total daily fiber

LDL cholesterol Cholesterol-transporting molecules in the blood ("bad cholesterol").

HDL cholesterol Cholesterol-transporting molecules in the blood ("good cholesterol").

Reverse cholesterol transport A process in which HDL molecules attract cholesterol and carry it to the liver, where it is changed to bile and eventually excreted in the stool.

Oxygen free radicals Substances, formed during metabolism, that attack and damage proteins and lipids, in particular the cell membrane and DNA, leading to the development of diseases such as heart disease, cancer, and emphysema.

intake must be in the range of 25 to 30 grams per day, total fat consumption must be significantly lower than the current 30 percent of total daily caloric intake guideline, saturated fat consumption has to be under 10 percent of the total daily caloric intake, and the average cholesterol consumption should be much lower than 300 mg per day.

Most people's fiber intake in the United States averages less than 12 grams per day. Fiber, in particular the soluble type, has been shown to lower cholesterol. Soluble fiber dissolves in water and forms a gel-like substance that encloses food particles. This property helps bind and excrete fats from the body. The incidence of heart disease is very low in populations where daily fiber intake exceeds 30 grams per day. Further, a 1996 Harvard University Medical School study on 43,000 middle-aged men who were followed for more than 6 years showed that increasing fiber intake to 30 daily grams resulted in a 41 percent reduction in heart attacks.[16]

| Low-Fat Diets |

Research on the effects of a 30 percent-fat diet have shown that it has little or no effect in lowering cholesterol and that CHD actually continues to progress in people who have the disease. The good news came in a study published in the *Archives of Internal Medicine*.[17] Men and women in the study lowered their cholesterol by an average of 23 percent in only 3 weeks following a 10 percent or less fat-calorie diet combined with a regular aerobic exercise program, primarily walking. In this diet, cholesterol intake was less than 25 mg/day. The author of the study concluded that the exact percent-fat guideline (10 or 15 percent) is unknown (it also varies from individual to individual), but that 30 percent total fat calories is definitely too much when attempting to lower cholesterol.

A daily 10 percent-total-fat diet requires the person to limit fat intake to an absolute minimum. Some health care professionals contend that a diet like this is difficult to follow indefinitely. People with high cholesterol levels, however, may not have to follow that diet indefinitely but should adopt the 10 percent-fat diet while attempting to lower cholesterol. Thereafter, eating a 20 to 30 percent fat diet may be adequate to maintain recommended cholesterol levels.

A drawback of very low-fat diets (less than 25 percent fat) is that they tend to lower HDL cholesterol and increase triglycerides. If HDL cholesterol is already low, monounsaturated and polyunsaturated fats should be added to the diet. Nuts and olive, canola, corn, and soybean oils high in monounsaturated fats and polyunsaturated fats. A specialized nutrition book should be consulted to determine other food items that are high in monounsaturated and polyunsaturated fats.

The NCEP guidelines recommend that people consider drug therapy if, after 6 months on a low-cholesterol, low-fat diet, cholesterol remains unacceptably high. An unacceptable level is an LDL cholesterol above 190 mg/dl for people with fewer than two risk factors and no signs of heart disease. For people with more than two risk factors and with a history of heart disease, LDL cholesterol above 160 mg/dl is unacceptable.

HIGH TRIGLYCERIDES

Triglycerides are also known as **free fatty acids**. They make up most of the fat in our diet and most of the fat that circulates in the blood. In combination with cholesterol, triglycerides speed up formation of plaque in the arteries. Triglycerides are carried in the bloodstream primarily by very low-density lipoproteins (VLDLs) and **chylomicrons**.

Although they are found in poultry skin, lunch meats, and shellfish, these fatty acids are manufactured mainly in the liver from refined sugars, starches, and alcohol. High intake of alcohol and sugars (honey and fruit juices included) significantly raises triglyceride levels. Triglycerides can be lowered by cutting down on these foods and overall fat consumption, quitting smoking, reducing weight (if overweight), and doing aerobic exercise. An optimal blood triglyceride level is less than 125 mg/dl (see Table 11.2). For people with cardiovascular problems, this level should be below 100 mg/dl.[18]

Some people consistently have slightly elevated triglyceride levels (above 140 mg/dl) and HDL cholesterol levels below 35 mg/dl. About 80 percent of these people have a genetic condition called LDL phenotype B (approximately 40 percent of the U.S. population falls in this category). Although the blood lipids may not be notably high, these people are at higher risk for atherosclerosis and CHD.[19]

ELEVATED HOMOCYSTEINE

Clinical data indicating that many heart attack and stroke victims have normal cholesterol levels has led researchers to look for other risk factors that may contribute to atherosclerosis. Although it is not a blood lipid, a high concentration of the amino acid **homocysteine** in the blood is

A single cholesterol test may not be a true indicator of a person's regular cholesterol values.

TABLE **11.2**   TRIGLYCERIDES GUIDELINES

Amount	Rating
<125 mg/dl	Desirable
126–499 mg/dl	Borderline high
≥500 mg/dl	High risk

BLOOD CHEMISTRY TEST GUIDELINES

People who have never had a blood chemistry test should do so to establish a baseline for future reference. The blood test should include total cholesterol, LDL-cholesterol, and HDL-cholesterol.

Following an initial normal baseline test no later than age 20, for a person who adheres to the recommended dietary and exercise guidelines, a blood analysis at least every 5 years prior to age 40 should suffice. Thereafter, a blood lipid test is recommended every year, in conjunction with a regular preventive medical examination.

A single baseline test is not necessarily a valid measure. Cholesterol levels vary from month to month and sometimes even from day to day. If the initial test reveals cholesterol abnormalities, the test should be repeated within a few weeks to confirm the results.

thought to enhance plaque formation and subsequent blockage of the arteries.[20]

The body uses homocysteine to help build proteins and carry out cellular metabolism. It is an intermediate amino acid in the interconversion of two other amino acids—methionine and cysteine. This interconversion requires the B vitamin folate (folic acid) and vitamins B_6 and B_{12}. Typically, homocysteine is metabolized rapidly, so it does not accumulate in the blood or damage the arteries.

Many people, however, have high blood levels of homocysteine. This might result from either a genetic inability to metabolize homocysteine or a deficiency in the vitamins required for its conversion. Homocysteine is typically measured in micromoles per liter (μmol/l). In a 10-year follow-up study of people with high homocysteine levels, the data showed that those individuals with a level above 14.25 μmol/l had almost twice the risk of stroke compared with individuals whose level was below 9.25 μmol/l.[21] It is theorized that homocysteine accumulation is toxic because it may

1. cause damage to the inner lining of the arteries (the initial step in the process of atherosclerosis),

2. stimulate the proliferation of cells that contribute to plaque formation, and
3. encourage clotting that may completely obstruct an artery and lead to a heart attack or stroke.

Keeping homocysteine from accumulating in the blood seems to be as simple as eating the recommended daily servings of vegetables, fruits, grains, and some meat and legumes. Increasing evidence that folate can prevent heart attacks has led to the recommendation that people consume 400 mcg per day. Unfortunately, estimates indicate that less than 88 percent of Americans get 400 daily mcg of folate.[22] Five servings of fruits and vegetables daily can provide sufficient levels of folate and vitamin B_6 to remove homocysteine from the blood. People who consume five servings are unlikely to derive extra benefits from a vitamin B complex supplement (400 mcg of daily folate also are recommended for women of child-bearing age to prevent birth defects).

Vitamin B_{12} is found primarily in animal flesh and animal products. Vitamin B_{12} deficiency is rarely a problem, given that 1 cup of milk or an egg provides the daily requirement. The body also recycles most of this vitamin; therefore, a deficiency takes years to develop.

For people who have elevated cholesterol, 500 mg of niacin (also a B vitamin) daily can help lower cholesterol. Niacin supplementation, nonetheless, may produce side effects such as flushing, tingling, and itching. These symptoms usually disappear in a few days but may return if the dose is altered or the supplement is not taken at the same time each day. Supplements, nonetheless, are not a replacement for a diet with ample amounts of daily fruits, vegetables, and whole grains.

HIGH BLOOD PRESSURE (HYPERTENSION)

Blood pressure is a measure of the force exerted against the walls of the blood vessels by the blood flowing through them. Blood pressure is assessed using a **sphygmomanometer** and a stethoscope.

The sphygmomanometer consists of an inflatable

Triglycerides Fats formed by glycerol and three fatty acids. Also known as "free fatty acids."

Free fatty acids (FFA) Fats formed by glycerol and three fatty acids. Also known as "triglycerides."

Chylomicrons Triglyceride-transporting molecules in the blood.

Homocysteine An amino acid that, when allowed to accumulate in the blood, may lead to plaque formation and blockage of arteries.

Blood pressure A measure of the force exerted against the walls of blood vessels by the blood flowing through them.

Sphygmomanometer An inflatable bladder contained within a cuff and a mercury gravity manometer (or an aneroid manometer) from which the blood pressure is read.

TABLE 11.3 BLOOD PRESSURE GUIDELINES

Rating	Systolic	Diastolic
Optimal	≤120	≤80
Normal	121–129	81–84
High normal	130–139	85–89
Stage 1 Hypertension	140–159	90–99
Stage 2 Hypertension	160–179	100–109
Stage 3 Hypertension	≥180	≥110

Source: National Heart, Lung, and Blood Institute.

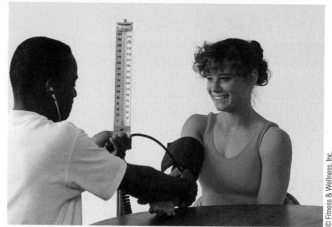

Blood pressure assessment using a mercury gravity manometer.

bladder contained within a cuff and a mercury gravity manometer or an aneroid manometer from which the pressure is read. The pressure is measured in milliliters of mercury and usually expressed in two numbers. Ideal blood pressure should be 120/80 or below (see Table 11.3). The first (higher) number reflects the pressure exerted during the forceful contraction of the heart or systole (hence the name **"systolic" pressure**), and the second (lower) number, or **diastolic pressure**, is taken during the heart's relaxation, when no blood is being ejected.

Based on current American Heart Association estimates, about 50 million people in the United States are hypertensive. **Hypertension** has been viewed as the point at which the pressure doubles the mortality risk, about 160/96. Statistical evidence clearly indicates, however, that blood pressure readings above 140/90 increase the risk of disease and premature death. Therefore, the American Heart Association considers all blood pressures above 140/90 to be hypertension.

All inner walls of arteries are lined by a layer of smooth endothelial cells. Blood lipids cannot penetrate the healthy lining and start to build up on the walls unless damage is done to the cells. High blood pressure is thought to be a leading contributor to destruction of this lining. As blood pressure rises, so does the risk for atherosclerosis. The higher the pressure, the greater is the damage to the arterial wall, making the vessels susceptible to fat deposits, especially if serum cholesterol also is high. Blockage of the coronary vessels decreases blood supply to the heart muscle and can lead to heart attacks. When brain arteries are involved, strokes may follow.

Even though the threshold for hypertension has been set at 140/90, many experts believe that the lower the blood pressure, the better. Even if the pressure is as low as 90/50, as long as individuals do not have any symptoms of low blood pressure or hypotension, they do not need to be concerned. Typical hypotension symptoms are dizziness, lightheadedness, and fainting.

Blood pressure may fluctuate during a regular day. Many factors affect blood pressure, and a single reading may not be a true indicator of your real pressure. For example, physical activity and stress increase blood pressure, whereas rest and relaxation decrease it. Consequently, several measurements should be taken before diagnosing elevated pressure.

Hypertension has been called "the silent killer." It does not hurt, it does not make you feel sick, and unless you check it, years may go by before you even realize you have a problem. High blood pressure is a risk factor not only for CHD but also for congestive heart failure, strokes, and kidney failure.

DIABETES

In **diabetes mellitus**, blood glucose is unable to enter the cells because the pancreas totally stops producing **insulin**, or it does not produce enough to meet the body's needs, or the cells develop **insulin resistance**. The role of insulin is to "unlock" the cells and escort glucose into the cell. Diabetes affects more than 16 million people in the United States, and the National Institutes of Health estimate the cost of diabetes at $98 billion annually.

The incidence of cardiovascular disease and death in the diabetic population is quite high. More than 80 percent of people with diabetes mellitus die from cardiovascular disease. People with chronically elevated blood glucose levels may have problems metabolizing fats, which can make them more susceptible to atherosclerosis, coronary heart disease, heart attacks, high blood pressure, and strokes. Diabetics also have lower HDL cholesterol and higher triglyceride levels.

Chronic high blood sugar can also lead to nerve damage, vision loss, kidney damage, and decreased immune function (making the individual more susceptible to infections). Diabetics are 4 times more likely to become blind and 20 times more likely to develop kidney failure. Nerve damage in the lower extremities decreases the person's awareness of injury and infection. A small, untreated sore can cause severe infection, gangrene, and even lead to an amputation.

An 8-hour fasting blood glucose level above 126 mg/dl on two separate tests confirms a diagnosis of diabetes (see Table 11.4). A level of 126 or higher should be brought to the attention of a physician.

Diabetes is of two types: **Type I**, or insulin-dependent diabetes (IDDM), and Type II, or non-insulin-dependent diabetes (NIDDM). Type I also is called "juvenile diabetes" because it is found mainly in young people. With Type I, the pancreas produces little or no insulin. With **Type II**, the pancreas either does not produce sufficient insulin or it produces adequate amounts but the cells become insulin-resistant, thereby keeping glucose from entering the cell. Type II accounts for 90 to 95 percent of all diabetes cases.

Although diabetes has a genetic predisposition, Type II, or adult-onset diabetes, is related closely to overeating, obesity, and lack of physical activity. Type II diabetes, once limited primarily to overweight adults, now accounts for almost one-half of the new cases diagnosed in children. More than 80 percent of all Type II diabetics are overweight or have a history of excessive weight. In most cases this condition can be corrected through a special diet, a weight-loss program, and a regular exercise program.

Aerobic exercise helps prevent diabetes in middle-aged men.[23] The protective effect is even greater in those with risk factors such as obesity, high blood pressure, and family propensity. The preventive effect is attributed to less body fat and better sugar and fat metabolism resulting from the regular exercise program. At 3,500 calories per week, the risk was cut in half, as compared to sedentary men. This preventive effect, according to one of the authors of the study, should hold for women, too.

Both moderate-intensity and vigorous physical activity are associated with increased insulin sensitivity and decreased risk for diabetes. The key to increase and maintain proper insulin sensitivity, however, is regularity of the exercise program. Failure to maintain habitual physical activity voids these benefits.

A diet high in complex carbohydrates and water-soluble fibers (found in fruits, vegetables, oats, and beans), low in saturated fat, and low in sugar is helpful in treating diabetes. A simple aerobic exercise program (walking, cycling, or swimming four to five times per week) is often prescribed because it increases the body's sensitivity to insulin. Aggressive weight-loss, especially if combined with exercise, often allows diabetic patients to normalize their blood sugar level without the use of medication. Individuals who have high blood glucose levels should consult a physician to decide on the best treatment. (Exercise guidelines for diabetic patients are discussed in detail in Chapter 7 on page 145.)

Although complex carbohydrates are recommended in the diet, diabetics need to pay careful attention to the glycemic index (explained in Chapter 10, page 247). Refined and starchy foods have a high glycemic index (small-particle carbohydrates which are quickly digested); whereas grains, fruits, and vegetables are low-glycemic foods. Foods with a high glycemic index cause a rapid increase in blood sugar. A diet that includes many high-glycemic foods increases the risk for cardiovascular disease in people with high insulin resistance and **glucose intolerance**.[24] Combining a moderate amount of high-glycemic foods with low–glycemic index foods or with some fat and protein, however, can bring the average index down.

Systolic pressure Pressure exerted by the blood against the walls of the arteries during the forceful contraction (systole) of the heart.

Diastolic pressure Pressure exerted by the blood against the walls of the arteries during the relaxation phase (diastole) of the heart.

Hypertension Chronically elevated blood pressure.

Diabetes mellitus A disease in which the body doesn't produce or utilize insulin properly.

Insulin Hormone secreted by the pancreas; essential for proper metabolism of blood glucose (sugar) and maintenance of blood glucose level.

Insulin resistance The inability of the cells to respond appropriately to insulin.

Type I diabetes Insulin-dependent diabetes mellitus (IDDM), a condition in which the pancreas produces little or no insulin. Also known as juvenile diabetes because it is seen primarily in young people.

Type II diabetes Non-insulin-dependent diabetes mellitus (NIDDM), a condition in which insulin is not processed properly. Also known as adult-onset diabetes.

Glucose intolerance A condition characterized by slightly elevated blood glucose levels.

TABLE 11.4 BLOOD GLUCOSE GUIDELINES

Amount	Rating
≤126 mg/dl	Desirable
127–149 mg/dl	High
≥150 mg/dl	Very high

SMOKING

More than 48 million adults and 3.5 million adolescents in the United States smoke cigarettes. Cigarette smoking is the single largest preventable cause of illness and premature death in the United States. If we include all related deaths, tobacco is responsible for over 430,000 unnecessary deaths per year—enough deaths to wipe out the entire population of Miami and Miami Beach in a single year. About 50,000 of those who die are nonsmokers who were exposed to second-hand smoke.

Smoking has been linked to cardiovascular disease, cancer, bronchitis, emphysema, and peptic ulcers. In relation to coronary disease, not only does smoking speed up the process of atherosclerosis, but the risk of sudden death following a myocardial infarction also increases threefold.

> Smoking actually presents a much greater risk of death from heart disease than from lung disease.

Smoking allows the release of nicotine and another 1,200 toxic compounds or so into the bloodstream. Similar to hypertension, many of these substances destroy the inner membrane that protects the walls of the arteries. Once damage to the lining occurs, cholesterol and triglycerides can be deposited readily in the arterial wall. As the plaque builds up, it obstructs blood flow through the arteries.

Furthermore, smoking encourages the formation of blood clots, which can completely block an artery already narrowed by atherosclerosis. In addition, carbon monoxide, a byproduct of cigarette smoke, decreases the blood's oxygen-carrying capacity. A combination of obstructed arteries, nicotine, and less oxygen in the heart muscle heightens the risk for a serious heart problem.

Smoking also increases heart rate, raises blood pressure, and irritates the heart, which can trigger fatal **cardiac arrhythmias** (irregular heart rhythms). Another harmful effect is a decrease in HDL cholesterol, the "good" type that helps control blood lipids. Smoking actually presents a much greater risk of death from heart disease than from lung disease.

Pipe and cigar smoking and chewing tobacco also increase the risk for heart disease. Even if no smoke is inhaled, toxic substances are absorbed through the membranes of the mouth and end up in the bloodstream.

EXCESSIVE BODY FAT

Body composition is the ratio of lean body weight to fat weight. If the body contains too much fat, the person is considered obese. Although some experts recognize obesity as an independent risk factor for CHD, the risks attributed to obesity may actually be caused by other risk factors that usually accompany excessive body fat. Risk factors such as high blood lipids, hypertension, and diabetes, usually improve with increased physical activity. Overweight people who are physically active do not appear to be at increased risk for premature death.

Attaining recommended body composition helps improve some of the CHD risk factors and also yields a better state of health and wellness. People with a weight problem who desire to achieve recommended weight can do so by

- increasing their daily physical activity and exercise habits (both aerobic and strength training)
- consuming a diet low in fat and refined sugars and high in complex carbohydrates and fiber
- moderately reducing their total caloric intake but still consuming all of the necessary nutrients to sustain normal body functions.

Recommendations for weight management are discussed in Chapter 10.

PERSONAL AND FAMILY HISTORY

Individuals who have had cardiovascular problems are at higher risk than those who never have had a problem. People with this history should control the other risk factors as much as they can. Because most risk factors are reversible, this will greatly decrease their risk for future problems. The more time that has passed since the cardiovascular problem occurred, the lower the risk for recurrence.

Genetic predisposition toward heart disease has been clearly demonstrated and seems to be gaining in importance. All other factors being equal, a person with blood relatives who have or had heart disease before age 60 runs a greater risk than someone who has no such history. The younger the age at which the incident happened to the relative, the greater the risk for the disease.

In many cases, we have no way of knowing whether a person's true genetic predisposition or simply poor lifestyle habits led to a heart problem. A heart attack victim may have been physically inactive, overweight, and a smoker with bad dietary habits. Because we cannot differentiate these factors' effects reliably, anyone with a family history of cardiovascular problems should watch all other factors closely and maintain the lowest risk level possible. In addition, an annual blood chemistry analysis is strongly recommended to make sure the body is handling blood lipids properly.

TENSION AND STRESS

Tension and stress (discussed in Chapter 3) have become a normal part of life. Everyone has to deal daily with goals, deadlines, responsibilities, pressures. Almost everything in life (whether positive or negative) is a source of stress. The stressor itself is not what creates the health hazard but, rather, the individual's response to it.

The human body responds to stress by producing more catecholamines (hormones) to prepare the body for fight or flight. These hormones elevate heart rate, blood pressure, and blood glucose levels, enabling the person to take action.

If the person "fights or flees"—that is, takes physical action—the higher levels of catecholamines are metabolized, and the body returns to a "normal" state. But, if a person is under constant stress and unable to take physical action (such as with the death of a close relative or friend, loss of a job, trouble at work, or financial insecurity), the catecholamines remain elevated in the bloodstream.

People who are unable to relieve stress put a constant low-level strain on their cardiovascular system that could manifest itself in heart disease. In addition, when a person is in a stressful situation, the coronary arteries that feed the heart muscle constrict, reducing the oxygen supply to the heart. If the blood vessels are significantly blocked by atherosclerosis, abnormal heart rhythms or even a heart attack may follow.

AGE

Age is a risk factor because of the greater incidence of heart disease in older people. This tendency may be induced partly by other factors stemming from changes in lifestyle as we get older (less physical activity, poor nutrition, obesity, and so on).

However, young people should not think they will escape heart disease. The process begins early in life. This was clearly shown in American soldiers who died during the Korean and Vietnam conflicts. Autopsies conducted on soldiers killed at 22 years of age and younger revealed that approximately 70 percent had early stages of atherosclerosis. Other studies have found elevated blood cholesterol levels in children as young as 10 years old.

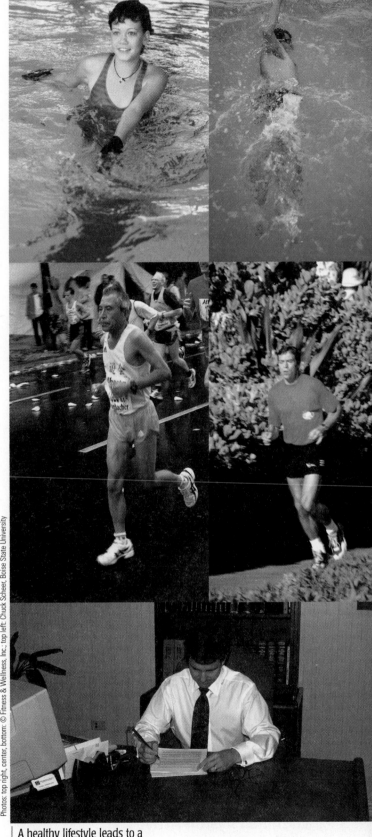

Photos: top right, center, bottom: © Fitness & Wellness, Inc.; top left: Chuck Scheer, Boise State University

A healthy lifestyle leads to a higher functional capacity throughout life.

Cardiac arrhythmias Irregular heart rhythms.

Even though the aging process cannot be stopped, it can certainly be slowed down. Physiological versus chronological age is an important concept in preventing disease. Some individuals in their 60s or older have the body of a 20-year-old. And 20-year-olds often are in such poor condition and health that they almost seem to have the body of a 60-year-old. Risk factor management and positive lifestyle habits are the best ways to slow down the natural aging process.

OTHER FACTORS

Additional evidence points to a few other factors that may be linked to coronary heart disease.

Gum Disease

One of these factors is gum disease. The oral bacteria that builds up with dental plaque can enter the bloodstream and contribute to blood vessel plaque formation, increase blood clots, and thus increase heart attack risk. Daily flossing for 1 to 2 minutes is the best way to prevent gum disease.

Snoring

Loud snoring has also been linked to cardiovascular disease. People who snore heavily may suffer from sleep apnea, a sleep disorder in which the throat closes for a brief moment, causing breathing to stop. In one study, individuals who snored heavily tripled their risk of a heart attack and quadrupled their risk of a stroke.[25]

GUIDELINES FOR PREVENTING CARDIOVASCULAR DISEASE

As discussed, most cardiovascular risk factors are preventable and reversible. Overall risk factor management is the best guideline to lower the risk. A regular aerobic exercise program in combination with proper nutrition, avoidance of tobacco, blood pressure control, stress management, and weight control are the key elements in preventing disorders of the cardiovascular system.

Lifetime Physical Activity

An active lifestyle combined with a systematic aerobic exercise program are two of the most important activities you can do to prevent and reduce the risk of cardiovascular problems. The basic principles for cardiorespiratory exercise are given in Chapter 7.

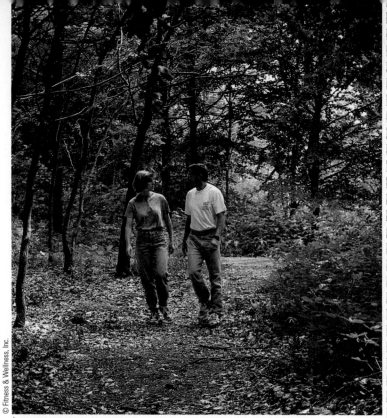

© Fitness & Wellness, Inc.

Moderate intensity activities greatly reduce the risk for premature cardiovascular death.

Although greater benefits are obtained at higher intensity levels, even a moderate-intensity aerobic exercise program can reduce cardiovascular risk considerably[26] (see Figure 11.4, page 283). A simple 40-minute walking (or equivalent) program, six to seven times per week, seems to have a strong inverse relationship with premature cardiovascular mortality. The minimum amount of exercise recommended for adults to achieve moderate fitness is presented in Table 11.5. Program 1 is of higher intensity than Program 2, thus only a minimum of three exercise sessions per week are required for Program 1 (as compared to a minimum of five to six for Program 2).

TABLE 11.5 MINIMUM AEROBIC EXERCISE FOR MODERATE FITNESS

Program 1	Days/ Week	Distance (miles)	Time (min)
Women	≥3	2	≤30
Men	≥3	2	≤27
Program 2			
Women	5–6	2	30–40
Men	6–7	2	30–40

From S. N. Blair, *Fitness and Mortality* (Dallas: Aerobics Research Center, 1991).

Nutrition Recommendations

The diet should contain ample amounts of fruits, vegetables, and grains. Because of their antioxidant effect, foods high in vitamins C and E and beta-carotene should be a regular part of the diet. Foods high in sugar and salt should be avoided. Alcohol should only be consumed in moderation. (See Chapter 8 for more specific recommendations.)

To lower total and LDL cholesterol levels, the following general dietary guidelines are recommended:

- Consume between 25 and 30 grams of fiber daily, including a minimum of 10 grams of soluble fiber (good sources are oats, fruits, barley, and legumes).
- Consume 25 grams of soy protein a day.
- Consume red meats (3 ounces per serving) fewer than three times per week, and avoid organ meats (such as liver and kidneys).
- Do not eat commercially baked foods.
- Avoid foods that contain transfatty acids, hydrogenated fat, or partially hydrogenated vegetable oil.
- Drink low-fat milk (1 percent or less fat, preferably) and use low-fat dairy products.
- Do not use coconut oil, palm oil, or cocoa butter.
- Limit egg consumption to less than three eggs per week (this applies only to people with high cholesterol, others may consume eggs in moderation).
- Eat fish instead of red meat.
- Bake, broil, grill, poach, or steam food instead of frying.
- Refrigerate cooked meat before adding it to other dishes. Remove fat hardened in the refrigerator before mixing the meat with other foods.
- Avoid fatty sauces made with butter, cream, or cheese.
- Maintain recommended body weight.

Soy protein is recommended to lower total and LDL cholesterol because a diet low in saturated fat and cholesterol that includes 25 grams of soy protein a day will lower cholesterol by an additional 5 to 7 percent, versus the same diet without the soy protein. This benefit is seen primarily in people with total cholesterol levels above 200 mg/dl. Some people may have to consume up to 60 grams a day to see an effect.

Margarines and salad dressings are now on the market that contain stanol ester, a plant-derived compound that lowers cholesterol. Over the course of several weeks, about 3 grams of margarine or 6 tablespoons of salad dressing containing stanol ester lowers LDL cholesterol by 14 percent.

The combination of a healthy diet, a sound aerobic exercise program, and weight control is the best prescription for controlling blood lipids. If this does not work, a physician can administer a blood test to break down the lipoproteins into their various subcategories. Most U.S. laboratories do not conduct these tests, but the American Heart Association has established six Lipid Disorder Training Centers that administer comprehensive blood tests. Your local American Heart Association can provide further information.

Smoking Cessation

Cigarette smoking is one of the six major risk factors for CHD. Nonetheless, the risk for both cardiovascular disease and cancer starts to decrease the moment you quit smoking. The risk for these two diseases approaches that of a lifetime nonsmoker 10 and 15 years, respectively, after cessation.

Quitting cigarette smoking is no easy task. Only about 20 percent of smokers who try to quit for the first time succeed each year. The addictive properties of nicotine and smoke make quitting difficult. Smokers have physical and psychological withdrawal symptoms when they stop smoking. Even though giving up smoking can be extremely difficult, it is by no means impossible.

The most crucial factor in quitting cigarette smoking is the person's sincere desire to do so. More than 95 percent of the successful ex-smokers have been able to quit on their own, either by quitting cold turkey or by using self-help kits available from organizations such as the American Cancer Society, the American Heart Association, and the American Lung Association. Only 3 percent of ex-smokers have quit as a result of formal "stop smoking" programs. A six-step plan to help people stop smoking is contained in Chapter 13.

Blood Pressure Control

Of all hypertension, 90 percent has no definite cause. Referred to as **essential hypertension**, this type is treatable. Aerobic exercise, weight reduction, a low-sodium/high-potassium diet, stress reduction, no smoking, a diet designed to decrease blood lipids, lower caffeine and alcohol intake, and antihypertensive medication have been used effectively to treat essential hypertension. The other 10 percent of hypertension is caused by pathological conditions such as narrowing of the kidney arteries, glomerulo-nephritis (a kidney disease), tumors of the adrenal glands, and narrowing of the aortic artery. With this type of

Essential hypertension
Persistent high blood pressure, having no known cause.

hypertension, the pathological cause has to be treated first to correct the blood pressure problem.

A factor contributing to high blood pressure in about half of all hypertensive people is too much sodium in the diet (salt, or sodium chloride, contains approximately 40 percent sodium). With high sodium intake, the body retains more water, which increases the blood volume and, in turn, drives up blood pressure. Although sodium is essential for normal body functions, only 200 mg, or one-tenth of a teaspoon of salt, is required daily. Even under strenuous conditions of job and sports participation that produce heavy perspiration, the amount of sodium required is seldom more than 3,000 mg per day. Yet, sodium intake in the typical American diet ranges between 6,000 and 20,000 mg per day!

When treating high blood pressure (unless it is extremely high), many physicians suggest trying a combination of aerobic exercise, weight loss, smoking cessation (if the person smokes), and reduced sodium before they recommend medication. In most instances, this treatment brings blood pressure under control.

Aerobic exercise is often prescribed for hypertensive patients. Studies have indicated that hypertensive patients who begin a moderate aerobic exercise program can expect a notable decrease in blood pressure after only a few weeks of training. The exercise-related drop in blood pressure may contribute to a 40 percent decrease in the risk for stroke and a 15 percent reduction in the risk for coronary heart disease.[27] Even in the absence of any decrease in resting blood pressure, hypertensive individuals who exercise have a lower risk of all-cause mortality compared with hypertensive/sedentary individuals.[28] The research data also show that exercise, not weight loss, is the major contributor to lower blood pressure. If aerobic exercise is discontinued, these changes are not maintained.

The best tip, though, is to take a preventive approach. Keeping blood pressure under control is easier than trying to bring it down once it is high. Blood pressure should be checked regularly, regardless of whether it is elevated. Regular physical exercise, weight control, a low-salt diet, no smoking, and stress management are the basic guidelines for blood pressure control.

STRESS MANAGEMENT

Individuals who are under a lot of stress and do not cope well with it need to take measures to counteract the effects of stress in their lives. One of the best suggestions is to identify the sources of stress and learn how to cope with them. People need to take control of themselves,

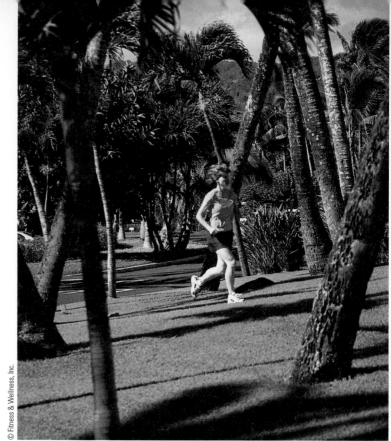

© Fitness & Wellness, Inc.

| Physical activity is an excellent tool to control stress. |

examine and act upon the things that are most important in their lives, and ignore less meaningful details. Relaxation techniques for stress management are presented in Chapter 3.

Physical exercise is one of the best ways to relieve stress. When a person takes part in physical activity, the body metabolizes excess catecholamines and is able to return to a normal state. Exercise also steps up muscular activity, which leads to muscular relaxation after completing the physical activity. Many executives prefer the evening hours for their physical activity programs, stopping after work at a health or fitness club. By doing this, they are able to burn up the excess tension accumulated during the day and enjoy the evening hours.

RESTING AND STRESS ELECTROCARDIOGRAMS

The electrocardiogram provides a valuable measure of the heart's function, recording the electrical impulses that stimulate the heart to contract. An ECG shows five general areas of heart function: heart rate, heart rhythm, the heart's axis, enlargement or hypertrophy of the heart, and myocardial infarction or heart attack.

On a standard 12-lead ECG, 10 electrodes are placed on the person's chest. From these 10 electrodes, 12 "pictures" or tracings of electrical impulses are studied from 12 different positions as they travel through the heart muscle (myocardium).

By looking at ECG charts, abnormalities in heart functioning can be identified. Based on the findings, the ECG may be interpreted as normal, equivocal, or abnormal. An ECG does not always identify problems, so a normal tracing is not an absolute guarantee. On the other hand, an abnormal tracing does not necessarily signal a serious condition.

ECGs are taken at rest, during stress of exercise, and during recovery. An **exercise ECG** is also known as a "graded exercise stress test" or a "maximal exercise tolerance test." Similar to a high-speed road test on a car, a stress ECG reveals the heart's tolerance to high-intensity exercise. It is a much better test to discover CHD than a resting ECG.

Stress ECGs are also used to assess cardiorespiratory fitness levels, screen individuals for preventive and cardiac rehabilitation programs, detect abnormal blood pressure response during exercise, and establish actual or functional maximal heart rate for exercise prescription.

At times the stress ECG has been questioned as a reliable predictor of CHD. Even so, it remains the most practical, inexpensive, noninvasive procedure available to diagnose latent (undiagnosed/unknown) CHD. The test is accurate in diagnosing CHD about 65 percent of the time. Part of the problem is that many times those who administer stress ECGs do it without clearly understanding the test's indications and limitations.

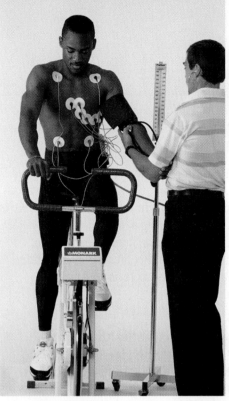

Graded treadmill exercise tolerance test with electro-cardiographic monitoring (exercise stress test).

© Fitness & Wellness, Inc.

The sensitivity of a stress test increases with the severity of the disease. More accurate results also are found for people at high risk for cardiovascular disease, in particular men over 45 and women over 55 with a poor cholesterol profile, high blood pressure, or a family history of heart disease. Test protocols, number of leads, electrocardiographic criteria, and the skill of the technicians administering the test also affect its sensitivity. Despite its limitations, a stress ECG test is still a useful tool for identifying people at high risk for exercise-related sudden death.

A FINAL WORD

Most of the risk factors for CHD are reversible and preventable. The fact that a person has a family history of heart disease and possibly some of the other risk factors because of neglect in lifestyle does not mean this person is doomed. A healthier lifestyle—free of cardiovascular problems—is something over which you have much control. You are encouraged to be persistent. Willpower and commitment are necessary to develop patterns that eventually will turn into healthy habits and contribute to your total well-being.

CRITERIA FOR STRESS ECG

Not every adult who wishes to start or continue an exercise program needs a stress ECG. The following criteria can be applied to determine when this type of test should be administered:

- Men over age 45 and women over age 55
- A total cholesterol level above 200 mg/dl or an HDL cholesterol below 35 mg/dl
- Hypertensive and diabetic patients
- Cigarette smokers
- Individuals with a family history of CHD, syncope, or sudden death before age 60
- Hypertensive and diabetic patients
- People with an abnormal resting ECG
- All individuals with symptoms of chest discomfort, dysrhythmias, syncope, or chronotropic incompetence (a heart rate that increases slowly during exercise and never reaches maximum)

Exercise ECG An exercise test during which workload is increased gradually (until the subject reaches maximal fatigue) with blood pressure and 12-lead electrocardiographic monitoring throughout the test.

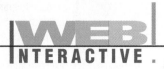

WEB ACTIVITIES

■ **American Heart Association** This comprehensive site features information on a variety of cardiovascular topics, including heart health and disease. There is a reference guide, featuring a heart and stroke guide from A to Z, warning signs, family heart health, exercise, nutrition, and other lifestyle interventions. This site is used by consumers as well as health professionals.
http://www.americanheart.org

■ **Improving Cardiovascular Health in African Americans** A series of seven brochures from the National Heart, Lung, and Blood Institute that you can download or read on-line.
http://www.nhlbi.nih.gov/health/public/heart/other/chdblack/index.htm

■ **Check Your Healthy Heart IQ** This site is sponsored by the National Heart, Lung, and Blood Institute. Test your knowledge about heart disease and its risks (high blood pressure, high blood cholesterol, smoking, and overweight) and ways to reduce your risk.
http://www.nhlbi.nih.gov/health/public/heart/other/hh_iq_ab.htm

■ **Heart Disease from Dr. Koop.com** This site features a comprehensive library containing a variety of heart disease topics, including angina, cholesterol, heart failure, coronary artery disease, and heart disease in women.
http://www.drkoop.com/conditions/heart_disease

InfoTrac

You can find additional readings related to wellness via InfoTrac College Edition, an on-line library of more than 900 journals and publications. Follow the instructions for accessing InfoTrac that came packaged with your textbook, then search for articles using a key word search.

Suggested Reading Janet Raloff, "Chocolate Hearts: Research Indicates Chocolate Contains Antioxidants Called Flavonoids that Reduce Risk of Cardiovascular Disease," *Science News* 157, no. 12 (March 18, 2000): 188.

1. Why do chocolate and cocoa seem to possess antioxidant properties?

2. Physiologically, how do the antioxidants found in chocolate promote vascular health?

3. Based on the above research, what happens to the body's cholesterol levels and platelet function after ingestion of chocolate and cocoa?

Web Activity
Texas Heart Institute Risk Factor Assessment
http://www.texasheartinstitute.org/heartest.html

Sponsor The Texas Heart Institute at St. Luke's Episcopal Hospital in Houston, Texas.

Description Risk factors are your personal characteristics, genetic makeup, and lifestyle behaviors that may increase your chances of having a heart attack or stroke. Some you can't change or control (age, gender, genetics); some you can, by making a few changes in your daily habits. Are you at risk? Find out by taking this short interactive quiz.

Available Activities

1. The site features ten simple questions about your personal characteristics and habits designed to determine your personal risk of having a heart attack or stroke.

2. The questions assess your risk based on age, family history, smoking habits, blood cholesterol level, blood pressure, physical activity, weight, diabetes, and past medical history of heart conditions.

Web Work

1. From the home page, answer all ten questions honestly by clicking on the appropriate radio button or typing in the information requested.

2. Question 4 allows you to calculate your body mass index (BMI) by entering your height and weight. Click on "calculate" button to receive your BMI.

3. When quiz is completed, click the "Submit" button to receive your relative risk and specific information on how to decrease your risks.

Helpful Hints

1. If you check more than three of the ten risk factors, you should see a health care provider for a complete assessment of your risks!

2. The evaluation you receive is comprehensive and provides practical guidelines on prevention of heart disease through risk factor reduction.

For additional Web activities, links, and suggested readings, visit our Health, Fitness, and Wellness Resource Center at http://health.wadsworth.com.

NOTES

1. American Heart Association, *2000 Heart and Stroke Facts Statistical Update* (Dallas: AHA, 1999).

2. U.S. Department of Health and Human Services, Centers for Disease Control and Prevention, National Center for Health Statistics, National Vital Statistics System: *Deaths: Final Data for 1998* 48, no. 11 (July, 24, 1998).

3. American Heart Association, *1999 Heart and Stroke Facts Statistical Update* (Dallas: AHA, 1998).

4. See note 1.

5. See note 2.

6. See note 3.

7. S. N. Blair, H. W. Kohl III, R. S. Paffenbarger Jr., D. G. Clark, K. H. Cooper, and L. W. Gibbons, "Physical Fitness and All-Cause Mortality: A Prospective Study of Healthy Men and Women," *Journal of the American Medical Association* 262 (1989): 2395–2401.

8. R. S. Paffenbarger Jr., R. T. Hyde, A. L. Wing, I. Lee, D. L. Jung, and J. B. Kampert, "The Association of Changes in Physical-Activity Level and Other Lifestyle Characteristics with Mortality Among Men," *New England Journal of Medicine* 328 (1993): 538–545.

9. P. A. Romm, M. K. Hong, and C. E. Rackley, "High-Density-Lipoprotein Cholesterol and Risk of Coronary Heart Disease," *Practical Cardiology* 16 (1990): 28–40.

10. C. J. Gluek, "Nonpharmacologic and Pharmacologic Alteration of High Density Lipoprotein Cholesterol: Therapeutic Approaches to Prevention of Atherosclerosis," *American Heart Journal* 110 (1985): 1107–1115.

11. J. M. Gaziano and C. H. Hennekens, "A New Look at What Can Unclog Your Arteries," *Executive Health Report* 27, no. 8 (1991): 16.

12. See note 11.

13. See note 9.

14. See note 1.

15. M. L. Stefanick et al., "Effects of Diet in Men and Postmenopausal Women with Low Levels of HDL Cholesterol and High Levels of LDL Cholesterol," *New England Journal of Medicine* 339 (1998): 12–20.

16. E. B. Rimm, A. Ascherio, E. Giovannucci, D. Spiegelman, M. J. Stampfer, and W. C. Willett, "Vegetable, Fruit, and Cereal Fiber Intake and Risk of Coronary Heart Disease Among Men," *Journal of the American Medical Association* 275 (1996): 447–451.

17. R. J. Barnard, "Effects of Lifestyle Modification on Serum Lipids," *Archives of Internal Medicine* 151 (1991): 1389–1394.

18. W. Castelli, "Smart Heart Strategies: Best Ways to Beat Heart Disease," *Bottom Line/Personal Health* 19, no. 4 (1998): 1–3.

19. R. Superko, "Platelets and Lipid Interaction with a Vessel Wall," (paper presented in symposium at American College of Sports Medicine Annual Meeting, 1991).

20. O. Nygard, J. E. Nordreahaug, H. Refsum, P. M. Ueland, M. Farstad, and S. E. Vollset, "Plasma Homocysteine Levels and Mortality in Patients with Coronary Heart Disease," *New England Journal of Medicine* 337 (1997): 230–236.

21. "The Homocysteine-CVD Connection," *HealthNews* (October 25, 1999).

22. C. J. Boushey, S. A. A. Beresford, G. S. Omenn, and A. G. Motulsky, "A Quantitative Assessment of Plasma Homocysteine as a Risk Factor for Vascular Disease," *Journal of the American Medical Association* 274 (1995): 1049–1057.

23. S. P. Helmrich, D. R. Ragland, R. W. Leung, and R. S. Paffenbarger, "Physical Activity and Reduced Occurrences of Non-Insulin-Dependent Diabetes Mellitus," *New England Journal of Medicine* 325 (1991): 147–152.

24. S. Liu et al., "A Prospective Study of Dietary Glycemic Load, Carbohydrate Intake, and Risk of Coronary Heart Disease in U.S. Women," *American Journal of Clinical Nutrition* 71 (2000): 1455–1461.

25. "Checkup for the New Millennium," *Consumer Reports on Health* (December, 1999).

26. See note 7.

27. R. Collins et al., "Blood Pressure, Stroke, and Coronary Heart Disease; Part 2, Short-term Reductions in Blood Pressure: Overview of Randomized Drug Trials in Their Epidemiological Context," *Lancet* 335 (1990): 827–838.

28. S. N. Blair et al., "Influences of Cardiorespiratory Fitness and Other Precursors on Cardiovascular Disease and All-cause Mortality in Men and Women," *Journal of the American Medical Association* 276 (1996): 205–210.

CARDIOVASCULAR DISEASE RISK ANALYSIS

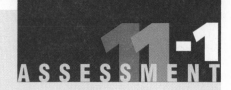

Name: _____   Date: _____   Grade: _____

Instructor: _____   Course: _____   Section: _____

Necessary Lab Equipment
None required.

Objective
Evaluate family and lifestyle factors that may affect your risk for cardiovascular disease and cancer.

Instructions
Read Chapter 12 prior to this lab so you may become familiar with normal blood lipids, blood glucose, and blood pressure values, as well as the seven warning signals for cancer..

Cardiovascular Disease

		Yes	No
1.	I accumulate at least 30 minutes of physical activity on most days of the week.	☐	☐
2.	I exercise aerobically a minimum of three times a week in the appropriate target zone for at least 20 minutes per session.	☐	☐
3.	I am at or slightly below the health-fitness recommended percent body fat (see Table 9.9, page 233).	☐	☐
4.	My blood lipids are within normal range.	☐	☐
5.	I get at least 25 grams of fiber in my daily diet.	☐	☐
6.	I eat more than five servings of fruits and vegetables every day.	☐	☐
7.	I limit total fat, saturated fat, and cholesterol in my daily diet.	☐	☐
8.	I am not a diabetic.	☐	☐
9.	My blood pressure is normal.	☐	☐
10.	I do not smoke cigarettes or use tobacco in any other form.	☐	☐
11.	I manage stress adequately in daily life.	☐	☐
12.	I do not have a personal or family history of heart disease.	☐	☐
13.	I am not over 45 years of age.	☐	☐

Evaluation

Risk Category	Number of "no" Answers
Very Low Risk	0
Low Risk	1 or less
Moderate Risk	2
High Risk	3
Very High Risk	4 or more

12 CANCER PREVENTION AND WELLNESS

- Know the differences in characteristics of benign and malignant tumors.

- Differentiate the major types of cancer.

- Recognize precancerous conditions and warning signs of cancer.

- Identify the three basic kinds of skin cancers.

- Learn about the gender-specific cancers, their incidence, and their risk factors.

- List guidelines for preventing cancer, including dietary guidelines.

- Understand the role of self-examinations (and how to conduct them) and examination by physicians.

301

CANCER IS THE SECOND LEADING CAUSE of death in the United States, accounting for about 23 percent of all deaths on a yearly basis. Unlike cardiovascular disease, the mortality rate for cancer has increased steadily since cancer statistics began to be kept in the 1930s.[1] In 1996, however, the cancer rate declined slightly for the first time. This decline was attributed to improved prevention and treatment, most markedly a reduction in cigarette smoking. Although cancer is second only to heart disease as the leading killer in the United States, it is the number-one health fear of the American people.

From 1991 to 1995,

- Deaths from lung cancer among men declined 6.7 percent (though it increased 6.4 percent among women).
- Colorectal cancer deaths fell 7 percent in men and 4.8 percent in women.
- Prostate cancer deaths dropped 6.3 percent.
- Breast cancer deaths fell 6.3 percent, and deaths from ovarian cancer declined by 4.8 percent.

Although the decline in deaths is certainly good news, the American Cancer Society states that we need to redouble our efforts to get people to stop smoking and to eat a healthier diet.

DEVELOPMENT OF CANCER

Cancer starts when an initiator alters DNA, the cell's basic genetic material, in a way that allows the cell to dictate its own rate of growth. The alteration can occur in minutes or days. Initiators include radiation, chemicals, and viruses. Having a cell with altered DNA, however, does not guarantee cancer. Fortunately, special enzymes travel up and down the DNA to repair breaks and changes in it.

Anything that speeds up the rate of cell division lessens the chance that repair enzymes will find the altered part of the DNA in time. Once a cell multiplies and incorporates its newly altered DNA into its genetic instructions, the cell no longer realizes its DNA has been changed.

Compounds that increase cell division are called "promoters." They are thought to promote cancer either by reducing the time available for repair enzymes to act or by encouraging cells with altered DNA to develop and grow. Development and growth of these altered cells may take up to 20 years. Common promoters are thought to be estrogen, alcohol, and dietary fat in excess.

Even after an altered cell has multiplied, cancer does not necessarily result. First, a cell mass must grow large enough to affect body metabolism. During this initial stage of growth, the immune system may find the altered cells and destroy them. Or the cancer cells themselves may be so defective that their own DNA limits their ability to grow, and they die anyway.

Actually, most of us probably have cancerous or **precancerous** cells in our bodies at some time. Many of them die because of mutation. Many more are destroyed by a healthy immune system. Occasionally, though, the immune system is unable to dominate, and cancer develops.

Benign and **malignant** tumors differ in the following ways:

1. Benign tumors resemble the normal tissues that surround them; malignant tumors do not.
2. The cells of benign tumors do not break off and metastasize; the cells of malignant tumors do.
3. Benign tumors do not invade surrounding tissues; malignant tumors do.
4. Benign tumors can be controlled by normal methods used to control any tissue growth; malignant tumors cannot.
5. Almost all benign tumors are encased (contained) in a fibrous capsule; very few malignant tumors are.
6. Benign tumors are not dangerous unless they interfere with blood flow; malignant tumors are fatal if untreated.

Survival depends on how early the cancer is diagnosed, what tissues are involved, the strength of the immune system, and potential treatment options. Cures have been discovered for some kinds of cancer. Equally important is that more than 8.4 million Americans with a history of cancer were alive in 2000. Currently, 4 of 10 people diagnosed with cancer are expected to be alive 5 years from the initial diagnosis.[2]

INCIDENCE OF CANCER

Someone in the United States dies of cancer every minute. It strikes people of all ages and is the leading killer of children between ages 3 and 14. More than half a million people in the United States die from cancer each year, and more than a million are diagnosed each year. One of every five deaths from any cause in the United States is from cancer.[3]

The incidence of cancer varies slightly between men and women. The most common cancers in men are prostate, lung, colon/rectal, and urinary/bladder, in that order. The most common cancers in women are lung, breast, colon/rectal, uterine, and ovarian. Leading sites and deaths from cancer in men and women are shown in Figure 12.1.

FIGURE **12.1** 2001 CANCER INCIDENCE AND DEATHS BY SITE AND SEX.

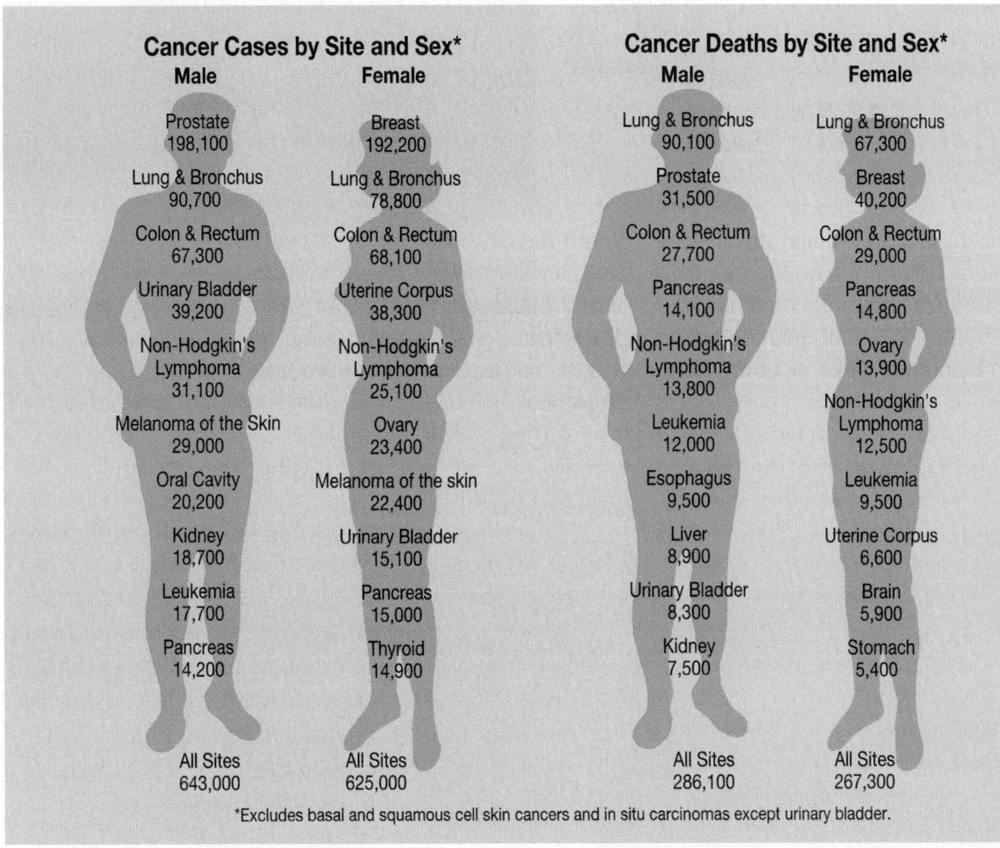

Cancer Cases by Site and Sex*

Male

Prostate
198,100

Lung & Bronchus
90,700

Colon & Rectum
67,300

Urinary Bladder
39,200

Non-Hodgkin's
Lymphoma
31,100

Melanoma of the Skin
29,000

Oral Cavity
20,200

Kidney
18,700

Leukemia
17,700

Pancreas
14,200

All Sites
643,000

Female

Breast
192,200

Lung & Bronchus
78,800

Colon & Rectum
68,100

Uterine Corpus
38,300

Non-Hodgkin's
Lymphoma
25,100

Ovary
23,400

Melanoma of the skin
22,400

Urinary Bladder
15,100

Pancreas
15,000

Thyroid
14,900

All Sites
625,000

Cancer Deaths by Site and Sex*

Male

Lung & Bronchus
90,100

Prostate
31,500

Colon & Rectum
27,700

Pancreas
14,100

Non-Hodgkin's
Lymphoma
13,800

Leukemia
12,000

Esophagus
9,500

Liver
8,900

Urinary Bladder
8,300

Kidney
7,500

All Sites
286,100

Female

Lung & Bronchus
67,300

Breast
40,200

Colon & Rectum
29,000

Pancreas
14,800

Ovary
13,900

Non-Hodgkin's
Lymphoma
12,500

Leukemia
9,500

Uterine Corpus
6,600

Brain
5,900

Stomach
5,400

All Sites
267,300

Source: 2001 *Cancer Facts and Figures.*
American Cancer Society (New York: ACS, 2001).

*Excludes basal and squamous cell skin cancers and in situ carcinomas except urinary bladder.

RISK FACTORS

In more than half of all diagnosed cases, the cancer has metastasized, making treatment more difficult. The American Cancer Society estimates that 2 of every 5 people who die from cancer could have been saved if they had been diagnosed sooner. In addition, we can go a long way toward preventing cancer by changing our behaviors.

The probable causes of cancer are many. We know that cancer is caused by certain substances in the environment. We also know that cigarette smoking and dietary factors play a role. So do heredity (the inherited tendency for certain kinds of cancers) and race. Some cancers can be caused by viruses. Viruses that increase the risk for cancer include Epstein-Barr, human papilloma, Hepatitis B, and T-cell leukemia/lymphoma. Although some controversy still surrounds the notion, increasing evidence suggests that attitudes and emotions might increase susceptibility to cancer and could cause physiological changes in the body that can lead to the development of cancer.

Table 12.1 shows the probability of developing invasive cancers. You can't control some causes of cancer —heredity and race, for instance—but you can actively reduce many identified risk factors and help beat the odds of developing cancer (see Figure 12.2). Proven, general risk factors are discussed next.

Tobacco

Cigarette smoking has been called the number-one preventable cause of death in the United States. It is estimated to directly cause approximately 28 percent of all cancers in the United States and approximately 87 percent of all lung cancers among Americans. It also is a leading cause of bladder cancer.[4]

Smoking—which also contributes to other serious diseases, including emphysema, heart disease, and stroke —introduces carbon monoxide and lethal **carcinogens** into the body. Your chance of getting

Cancer A group of more than a hundred diseases in which cells grow at an uncontrolled rate, mature in an abnormal way, and invade nearby tissues.

Precancerous A condition in which a benign (noncancerous) condition has the potential to become cancerous.

Benign Noncancerous.

Malignant Cancerous.

Carcinogens Cancer-causing substances.

TABLE **12.1** CHANCES OF DEVELOPING INVASIVE CANCERS

Site	Sex	Birth to 39 Years	40 to 59 Years	60 to 79 Years	Ever (Birth to Death)
All sites	Male	1 in 58	1 in 13	1 in 3	1 in 2
	Female	1 in 52	1 in 11	1 in 4	1 in 3
Breast	Female	1 in 217	1 in 26	1 in 15	1 in 8
Colon and Rectum	Male	1 in 1,667	1 in 108	1 in 23	1 in 16
	Female	1 in 2,000	1 in 137	1 in 30	1 in 17
Prostate	Male	<1 in 10,000	1 in 103	1 in 8	1 in 6

Source: *CA — A Cancer Journal for Clinicians*, 45, no. 1.

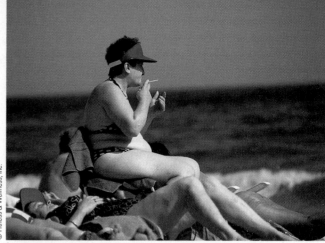

Cigarette smoking, obesity, and excessive sun exposure are major risk factors for cancer.

FIGURE **12.2** ESTIMATE OF THE RELATIVE ROLES OF THE MAJOR CANCER-CAUSING FACTORS.

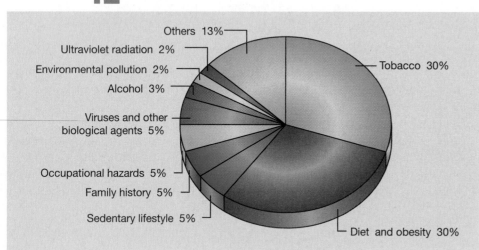

Others 13%
Ultraviolet radiation 2%
Environmental pollution 2%
Alcohol 3%
Viruses and other biological agents 5%
Occupational hazards 5%
Family history 5%
Sedentary lifestyle 5%
Tobacco 30%
Diet and obesity 30%

Diet

According to the American Cancer Society, diet is a major factor in about 30 percent of all cancers. Some scientists believe the role of diet may be equivalent to that of cigarette smoking in boosting the risk of developing cancer. A diet high in saturated fats increases the risk for cancer. Specific culprits are tropical oils (such as coconut oil and palm oil) and animal fats (fatty meats, whole milk, cheese, and other animal-source foods). The cancer risk increases substantially if more than 30 percent of daily calories comes from fat and more than 10 percent comes from saturated fats.

Also, if the diet doesn't contain enough fiber, the risk of certain kinds of cancers, especially cancer of the colon, may increase significantly. Other dietary factors that increase the risk of cancer include

- foods cured or pickled with salt or nitrites, such as luncheon meats,
- smoked foods,
- charcoal-broiled foods,
- foods containing cyclamates (a type of artificial sweetener),
- vitamin and mineral deficiency, and
- excessive alcohol consumption.

Environmental Carcinogens

Carcinogens include atmospheric agents ranging from electromagnetic radiation and radon gas to chemicals,

> More than 50 carcinogenic chemicals have been identified in tobacco smoke.

cancer as a result of cigarette smoking is related to how long you have smoked, how many packs a day you smoke, and how deeply you inhale the smoke.

Smokeless tobacco also poses significant risk for cancer, despite the persistent myth that it's okay to "chew" as long as you don't smoke. Smokeless or chewing tobacco is a leading cause of cancer of the mouth, throat, esophagus, and larynx.

Also of concern is **secondhand smoke**. Children are at particular risk for lung diseases such as bronchitis.[5] Nonsmokers who live with smokers have been found to develop lung cancer at a higher rate than other nonsmokers.

POSSIBLE CARCINOGENS (CANCER-CAUSING SUBSTANCES)

- Aflatoxins (in rotting peanuts)
- Alcohol
- Alkylating agents
- Anabolic steroids
- Arsenic
- Asbestos
- Benzene
- Benzo(a)pyrene (in tobacco smoke)
- Beryllium
- Betel nuts
- Cadmium
- Chlornaphazine
- Chrome ores
- Chrysene (in tobacco smoke)
- Coke (a type of coal)
- Creosote oil
- Cyclamates
- Diethylstilbestrol (DES)
- Estrogen (synthetic)
- Ionizing radiation
- Immunosuppressive drugs
- Isopropyl oil
- Mesothorium
- Nickel carbonyl
- Nickel ores
- Nitrates
- Nitrites
- Nitrosamines
- Oral contraceptives
- Paraffin oil (crude)
- Penacetin
- Radiation
- Radium
- Radioactive dust/gas
- Radon
- Soots
- Tars
- Tar fumes
- Tobacco
- Ultraviolet light
- Vinyl chloride
- Wood dust
- X-rays

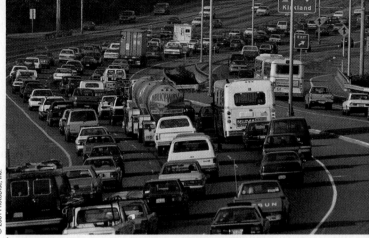

© 2001 PhotoDisc, Inc.

Automobile exhaust was a leading source of environmental carcinogens before the advent of catalytic converters.

Medical Substances

Cancer can follow exposure to certain medical substances such as drugs, agents used in chemotherapy, medications used to suppress the immune system, hormones, and x-rays. For example, the drug diethylstilbestrol (DES)—used to treat complications and prevent miscarriages until the mid-1960s—has been found to cause cancer of the female reproductive organs in the daughters of women who took the drug.

Cancer caused by x-rays is rare, but it can happen from exposure to large doses of radiation. Precise calibration of x-ray equipment has helped prevent accidental exposure to large doses in most cases. The effects of radiation are cumulative, so repeated small doses over a long period may be a cause for concern. Lead shields are used to protect parts of the body that are not being x-rayed from accidental exposure.

Viruses

The first virus known to cause cancer was identified in 1911 by a scientist who injected it into chickens, causing cancerous tumors. Since that time, exhaustive research has been conducted in the attempt to identify viruses that may cause cancers in humans.

One group of viruses—three variants of the human papilloma virus (HPV), which causes genital warts—is suspected of causing cervical cancer and other genital malignancies. These cancer-causing viruses can be sexually transmitted.[6]

Approximately 2 percent of all cancers in the United States may be related to viruses. In some cases the virus may be responsible for causing or initiating the cancer; once the disease takes hold, the virus no longer is in the picture. In other situations, the viruses may not actually

such as vinyl chloride and arsenic. In most cases, the risk of cancer is related to the dose. A one-time massive exposure to a carcinogen may cause cancer, as can prolonged, long-term exposure to small amounts.

As carcinogens are identified, policies are instituted to protect the public from exposure. For example, strict building codes now ban the use of asbestos. Accidental exposure still occurs, however, when demolishing or remodeling old buildings. Schools, in particular, have to take extreme measures to prevent children from being exposed to the asbestos, which was formerly used for fireproofing.

The chemicals in the water we drink, the hydrocarbons emitted in automobile exhaust, and the agents in some insecticides and pesticides have been shown to cause cancer at certain levels. Few people are exposed to a high level of these pollutants, but the effects of chronic, low-level exposure are being studied.

Secondhand smoke A mixture of smoke exhaled by smokers and smoke from the burning portion of a cigarette, pipe, or cigar.

cause the cancer but may increase the risk of developing cancer.

Scientists also have identified a particular kind of virus called **retroviruses**. The human immunodeficiency virus (HIV), which causes AIDS, is a retrovirus.

Controversy still surrounds the notion of cancer-causing viruses. Most scientists conclude that certain viruses may cause cancer only under certain circumstances. For example, Epstein-Barr virus (EBV), which causes mononucleosis in the United States, causes a cancer called Burkitt's lymphoma among children in Africa. Scientists now are researching the possibility that EBV, or similar viruses responsible for herpes, may sharply increase the risk of Hodgkin's disease, cervical cancer, and some forms of leukemia.

Heredity

Heredity is a factor in an estimated 10 percent of all cancers in the United States. Approximately 14 million Americans are at risk because they inherited the tendency for certain malignancies.[7] Cancers caused by hereditary factors often begin in childhood. Such factors can increase the likelihood of developing the cancer by as much as 30 times normal odds.

> Heredity is a factor in an estimated 10 percent of all cancers in the United States.

Certain genetic markers called **oncogenes** can be used to predict cancer in some cases. Cancer also can be predicted if **suppressor genes**, which protect against cancer, are missing from certain genetic material.

In a few cases, the cancer itself is inherited. One example is retinoblastoma, a cancer of the eye that occurs in infants and young children. More often, what is inherited is not the actual cancer but, rather, the predisposition for (or the tendency to develop) that cancer. Exciting new research has identified, for example, a gene that predisposes its carriers to cancer of the colon. Once the gene is identified, a person carrying the gene can take certain precautions and undergo aggressive early screening to improve the odds of preventing or successfully treating the disease.

The risk for certain leukemias can be genetically passed from parent to child. The tendency for lung, colon, breast, uterine, prostate, bone, brain, stomach, and adrenal gland cancers also can be inherited.

Stress

An individual's response to stress has been linked to the risk for developing cancer, as well as certain other diseases, such as heart disease. Chronic stress and the hormones it unleashes on the body interfere with the immune system's ability to recognize cancerous cells and destroy them.

Joseph G. Courtney, of the University of California, Los Angeles, School of Public Health, and his co-workers joined forces with researchers in Sweden to analyze their large database of Stockholm-area patients with colorectal cancer. Courtney's team confirmed that on-the-job aggravation seems to put people at higher risk for developing colon and rectal cancers. Those who reported a history of workplace problems over the past 10 years faced 5.5 times the colorectal cancer risk versus adults who reported no such problems.[8]

Although controversy still surrounds the idea, researchers have also identified a "cancer-prone" personality, a collection of traits that seem to occur in people who later develop cancer. Called the "Type C" personality, it is characterized by unusual compliance and the tendency to internalize conflict. It also is marked by the individual's inability to deal with stress in a healthy way.

Chronic Irritation

Evidence indicates that chronic irritation of cells or tissues can lead to the development of cancer. Linked to certain kinds of cancers and increased risk for cancer are the following:

- chronic low-grade infections
- repeated bladder infections
- repeated ulceration of tissues
- chronic infection of scar tissue
- constant irritation of a mole or other benign growth
- certain kinds of injuries

SIGNS OF INHERITED CANCER

Four patterns generally identify hereditary cancers:

1. Many family members develop the same kind of cancer.
2. The cancer strikes victims at an earlier age than usual. (Breast cancer, for example, typically occurs in the 60s but may strike a woman in her 40s who inherited the tendency.)
3. The cancer strikes more than once (in both breasts, for example, or in two different places in the liver).
4. The person has an unusual gender pattern. (For example, a cancer unusual in women will affect all the women in a family.)

- long-term irritation of gallstones against the gallbladder

Estrogen-Replacement Therapy

When the level of estrogen, normally produced by the ovaries, tapers off as a woman reaches menopause, physicians often prescribe estrogen-replacement therapy to ease or delay the troublesome symptoms of menopause. Evidence shows that estrogen-replacement therapy also helps to prevent osteoporosis, a loss of bone tissue that affects mostly older women. Estrogen-replacement therapy, however, increases the risk of endometrial cancer (a cancer of the lining of the uterus) and may increase the risk of breast cancer.

TYPES OF CANCER

In addition to being familiar with general risk factors, knowing the specific risk factors for certain kinds of cancers can help you reduce the odds of developing one of the more common cancers.

Cancers have been classified according to six general types:

1. **Carcinomas.** Spread through the bloodstream and lymph system, carcinomas—the most common kind of cancers—affect the tissues that line most body cavities and cover body surfaces. Examples are lung cancer, breast cancer, skin cancer, colon cancer, and uterine cancer. (If the cancer occurs in a gland, it is called an adenocarcinoma.)

2. **Sarcomas.** Spread through the bloodstream, sarcomas affect the connective tissues of the body, such as the muscles, bones, and cartilage. Sarcomas are not as common as carcinomas, but they grow and spread more quickly and form more solid tumors.
3. **Lymphomas.** Spread through the lymph system, lymphomas are cancers of the lymphatic, or infection-fighting, cells. Lymph nodes in the groin, armpits, and neck can be affected. An example of lymphoma is Hodgkin's disease.
4. **Melanomas.** Spread through the bloodstream, melanomas affect the skin. They generally begin as a mole that later becomes cancerous. They grow and spread rapidly.
5. **Leukemias.** Spread through the bloodstream, leukemias affect the tissues that manufacture blood, especially the spleen and the bone marrow.
6. **Neuroblastomas.** Spread through the bloodstream, neuroblastomas affect the nervous system or the adrenal glands. Relatively uncommon, they occur most often in children under age 10.

CANCER SITES

Following are some common cancer sites, and Table 12.2 summarizes pertinent data on these cancers.

Skin Cancer

More than 1.3 million Americans were diagnosed with some form of skin cancer in the year 2000. Skin cancer is probably the most underrated type of cancer: It accounts for approximately 40 percent of all cancers, and is the fastest-growing type of cancer in men over 50.[9] The sharp increase in the incidence of skin cancer is alarming. Over the past decade, it has increased about 90 percent. As many as 1 in every 90 Americans have some type of skin cancer.

The three basic kinds of skin cancers are

1. **Basal cell carcinoma.** This is the most common, and least serious, of the skin cancers. It usually does not spread, and it grows slowly. Most basal cell carcinomas occur on the face, neck, and hands—areas of frequent exposure to the sun.
2. **Squamous cell carcinoma.** This type of cancer grows faster than

Retroviruses Viruses that invade a cell's genetic structure and are passed on to each succeeding generation of cells as the cells divide.

Oncogenes Pieces of genetic material that serve as markers to predict later mutation and development of certain cancers, probably by encouraging mutation of related cells.

Suppressor genes Pieces of genetic material that are part of a cell's normal protective mechanism against development of cancer.

TABLE **12.2** COMMON CANCERS

	Risk Factors	Warning Signals	Early Detection	Treatment	5-Year Survival with Treatment
Lung cancer (est. 164,000 new cases a year; 156,900 deaths)	Cigarette smoking for 20 or more years; exposure to certain industrial substances, particularly asbestos; secondhand smoke; radiation; radon.	Persistent cough, sputum streaked with blood, chest pain, recurring bronchitis or pneumonia.	Difficult to detect early. Diagnosis based on chest x-ray, sputum testing, fiberoptic bronchoscopy (direct examination of the lungs by means of a specially lighted tube).	Surgery, radiation therapy, chemotherapy.	The leading cause of cancer death among both men and women.
Breast cancer (est. 184,200 new cases a year; 41,200 deaths)	Over age 50, personal or family history of breast cancer, no children or first child after age 30, dense breast tissue, obesity, high fat intake, alcohol, estrogen replacement therapy after menopause.	Breast changes: lumps, thickening, swelling, puckering, dimpling, skin irritation, nipple distortion, scaliness, discharge, pain, tenderness.	Monthly breast self-examination. Professional breast exam every 3 years for women ages 20–40 and every year over age 40. Yearly mammography for all women over 50, every 1 or 2 years for women 40–49; baseline mammogram for those 35–39. Tissue biopsy confirms diagnosis.	Surgery, from lumpectomy (local removal of tumor) to a modified radical mastectomy (removal of breast and lymph glands, leaving underlying muscle intact); radiation; chemotherapy; or all three. For metastatic breast cancer, autologous bone marrow transplantation.	Until recently, the leading cause of cancer death in women; now surpassed by lung cancer.
Uterine and cervical cancer (48,900 new cases a year; 11,100 deaths)	For cervical cancer: early age of first intercourse, multiple sex partners, genital herpes, human papilloma virus infection, significant exposure to secondhand smoke. For uterine cancer: infertility, failure to ovulate, prolonged estrogen therapy, obesity.	Unusual vaginal bleeding or discharge.	Pap smear every 3 years after two initial negative tests 1 year apart.	Surgery, radiation, or a combination of the two. In precancerous stages, cervical cells may be destroyed by extreme cold or intense heat. Precancerous endometrial changes are treated with the hormone progesterone.	Cervical cancer mortality has declined 70% during the last 40 years with wider application of the Pap smear. Postmenopausal women with abnormal bleeding should be checked.
Ovarian cancer (est. 23,100 new cases a year; 14,000 deaths)	Family history of ovarian cancer; personal history of breast cancer; obesity; infertility (because the abnormality that interferes with conception may also play a role in cancer development); low levels of transferase, an enzyme involved in metabolism of dairy foods.	Often no obvious symptoms until advanced stages. Painless swelling of abdomen; irregular bleeding; lower abdominal pain; digestive and urinary abnormalities; fatigue; backache; bloating; weight gain.	Women with family history: annual pelvic and abdominal exams; blood test for a tumor marker called CA125 every 6 months; annual pelvic ultrasound. (In cases of very high risk, some oncologists recommend prophylactic removal of ovaries no later than age 35.)	Surgery, sometimes in combination with chemotherapy or radiation.	85% if detected and treated early; 23% in advanced cases.

Cancer	Risk factors	Symptoms	Detection	Treatment	Notes
Colon and rectum cancer (est. 130,200 new cases a year; 56,300 deaths)	Personal or family history of colon and rectal cancer or polyps (growths) in the colon or rectum; inflammatory bowel disease; high-fat, low-fiber diet.	Unusual bleeding from rectum, blood in stool, a change in bowel habits.	Digital rectal exam (once a year after age 40); stool-blood slide test that detects blood in feces (every year after age 50); proctosigmoidoscopy, a rectal exam using a hollow, lighted tube (every 3–5 years after age 50, following 2 consecutive normal annual exams). Diagnosis may require a colonoscopy (viewing the entire colon) or a barium enema.	Surgery, sometimes in combination with chemotherapy or radiation.	Considered a highly curable disease when digital and proctoscopy examinations are included in routine checkups.
Skin cancer (melanoma) (est. 47,700 new cases a year; 7,700 deaths)	Excessive exposure to sun, fair complexion, occupational exposure to carcinogens. (Inherited skin disorders, such as xeroderma pigmentosum and familial atypical multiple mole melanoma, account for 10% of cases.)	Unusual skin condition, especially a change in size or color of a mole; appearance of darkly pigmented growth or spot; oozing, scaliness, bleeding; appearance of a bump; change in sensation, itchiness, tenderness, or pain.	Examine moles on your skin once a month.	Surgery, radiation, electrodesiccation (tissue destruction by heat), cryosurgery (tissue destruction by cold), or a combination of therapies.	Melanoma is readily detected by observation and diagnosed by simple biopsy.
Oral cancer (including pharynx) (est. 30,200 new cases a year; 7,800 deaths)	Heavy smoking of cigarettes, cigars, pipes; excessive drinking; use of chewing tobacco.	A sore that bleeds easily and doesn't heal; a lump or thickening; a reddish or whitish patch; difficulty chewing, swallowing, or moving the tongue or jaws.	Regular exams by your dentist or primary-care physician.	Surgery and radiation.	Many more lives should be saved because the mouth is easily accessible to visual examination by physicians and dentists.
Leukemia (est. 30,800 new cases a year; 21,700 deaths)	Down syndrome and other inherited abnormalities; excessive exposure to radiation and to certain chemicals, such as benzene.		Difficult to detect early because its symptoms are often similar to those of less serious conditions, such as flu. Diagnosis is based on blood tests and bone-marrow biopsy.	Chemotherapy, drugs, blood transfusions, and antibiotics; bone-marrow transplants.	Leukemias are cancers of blood-forming tissues and are characterized by the abnormal production of immature white blood cells. Acute leukemia strikes mainly children and is treated by drugs that have extended life from a few months to as much as 10 years. Chronic leukemia strikes usually after age 25 and progresses less rapidly.
Testicular cancer (6,900 new cases a year; 300 deaths)	Young men under age 35.		Testicular self-examinations.	Surgical removal of the diseased testis, radiation therapy, chemotherapy, removal of nearby lymph nodes.	96% if the cancer is localized; 89% overall.
Prostate cancer (est. 180,400 new cases a year; 31,900 deaths)	Risk increases with age. African-American men more susceptible than whites. Suspected risk factors: family history, high-fat diet, exposure to heavy metal cadmium, high number of sexual partners, history of frequent STDs.	Frequent urination, difficulty urinating, blood in the urine, lower back pain.	Rectal exam; PSA blood test available.	Surgical removal of prostate, conventional radiation, or implanting "seeds" of radioactive iodine in the prostate; hormone therapy.	Occurs mainly in men over 60; can be detected by digital rectal exam at annual checkup.

Adapted from the American Cancer Society, *Cancer Facts and Figures* (2000).

the basal cell type and involves deeper layers of skin, but it rarely spreads to other parts of the body.

3. **Malignant melanoma**. This rapidly growing cancer is the most dangerous skin cancer and almost always spreads to other organs. Of the 9,600 people who die from skin cancer each year, approximately 7,700 succumb to malignant melanoma. It is the number-one cancer killer of American women ages 25 to 29 and number two for women ages 30 to 34.

> Malignant melanoma is the number-one cancer killer of American women ages 25 to 29 and number two for women ages 30 to 34.

Basal and squamous cell carcinomas are detected and treated quite easily. Malignant melanoma can be treated successfully if it is diagnosed and treated early. If not treated early, **metastasis** makes treatment extremely difficult.

The risk factors for skin cancer include

- sun exposure (most dangerous are ultraviolet B rays, at their strongest between 10 A.M. and 3 P.M.)
- fair skin that burns easily and rarely tans,
- blonde and red hair,
- artificial sources of ultraviolet rays, such as tanning booths and sunlamps,
- history of one or more severe sunburns,
- a dark brown or black wart,
- birthmarks and congenital moles (although these do not always become cancerous, they should be watched closely and removed if they begin to grow or change in appearance);

PRECANCEROUS SKIN CONDITIONS

Precancerous conditions are those in which a benign, or noncancerous, condition becomes cancerous for one reason or another. Generally, physicians recommend that the following precancerous skin conditions be surgically removed or repaired to prevent their becoming cancerous, regardless of how low the risk may be:

- Benign tumors
- Chronic scaly patches on the skin
- Brown or black warts
- Moles subject to chronic irritation (such as those on the waist that are constantly rubbed by a waistband or belt)
- A lump on the lip, tongue, or inside the cheek
- A scaly patch on the inside of the cheek

SKIN TYPES

A fair-skinned person (Type 1) in the sun at noon and at an elevation of about 5,000 feet stands a good chance of beginning to burn within 10 minutes. The times are determined by multiplying the sun-protection factor (SPF) number by 10 minutes. For example, SPF 15 $\times$ 10 min = 150 min = 2 hrs 30 min. To determine how long a given SPF will protect your skin, this six-point standard scale used by dermatologists gives guidelines for your exposure limits.

Type 1—Fair skin with blue or green eyes and light blond or red hair; typical time for skin to burn: 10–20 minutes.

Type 2—Fair skin with deep blue, hazel, or brown eyes and ash blond, deep red, or light brown hair; typical burn time: 15–30 minutes.

Type 3—Medium skin with brown eyes and brown hair; typical burn time: 20–40 minutes.

Type 4—Light to medium brown skin with dark brown eyes and hair; typical burn time: 25–50 minutes.

Type 5—Light to golden brown skin with dark brown eyes and black hair; typical burn time: 30–60 minutes.

Type 6—Brown to deepest brown skin with dark brown eyes and black hair; typical burn time: 40–75 minutes.

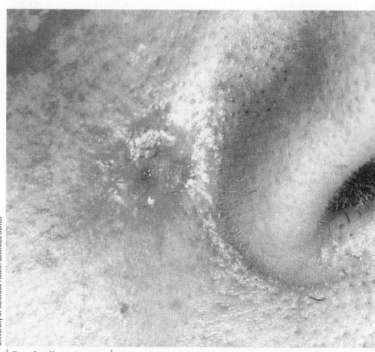

University of Colorado Health Sciences Center

Basal cell carcinoma.

- moles that are irritated chronically (moles at the waistline, bra line, or other areas where clothing rubs them constantly); and
- occupational exposure to creosote, coal tar, pitch, arsenic, or radium.

Danger signs of skin cancer are given in Figure 12.3.

FIGURE **12.3** DANGER SIGNS OF CANCER.

The American Academy of Dermatology advises: Know your spots and do a spot check. Also, have your skin checked by a doctor for any changes once a year. If you notice one of the following changes in your skin, you should see your family doctor or dermatologist immediately:

- Basal-cell or squamous-cell carcinomas: any lesion that is new, starts growing, starts changing, bleeds, is scabby, or doesn't heal.
- Melanoma:
  A. *Asymmetry:* One half of a mole or lesion doesn't look like the other half.
  B. *Border:* A mole has an irregular, scalloped, or not clearly defined border.
  C. *Color:* The color varies or is not uniform from one area of a mole or lesion to another, whether the color is tan, brown, black, white, red, or blue.
  D. *Diameter:* The lesion is larger than 6 millimeters (one-quarter inch) or larger than a pencil eraser.
- Actinic keratosis: a precancerous skin lesion that is dry, scaly, reddish, and slightly raised.

Melanoma Warnings

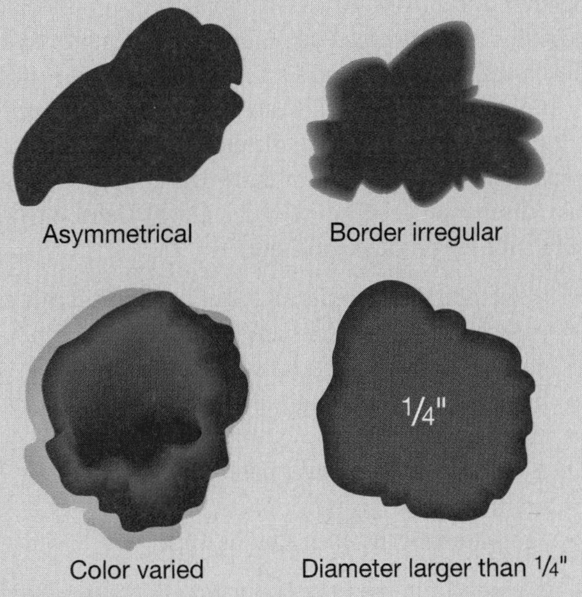

Asymmetrical

Border irregular

Color varied

Diameter larger than 1/4"

Adapted from *FDA Consumer*, May 1991.

THE UV INDEX

The Ultraviolet Index is a measure of the sun's damaging ultraviolet rays during the hottest part of the day. This chart can help you interpret the UV Index the next time you see one:

Solar-hazard Rating	Health Risk	Time to Burn*
0–2	Very low	More than 30 minutes
3–4	Low	15 to 90 minutes
5–6	Moderate	10 to 60 minutes
7–9	High	7 to 35 minutes
10 & over	Very high	5 to 30 minutes

* The "time to burn" ranges are based on the amount of time it takes for a person to sunburn and varies widely by skin type.

Lung Cancer

The leading cancer killer among both men and women, lung cancer caused an estimated 156,900 deaths in 2000. Lung cancer occurs almost exclusively among cigarette smokers. According to the U.S. Department of Health and Human Services, the cellular changes and tissue damage that lead to lung cancer have been observed in 93 percent of active smokers and 6 percent of former smokers, but in only 1 percent of those who have never smoked. Researchers estimate that close to 90 percent of all lung cancer could be eliminated if people did not smoke.[10]

Once a disease affecting men predominantly, lung cancer in women has risen along with higher smoking rates among women. Today, lung cancer is decreasing steadily in men while increasing steadily in African Americans, teenagers, and women. Lung cancer now surpasses breast cancer as the leading cause of cancer deaths in women.

Lung cancer spreads rapidly, and it is rarely detected early, because it usually does not cause symptoms or show up on an x-ray until it is quite advanced. By that time, the damage usually is too extensive to treat successfully. The 5-year survival rate of lung cancer patients is only about 14 percent.

When symptoms do arise, they might be manifested by persistent hoarseness, a nagging cough, repeated bouts

Metastasis The process that occurs when cancer cells from one growth break off, enter the bloodstream or lymph system, and are carried to a distant part of the body, where they cause another cancerous growth to begin.

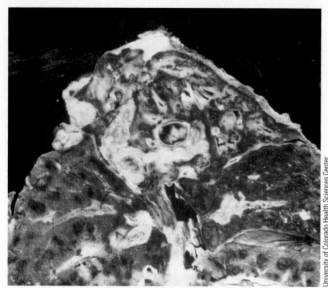

| Lung cancer is the frequent result of smoking. |

of pneumonia or bronchitis, or spitting up blood. Treatment consists of surgery for localized cancers combined with radiation treatment and chemotherapy for lung cancer that has spread.

The number-one risk factor for lung cancer is cigarette smoking. Most at risk are those who have smoked more than 20 years. Secondhand smoke inhaled by nonsmokers who live or work with smokers also increases the risk of lung cancer significantly. The Centers for Disease Control and Prevention estimate that 3,000 nonsmokers die each year from lung cancer caused by secondhand tobacco smoke. Other risk factors for lung cancer include

- exposure to asbestos,
- high-level air pollution,
- exposure to carcinogenic chemicals,
- exposure to certain metals (cadmium, cobalt, chromium, silver, nickel, steel),
- exposure to arsenic or radioactive ores, and
- exposure to radon gas.

All other risk factors for lung cancer are much more marked if the individual also smokes.

| Colon and Rectal Cancer |

Cancer of the colon and rectum—also called colorectal cancer—is the third leading cancer killer in the United States among both men and women. About 132,000 new cases are diagnosed each year, and almost 56,000 Americans die of colorectal cancer annually. If detected early, colorectal cancer usually can be treated successfully because it grows and spreads quite slowly. Treatment usually consists of radiation or surgery.

Changes in bowel habits and bleeding from the rectum not attributable to hemorrhoids are the most common signs of colorectal cancer. Bright red blood in the stools that is not attributable to hemorrhoids is another sign. Risk factors include

- a personal or family history of polyps (benign growths) in the colon or rectum,
- a family history of colorectal cancer,
- a diet high in fats and low in fiber, and
- inflammatory bowel problems, such as colitis.

Age also is considered a risk factor. The risk for colorectal cancer increases sharply after age 40. Researchers believe that at least half, and possibly all, cases of colorectal cancer can be attributed to a genetic tendency for polyps in the colon or rectum combined with a high-fat, low-fiber diet.

The American Cancer Society recommends a colon exam called a flexible sigmoidoscopy every 5 years for men and women beginning at age 50. The test should be started at age 40 for those with a family history of colorectal cancer or ulcerative colitis.

| Breast Cancer |

The second leading killer of women, breast cancer kills almost 41,000 American women and 400 men each year. Approximately 183,000 women in the United States were diagnosed with breast cancer in the year 2000. American Cancer Society estimates are that 1 in 8 American women will develop breast cancer at some time in her life.

Early detection is the key. With early detection and treatment, the 5-year survival rate for breast cancer can be over 90 percent. Heightened awareness of the disease together with breast self-examination and regular mammograms beginning at a younger age have improved survival rates, because cancers are being diagnosed earlier.

General symptoms of breast cancer include a thickening or lump in the breast; distortion or dimpling of a breast; swollen lymph nodes under the arm; or retraction, pain, discharge, or scaliness of the nipple. General risk factors for breast cancer include

- a grandmother, mother, or sister with breast cancer,
- early onset of menstruation (before age 12),
- delayed onset of menopause (after age 55),
- first pregnancy after age 30,
- obesity,
- a woman who has never been pregnant,
- a woman who has never breastfed, and
- age (dramatic increase after age 50).

A report from the Utah Population Database suggests that 17 to 19 percent of breast cancer cases may be attributable to a family history of the disease. Also, women with a first-degree relative with colon cancer had a 30 percent increase in risk for breast cancer. A family history of breast cancer, however, does not necessarily affect the prognosis or outcome adversely.

Hormone replacement therapy (HRT), usually for post-menopausal women, may be associated with a higher risk, although the available data are difficult to interpret. Some researchers believe the progestin component of HRT may have a greater impact on risk than the estrogen component. The studies of oral contraceptives, which contain the same hormones, show no significant increase in risk. Because of the remaining uncertainty, though, some gynecologists advise against long-term use of oral contraceptives in young women who have not borne children.

Despite earlier findings that a high-fat diet raises the risk, more recent studies have found little support for a role of dietary fat in the onset of breast cancer. Evidence is mounting that daily alcohol consumption does increase the risk, however. Daily consumption of vitamin A—as little as one carrot or less—may reduce the risk.

Exercise also may reduce the risk of breast cancer. Some researchers think exercise may change the proportions of estrogen and progesterone produced during the menstrual cycle, which may affect the risk.

Other studies reveal interesting findings, but these have not been confirmed yet. According to one of these, the longer a woman breastfeeds and the more babies she nurses, the less is her risk for breast cancer.[11] Diethylstilbestrol (DES) taken during pregnancy increases a woman's risk for breast cancer later in life, but this risk probably is small and does not increase with time. Environmental factors—specifically, pesticide residues in food—also have been implicated, but this is difficult to study systematically.

> The American Cancer Society estimates that only 5 to 10 percent of breast cancer is inherited.

Many factors probably contribute to a woman's risk of developing breast cancer, but the known risk factors account for only a small percentage of breast cancer cases. The majority of patients (60 to 70 percent) have no known risk factors for the disease except older age. Thus, age is the most influential known risk factor.

| Cervical Cancer |

More than half of all uterine cancers start in the cervix, the neck of the uterus that protrudes into the top end of the vagina. The death rate from cancer of the cervix has decreased more than 70 percent during the past four decades because of early detection, mainly in the form of Pap smears (especially among younger women) and regular gynecological examinations.

Today, approximately 13,000 women are diagnosed with invasive cervical cancer each year in the United States. With early diagnosis, treatment is usually successful because the cancer has not spread. Unusual vaginal bleeding or discharge is often an early symptom. Risk factors for cervical cancer can be

- early age at first intercourse,
- multiple sex partners,
- a history of viral genital infections, especially herpes and the human papilloma virus, and
- cigarette smoking.

| Uterine Cancer |

Uterine cancer, which involves the endometrium, or lining, of the uterus, strikes approximately 36,000 women in the United States each year. Because of improved early detection, the death rate from uterine cancer has fallen dramatically. Only about 6,500 deaths a year in this country are attributed to uterine cancer. With early detection, treatment generally is successful. Symptoms of uterine cancer might be unusual vaginal discharge, unusual vaginal bleeding, or bleeding between menstrual periods. Risk factors for uterine cancer include

- late onset of menopause,
- history of infertility/failure to ovulate,
- prolonged estrogen replacement therapy,
- obesity, and
- diabetes.

| Ovarian Cancer |

Although ovarian cancer claims a relatively few 14,000 American women each year, it is a particularly difficult cancer because it typically reveals no symptoms until in its latest stages, and it can be difficult to diagnose. The survival rate 5 years after diagnosis averages 40 percent. Late symptoms include abdominal swelling or bloating (the most common sign), persistent abdominal gas, and unexplained stomachaches or indigestion.

Age is a factor. The risk increases with age and is highest for women in their 60s. For unknown reasons, the rates are higher in Jewish women. This form of cancer also strikes Americans, Scandinavians, and Scots at three times the rate of occurrence in Japanese women.

Other risk factors include

- a grandmother, mother, or sister with ovarian cancer,
- never had children (doubles the risk),

- use of oral contraceptives,
- occurrence of colorectal, breast, or uterine cancer (doubles the risk), and
- early onset of ovulation.
- A diet high in fat may be a risk factor for ovarian cancer, though more research is needed.

Prostate Cancer

The leading cancer in American men and the second leading cause of cancer death in men (after lung cancer), prostate cancer strikes more than 180,000 men in the United States every year. About 32,000 die from it.

Prostate cancer often is detected early because it generally provokes an array of symptoms fairly early in its development. The symptoms, however, can be mistaken for signs of other, more common ailments, such as an enlarged prostate or bladder infection. If detected early, prostate cancer can be treated successfully about 84 percent of the time. A blood test that measures the amount of prostate-specific antigen (PSA) in the blood can be used to help diagnose prostate cancer. The test is recommended for men beginning at age 50.

Signs and symptoms of prostate cancer include pain in the pelvis, lower back, or upper thighs; blood in the urine or semen; pain or burning during urination; frequent urination; and weak or interrupted urine, difficulty starting or stopping the flow of urine, or inability to urinate.

The risk of prostate cancer increases with age. For that reason, the American Cancer Society recommends an annual prostate exam beginning at age 50. At highest risk are men over age 65, in whom more than 80 percent of all prostate cancers are diagnosed. Another substantial risk factor is race: African-American men have the highest rate of prostate cancer in the world (30 percent higher than for whites). Oddly enough, the cancer is relatively rare in Africa and is much more common in North America and northwest Europe than it is in Central and South America or the Near East.

Other risk factors include

- a family history of prostate cancer,
- occupational exposure to cadmium, and
- a high-fat diet.

Testicular Cancer

Although testicular cancer is not one of the most common types of cancer in the United States, it is the most common cancer in young men between ages 17 and 34. Of all cancer deaths in that age group, 12 percent are from testicular cancer. For unknown reasons, the incidence of testicular cancer in this age group has been increasing

steadily. If this cancer is found in its early stages, the chances for cure are nearly 100 percent.

Early detection is the key to successful treatment. Many men discover the cancer themselves through self-examination. The major warning sign is an often-painless thickening or hard lump in the testicle. Other signs include pain or a sensation of heaviness in the affected testicle, an accumulation of fluid or blood in the scrotum, and a dull ache in the groin that may involve the lower abdomen. Although the exact cause of testicular cancer is not known, identified risk factors for testicular cancer include

- an undescended testicle (risk can be 40 times as high),
- a testicle that did not descend until after age 6 (risk can be 40 times as high), and
- a grandfather, father, or brother with testicular cancer.

Bladder Cancer

Approximately 53,000 new cases of bladder cancer are diagnosed each year in the United States, and more than 12,000 Americans die from it each year. If the cancer is detected while it is still confined to the bladder—before it has metastasized to involve other organs—almost 9 in 10 can be cured. A new test called "flow cytometry" currently is being evaluated as an early detection tool for bladder cancer.

The most common signs of bladder cancer are more frequent urination and blood in the urine. The cancer is four times more common in men than in women. Other risk factors include

- cigarette smoking (smoking is believed to cause almost half the bladder cancers in men and approximately 40 percent of the bladder cancers in women),
- occupational exposure to leather and rubber,
- occupational exposure to dyes, and
- living in an urban area.

Pancreatic Cancer

Although pancreatic cancer is not one of the most common cancers, its incidence has more than doubled in the past two decades, making it the fourth most common cancer killer in American men and the fifth most common cancer killer among American women.

About 28,300 new cases are diagnosed in the United States each year, and 28,200 Americans die each year of pancreatic cancer. The survival rate from pancreatic cancer is low because the disease spreads rapidly. Few patients with pancreatic cancer survive more than 3 years. In addition, pancreatic cancer is a "silent" disease, usually progressing without symptoms until extremely advanced stages.

The risk for pancreatic cancer increases with age. The highest risk is between ages 65 and 79. More men die of pancreatic cancer each year, but women are diagnosed in higher numbers. African Americans are at higher risk than people of other races. Other risk factors include

- smoking cigarettes,
- consuming alcohol,
- eating a high-fat diet, and
- being exposed to gasoline or some chemical cleaners on the job.

| Oral Cancer |

Oral cancer has increased substantially over the past two decades, which correlates with the popularity of smokeless tobacco, or chewing tobacco. Twice as many men as women get oral cancer. More than 30,000 Americans are diagnosed with oral cancer each year, and approximately 8,500 die.

Oral cancer can develop anywhere in the oral cavity. Most often it develops on the lining of the cheeks, the lips, the gums, and the floor of the mouth. Signs of oral cancer generally include a sore that fails to heal or that bleeds easily; a whitish patch that does not go away (called leukoplakia); a lump or thickening in the cheek, tongue, or lips; and difficulty chewing or swallowing.

The most common risk factor is the use of smokeless tobacco (chewing tobacco). Other risk factors are smoking cigarettes, cigars, or a pipe, and excessive alcohol consumption.

| Leukemia |

Leukemia, a cancer of the blood-forming tissues (such as the spleen and the bone marrow), can strike people of all ages. Though most people believe it is more common among children, it actually strikes 12 times more adults than children. Approximately 30,800 people (2,600 of them children) are diagnosed with leukemia each year in the United States. With advances in treatment, survival rates have improved dramatically over the past three decades.

Leukemia can be chronic or acute, and it has a number of varieties. Two of the known risk factors for leukemia are excessive exposure to radiation and exposure to benzenes and other hydrocarbons.

Many forms of leukemia develop slowly and cause few, if any, symptoms. As the immature white blood cells progressively crowd out the red blood cells, normal white blood cells, and platelets, symptoms begin to develop. Leukemia often is misdiagnosed in adults because the most common initial symptom is fatigue, which is a symptom of a number of conditions. Leukemia usually is diagnosed much more quickly in children because additional symptoms—such as weight loss, paleness, frequent nosebleeds, easy bruising, and repeated infections—tend to develop suddenly and rapidly in children.

GUIDELINES FOR PREVENTING CANCER

As much as 85 percent of all cancer is related to lifestyle and environmental factors over which we have control. Table 12.3 summarizes major preventive measures. By changing your lifestyle and taking control over your environment, you have a pretty good chance to avoid cancer. Your general risk for cancer can be cut dramatically if you do the following:

- avoid substances known to cause cancer, such as tobacco and overuse of alcohol,
- avoid overexposure to sunlight,
- avoid overeating and eat an anti-cancer diet,
- do appropriate self-examinations, and
- get regular checkups to boost your chances of early detection.

> As much as 85 percent of all cancer is related to lifestyle and environmental factors over which we have control.

| Smoking Cessation |

According to former U.S. Surgeon General C. Everett Koop, the single best thing you can do to lower your risk for cancer is to stop smoking. Smoking causes 87 percent of all lung cancers and 3 of 10 cancers overall. If you don't smoke, don't start. If you're smoking now, stop. That holds true for any tobacco in any form, not just cigarette smoking.

Your lungs will start to heal as soon as you stop smoking. Your risk will be slightly higher than if you never smoked, but eventually the risk can be the same as nonsmokers. A smoking cessation program is presented in Chapter 13.

Even if you don't smoke, you should limit the amount of cigarette smoke you are exposed to.

TABLE 12.3 PREVENTING CANCER

Stop smoking	Cigarette smoking is responsible for 85% of lung cancer cases among men and 75% among women—about 83% overall. Smoking accounts for about 30% of all cancer deaths. Those who smoke two or more packs of cigarettes a day have lung cancer mortality rates 15 to 25 times greater than nonsmokers.
Limit sunlight exposure	Almost all of the more than 600,000 cases of nonmelanoma skin cancer diagnosed each year in the United States are considered to be sun-related. Sun exposure is a major factor in the development of melanoma, and the incidence increases for those living near the equator and at high altitudes.
Limit alcohol intake	Oral cancer and cancers of the larynx, throat, esophagus, and liver occur more frequently among heavy drinkers of alcohol.
Avoid smokeless tobacco	Use of chewing tobacco or snuff increases risk of cancer of the mouth, larynx, throat, and esophagus and is highly habit-forming.
Monitor estrogen intake	For mature women, estrogen treatment to control menopausal symptoms increases risk of endometrial cancer. Estrogen use by menopausal women calls for careful discussion between the woman and her physician.
Monitor radiation exposure	Excessive exposure to ionizing radiation can increase cancer risk. Most medical and dental x-rays are adjusted to deliver the lowest dose possible without sacrificing image quality. Excessive radon exposure in homes may increase risk of lung cancer, especially in cigarette smokers. If levels are found to be too high, remedial actions should be taken.
Avoid occupational hazards	Exposure to several different industrial agents (nickel, chromate, asbestos, vinyl chloride, etc.) increases risk of various cancers. Risk from asbestos is greatly increased when combined with cigarette smoking.
Improve nutrition	Risk for colon, breast, and uterine cancers increases in obese people. High-fat diets may contribute to the development of cancers of the colon and prostate. High-fiber foods may help reduce risk of colon cancer. A varied diet containing plenty of vegetables and fruits rich in vitamins A and C may reduce risk for a wide range of cancers. Salt-cured, smoked, and nitrite-cured foods have been linked to esophageal and stomach cancer. Heavy use of alcohol, especially when accompanied by cigarette smoking or chewing tobacco, increases risk of cancers of the mouth, larynx, throat, esophagus, and liver.
Increase physical activity	Accumulate at least 30 minutes of moderate intensity physical activity on most days of the week.
Monitor body weight	Stay within your recommended (healthy) body weight range.

Adapted from the American Cancer Society.

Nonsmokers who are forced to breathe the cigarette smoke of others run an increased risk of developing cancer.

| Limit Sun Exposure |

The major cause of skin cancer is too much sun, so if you want to lower your risk for developing skin cancer, limit your exposure to the sun. Sunscreens protect against the ultraviolet rays of the sun. The sun protection factor (SPF) tells you the protection you're getting. An SPF of 10, for example, lets you stay in the sun 10 times as long as you normally would without burning. If your skin normally starts to redden after 20 minutes, a sunscreen with an SPF of 10 lets you stay in the sun 200 minutes before you start to burn. After that time, you'll begin to burn. You can't simply apply more and expect longer protection.

Always use a sunscreen if you're going outside for longer than 15 minutes, even if you think you won't be getting that much sun exposure. Choose a sunscreen that provides adequate protection for your skin type. Choose a broad-spectrum sunscreen that protects against both UVA and UVB radiation. Apply it at least 30–45 minutes before exposure to the sun. Apply the sunscreen frequently if you're in and out of the water (look for a waterproof or water-resistant sunscreen). Apply the screen heavily to areas where your skin is thin, such as your nose, face, neck, and hands. Use sunscreen even on cloudy days (clouds don't block the ultraviolet rays) and during the winter when you're outside. Sunscreen is increasingly important the closer you are to the equator and the higher the altitude where you live or visit: Both situations afford less atmospheric protection from UV rays.

To further cut your risk for overexposure to the sun, do the following:

- Even when using a sunscreen, avoid being in the sun between 10 A.M. and 3 P.M., when UV rays are at their most intense. If your shadow is shorter than your

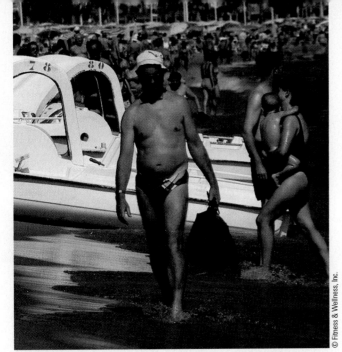

| Sunburns pose a risk for skin cancer from overexposure to ultraviolet rays of the sun. |

height, the sun is strong enough to quickly burn your skin. You can burn even if you're sitting in the shade. Plan outdoor activities during the early morning or early evening hours, when sun is less intense and temperatures are cooler.

- Even if you are using a sunscreen, avoid long sun exposure whenever possible.
- If you have to stay outside for long periods, wear protective clothing—long pants, a long-sleeved shirt, a hat with a brim or visor. Wear tightly woven cottons and avoid white or thin fabrics. Don't sit in the sun in wet clothing.
- Don't assume that because your skin isn't red, it isn't getting burned. A sunburn becomes most evident 6 to 24 hours after being in the sun.
- Avoid surfaces that reflect the sun's rays more intensely: concrete, snow, expanses of metal, expanses of sand.
- Stay out of the sun or take extra precautions if you are taking antibiotics (especially penicillin or tetracycline), birth control pills, insulin (especially oral insulin), diuretics, and some medications used to lower blood pressure. They increase the damage from ultraviolet rays.
- Don't drink alcohol if you will be exposed to sunlight. Alcohol, too, increases the damage from ultraviolet rays.
- Don't patronize tanning salons or booths and don't use a sunlamp. Tanned skin is damaged skin. There is no such thing as a "safe" tan.

Most important, do whatever you can to avoid a sunburn. The risk of skin cancer from exposure to

sunlight is cumulative. Each time you are unprotected and exposed to sunlight, some amount of damage accrues. With increasing damage, you also increase your risk of developing skin cancer. Sunburns are especially dangerous. Experts say that even one bad sunburn during childhood can double your risk for getting skin cancer later on.

Anti-Cancer Diet

The first specific recommendations relating to an "anti-cancer diet" were published 20 years ago, when the National Academy of Sciences issued a report stating that certain changes in diet could reduce the risk of cancer. Since then, the National Institutes of Health, the U.S. Surgeon General, the U.S. Department of Agriculture, and the U.S. Department of Health and Human Services have joined the National Academy of Sciences in continuing research on the link between diet and cancer. They conclude that at least 35 percent of cancer deaths are caused by what people eat.

Food affects the risk of cancer in at least three ways:

1. Some foods protect against cancer. These foods contain chemicals (phytochemicals) and other compounds that actually can stop or reverse steps in the development of cancer. These chemicals also boost the body's natural defenses against various carcinogens.
2. Some foods (such as smoked foods) contain carcinogens. Others contain chemicals (such as nitrite) that are converted into carcinogens during the digestive process.

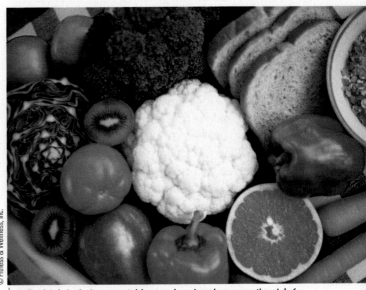

| A diet high in fruits, vegetables, and grains decreases the risk for cancer. |

3. Eaten regularly for long periods, certain foods, especially those high in fat, provide an environment in which cancer cells can grow more readily.

Based on research by the U.S. Surgeon General and a variety of scientific agencies, the American Institute for Cancer Research has issued a four-part dietary guideline to reduce the risk of cancer:

1. Reduce total dietary fat to no more than 30 percent of total calories. In particular, reduce saturated fat (fat that is solid at room temperature) to less than 10 percent of total calories.
2. Eat more fruits, vegetables, and whole grains.
3. Eat salt-cured, salt-pickled, and smoked foods rarely.
4. Drink alcoholic beverages in moderation or not at all.

The American Cancer Society and the National Academy of Science have jointly released the following detailed dietary guidelines for reducing cancer risk:

- Maintain a normal weight. A 12-year study involving almost a million Americans showed that those who were overweight—especially those who were 40 percent or more overweight—ran substantially higher risks for cancer. According to the study, those who are obese run a one-and-a-half times greater risk for cancer of the breast and colon, two times higher risk for cancer of the prostate, three times greater risk for cancer of the gallbladder, and five times greater risk for uterine cancer. The American Cancer Society recommends limiting calories and increasing exercise to maintain recommended weight.
- Reduce the amount of fat you eat. Major sources of fat in the American diet are visible fats (the fats we add to foods, such as butter, mayonnaise, and salad dressings) and the less visible fats that are found in eggs, dairy foods, meats, and baked goods. Cut down on foods high in fats, such as red meats, whole milk and whole milk products, cheeses, butter, pastries, candies, and oils. Trim all visible fat from your meat before cooking it, and remove skin and fat from chicken before cooking. Instead of frying foods, use low-fat methods of cooking such as broiling, steaming, baking. Use less cooking oil than a recipe calls for. Skim all visible fats from soups, stews, and gravies; if you can, refrigerate them overnight, then remove the hardened fat that rises to the surface. Cut back on the use of cream, butter, margarine, shortening, mayonnaise, and salad dressing. Substitute foods naturally low in fat, such as whole grains, legumes, fruits, and vegetables.
- Eat a wide variety of more high-fiber foods, such as whole grain cereals, whole grain breads, bran cereals, legumes (including kidney beans), lima beans, pinto beans, rice, popcorn, and brown rice. Leave well-scrubbed skins on fruits and vegetables. Eat foods with visible hulls, seeds, and textured skins, such as strawberries, raspberries, and peaches.

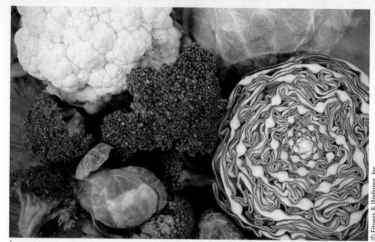

Cruciferous vegetables are recommended in a cancer-prevention diet.

- Eat food rich in vitamins A and C every day. Good sources of vitamin A are fresh foods that are dark green or deep yellow in color: spinach, broccoli, carrots, sweet potatoes, squash, apricots, and peaches. Good sources of vitamin C are citrus fruits (such as oranges, grapefruit, and tangerines), strawberries, cantaloupes, tomatoes, and green peppers. Many of these foods also are rich in beta-carotene.
- Eat cruciferous vegetables such as cabbage, broccoli, cauliflower, Brussels sprouts, and kohlrabi.
- Cut down on salt-cured, smoked, and nitrite-cured foods. Nitrites in salt-cured and salt-pickled foods become carcinogenic during the digestive process. Limit the amount of bacon, ham, hot dogs, beef jerky, smoked fish, smoked meats, and salt-cured fish you eat. If you barbecue often, cook food at lower temperatures or a greater distance from the flame so food doesn't get charred.
- If you drink, use alcohol in strict moderation. Alcohol significantly increases your risk for a number of cancers, especially if you also smoke cigarettes. Besides the harmful effects of the alcohol itself, alcohol can interfere with eating a healthy, balanced diet.

In addition to these guidelines, the following dietary suggestions can further reduce your risk of cancer:

- Get plenty of calcium. It seems to help neutralize carcinogenic substances in the digestive tract. Early studies indicate calcium may help prevent colon cancer. Low-fat milk and nonfat milk and dairy products are good sources, as are dark-green vegetables, and foods that have been fortified with calcium.

© Fitness & Wellness, Inc.

- Avoid foods that have been treated heavily with chemicals or pesticides or processed with large amounts of additives. Wash fruits and vegetables well before you eat them.
- Refrigerate foods that need it, especially fruits and vegetables. Fruits and vegetables naturally produce nitrites, a process that refrigeration slows down.

Table 12.4 summarizes the dietary measures that may lower your risk for cancer. The key seems to be variety and moderation.

TABLE 12.4 ANTI-CANCER DIETARY MEASURES

Substance	Associated Cancers	Comments	Steps to Take
Fiber	May *decrease* risk of colorectal cancer.	Different types of fiber may affect cancer risk differently. Benefits also may be due to lower fat intakes usually associated with high-fiber diets.	Eat 4 to 5 servings a day of a variety of vegetables, fruits, whole-grain cereals, and legumes. Maximize fiber in vegetables and fruits by eating them unpeeled.
Fruits and vegetables	May *decrease* risk of colorectal and breast cancers.	Eat good sources of fiber (see above). Cruciferous vegetables, such as broccoli, cabbage, and Brussels sprouts, also contain indoles—nitrogen compounds that, in some studies, have knocked out carcinogens that can lead to breast cancer.	To maximize indole intake, eat vegetables raw, steamed, or microwaved; boiling leaches up to half the indoles.
Fat	May *increase* risk of breast, colon, and prostate cancers.	Lowering fat intake will almost automatically lower caloric intake and boost fiber intake—steps that will also lower cancer risk.	Decrease calories from fat to 25% to 30% of total daily calories. (Current average intake is 40% of total calories.)
Alcohol	Heavy use *increases* risk of cancers of the oral cavity, larynx, and esophagus; moderate use may *increase* breast cancer risk.	Cigarette smoking in conjunction with alcohol drinking greatly increases cancer risk. Alcohol use also can cause liver cirrhosis, which may lead to liver cancer.	Drink only occasionally and sparingly.
Salt-cured, smoked, barbecued, and nitrite-preserved foods	May *increase* risk of stomach, esophageal, and lung cancers.	Smoking and charcoal-grilling foods produces tars that are similar to those in cigarette smoke and are absorbed by the food. Manufacturers have substantially decreased nitrites used in meat preservation.	Opt for other cooking methods; limit intake of salt-cured and nitrite-preserved foods.
Beta-carotene and antioxidant vitamins (A, C, and E)	Inconclusive	Vitamin E and beta-carotene have been associated with lower rates of cancer in humans; a lesser effect has been noted with the other antioxidant nutrients. More research is needed.	Eat a balanced and varied diet to ensure that you get the RDA for all vitamins; do not take megadose vitamin supplements.
Selenium	Inconclusive	Limited evidence shows this trace element may protect against breast and colon cancers; however, it is highly toxic in high doses.	Taking selenium supplements can be dangerous; you get all the selenium you need from a varied diet.
Artificial sweeteners	Inconclusive	High levels of saccharin cause bladder cancer in rats, but no evidence of this in humans. Long-term effects of aspartame are unknown.	Moderate use poses no risk.
Coffee and caffeine	None	Both coffee and caffeine have received a clean bill of health.	Moderate use of coffee and caffeine does not appear to be a risk.
Food additives	None	Chemical additives found to be carcinogenic in animals have been banned; insufficient evidence that additives currently in use have any cancer risk or benefit.	None

Reprinted with permission of the *Johns Hopkins Medical Letter Health After 50*, © MedLetter Associates, 1992.

APPROPRIATE SELF-EXAMS

One of the keys to successful cancer treatment is early detection. You should examine yourself regularly for skin and breast or testicular cancer.

Skin Self-Exams

One of the easiest and quickest self-exams is a brief survey to detect possible skin cancers (see Figure 12.4). A simple skin self-exam can reduce deaths from melanoma by as much as 63 percent, saving as many as 4,500 lives in the United States each year.

- Make a drawing of yourself. Include a full front view, a full back view, and close-up views of your head (both sides), the soles of your feet, the tops of your feet, and the backs of your hands.
- After you get out of the bath or shower, examine yourself closely in a full-length mirror. On your sketch make note of any moles, warts, or other skin marks you find anywhere on your body. Pay particular attention to areas that are exposed to the sun constantly, such as your face, the tops of your ears, and your hands.
- Briefly describe each mark on your sketch: its size, color, texture, and so on.
- Repeat the exam about once a month. Watch for changes in the size, texture, or color of moles, wart, or other skin mark. If you notice any difference, contact your physician. You also should contact a doctor if you have a sore that does not heal.

Breast Self-Exams

Early detection of breast cancer is vital to successful treatment, and a woman who performs regular monthly self-exams has a much better chance of detecting changes that could indicate problems. When you're doing self-exams regularly, you can detect a growth when it's about the size of a pea; a physician doing a breast exam probably won't detect it until it's two to three times that size.

Perform the exam on both breasts regularly, once a month. A week after your menstrual period is the best time, as your breasts won't be subject to the swelling that sometimes precedes menstruation, and it will be a regular reminder. If you don't have periods, pick a day you can remember easily (such as the first day of the month). See Figure 12.5.

The key to breast self-examination is to do the exam regularly. Cancer is detected soonest when you notice a change from one month to the next. Immediately report to your doctor any changes or anything unusual. And don't forgo your yearly medical exam.

FIGURE 12.4 SELF-EXAM FOR SKIN CANCER.

1 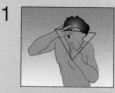 Examine your face, especially the nose, lips, mouth, and ears—front and back. Use one or both mirrors to get a clear view.

2 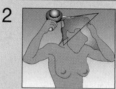 Thoroughly inspect your scalp, using a blow dryer and mirror to expose each section to view. Get a friend or family member to help, if you can.

3 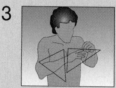 Check your hands carefully: palms and backs, between the fingers, and under the fingernails. Continue up the wrists to examine both front and back of your forearms.

4 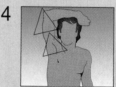 Standing in front of a full-length mirror, begin at the elbows and scan all sides of your upper arms. Don't forget the underarms.

5 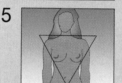 Next focus on the neck, chest, and torso. Women should lift breasts to view the underside.

6 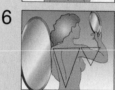 With your back to the full-length mirror, use the hand mirror to inspect the back of your neck, shoulders, upper back, and any part of the back of your upper arms you could not view in step 4.

7 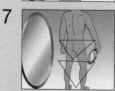 Still using both mirrors, scan your lower back, buttocks, and backs of both legs.

8 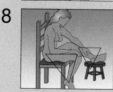 Sit down; prop each leg in turn on another stool or chair. Use the hand mirror to examine the genitals. Check front and sides of both legs, thigh to shin; ankles, tops of feet, between toes, and under toenails. Examine soles of feet and heels.

Reprinted with permission from *Family Practice Recertification*, 14, no. 3, (March, 1992).

FIGURE **12**.5 BREAST SELF-EXAM.

1 Raising one arm at a time over your head, use the fingertips of the opposite hand to check for any changes, lumps, or thickening.

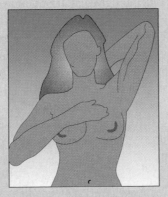

2 Start near the nipple and work outward in widening circles.

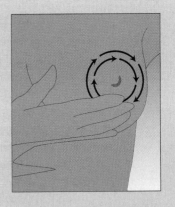

3 Visually examine your breasts in a mirror with your arms at your sides.

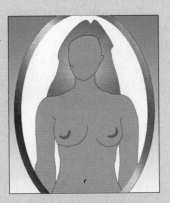

4 Visually examine your breasts in a mirror with your arms raised above your head.

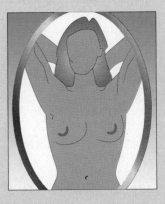

5 Check your nipples by squeezing them gently. Unless you have recently had a baby, any discharge is abnormal.

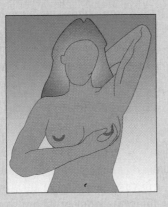

6 Place a pillow under your shoulder and your arm under your head. With your other hand, feel your breast and armpit for lumps, thickening, or other changes.

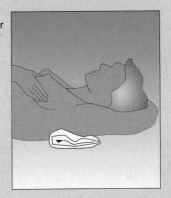

Adapted from *Family Practice Recertification* 14(3), March 1992. Used by permission.

| Testicular Self-Exam |

Testicular cancer detected early can be treated successfully a good deal of the time. The key to early detection is a simple, 3-minute self-exam done once a month. Choose a particular day each month that is easy to remember (such as the first of the month) and do the exam as soon as you get out of a warm bath or shower, because your testicles and scrotal skin are most relaxed then. You need to examine both testicles one at a time as demonstrated in Figure 12.6.

- Using both hands, roll the testicle gently between your thumbs and fingers. You'll feel a rope-like structure toward the back of the testicle. That's the epididymis, and it's normal. Most cancers occur toward the front of the testicle, and they will feel like a pea-sized lump or hard knot.
- Repeat the exam on the other testicle.
- Immediately report to your doctor any nodules or lumps.

FIGURE **12.6** TESTICULAR SELF-EXAM.

Checking yourself for testicular cancer

Cancer of the testicle is a disease that usually strikes men between ages 15 and 34, although it can start at any age. All men are at risk, but if you have a testicle that did not come down into the scrotum normally or if you have a brother or father with the disease, your risk is higher. Fortunately, this is among the most curable of cancers—if it is caught early. Many doctors recommend that all men examine their testicles on a regular basis.

How do I do the examination?

- Set aside a few minutes to do the examination while you're in the shower.
- Roll each testicle between your thumb and fingers several times (see the illustration).

What should I feel?

- A normal testicle is most often compared to a hard-boiled egg. It should be egg-shaped and have a smooth surface.
- In back of each testicle lies the epididymis. This is a small cord that has the same shape as a small candy cane or comma.

What is abnormal?

Promptly make an appointment with your doctor if you have any of the following:

- A usually painless lump on one testicle
- Swelling in a testicle
- A persistent ache or dragging feeling in the groin.

What if it's cancer?

No man wants to face the possibility of testicular cancer. Remember, not all lumps in scrotum are cancerous—but only your doctor can help you find out. Other possibilities include infections and cysts.

If it turns out that you do have testicular cancer, you should know that it is highly curable. Most men are cured even if the cancer has started to spread. In addition, most men who want to have children now are able to do so after treatment.

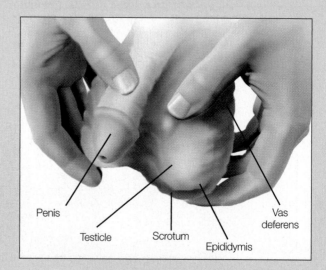

Penis
Testicle
Scrotum
Epididymis
Vas deferens

Reprinted with permission from *Patient Care* (May 30, 2000), Medical Economics, and Tim Phelps.

| Age-Appropriate Checkups |

In addition to self-exams you do at home, your physician can do examinations and tests to enable early detection of cancer. The exams in Table 12.5 are the final weapon in your arsenal against cancer.

If you are at high risk for a certain cancer, you should have screening tests more often. Check with your physician. Sexually active women should have annual Pap smears and pelvic exams as soon as sexual activity begins. Women also should have a mammography. Recent findings indicate that mammograms should begin while a woman is in her 40s—not in her 50s, as has been recommended routinely by federal agencies since 1993. One of the advantages of earlier mammograms is that almost half the breast cancers in women under age 50 are noninvasive forms that are virtually 100 percent curable if detected early. Left undetected and untreated, these cancers progress into invasive cancers that are more difficult to cure.

To get the best reading from your mammogram, make sure the x-ray technician is certified by the American Registry of Radiological Technologists or a state licensing board; that the technician has mammogram training; and that the facility is accredited by the American College of Radiology (ACR).

In addition to monthly breast self-exams, the ACS recommends a breast exam by a physician every 3 years for women ages 20 to 40 and annual exams by a physician every year beginning at age 40.

TABLE 12.5 RECOMMENDED MEDICAL CHECKUPS

Site	Recommendation
Cancer-related Checkup	A cancer-related checkup is recommended every 3 years for people aged 20–40 and every year for people age 40 and older. This exam should include health counseling and depending on a person's age, might include examinations for cancers of the thyroid, oral cavity, skin, lymph nodes, testes, and ovaries, as well as for some nonmalignant diseases.
Breast	Women 40 and older should have an annual mammogram, an annual clinical breast examination (CBE) by a health-care professional, and should perform monthly breast self-examination (BSE). The CBE should be conducted close to and preferably before the scheduled mammogram.
	Women aged 20–39 should have a clinical breast examination by a health-care professional every three years and should perform monthly BSE.
Colon & Rectum	Beginning at age 50, men and women at average risk should follow one of the examination schedules below: • Fecal occult blood test (FOBT) every year, or • Flexible sigmoidoscopy every five years,* or • FOBT every year and flexible sigmoidoscopy every 5 years,* or • Double-contrast barium enema every 5 years,* or • Colonoscopy every 10 years.* } Of these 3 options, the American Cancer Society prefers the third option, annual FOBT and flexible sigmoidoscopy every 5 years. * A digital rectal exam should be done at the same time as sigmoidoscopy, colonoscopy, or double-contrast barium enema. People who are at increased or high risk for colorectal cancer should talk with a doctor about a different testing schedule.
Prostate	Beginning at age 50, the prostate-specific antigen (PSA) test and the digital rectal exam should be offered annually to men who have a life expectancy of at least 10 years. Men at high risk (African-American men and men who have a first-degree relative who was diagnosed with prostate cancer at a young age) should begin testing at age 45. Patients should be given information about the benefits and limitations of tests so they can make an informed decision.
Uterus	Cervix: All women who are or have been sexually active or who are 18 and older should have an annual Pap test and pelvic examination. After three or more consecutive satisfactory examinations with normal findings, the Pap test may be performed less frequently. Discuss the matter with your physician.
	Endometrium: Beginning at age 35, women with or at risk for hereditary non-polyposis colon cancer should be offered endometrial biopsy annually to screen for endometrial cancer.

Cancer Facts and Figures. © 2001, American Cancer Society, Inc. Used by permission.

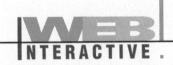

WEB ACTIVITIES

■ **American Cancer Society** This site features current topics, research, statistics and information concerning prevention and early detection. It offers links to community American Cancer Society organizations, a calendar of local events and an extensive resources section.
http://www.cancer.org

■ **National Cancer Institute** This comprehensive site features information on different types of cancers,

treatments, clinical trials, statistics, publications, and health risk factors.
http://www.nci.nih.gov

■ **Types of Cancers** This site is a searchable database of all major types of cancers, sponsored by the National Cancer Institute. Information concerning known causes, prevention, detection, and treatment is available.
http://cancernet.nci.nih.gov/cancertypes.html

■ **Cancer Quiz: Test Your Prevention Smarts** Take this seven-question quiz to assess your knowledge regarding cancer prevention.
http://mayohealth.org/mayo/0003/htm/cancer/cancer_q.htm

■ **National Center for Chronic Disease Prevention and Health Promotion, Cancer Prevention and Control** This site, sponsored by the Centers for

Disease Control and Prevention (CDC), features current information on cancer of the breast, cervix, prostate, skin, and colon. The site also provides monthly spotlights on specific cancers, as well as links to the National Comprehensive Cancer Control Program and the National Program of Cancer Registries.

http://www.cdc.gov/cancer/index.htm

InfoTrac

You can find additional readings related to wellness via InfoTrac College Edition, an on-line library of more than 900 journals and publications. Follow the instructions for accessing InfoTrac that came packaged with your textbook, then search for articles using a key word search.

Suggested Reading Andrea D. Platzman, "Preventing Cancer: What to Eat, What to Do, What to Avoid to Lower Your Risk," *Environmental Nutrition* 22, no. 10 (Oct. 1999): 1.

1. What is the recommended daily intake of fiber to help prevent colon cancer?
2. What roles do folic acid and selenium play in cancer prevention?
3. How does green tea protect against cancer?

Web Activity

Breast Cancer Interactive

http://www.tricaresw.af.mil/breastcd/index.html

Sponsor Health Net: TriCare Southwest—A large publicly-traded managed health care company.

Description This site features an excellent personal breast cancer risk analysis, as well as several multimedia links, including a layman site, self-exam video, clinical exam video, and a mammogram video. The site also contains teaching aids and resources.

Available Activities

1. Personalized breast cancer risk analysis
2. Layman's electronic textbook
3. Clinical details textbook
4. Listen to or read breast cancer survivor stories
5. Access to nursing and social support services
6. Frequently asked questions and a glossary

Web Work:

1. From the home page, click on the "decision tree" button and answer the five simple questions pertaining to your history.
2. Once completed, you will be given a risk assessment with several links based on your responses. Click on one or more of these URLs to learn more about your particular risk factor or condition.
3. Upon completion, click on the "Health Clinic" link to take you to the following interactive sections: layman's textbook, breast self-exam video, clinical exam video, or the mammogram video.

Helpful Hints:

1. Before you complete your own personalized breast cancer risk analysis, first click on the example decision tree link so you can learn how the decision tree works for two imaginary women.
2. Upon completion of the survey, make certain you check out the various resources as well as the breast self-exam, the clinical exam, and the mammogram videos.

For additional Web activities, links, and suggested readings, visit our Health, Fitness, and Wellness Resource Center at http://health.wadsworth.com.

NOTES

1. National Cancer Institute.
2. American Cancer Society, *Cancer Facts & Figures, 2000* (Atlanta: American Cancer Society, 2000).
3. See note 2.
4. See note 2.
5. American Lung Association.
6. R. Lowry, D. Holtzman, B. I. Truman, L. Kann, J. L. Collins, and L. J. Kolbe, "Substance Use and HIV-Related Sexual Behaviors Among U.S. High School Students," *American Journal of Public Health* 84 (1994): 1116–1120.
7. American Cancer Society, *Cancer Facts & Figures, 1994* (Atlanta: American Cancer Society, 1994).
8. *Epidemiology* (Sept. 1993)
9. See note 7.
10. See note 7.
11. See note 7.

WHAT IS YOUR RISK
OF DEVELOPING CERTAIN CANCERS?

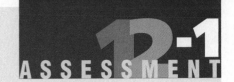

Name: _____   Date: _____   Grade: _____

Instructor: _____   Course: _____   Section: _____

Instructions

For each question, select the response that best describes you; record the point value in the space provided. Total your points for each section separately.

Lung Cancer

1. Sex _____
   - 2   Male
   - 1   Female

2. Age _____
   - 1   39 or younger
   - 2   40–49
   - 5   50–59
   - 7   60 and over

3. 8   Smoker _____
   - 1   Nonsmoker

4. Type of smoking _____
   - 10   Current smoker of cigarettes or little cigars
   - 3   Pipe and/or cigar, but not cigarettes
   - 2   Ex-cigarette smoker
   - 1   Nonsmoker

5. Amount of cigarettes smoked per day _____
   - 1   0
   - 5   Less than 1/2 pack
   - 9   1/2–1 pack
   - 15   1–2 packs
   - 20   2 or more packs

6. Type of cigarette* _____
   - 10   High tar/nicotine
   - 9   Medium tar/nicotine
   - 7   Low tar/nicotine
   - 1   Nonsmoker

7. Duration of smoking _____
   - 1   Never smoked
   - 3   Ex-smoker
   - 5   Up to 15 years
   - 10   15–25 years
   - 20   25 or more years

*Tar/nicotine levels:
High: 20+ mg tar/1.3+ mg nicotine
Medium: 16–19 mg tar/1.1–1.2 mg nicotine
Low: 15 mg or less tar/1.0 mg or less nicotine

8. Type of industrial work _____
   - 3   Mining
   - 7   Asbestos
   - 5   Uranium and radioactive products

   Lung total _____

Colon and Rectal Cancer

1. Age _____
   - 10   39 or younger
   - 20   40–59
   - 50   60 and over

2. Has anyone in your immediate family ever had: _____
   - 20   Colon cancer
   - 10   One or more colon polyps
   - 1   Neither

3. Have you ever had: _____
   - 100   Colon cancer
   - 40   One or more colon polyps
   - 20   Ulcerative colitis
   - 10   Cancer of the breast or uterus
   - 1   None

4. Bleeding from the rectum (other than obvious hemorrhoids or piles) _____
   - 75   Yes
   - 1   No

   Colon and rectal total _____

Skin Cancer

1. Frequently work or play in the sun _____
   - 10   Yes
   - 1   No

2. Work in mines, around coal tars, or around radioactivity _____
   - 10   Yes
   - 1   No

3. Complexion—fair skin or light skin _____
   - 10   Yes
   - 1   No

   Skin total _____

Breast Cancer (women only)

1. Age group _____
   - 10   20–34
   - 40   35–49
   - 90   50 and over

2. Racial group _____
   - 5   Asian American
   - 20   African American
   - 25   Non-Hispanic White
   - 10   Hispanic American

3. Family history _____
   - 30   Mother, sister, aunt, or grandmother with breast cancer
   - 10   None

4. Your history _____
   - 25   Previous lumps or cysts
   - 10   No breast disease
   - 100   Previous breast cancer

5. Maternity _____
   - 10   First pregnancy before age 25
   - 15   First pregnancy after age 25
   - 20   No pregnancies

                          Breast total _____

Cervical Cancer (women only)

1. Age group _____
   - 10   Younger than 25
   - 20   25–39
   - 30   40–54
   - 30   55 and over

2. Racial group _____
   - 10   Asian American
   - 20   African American
   - 10   Non-Hispanic White
   - 20   Hispanic American

3. Number of pregnancies _____
   - 10   0
   - 20   1 to 3
   - 30   4 or more

4. Viral infections _____
   - 10   Herpes and other viral infections or ulcer formations on the vagina
   - 1   Never

5. Age at first intercourse _____
   - 40   Younger than 15
   - 30   15–19
   - 20   20–24
   - 10   25 and over
   - 5   Never

6. Bleeding between periods or after intercourse _____
   - 40   Yes
   - 1   No

                          Cervical total _____

Endometrial Cancer (women only)

(Body of uterus. These questions do not apply to a woman who has had a total hysterectomy.)

1. Age group _____
   - 5   39 or less
   - 20   40–49
   - 60   50+

2. Race _____
   - 10   Asian American
   - 10   African American
   - 20   White
   - 10   Hispanic American

3. Births _____
   - 15   None
   - 7   1 to 4
   - 5   5 or more

4. Weight _____
   - 50   50 or more pounds overweight
   - 15   20–49 pounds overweight
   - 10   Underweight for height
   - 10   Normal

5. Diabetes (elevated blood sugar) _____
   - 3   Yes
   - 1   No

6. Estrogen hormone intake _____
   - 15   Yes, regularly
   - 12   Yes, occasionally
   - 10   None

7. Abnormal uterine bleeding _____
   - 40   Yes
   - 1   No

8. Hypertension (high blood pressure) _____
   - 3   Yes
   - 1   No

                          Endometrial total _____

Source: From American Cancer Society, Texas Division, Inc.

Analysis

If your LUNG total is:

24 or less	You have a low risk for lung cancer.
24–49	You may be a light smoker and would benefit from quitting.
50–74	As a moderate smoker, your risks for lung and upper respiratory tract cancer are increased. If you stop smoking now, these risks will decrease.
75 or over	As a heavy cigarette smoker, your risks for lung and upper respiratory tract cancer are greatly increased. You should stop smoking now. See your physician if you have possible signs of lung cancer (nagging cough, hoarseness, persistent sore in the mouth or throat).

If your COLON AND RECTAL total is:

29 or less	You are at low risk for colon and rectal cancer.
30–69	You are at moderate risk. Testing by your physician may be indicated.
70 or over	You are at high risk. You should see your physician for the following tests: digital rectal exam, stool occult blood test, and (where applicable) proctoscopic exam.

Your SKIN CANCER risk:

Numerical risks for *skin* cancer are difficult to state. For instance, a person with a dark complexion can work longer in the sun and be less likely to develop cancer than a light-complected person. Furthermore, a person wearing a long-sleeved shirt and wide-brimmed hat may work in the sun and be less at risk than a person who wears a bathing suit for only a short period. The risk goes up greatly with age. If you answered "yes" to any question, you need to protect your skin from the sun or any other toxic material. Changes in moles, warts, or skin sores are important and should be seen by your physician.

If your BREAST total is:

100 or less	You are at low risk. You should do monthly breast self-examination (BSE) and have your breasts examined by a physician as part of a cancer-related checkup.
100–199	You are at moderate risk. You should practice monthly BSE and have your breasts examined by a physician as part of a cancer-related checkup. Periodic mammograms should be included, as directed by your physician.
200 or over	You are at high risk. You should practice monthly BSE and have professional examinations more often. See your physician for the examinations recommended for you.

If your CERVICAL total is:

40–69	You are at low risk. Your physician will advise you about how often you should have a Pap test.
70–99	You are at moderate risk. More frequent Pap tests may be required.
100 or more	You are at high risk. You should have a Pap test and pelvic exam as advised by your physician.

If your ENDOMETRIAL Total is:

49–59	You are at low risk for developing endometrial cancer.
60–99	Your risks are slightly higher (moderate risk). Report any abnormal bleeding immediately to your doctor. Tissue sampling at menopause is recommended.
100 or over	Your risks are much greater (high risk). See your doctor for tests as appropriate.

Personal Interpretation

In the space provided below, discuss the results of your cancer questionnaire, state your feelings about cancer, and discuss any experiences that you have had with a cancer patient.

_____
_____
_____
_____
_____
_____
_____
_____
_____
_____
_____
_____

Discuss lifestyle changes that you can implement to help decrease your personal risk of developing cancer.

_____
_____
_____
_____
_____
_____
_____
_____
_____
_____
_____
_____

13 ADDICTIVE BEHAVIOR AND WELLNESS

OBJECTIVES

Define addiction and differentiate it from habit.

Delineate the difference between physiological addiction and psychological addiction.

Cite the threats of addiction to the dimensions of wellness.

Define the addictive personality.

Discuss addictive personality traits.

List the major risk factors of addiction.

Cite some guidelines for managing and changing addictive behavior.

Describe the harmful health effects of tobacco, alcohol, and other drug use and abuse.

© Jim Ackerman, CORBIS

329

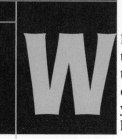

E ALL HAVE HABITS. You might have the habit of flopping down in front of the television as soon as you get home every day, or biting your nails when you are bored. Most habits are harmless, but when a habit escalates into an addiction, it threatens wellness.

Broadly defined, an **addiction** is an abnormal or disordered relationship with an object (such as tobacco or alcohol) or an event or behavior (such as shoplifting or gambling). Continued involvement with the object or activity may have harmful consequences. Addiction is a process that evolves over time. It almost always begins as a pleasurable, voluntary activity but ends by causing continuous disruption in an addict's life. Typical characteristics of addictive behavior are

- a compulsive need to do a particular thing,
- loss of control of actions, and

SIGNS OF ADDICTIVE BEHAVIOR

- No matter how much you get, it's never enough. You're frustrated constantly by the need to do more or get more. (That frustration, incidentally, is much different from the motivation that stems from challenge and determination.)
- You don't get pleasure from the behavior. It doesn't contribute to an overall sense of well-being.
- The behavior becomes predictable. You know you'll do a certain thing a certain way. The pattern doesn't change.
- You become inflexible about the behavior. For example, you run 2 miles before class every morning and balk at a friend's suggestion that you play tennis instead. If your friend won't run with you, you run anyway—either before you play tennis or instead of playing tennis.
- You have a lower sense of self-worth or self-esteem because of what you're doing, but you can't seem to stop.
- Even if you don't enjoy the behavior, you feel driven to do it anyway. For example, you might be disgusted by your obsession to look at pornographic magazines and think it's a dirty habit, but you can't seem to stop. Your behavior even might make you sick, but you can't seem to change.
- You stay locked in the behavior as a way of escaping demands or stresses, not because you see the behavior as an exhilarating challenge.
- The behavior dulls your senses, provides an escape, or otherwise helps you get away from stress, unhappiness, boredom, or frustration. Whenever you get a chance for challenge or reward, you resort to the addictive behavior instead of taking a chance on some other behavior.

FIGURE 13.1 THE DOWNWARD SPIRAL OF PHYSIOLOGICAL ADDICTION.

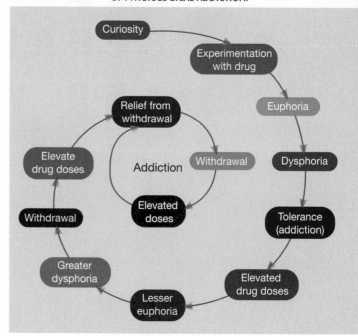

- repeating the action even though the results are harmful.

Most people with addictions deny they have a problem. Denial, a common component of addiction, is the refusal to admit, or failure to see, that a problem exists. Addicts cannot see it even though people around them see it clearly. Denial prevents people from seeking treatment long after their problems have become unmanageable. Assessment 13-1 can provide you with insight about addiction.

Addiction can be either physiological or psychological. Physiological addiction is a change in the body's biochemistry so that it demands the presence of a substance (a drug), not for pleasure, but in order to function normally. As the body begins to clear the substance from its system, the altered body chemistry disrupts normal functioning, and the symptoms of withdrawal ensue. Withdrawal is extremely unpleasant and creates an urgent need for another dose of the drug. By this time in the addictive process, the drug may be producing little or no euphoria. See Figure 13.1 for a description of the downward negative spiral of drug addiction. The withdrawal is so miserable that suicidal behavior sometimes occurs.[1]

A drug is a substance that modifies one or more of the body's functions. Drugs that produce euphoria (an enhanced feeling of well-being) are more likely to be abused. To be addictive, a substance must be able to produce a change in mood. A drug is physiologically addictive when its use results in tolerance, that is, when ever-larger doses are needed to achieve the effect. When a person is addicted to a drug and the drug is withheld, brainwave patterns change, mood alters, and drug-seeking behavior follows.

Physiological addiction also has a psychological component—a strong craving for the drug. But psychological addiction can occur without physiological addiction, and the craving can be for some other habit or behavior. People can become addicted to gambling,[2] computers, exercise, television, work, sex, cleanliness, or over-the-counter medications. College students are at risk for developing addictions to the Internet.[3] A person may switch addictions from one object or behavior to another.

People with psychological addiction have not learned healthy ways to cope with emotional pain. They crave relief from emotional hurt and use a substance or behavior to distract themselves. The underlying motive is the same, regardless of the behavior used to relieve pain. People who use behaviors or drugs this way achieve temporary numbness and short-term relief, but if the behavior is destructive, or if involvement in the behavior keeps a person from taking care of themselves, they experience negative consequences. If the person repeatedly turns to the behavior or substance, they are caught up in the cycle depicted in Figure 13.2.

Addiction is a staggering problem in the United States.[4] Drug addiction is alarmingly widespread.[5] Addiction threatens all six dimensions of wellness—physical, emotional, social, intellectual, spiritual, and occupational—as follows:

1. Physical wellness. People who are addicted to an object or an event typically fail to take good care of themselves because they are preoccupied with the addictive behavior. They might not get enough sleep, may skip meals, and could even put themselves in dangerous situations. Certain addictive behaviors damage the body itself. As examples, bulimia damages the throat and alcoholism damages the liver. The stress accompanying some addictions can injure virtually every organ and system in the body. Addictions can result in death either from intentional or unintentional drug overdose.

2. Emotional wellness. Addictive behavior lowers self-esteem. The addict usually feels guilty, anxious, angry, depressed, and ashamed. Many addicts have unexplained mood swings or episodes of rage and violence.

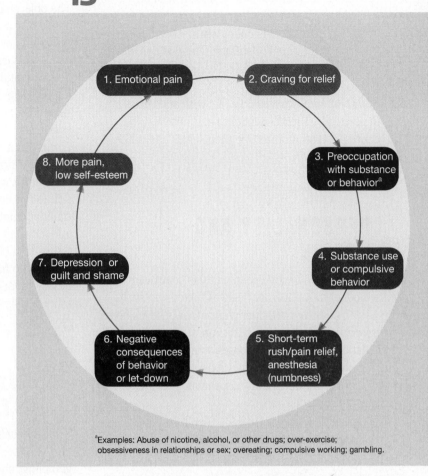

FIGURE 13.2 THE CYCLE OF PSYCHOLOGICAL ADDICTION.

1. Emotional pain
2. Craving for relief
3. Preoccupation with substance or behavior[a]
4. Substance use or compulsive behavior
5. Short-term rush/pain relief, anesthesia (numbness)
6. Negative consequences of behavior or let-down
7. Depression or guilt and shame
8. More pain, low self-esteem

[a]Examples: Abuse of nicotine, alcohol, or other drugs; over-exercise; obsessiveness in relationships or sex; overeating; compulsive working; gambling.

3. Social wellness. Other than the interaction the addiction requires, an addict usually is a loner who gradually cuts off relationships with family members, friends, colleagues, or classmates. Addiction brings with it a powerful preoccupation that takes priority over people, places, and events outside of the addictive behavior.

4. Mental wellness. Addiction impairs reasoning, judgment, and logic. Things that used to provide intellectual challenge or stimulation—coursework in a class, exploration of nearby geological sites, debates over a current topic—no longer matter.

5. Spiritual wellness. Because of the time and energy demands of an addiction, addicts have difficulty maintaining the same priorities and values they once had. Addicts gradually lose a sense of self and a feeling of being connected to the people and the world around them. They can't focus on something other than themselves, nor can they appreciate themselves in a meaningful way.

Addiction An abnormal or disordered relationship with an object, event, or behavior.

6. Occupational wellness, which some models also consider a sixth dimension. A person with an addiction is focused on the addictive behavior; this leaves little time for school or work. Absenteeism increases; work quality suffers; relationships with professors, other students, colleagues, and supervisors are impaired.

7. Environmental wellness. People with addictions are distracted by their dependence and unable to be concerned about protecting themselves and others against hazards.

PERSONALITY AND ADDICTION

The notion of an addictive personality is controversial. One school of thought flatly believes there is no such thing as an addictive personality. Another believes no set of personality traits leads to addiction but has identified a constellation of traits that disposes someone to addiction. The more of these characteristics a person has, and the stronger each trait or condition is, the more vulnerable that person is to addiction.

The Non-Addictive Personality

Some traits of people who are less likely to show addictive behavior include the ability to face problems head-on with optimism and realism. They work to overcome their problems. They recognize their own limitations and pace themselves accordingly to maximize their ability to cope.

The person who is less prone to addictions has the ability to look at their circumstances realistically. They set realistic goals and work toward achieving their goals in a structured, reasonable way. They are not too hard on themselves when they don't achieve a goal. They recognize their limitations and weaknesses and also appreciate their strengths and good qualities.

> Most people with addictions deny their problems.

People who are less likely to become addicted have a keen interest in other people, allow others the freedom to pursue their own interests, and have at least a few deep relationships with other people. They have the ability to love and be loved and consider others' feelings, desires, and needs. They are not controlled by others but at the same time are sensitive to others.

The Addictive Personality

The objects, events, or behaviors involved in some addictions may not be harmful, but an addict has an unhealthy or abnormal relationship with those objects, events, or behaviors. For example, food provides us with nutrition and energy, but food addicts eat compulsively and endanger their health. Sex provides intimacy, but a sex addict becomes preoccupied with pornography or an ever-expanding gamut of sexual partners. Drugs can treat disease, but drug addicts harm themselves by abusing the substance.

People who are emotionally unhealthy are at greater risk for addiction (see Chapter 2 for more details about traits of emotionally unhealthy people). Low self-esteem and a strong need for immediate gratification are two key traits often observed in addicts. The addictive personality is one who has learned not to trust people, does not have healthy relationships, and never has learned to connect to other people, his or her own emotions, or the surrounding world.[6]

RISK FACTORS FOR ADDICTION

Addictive behavior covers a wide spectrum—use of the Internet,[7] sexual addiction,[8] eating disorders, compulsive gambling, shoplifting, compulsive spending, and alcoholism, to name a few. Factors leading to addiction include the following:

- The behavior is reinforced.
- The addiction is an attempt to meet basic human needs, such as physical needs, the need to feel safe, the need to belong, the need to feel important, or the need to reach one's potential.
- The addiction seems to temporarily relieve stress.
- The addiction can be present within the person's value system (a person whose values wouldn't let him or her shoot heroin may be able to rationalize compulsive eating or obsessive television watching, for example).
- A serious physical illness is present, and the addiction provides escape from pain or the fear of disfigurement.
- There is pressure to perform or succeed.
- The person hates himself or herself.
- Society allows addiction. Advertising even encourages it.

Most people with addictions deny their problem. Even when the addiction is clear to people around them, they continue to deny that the addiction exists. Instead, they tend to get angry when someone tries to talk about the behavior and are likely to make excuses for their actions. Many addicts will also blame others for the problem. In some cases, an addict will admit the problem, but fail to take any steps to change.

Drug addiction is unexpected. Probably no one who starts out using a substance intends to get hooked, but it happens nevertheless. A person tries a drug for one reason but continues taking it because addiction has set in. People who experiment with drugs often want to believe that addiction will not happen to them, only to others who are somehow inferior. The truth is no one is exempt. The only way to escape drug addiction is to refrain from experimenting with drugs that produce it.

The same general experience and behaviors are involved in all kinds of addictions, whether they involve food, sex, gambling, shopping, alcohol, or other drugs. The following sections present information regarding addictions to tobacco, alcohol, marijuana, and cocaine.

TOBACCO

Tobacco products—cigarettes, cigars, pipes, smokeless tobacco—all contain the addictive drug **nicotine**. The dysphoria (unpleasant mood that occurs when the drug wears off) associated with nicotine withdrawal is so intense that quitting tobacco use is extremely difficult. For this reason, it is wise to never start smoking.

The percentage of the U.S. population that smokes has declined over the last three decades, although the percentage of young people who smoke remains high.[9] Adults with less than a 12th-grade education are more than twice as likely to smoke as are those with a college degree. About 35 percent of students in grades 9–12 smoke cigarettes, whereas only 25 percent of adults smoke.

| Health Risks |

People who engage in any form of tobacco use put themselves at tremendous risk. They die earlier, and they experience diseases and suffering. The most commonly known disease is lung cancer. Approximately 90 percent of all lung cancer is caused directly by cigarette smoking, and of the 10 percent that occurs in nonsmokers, 1 in 5 results from inhaling secondary cigarette smoke. The particulates in tobacco smoke are 500,000 times greater than the most heavily polluted air in the world. Lung cancer is the leading cause of cancer death in the United States, killing more than 153,000 Americans every year.

Another risk to health is exposure to carbon monoxide, which reduces the ability of red blood cells to carry oxygen. The concentration of carbon monoxide in tobacco smoke is 800 times higher than the level considered safe by the U.S. Environmental Protection Agency.

Other cancers are observed in smokers. Oral cancer (cancer of the mouth, palate, larynx, pharynx, and esophagus are commonly observed in cigarette smokers; cancer of the lip, tongue, and jaw are seen in pipe smokers). Seventy percent of all oral cancer cases are caused by

Nicotine A poisonous, addictive component of tobacco, inhaled by smokers or absorbed through the lining of the mouth by people who chew it.

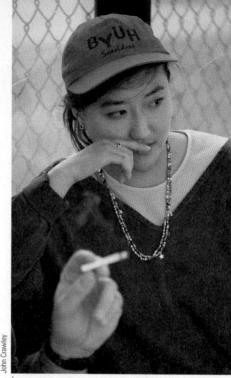

Protecting non-smokers' health is important.

John Crawley

disease each year (half of those who die from heart disease) are attributed directly to cigarette smoking. Smokers have a 70 percent higher death rate from heart disease; heavy smokers, a 200 percent higher death rate than moderate smokers.

More bad news about smoking: increased risk of peptic ulcer, miscarriage, stillbirths, death during infancy, low birth weight babies, sudden infant death syndrome (SIDS) among babies born to mothers who smoke, and higher rates of asthma and middle-ear infections among children of smoking parents.

Smoking is considered the leading preventable cause of death and disability in the United States,[10] yet many college students are unaware of the magnitude of this problem. College students are surprisingly uninformed regarding the devastating and harmful outcomes related to smoking.[11] Smoking not only drastically shortens life, but it also reduces the years of healthy life. Many smokers experience years of pain and suffering from smoking-related illnesses.

Years ago, smoking was socially acceptable. But currently, as more people become informed regarding the vast negative health effects, smoking is viewed negatively by society. In this way, smoking can limit social opportunities. To the majority of nonsmokers, smoking is offensive. Smoking discolors teeth and leaves unpleasant odors in clothes, mouth, hair, furniture, and dwelling. Nonsmokers are also concerned about the health risks of being around a smoker.

Another health concern regarding smoking is that nicotine is considered a "gateway" drug. For example, people do not begin drug abuse with heroin or cocaine. When past drug use patterns of heavy drug abusers are studied, a trend is obvious: These abusers started using tobacco.[12] Tobacco use creates a gateway or path to other drug use and abuse. People who use tobacco often experiment with other, more dangerous drugs.[13] Researchers attribute the gateway effect to social and pharmacologic factors related to nicotine.[14]

cigarettes or chewing tobacco. Cancer of the pancreas, bladder, and cervix are also associated with smoking.

Chronic obstructive pulmonary diseases, including emphysema, asthma, and chronic bronchitis, are 25 times greater among smokers. Smoking also damages the respiratory system, increasing the risk of pneumonia, influenza, and colds. Smoke destroys the air sacs in the lungs, reducing their ability to absorb oxygen and eliminate carbon dioxide. Smokers are 18 times more likely than nonsmokers to die of lung disease.

Smokers have greater frequency of heart attacks, strokes, and coronary artery disease, including damage to the inner surface of coronary arteries. Smoking reduces the amount of oxygen that gets to the heart, weakening it. Smokers are twice as likely to have a stroke. Smoking also adds an estimated 10 years of aging to the arteries. More than a quarter of a million deaths from heart

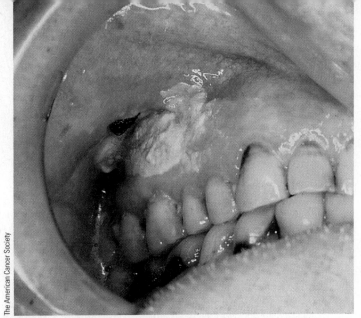

Oral cancer (white growth) and gum and teeth damage caused by smokeless tobacco.

The American Cancer Society

Another issue of concern about tobacco is that smoking is associated with other negative health behaviors.[15] Adolescents who smoke are more likely to abuse alcohol, eat poorly, and be physically inactive.[16] Smoking behavior often precedes other drug abuse.[17] Adolescents who use tobacco are also more likely to be involved in reckless and aggressive behaviors, and more likely to have larger number of sex partners[18] and take other sexual risks.[19] Smoking appears to be associated with a risk-taking personality.[20]

Smokeless Tobacco

The use of smokeless tobacco (chew and snuff) has increased dramatically over the past 2 decades. Nearly a third of the nation's 10 million users are under age 21. Almost 16 percent of high school males use smokeless tobacco.

To create chewing tobacco, tobacco leaves are treated with molasses and other flavorings. A plug of the tobacco is placed between the lower lip and the gums, where it is sucked to release the nicotine. A dip of chewing tobacco contains two to three times more nicotine than a cigarette. An average-sized dip held in the mouth for 30 minutes provides the same nicotine response as smoking four cigarettes. Someone who uses two cans of chewing tobacco a week gets as much nicotine as someone who smokes a pack and a half of cigarettes every day. Chew also contains cancer-causing nitrosamines at levels higher than foods may legally contain. Snuff is even more dangerous, because powdered tobacco releases more of its chemicals in the mouth.

Smokeless tobacco causes oral cancer as well as a variety of mouth and gum diseases, including loss of taste, bad breath, gingivitis, pyorrhea, tooth loss, unusual wear on tooth surfaces, tooth decay, receding gums, damage to the jawbone, and leukoplakia (precancerous thick, rough, leathery, white patches on the tongue, gums, or inner cheek). One in five people who develop leukoplakia is eventually diagnosed with oral cancer. Smokeless tobacco has also been shown to increase blood pressure and to interfere with the body's ability to use the nutrients in food effectively. Assessments 13-2 and 13-3 can provide insight about tobacco behavior.

ALCOHOL

The term "alcohol," as commonly used, refers to the active ingredient of alcoholic beverages—ethanol or ethyl alcohol. The percentage of alcohol in distilled liquor is stated as proof: "100-proof" liquor is 50 percent alcohol. A drink is a dose of any alcoholic beverage that delivers ½ ounce of pure ethanol, such as 3 to 4 ounces of wine, a 10 oz standard wine cooler, a 12 oz standard beer, or 1 oz of hard liquor (whiskey, gin, rum, or vodka).

Alcohol is toxic. Taken in large doses, it can be poisonous. However, sufficiently diluted and taken in small enough doses, alcohol produces euphoria, or a sense of well-being and pleasure, but not without risk. Alcohol is a drug that modifies one or more of the body's functions. Like other euphoria-producers, alcohol can be addicting. The cycle of addiction, both physiological and psychological, entraps about 1 out of every 10 users of alcohol and not only ruins their lives but also disrupts the lives of all who surround them in the family and on the job. Alcohol use becomes abuse when it interferes with family, work, school, or social life or when it involves any violation of the law (including drunk driving).

Alcohol use and abuse is increasing among teenagers.[21] Nationwide, half of all high school students reported alcohol consumption at least once a month. One-third reported **binge drinking**—the quick consumption of several alcoholic drinks in a short period of time for the purpose of becoming intoxicated. Binge drinking and participating in drinking games are popular on college campuses.[22] Drinking games are designed to ensure over-consumption of alcohol and are extremely life threatening.

People drink for many reasons: to celebrate, to unwind, to get high, or because they like the taste of alcoholic beverages. Many people drink because peer pressure demands it, and young people may drink because they think drinking shows their maturity. Still-younger people use it as a way of rebelling against authority. Some people use alcohol as a way of escaping life's pressures.

A common reason college students give for drinking alcohol is to overcome shyness. Many people long to have the courage to meet new friends, particularly members of the other sex, but have not developed the social skills or confidence to do so with ease. They claim drinking alcohol makes them feel more confident, and they are able to be outgoing, carefree, and bold under its influence. They do add, however, that some problems often result: They become intoxicated, embarrass themselves, and suffer bruised egos the next day. People who use "liquid courage" to help with socialization learn that they still do not have the skills necessary for successful social interaction.

> Many college students drink alcohol to be more social. This is unnecessary because social skills are better developed without alcohol.

Another way people are encouraged to drink is through the deceptive appeals of the alcohol industry. Billboards, magazines, ads, TV dramas, and movies project an image of the alcohol drinker in a variety of appealing ways to encourage excessive alcohol consumption and increase alcohol sales. All of these appeals have two things in common: First, they suggest that consuming alcohol can help people achieve the qualities they most desire, such as being sophisticated or more social, having sex appeal, or being athletic. These appeals and television situations portraying drunkenness as humorous do not show what happens in reality when people abuse alcohol.

Looked at with a rationale eye, alcohol use hinders the attainment of all the qualities used to promote it. A person striving for sophistication and for rewarding social and sexual interactions needs not to lose control, but to gain it by practicing social skills. A person seeking sports success will not find it by drinking beer, but by faithfully practicing the sport. The ads, though, deceive people by not mentioning that alcohol abuse causes accidents, impotence, other health problems and can destroy relationships. All such advertisements suppress facts and strengthen the emotional impulse to consume alcohol.

Another reason cited for drinking, especially heavy drinking or problem drinking, is the inability to cope with negative moods and distress. Some people have acquired better skills at handling or coping with unpleasant mood states. People who have poor self-regulating skills are more likely to engage in problem drinking behavior. Poor emotional health status also contributes to alcohol abuse. People are more likely to abuse alcohol if they are depressed, lonely, or have inadequate social support systems.[23]

| Health Risks |

Alcohol is involved in more than half of all fatal automobile accidents in the United States. Someone is injured every minute, and someone dies every 23 minutes from an alcohol-related accident. One in every two of us is projected to be involved in an alcohol-related accident at some time in our lives. Our entire society suffers the consequences of alcohol abuse in terms of crimes, medical expenses, and emotional health.

Binge drinking is a problem of concern because it has many serious health consequences, including death.[24] Students who participate in binge drinking and drinking games experience more alcohol-related ill effects than other students.[25] Students who are involved in drinking games are also more likely than others to be involved in situations of sexual victimization.[26]

Alcohol abuse impairs health status both in the short-term and the long-term. Short-term risks include dangers of acute intoxication (including alcohol poisoning that can cause death). In addition, people who become intoxicated are at higher risk of accidents, violence, rape, and other sexual victimization.

Short-term alcohol intoxication can cause fatty liver, which is the accumulation of fat in the liver cells. It interferes with the distribution of nutrients and oxygen to the liver cells. If drinking episodes are so close together that the liver cannot recover between times, liver disease develops. This is a common problem among people who drink excessively on the weekends.

The hangover, or the awful feeling of headache pain and nausea that one has the morning after drinking too much, is a mild form of drug withdrawal. The hangover is caused by dehydration of brain cells. When brain cells begin to rehydrate, nerve pain accompanies their swelling back to normal size. Another contributor to the hangover is the accumulation of formaldehyde, which is a byproduct of alcohol metabolism.

> Time alone can cure a hangover. Do not take Tylenol when drinking: It can cause toxic liver damage.

Time alone (to metabolize the alcohol) is the only cure for a hangover. Simple-minded remedies clearly will not work: for example taking vitamins, drinking more alcohol, drinking coffee. Taking Tylenol (or acetaminophen) when drinking can cause dangerous liver damage. The best cure actually is to drink less next time.

Like tobacco, alcohol is considered a gateway drug to use of other, more dangerous drugs.[27] In addition, alcohol abuse is linked to involvement in other harmful health behaviors.[28] Adolescents who abuse alcohol are more likely to take sexual risks, putting them at risk for pregnancy and for STDs including AIDS.[29]

Long-term risks associated with alcohol are many and are depicted in Figure 13.3. The most commonly observed effects include liver disease, nutritional deficiencies, and impotence.[30] In addition to the devastating physical harm alcohol abuse causes, it also results in considerable emotional and social damage.[31] Problem drinkers affect family, friends, fellow employees, and the community. Assessment 13-4 can help you determine if you may have a problem with alcohol.

| Fetal Alcohol Syndrome |

Women who drink throughout pregnancy run the risk of giving birth to a baby with **fetal alcohol syndrome** (FAS), the second leading cause of mental retardation in the United States and the third most common birth defect. Another more common condition is fetal alcohol effects (FAE), which occurs when babies are exposed to alcohol in the womb but do not have the classic signs of fetal alcohol syndrome. Even a few drinks during the entire term of a pregnancy or one episode of heavy drinking can be harmful to the fetus. Women who are pregnant should not consume any alcohol.

Tests show the blood alcohol content is much higher in the fetus than in the mother who drank the alcohol. The greatest

FIGURE **13.3** LONG-TERM RISKS ASSOCIATED WITH CHRONIC ALCOHOL USE.

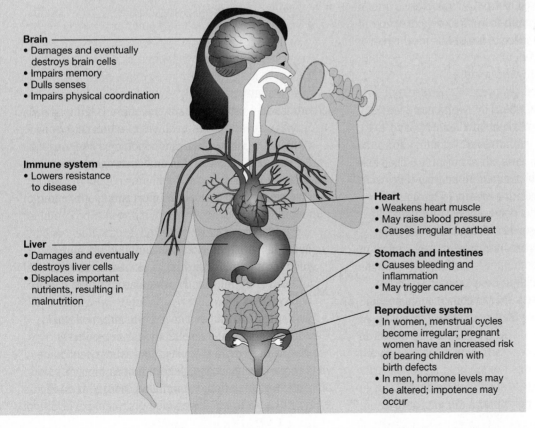

Brain
- Damages and eventually destroys brain cells
- Impairs memory
- Dulls senses
- Impairs physical coordination

Immune system
- Lowers resistance to disease

Liver
- Damages and eventually destroys liver cells
- Displaces important nutrients, resulting in malnutrition

Heart
- Weakens heart muscle
- May raise blood pressure
- Causes irregular heartbeat

Stomach and intestines
- Causes bleeding and inflammation
- May trigger cancer

Reproductive system
- In women, menstrual cycles become irregular; pregnant women have an increased risk of bearing children with birth defects
- In men, hormone levels may be altered; impotence may occur

Binge drinking Imbibing at least five alcoholic beverages in one sitting for men, and four for women.

Fetal alcohol syndrome A set of mental and physical characteristics in a newborn caused by moderate-to-heavy alcohol drinking during pregnancy.

harm probably is done during the first 3 months of pregnancy, when the fetus is most susceptible, but alcohol at any time during fetal development can cause damage. Generally, drinking during the first trimester damages organ development; during the last trimester, it damages development of the central nervous system.

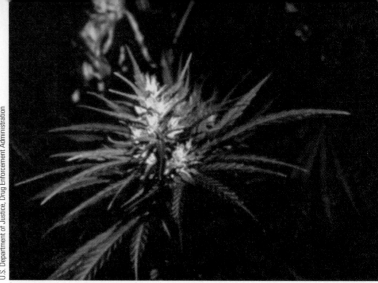

FAS is characterized by low birth weight, small head size, mental retardation, poor motor development, long-term developmental disabilities, and a distinctive set of facial malformations (short eye openings, low nasal bridge, thin upper lip, and absence of a groove above the upper lip).

| The flowering top of **Cannabis sativa**. |

> Women should not drink alcoholic beverages during pregnancy because of the risk of birth defects.

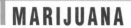

MARIJUANA

After a period of decline beginning in the late 1970s, marijuana use by teens is rising.[32] Nationwide, 47 percent of U.S. high school students reported using marijuana at some time in their lifetimes. Made from the dried, crushed leaves and flowers of the *Cannabis sativa* plant, marijuana—which looks a lot like tobacco—most often is rolled into papers and smoked like cigarettes. Some users pack it firmly into a pipe or smoke it through a water pipe. Less often, it is brewed into tea or baked in brownies. Although marijuana is a chemically complex plant with more than 400 identified substances, the one that has made marijuana popular is its chief psychoactive agent, **THC** (delta-9-tetrahydrocannabinol).

The marijuana that today's college students smoke is much more potent than that used by earlier generations. It is estimated that the plants cultivated today have three times the amount of THC as those cultivated just 10 years ago.

Marijuana is fat-soluble, stored in the fatty tissues of the brain, body, and reproductive organs. The immediate effects of marijuana intoxication are felt within 10 to 30 minutes and usually last several hours, and marijuana actually stays in the system as long as a month. The body has difficulty completely eliminating the THC, and the effects are cumulative, building up over time. What this means is that if you smoke a joint every weekend, which may not seem all that bad, your body is constantly permeated with the drug.

Marijuana has received a great deal of controversial media coverage. Publicity has ranged from scare tactics about the monstrous effects of the drug to a casual attitude that marijuana is not harmful. The immediate effects of use are bloodshot eyes, dry mouth and throat, coughing, and mild muscular weakness. Though marijuana may be considered less toxic than other illegal drugs, it has harmful effects on short-term memory and other cognitive functions.[33] Marijuana distorts perceptions of the passage of time and impairs depth perception. It alters perceptions and delays reaction time. For this reason it is dangerous to drive under its influence. In addition, marijuana use presents the following risks and long-term effects:

- Inhibited brain and motor functions.
- Changes in cell membranes, especially those in the brain and reproductive tracts, interfering with cells' ability to absorb energy.
- Interference with immunity, compromising the ability to fight infection.
- Faster heart rate and heightened blood pressure, leading to long-term cardiac damage (this is a problem particularly for people who already have arteriosclerosis, angina, or some other heart disease).
- Lung damage as much as four times that caused by inhaling the same amount of tobacco smoke. Marijuana is higher in tars and contains more carcinogens.
- Impaired oxygen and carbon dioxide exchange in the lungs.
- Depressed sex drive and impotence.
- Impaired male fertility because of lowered sperm count, reducing sperm motility (movement) and damaging sperm (causing irregularly shaped sperm).
- Reduced female fertility by inhibiting ovulation.
- Birth defects in babies born to mothers who smoke it during pregnancy (especially low birth weight, premature birth, and congenital deformities similar to those of fetal alcohol syndrome). Marijuana may cause breaks in both the ova and the sperm, resulting in birth defects.

Some people respond to long-term use by developing amotivational syndrome, or the loss of ambition and drive. Some people develop a psychological addiction to marijuana and require therapy to overcome dependence.

Perhaps one of the most serious risks from marijuana use is its status as a gateway drug to other drug use and abuse. Those who use marijuana regularly are much more likely to experiment with other, more dangerous drugs, such as cocaine, LSD and even heroin.[34]

Cocaine

Cocaine is not abused as often as alcohol and marijuana. In a national survey, slightly over 8 percent of students reported using some form of cocaine. Commonly known as "coke" and "snow," cocaine is a crystalline powder extracted from the leaves of the coca plant grown in Central and South America. It is probably the most powerfully addictive of any of the illicit drugs and can be injected, smoked (called "**freebasing**"), or inhaled through the nose. It acts as both a powerful local anesthetic and a central nervous system stimulant. In fact, mixtures of novocaine and caffeine have been sold on the street as cocaine.

The effects of cocaine can be immediate and devastating. Cocaine that is snorted reaches the brain within 3 minutes; when smoked or injected, it reaches the brain within seconds. Powdered cocaine that is snorted can destroy the sense of smell, damage the mucous membranes, destroy the septum of the nose, and cause sinusitis. Smoking cocaine causes lung and liver damage, weight loss, and an increase in blood pressure and heart rate. Injecting cocaine can damage the linings of the arteries, damage the heart, and cause skin infections. Cocaine has been known to cause sudden death.

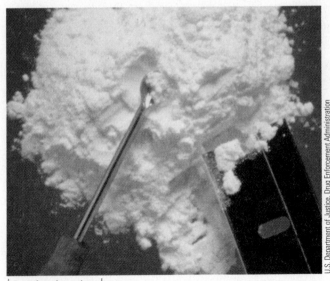

| Powdered cocaine. |

Crack

A particularly dangerous and addictive form of cocaine is **crack**, which derives its name from a popping or crackling sound that happens when it is smoked. Crack cocaine reaches the brain within 4 to 6 seconds, creating intense euphoria. Addiction to crack is so powerful that it has been defined as one of the most serious drug problems in the country.

HEALTH EFFECTS

Health effects of cocaine and crack cocaine include the following:

- Rapid increase in heart rate and blood pressure (can cause strokes or bleeding in the brain, even in young, healthy people).
- Increased breathing rate.
- Heart and respiratory failure, including fluid buildup in the lungs.
- Raised body temperature.
- Lowered immune system response.
- Damaged upper respiratory system (if inhaled).
- Reduced appetite (can lead to malnutrition).
- Liver damage.
- Impotence.
- "Cocaine psychosis," characterized by paranoia, delusions, and violence.

Babies born to cocaine users incur significant developmental problems before birth. Cocaine crosses the placenta, exposing the fetus to the drug. In addition, fluctuations in the mother's blood pressure cause blood vessels in the baby's brain to deteriorate, eventually resulting in strokes. Babies who are born cocaine-addicted experience jitteriness; inability to sleep; irritability; long-lasting emotional and social problems; brain damage; heart defects; kidney damage; possible malformed head, arms, fingers; and increased risk for sudden infant death syndrome (SIDS).

OTHER ADDICTIVE DRUGS AND CAUTIONS

Other drugs, legal and illegal, carry risk factors as well. Table 13.1 presents types of drugs and their short- and long-term effects. Two important issues concerning illegal drug use are first, the user risks problems with the law; second, illegal

THC (tetrahydrocannabinol) The psychoactive ingredient in marijuana.

Freebasing Smoking cocaine that has been separated from its hydrochloric salt by mixing it with a volatile chemical.

Crack A particularly dangerous and addictive form of cocaine.

TABLE 13.1 HOW DIFFERENT DRUGS AFFECT THE BODY

Type of Drug (Chemical)	Alcohol	Amphetamines ("speed," "bennies," "black beauties," "uppers")	Cocaine ("crack")	LSD (and other hallucinogens)
	• ethyl alcohol (ethanol), a clear liquid (in beer, wine, spirits)	• synthetically produced: amphetamine (speed), dextroamphetamine (dexedrine), methylamphetamine or "ice," methylphenidate (Ritalin), and so on.	• derived from South American coca bush (still chewed in Andes to offset fatigue)	• derived from mushrooms (psilocybin) or cactus (mescaline) or synthetically—e.g., lysergic acid (LSD or "acid") and phencyclidine (PCP or "hog," "angel dust")
	• made synthetically or from gain, fruit, or vegetables	• used as pills, inhaled or injected (speed)	• Crack is mixture of cocaine and baking soda.	• Structures resemble catecholamines—normal brain neurotransmitters.
	• favored for its relaxing, intoxicating properties	• CNS stimulants that resemble action of adrenaline (natural body hormone)	• Cocaine hydrochloride is white powder ("coke," "C," "flake," "snow").	• Hallucinogens can distort reality and produce severe delusions.
	• beers contain about 5% alcohol, wines to 12%, and spirits about 40% (about 13.6 g per drink)		• formerly used in many medicines (until 1920).	
	• a sedative-hypnotic and central nervous system (CNS) depressant		• stimulant action—like amphetamine, but now legally classed as a narcotic.	
Short-Term Effects (after a single dose)	Effects vary with user's size, sex, and amount of food in stomach: • initial relaxation and loss of inhibitions • increased sociability • impaired coordination • slowing down of reflexes and mental processes • attitude changes, increased risk-taking, and bad judgment/danger in driving car, operating machinery • sleepiness	• nervous system briefly stimulated • reduced appetite • increased energy, offsetting fatigue • talkative restlessness, greater alertness • faster breathing • rise in heart rate and blood pressure (with risk of burst blood vessels and heart failure) • raised temperature, dry mouth, sweaty skin • dilated pupils • alleviated nose stuffiness (original medicinal use)	• short-acting, powerful CNS stimulant, also a local anesthetic • effects vary depending whether drug is "snorted" (inhaled); injected; put in mouth, rectum, or vagina; or smoked (as crack) • transient euphoria and increased energy • appetite loss • rise in heart rate and breathing • dilated pupils • agitated, restless talkativeness • brief rise in sex drive	• unpredictable effects—at first, like amphetamine • excitation, arousal • raised temperature • altered sense of smell, shape, size, color, distance • exhilaration, perceived "mind expansion" or anxiety—depending on user • rapid pulse, dilated pupils, blank stare • exaggerated sense of power with possibly violent behavior • later, dramatic perceptual distortions • occasionally, convulsions
With Larger Doses and Longer Use	• blackouts (memory loss) • facial flushing, slurred speech • staggering gait, stupor • rise in blood pressure • pancreatitis, hepatitis, stomach ulcers, injuries (broken bones) • effects magnified by other depressants (e.g., opiates, barbiturates, tranquilizers, antihistamines, sleep aids, cold remedies) • alone or combined with other drugs can increase accident rates • overdose may be fatal, from respiratory distress	• bizarre behavior, talkativeness, restlessness, tremors, excitability • sense of power, superiority, aggression • illusions and hallucinations • some users become paranoid, suspicious, panicky, violent • raised blood pressure • insomnia	• permanently stuffy nose (if snorted) and risk of perforated nasal septum • brief euphoric effect followed by "crash"—depression • anesthetic effect can depress brain function • bizarre, erratic, perhaps violent actions • paranoid "psychosis" (disappears if drug is discontinued) • sensation of "crawling under the skin" • convulsions, disturbed heart action, even death	• anxiety, panic attacks, paranoid delusions, occasionally psychosis (like schizophrenia) • injury or accidents because of drug-induced delusions or distance misjudgment • increased risk of fetal abnormalities • Tolerance develops rapidly but also disappears fast with renewed drug sensitivity. • with PCP, high fever, muscle spasm, erratic behavior, psychosis lasting weeks or more
Long-Term Effects (prolonged repeated use)	• harms many body organs—pancreas, heart, liver, kidney, brain—and GI tract, blood circulation, • may produce liver cirrhosis, ulcers, memory loss, impotence • increased risk of cancers (mouth, larynx, throat, maybe breast) • depletes vitamins • damages offspring • dependence	• malnutrition, emaciation (owing to appetite loss) • anxiety states • "amphetamine-psychosis" (with schizophrenia-like hallucinations) • kidney damage • susceptibility to infection • sleep disorders • psychological dependence	• weight loss, malnutrition • destroyed nose tissues (if sniffed) • restlessness, mood swings, insomnia, extreme excitability, suspiciousness/paranoia, delusions ("psychosis") • depression • impotence • risk of heart attacks • strong psychological dependence	• long-term medical effects not known • may include muscle tenseness or "flashbacks"—brief, spontaneous recurrence of prior LSD (hallucinogenic) experiences • prolonged, profound depression • panic attacks • psychological dependence
Withdrawal Symptoms	• insomnia, headache • nausea • shakiness, tremors • sweating, seizures	• long sleep, chills • ravenous hunger • depression	• little or no withdrawal sickness; sleepiness • extreme exhaustion • possibly "cocaine blues" (depression)	• few withdrawal effects, possible "flashbacks," anxiety

Adapted from *Health News* (May 1990).

Nicotine	Caffeine	Cannabis (marijuana, "pot," "grass," hashish)	Narcotic (opioid) Analgesics (painkillers)	Solvents (Inhalants)
• derived from tobacco • used medicinally in South America • Tobacco smoke contains 4,000 chemicals, but nicotine is the most addictive. • A typical Canadian cigarette contains one mg nicotine, but amount absorbed varies with smoker. • CNS stimulant	• derived from tea, coffee beans, kola nuts, chocolate • used in many medicines (e.g., with painkillers, cold/cough, pain remedies, antihistamines) • Average cup of coffee contains 60–75 mg caffeine, colas about 35 mg (per 250 ml). • CNS stimulant	• derived from *cannabis sativa*, or hemp plant; preparations vary in potency; "hash" most potent, marijuana least • smoked in "joints" or chewed (sometimes with food) • medicinally used for epilepsy, glaucoma, against nausea • classed as hallucinogen	• poppy derivatives (opium, codeine, morphine, heroin) and synthetics (Demerol, Methadone, Dilaudid, Percodan) • smoked, eaten, or injected • ancient painkillers used medicinally • deaden pain, produce euphoria and drowsiness	• volatile organic hydrocarbons from petroleum and natural gas (e.g., gasoline, toluene, hexane, chloroform, carbon tetrachloride, nail polish remover or acetone, lighter fluid, paint thinners, cleaning fluid, airplane cement, plastic glue) • hallucinogenic effects
• increased pulse • increased, then reduced brain and nervous system activity • increased blood pressure • sense of relaxation • reduced urine output • impaired cleansing action of lung's cilia (hairs)	• stimulates brain, speeds nerve-cell transmission • elevated mood and alertness • stimulated mental activity • enhanced mental performance • reduced fatigue • shortened sleep • more urine output • increased stomach acidity • decreased appetite	• dreamlike euphoria, laughter, relaxation • altered sense of space, time • increased heart rate • reddened eyes • dreamy, "stoned" look • at later stages, users are quiet, reflective, sleepy. • combined with alcohol, increased effects, distorted behavior • impaired short-term memory, thinking, and ability to drive car or perform complex tasks	• briefly stimulated, then depressed higher brain centers • quick pleasure surge (for few minutes) then stupor (which mutes hunger, pain, sex drive) • taken by mouth, effects slower, no initial pleasure surge • pupils tiny, body warm, limbs heavy • dry mouth, itchy skin • users may "nod" off, alternately awake or asleep, oblivious to surroundings	• exhilaration, lightheadedness, excitability, disorientation • confusion, slurred speech, dizziness • distorted perception • visual and auditory hallucinations • impaired muscular control • possible nausea, increased saliva, sneezing • dampened reflexes • recklessness, feelings of power, invincibility
• lung damage • damaged blood circulation • slowed wound-healing • vitamin C depletion • shortness of breath • more upper respiratory infections • cancer-formation risks	• nervousness, hand tremors • delayed sleep onset, reduces "depth" of sleep, insomnia • abnormally rapid heartbeat • jitteriness • mild delirium possible • convulsions (rare)	• slowed digestive (gastrointestinal) activity • time misjudgment • sharpened or distorted sense of color, sound • slow and confused thinking • apathy, loss of motivation/drive • large doses can produce severe confusion, panic attacks. • hallucinations (even psychosis)	• heavy extremities • permanent drowsiness • pinpoint pupils • cold, moist, bluish skin • progressively slower breathing • depressed breathing • dangers increase with alcohol intake	• drowsiness and possible unconsciousness • severe disorientation • risks increase with fume concentration. • irregular heartbeat, heart action disturbed • large doses may cause heart failure (e.g., "sudden sniffing death" especially with spot removers or airplane cement)
• narrowed blood vessels, risk of heart attack, stroke • bronchitis, emphysema • raised risk of cancers of mouth, lung, larynx, throat, bladder, pancreas, possibly cervix • stomach ulcers • impairs fetal growth • strong dependence	• risk of stomach ulcers • possible damage to unborn baby • regular coffee use (more than 5 cups daily) can lead to dependence	• loss of drive, reduced energy • regular use increases risk of — bronchitis, lung cancer — reduced sex hormones — impaired learning — memory loss • decrease in immunity • psychological dependence	• constipation • moodiness • risk of endocarditis (heart infection) and other infections (AIDS) from needle sharing • hormone upsets (menstrual irregularities) • liver damage • damaged offspring • strong dependence	• pallor; thirst; nose, eye, or mouth sores • irritability, hostility, forgetfulness • may damage liver, kidney, and brain • nosebleeds, impaired blood-cell formation • depression, weight loss • other drugs compound damage • dependence possible
• anxiety, jitteriness • inability to concentrate • increased appetite	• severe headache • irritability • tiredness	• possible nausea, insomnia, anxiety, irritability	• striking withdrawal effects (4–5 hours after last dose): sweating, anxiety, diarrhea, "gooseflesh," shivering, tremors	• restlessness, anxiety, irritability, headaches • stomach upsets • delirium (rare)

drugs are not standardized. No watchdog agency, such as the Food and Drug Administration, screens illegal drugs for safety, purity, or concentration. Substances provided by an illicit source are of unpredictable composition, and they vary from batch to batch. Illegal drug sales provide a profit at each level of sale, so sellers tend to mix them liberally with extenders. For example, "consumer quality" cocaine is expected to contain some quantity of white powder other than pure cocaine, usually talcum powder or sugar lactose. However, some sellers of cocaine maximize profits by adding sugar then masking the weakened effect with cheaper drugs such as amphetamines, caffeine, or anesthetics that mimic some of cocaine's effects. Additionally, many illegal drugs are manufactured in

filthy basements and may contain rat droppings and other unsanitary products. As great a danger as the drugs themselves may pose to the users, greater still may be the dangers from unknown substances they contain.

Another important issue related to drug use is the **synergistic effect.** If you are taking any kind of medication—even over-the-counter drugs such as a cold medicine—you could get into serious trouble if you drink. Alcohol blocks the actions of some drugs and vastly increases the effects of many others, resulting in something similar to a severe overdose. We cannot list all the drugs here, but be especially cautious if you are taking any of the following:

- Pain pills, both narcotic (e.g., Darvon) and non-narcotic (e.g., aspirin),
- Over-the-counter cold medication,
- Antihistamines for colds or allergies,
- Antibiotics,
- Sleeping pills,
- Diet pills,
- Tranquilizers, or
- Medication for depression.

Alcohol also can have serious, even fatal, consequences if you drink while you are taking the medications commonly prescribed for high blood pressure, water retention, epilepsy, diabetes, hemophilia, or heart disease. To be safe, abstain from alcohol completely when taking medications. If you don't, talk to your doctor or pharmacist about possible drug-alcohol interactions before you have a drink.

THE MISERY OF DRUG ADDICTION

We drank for happiness
And became unhappy.
We drank for joy
And became miserable.
We drank for sociability
And became argumentative.
We drank for friendship
And made enemies.
We drank for sleep
And awakened without rest.
We drank for strength
And felt weak.
We drank "medicinally"
And acquired health problems.
We drank for relaxation
And got the shakes.
We drank for bravery
And became afraid.
We drank to make conversation easier
And slurred our speech.
We drank to feel heavenly
And ended up feeling like hell.
We drank to forget
And were forever haunted.
We drank for freedom
And became slaves.
We drank to erase problems
And saw them multiply.
We drank to cope with life
And invited death.

Source: An AA poem from **Professional Counselor** (December 1993).

OVERCOMING TOBACCO ADDICTION

If a person quits using tobacco, the benefits start almost immediately, and 15 years after quitting smoking, that

STRATEGIES FOR DEALING WITH WHY YOU SMOKE

	Why You Smoke	Substitutes
Stimulation	You smoke to keep from slowing down, for a lift, to pep you up.	Find something else to pep you up—a hobby, brisk walks, simple exercises.
Handling	You like the ritual of smoking and having something in your hands and mouth.	Pick something else to handle: coins, pen or pencil, "worry beads"; try doodling or chew on paper straws or minted toothpicks.
Relaxation	You enjoy smoking; it's a reward, a time you feel good about yourself.	Consider the harm cigarettes cause you and the reward of quitting. Substitute social or physical activity; prove self-control and feel good about yourself.
Crutch	You smoke to deal with problems and negative feelings.	Prove to yourself smoking doesn't solve problems. Reduce tension other ways: Take deep breaths, call a friend, talk over feelings. Work on keeping your "cool."
Craving	You feel "hooked" and begin to think of the next cigarette before you put out the present one. You're aware of the need to smoke.	Recognize that quitting will be difficult and prepare to see it through. Plan to try to stop cold turkey, abstaining completely. The day before quitting, smoke to the point of distaste.
Habit	You smoke automatically, often without realizing what you're doing.	Become aware of every cigarette you smoke and ask yourself why you're smoking and if you really want it. Wrap up your cigarettes or put them in a place difficult to access.

person's risk of death and disease will be no higher than if they had never smoked at all (assuming the person is not already ill when they quit). The risk of dying of heart attack is cut in half after only 1 year of not smoking. Some think that nothing else a person can do for health can have such immediate, far-reaching dividends as quitting smoking.

PRODUCTS TO HELP YOU QUIT SMOKING

The Food and Drug Administration has approved Nicotrol NS, a nicotine spray. This product is projected to be a big help to smokers in general and to heavier smokers in particular.

Nicotine gum (available over-the-counter) and nicotine patches (available by prescription) have been on the market for several years.

The advantage of the spray over the gum and patch is that the nicotine reaches the bloodstream faster. This means the spray provides more immediate relief from nicotine cravings. One squirt up each nostril equals 1 mg of nicotine.

Source: McNeil Consumer Products.

It is extremely difficult to quit smoking. A smoker not only must overcome the addiction to nicotine but also must break the habit of reaching for a cigarette at certain times. Further, nicotine withdrawal can be unpleasant, causing nausea, vomiting, restlessness, irritability, and an intense craving for tobacco.

No one method of quitting works for everyone. Your reasons for smoking and your habits are unique to you. So are your life circumstances. Some suggest that if you are severely depressed, going through a major life crisis, or having severe emotional problems, you should reduce the number of cigarettes you smoke instead of quitting completely until the problem is resolved. If you smoke two or more packs of cigarettes a day, you might do better by first trying to cut down the number of cigarettes you smoke, then gradually stopping the habit completely.

Some of the following techniques or suggestions may help in smoking cessation:

- There are no safe cigarettes and there is no safe way to smoke. While you are quitting, though, choose a brand lower in tar and nicotine than the brand you use now, smoke fewer

Synergistic effect A phenomenon in which the effects of using more than one drug simultaneously are different and greater than using any of the drugs alone.

QUIT SMOKING IN SIX STEPS

The following six-step plan has been developed as a guide to help you quit smoking. The total program should be completed in 4 weeks or less. Steps 1 through 4 should take no longer than 2 weeks. A maximum of 2 additional weeks are allowed for the rest of the program.

Step One   Decide positively that you want to quit. Prepare a list of the reasons you smoke and why you want to quit.

Step Two   Initiate a personal diet and exercise program. Exercise and reduced body weight create more awareness of healthy living and increase motivation for giving up cigarettes.

Step Three   Decide what approach you will use to stop smoking. You may quit cold turkey or gradually decrease the number of cigarettes you smoke daily. Many people have found that quitting cold turkey is the easiest way to do it. Although it may not work the first time, after several attempts all of a sudden smokers are able to overcome the habit without too much difficulty. Tapering off cigarettes can be done in several ways. You may start by eliminating cigarettes you do not necessarily need, switch to a brand lower in nicotine or tar every couple of days, smoke less of each cigarette, or simply cut down the total number of cigarettes you smoke each day.

Step Four   Set the target date for quitting. In choosing the target date, a special date may add a little extra incentive. An upcoming birthday, anniversary, vacation, graduation, family reunion—all are examples of good dates to free yourself from smoking.

Step Five   Stock up on low-calorie foods—carrots, broccoli, cauliflower, celery, popcorn (butter- and salt-free), fruits, sunflower seeds (in the shell), sugarless gum, and plenty of water. Keep such food handy on the day you stop and the first few days following cessation. Replace this food for cigarettes when you want one.

Step Six   This is the day you will quit smoking. On this day and the first few days thereafter, do not keep cigarettes handy. Stay away from friends and events that trigger your desire to smoke. Drink large amounts of water and fruit juices and eat low-calorie foods. Replace smoking time with new, positive substitutes that will make smoking difficult or impossible. When you desire a cigarette, take a few deep breaths and then occupy yourself by talking to someone else, washing your hands, brushing your teeth, eating a healthy snack, chewing on a straw, doing dishes, playing sports, going for a walk or bike ride, going swimming, and so on.

If you have been successful and stopped smoking, a lot of events can still trigger your urge to smoke. When confronted with such events, people rationalize and think, "One won't hurt." It will not work! Before you know it, you will be back to the regular nasty habit. Therefore, be prepared to take action in those situations. Find adequate substitutes for smoking. Remind yourself of how difficult it has been and how long it has taken you to get to this point. Keep in mind that it will only get easier rather than worse as time goes on.

From Werner W. K. Hoeger and Sharon A. Hoeger, **Fitness & Wellness**, 5th ed. (Belmont, CA: Thomson Learning, 2002). Used by permission.

cigarettes each day, inhale less deeply, and put out the cigarette after you've smoked only half of it.

- Set a goal. Determine a date when you want to quit smoking. Start now to quit, and tell those around you about it.
- Use an aid such as nicotine gum or a nicotine patch, which is applied to the skin and delivers a continuous flow of nicotine to the body 24 hours a day. The patch is used in decreasing strengths for 8 to 12 weeks, gradually weaning the user from nicotine. Possible side effects include dry mouth, nervousness, insomnia, and skin irritation where the patch is applied.
- Use relaxation techniques to help you overcome the urge to smoke and also to counteract the physical withdrawal symptoms and inability to sleep.

- Switch progressively to brands of cigarettes that have less and less nicotine. As your body's demand for nicotine diminishes, it will be easier to stop smoking without suffering difficult withdrawal symptoms.
- Change your brand of cigarettes. Buy a brand that doesn't taste good to you.
- Each time you resist smoking, put aside the money you would have spent on that pack of cigarettes. Keep it in a separate account. When you've succeeded in quitting, take a trip, buy a new stereo, or use the money for something you've always wanted.
- As you quit, you'll struggle with common withdrawal symptoms, such as irritability, headaches, dry mouth, hunger, constipation, and trouble going to sleep. Anticipate these symptoms and compensate for them.

SHORT-TERM BENEFITS OF SMOKING CESSATION

- For former smokers, the decline in risk of death compared with continuing smokers begins shortly after quitting.
- Smoking cessation halves the risks for cancers of the oral cavity and the esophagus, compared with continued smoking, as soon as 5 years after cessation, with further reduction over a longer period of abstinence.
- The risk of cervical cancer is substantially lower among former smokers in comparison with continuing smokers, even in the first few years after cessation.
- The excess risk of coronary heart disease (CHD) caused by smoking is reduced by about half after 1 year of smoking abstinence and then declines gradually.
- After smoking cessation, the risk of stroke returns to the level of lifetime nonsmokers; in some studies this has occurred within 5 years, but in others as long as 15 years of abstinence were required.
- For those without overt chronic obstructive pulmonary disease (COPD), smoking cessation improves pulmonary function about 5 percent within a few months after cessation.
- Pregnant smokers who stop smoking at any time up to the 30th week of gestation have infants with higher birth weight than do women who smoke throughout pregnancy. Quitting in the first 3 to 4 months of pregnancy and abstaining throughout the remainder of pregnancy protects the fetus from the adverse effects of smoking on birth weight.

Soak in a hot bath when you're feeling irritable or get a headache. Chew gum or sip fruit juice to moisten a dry mouth. To ease hunger, keep on hand plenty of low-fat, low-calorie snacks (such as raw fruits and vegetables or air-popped popcorn). Include plenty of fiber (such as whole-grain breads and cereals) in your diet.

- Have substitutes on hand for times when you want a cigarette. Chew sugarless gum, eat raw carrot sticks, suck on hard candy, or nibble on sunflower seeds.
- Avoid situations, people, and routines that have made it easy for you to smoke. If you always smoke after you eat a meal, for example, finish with a piece of fresh fruit instead, then swish out your mouth with a great-tasting mouthwash.
- Start a program of brisk exercise once a day.
- Many communities have smoking cessation programs and support groups. Consider joining a local group to get the support you need. Look in the yellow pages under "Smokers' Treatment," ask your physician to recommend a group, or call the local chapter of the American Cancer Society.

> "The only really stupid thing I did in my life was to start smoking."
> —Jack Ningana, actor, who had a vocal cord removed and now has a hoarse, strained voice.

OVERCOMING ALCOHOL ADDICTION

Alcoholism is a disease of addiction to alcohol. The sequence of symptoms in alcoholism are well defined. It typically progresses from the first drink, through increasing involvement with alcohol to a point where alcohol dominates the person's life, damaging family and relationships, work life, and physical health. Full-blown alcoholism typically takes from 3 to 10 years to develop after heavy drinking has begun. Problem drinking can often lead to alcoholism.

A key feature of alcoholism is denial: The person refuses to acknowledge it. As a result, a diagnosis made by someone else usually cannot lead to effective treatment, because the person with alcoholism will not cooperate. The best diagnosis for alcoholism, therefore, is self-diagnosis—which is why experts encourage the widespread use of self-tests, and why they emphasize certain symptoms that only the drinker can recognize. If you think you may have a drinking problem, here are some danger signs:

- You're preoccupied with drinking alcohol. You think about it or plan it even when you're not drinking.
- You drink to escape your problems or relieve stress.
- You need a drink to help you go to sleep.
- You need a drink to help you get going in the morning.
- You get drunk often or stay drunk several days at a time.
- You sneak drinks or drink alone.
- You make excuses for why you drink.
- You hide the amount you drink from your mate, children, friends.
- You gulp your drinks.
- You have had blackouts (periods during which you can't remember what happened).
- You've had frequent accidents because of drinking.
- You've been ill a lot because of drinking.

- You've missed work or school because of drinking.
- You've had financial or legal problems because of drinking.
- Your personality or behavior changes after you drink.
- Once you sober up, you regret the things you did while you were drinking.
- Other people tell you that you drink too much.
- You feel guilty about your drinking.
- You've tried to stop drinking but can't.
- You don't want to talk about the negative effects of drinking.

The causes of alcoholism are varied and not completely understood. Alcoholism appears to have a genetic component and also to be environmentally related. Why some people can drink socially for years without becoming addicted and others follow the downward spiral of alcoholism is not understood (Figure 13.4 describes the different fates of two drinkers).

Alcoholism is characterized by memory blackouts, which are episodes of temporary amnesia that occur after, not during, times when a person is drinking. During an event a person may function normally—not appear drunk and not pass out (a memory blackout in no way resembles passing out). Often people will not be able to tell that anything is wrong or even whether the drinker is drinking at the time. But afterward (typically the morning after), the drinker will remember nothing about the event. Blackouts are so striking that the discovery that one is having them is often enough to make a person quit drinking for life.

Alcoholism is not the addict's fault, but it is the addict's responsibility. If a person with alcoholism chooses to continue the addictive behavior, then that person alone should experience the negative consequences of their choices. Family members and friends should not cover up or fix problems the addict has caused (a response called "enabling"). Enabling is misguided helping that actually delays or fully hinders the alcohol addict from getting better.

Alcoholism is a complex problem that requires treatment. The first step is to break denial: The person has to admit they have a problem, take responsibility, and be willing to abstain from alcohol. Some people need to go to a treatment center, others are able to recover with the help of specific support groups such as Alcoholics Anonymous (AA). AA groups meet frequently in most communities.

AA programs are based on a 12-step program that begins with admitting there is a problem and, after healing and recovery, helping others with the disease. The 12-step program is very spiritual in nature and the most effective system for recovery.

Recovery from alcoholism is similar to recovery from any addiction. It involves two parts: first, learning to

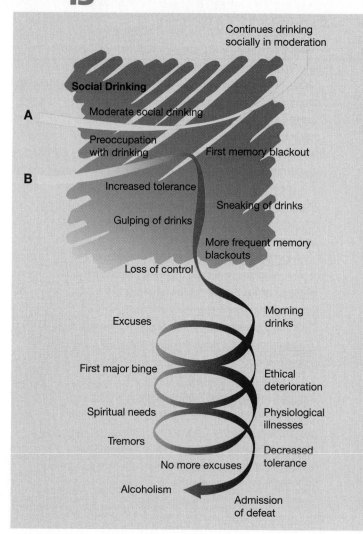

FIGURE 13.4 THE FATES OF TWO DRINKERS.

Continues drinking socially in moderation

Social Drinking

A — Moderate social drinking

Preoccupation with drinking

B — Increased tolerance

First memory blackout

Sneaking of drinks

Gulping of drinks

More frequent memory blackouts

Loss of control

Excuses

Morning drinks

First major binge

Ethical deterioration

Spiritual needs

Physiological illnesses

Tremors

Decreased tolerance

No more excuses

Alcoholism

Admission of defeat

abstain from the substance, and second, overcoming the problems that contributed to the addiction as well as the problems the addiction caused.

How to Drink and How to Refuse

Those who choose to drink need to learn to handle drinking responsibly. Those who choose to abstain may need to learn to do so gracefully.

Those who succeed in drinking moderately drink at appropriate times and in appropriate settings only. They limit their intake, and they prefer being in control. They acknowledge that they have responsibility not to damage themselves or society, and they know that being intoxicated is irresponsible drinking behavior.[35] Among the skills they report to be useful are the following:

"I get together with my friends and we decide ahead of time who will drive us home. The designated driver agrees not to drink at all at the party."

TYPICAL 12-STEP PROGRAM

1. We admitted we were powerless over the obsession or compulsion (such as drinking alcohol, using other drugs, gambling, overworking, overexercising, overeating, or excessively depending on other people)—that our lives had become unmanageable.
2. We came to believe that a power greater than ourselves could restore us to sanity.
3. We made a decision to turn our will and our lives over to the care of God as we understood Him.
4. We made a searching and fearless moral inventory of ourselves.
5. We admitted to God, to ourselves, and to another human being the exact nature of our wrongs.
6. We were entirely ready to have God remove all these defects of character.
7. We humbly asked Him to remove our shortcomings.
8. We made a list of all the persons we had harmed and became willing to make amends to them all.
9. We made direct amends to such people wherever possible, except when doing so would hurt them or others.
10. We continued to take personal inventory, and when we were wrong, promptly admitted it.
11. We sought through prayer and meditation to improve our conscious contact with God as we understood Him, praying only for knowledge of His will for us and the power to carry that out.
12. Having had a spiritual awakening as the result of these steps, we tried to carry this message to other people who suffer from the same compulsions and to practice these principles in all our affairs.

"I decide in advance how much I'm going to drink. I decide on 2 drinks and then I drink non-alcohol beverages."

"If they're serving beer by the pitcher, I still order it by the glass. Ordering beer by the pitcher tends to double a drinker's intake."

"I eat before and during a party, and then I drink slowly."

"I allow time to metabolize the alcohol I've drunk before I drive home."

"I sip my drinks; I add ice cubes or water; and if I'm thirsty, I drink water."

"I use fruit juices for mixers. They meet my calorie need and keep my blood sugar up."

"When I want dessert, I eat ice cream. A piña colada has too many calories."

"I don't accept drinks I don't want."

"I go slowly with unfamiliar drinks."

"I know my capacity and I don't exceed it."

Many people choose to not drink at all. They have the ability to socialize without alcohol, and they don't want to risk becoming addicted or experiencing any other negative effects of alcohol use. Sometimes drinkers pressure others to drink alcohol, and refusing can be challenging. People who abstained successfully have mastered many social skills to resist social pressure to drink.

Abstaining from alcohol or using it responsibly in moderation are the only two healthy alternatives. Excessive alcohol consumption results in short-term and

STRATEGIES: REFUSING A DRINK

To refuse an unwanted drink gracefully:

1. **Don't apologize.** It may take guts to say, "No, thanks." Say it calmly, casually, firmly. Keep it brief; don't give excuses, explanations, or arguments. A discussion period is a good time for explanations; a party is not.
2. **Expect others to respect your choice.** When you're confident of your own choice, you will take it for granted that your "No, thanks" will receive respect from others. Your firm manner will make your confidence clear to them, and respect is what you'll get. But if you're hesitant, you pave the way for others to tease or argue; they think you really want them to persuade you to accept.
3. **Respect the drinker's choice to drink.** Give the person who drinks the same acceptance you want to receive. If you don't—if you sneer or argue or shake your head sadly—you're backing the person into a corner. People who are cornered have to fight their way out; probably the person will try to embarrass you for your decision not to drink.
4. **Consider another group of friends.** If you continue to receive pressure to drink from those who are drinking, even after trying the above suggestions, consider developing other friendships. Those who push alcohol on nondrinkers are using alcohol irresponsibly, and they often are problem drinkers, uncomfortable if those around them are not drinking. If they base the friendship on your drinking behavior, you may benefit from looking elsewhere for quality friendships.

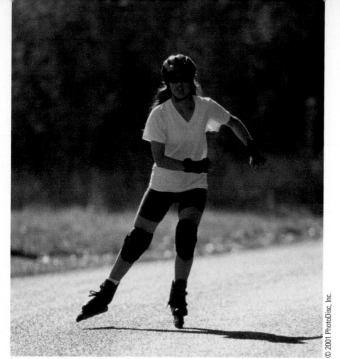

Life without the substance may be better.

long-term risks to health, family life, and society. Few addicts who attempt recovery make it all the way. This is why health professionals recommend never using drugs, including alcohol. Most people with addictions get caught in something like a revolving door: undergoing treatment, giving up the drug, getting out of treatment, taking the drug again, going back into treatment—and so on indefinitely. Consider drug-free alternatives. Being able to enjoy life without artificial highs is truly satisfying.

FINDING DRUG-FREE HIGHS

Pleasure is there for the taking, for those who know where to look. To get high, try any of the following:

1. Run, walk, or skip across an open field, through a park, or along a beach.
2. Ask one of your grandparents what life is about.
3. Play with a baby.
4. Give a friend a gift that you made with your own hands.
5. Get involved in worthwhile activities with groups in which you feel you are contributing and are needed.
6. Work hard at something and see it through to completion.
7. Have a good cry about that thing you have been hiding from for too long.
8. Learn to meditate.
9. Eat nourishing food.
10. Write some poetry for yourself (it doesn't have to rhyme).
11. Climb a mountain.
12. Visit a river.
13. Say "thank you" more often.
14. Beat the feathers out of a pillow next time you are very angry.
15. Stop biting your nails (or shed another bad habit).
16. Read a good book.
17. Give someone a long hug.
18. Call your parents and say, "I love you."

Source: Partially inspired by S. J. Levy, **Managing the Drugs in Your Life** (New York: McGraw-Hill, 1983): 104.

WEB INTERACTIVE.

WEB ACTIVITIES

■ **National Institute of Drug Abuse** This site, sponsored by the National Institutes of Health, provides information on a variety of abused drugs, research, and current events. The site features research on addictions and a link to additional information on club drugs and steroids.
http://www.nida.nih.gov

■ **Web of Addictions** This site features comprehensive and factual information on a variety of addictions, including alcohol and other drug abuse.
http://www.well.com/user/woa

■ **Truth: The Facts About Tobacco** This is a fun, creative site on tobacco education, designed for teens and young adults.
http://www.wholetruth.com/asp/truth/truth.asp

■ **The College Alcohol Study: Harvard University School of Public Health** This site describes the ongoing survey (1993, 1997, 1999, 2000, 2001) of over 15,000 students at 140 four-year colleges in 40 states. The CAS examines high-risk behaviors among college students, such as binge drinking, smoking, illicit drug use, violence, and other behavioral, social, and health problems. The principal investigator is Henry Wechsler, Ph.D.
http://www.hsph.harvard.edu/cas

- **Club Drugs** Information from the National Institute of Drug Abuse features factual information concerning these drugs: alcohol, LSD (acid), MDMA (ecstasy), GHB, GBL, ketamine (Special-K), Fentanyl, Rohypnol, amphetamines, and methamphetamine.
  http://www.nida.nih.gov/drugpages/clubdrugs.html

- **Drugs of Abuse Table** This site is arranged by drug classification. Information from the National Clearinghouse for Alcohol and Drug Information features factual information regarding descriptions, effects, symptoms of overdose, withdrawal symptoms, and indications of misuse.
  http://www.health.org/pubs/catalog/RP0s.htm

InfoTrac

You can find additional readings related to wellness via InfoTrac College Edition, an on-line library of more than 900 journals and publications. Follow the instructions for accessing InfoTrac that came packaged with your textbook, then search for articles using a key word search.

Suggested Reading Henry Wechsler, Ph.D., M.D. and Meichun Kuo, "College Students Define Binge Drinking and Estimate Its Prevalence: Results of a National Survey," *Journal of American College Health* 49, no. 2 (Sept. 2000): 57.

1. According to the results of this study, what major factor tends to shape the drinking habits of college students?
2. How do social norms programs at colleges and universities promote responsible use of alcohol and other drugs?
3. Define the term "binge drinker." Which students on campus are more likely to be binge drinkers?

Web Activity

Facts On Tap: Alcohol and Your College Experience:
http://www.factsontap.org

Sponsor The Children of Alcoholics Foundation and the American Council for Drug Education, two of the nation's leaders in substance abuse prevention education. The major funding sponsor is the Metropolitan Life Foundation.

Description This colorful and interactive Web site features a variety of activities and straightforward information written specifically for college students. Some of the topics include alcohol and the college experience, the effects of alcohol on the non-drinker, alcohol and the family, and a true/false quiz to test your knowledge about alcohol and its effects.

Available Activities Among the many informative links are three interactive activities to explore.
1. Under the "Alcohol and the College Experience" link is a quiz to reveal whether you have a problem with alcohol.
2. Another quiz to help you figure out if your relationship depends too heavily on alcohol is located under the "Risky Relationships" link.
3. A true/false quiz designed to test your alcohol knowledge is located under the "Naked Truth" link.

Web Work

1. From the home page, first click on the "College Experience" site to learn sobering statistics about the use of alcohol among college students, tips to help you cut down on or stop using alcohol, common misconceptions and the real truth, resources to go to for help, as well as a test to reveal if you have a problem with alcohol. Return to the home page.
2. Click on the link to take the short quiz to help you figure out if your relationship depends too heavily on alcohol.
3. From the home page, click on "The Naked Truth" link to go to a site that features a true/false quiz designed to test your alcohol knowledge. The site also includes information on how to determine your blood alcohol level and how your behavior changes as your blood alcohol level increases.
4. The "Non-Alcoholic Hangover" link features stories from students who were affected by someone else's drinking, as well as information on how to help a friend whose drinking is out of control.

Helpful Hint

1. There are also resources for college students, college staff, as well as links to college health centers that sponsor model alcohol education programs.

For additional Web activities, links, and suggested readings, visit our Health, Fitness, and Wellness Resource Center at http://health.wadsworth.com.

NOTES

1. J. R. Cornelius et al., "Cocaine Use Associated with Increased Suicidal Behavior in Depressed Alcoholics," *Addictive Behaviors* 23 (1998): 119–121.

2. G. M. Barnes et al., "Gambling and Alcohol Use Among Youth: Influences of Demographic, Socialization, and Individual Factors," *Addictive Behaviors* 24 (1999): 749–767.

3. J. R. Young, "Students Are Unusually Vulnerable to Internet Addiction, Article Says," *The Chronicle of Higher Education* 44 (1998): A25.

4. G. A. Marlatt, "Harm Reduction: Come As You Are," *Addictive Behaviors* 21 (1996): 779–788.

5. J. D. Kassel, "Generalized Expectancies for Negative Mood Regulation and Problem Drinking Among College Students," *Journal of Studies on Alcohol* 61 (2000): 332–337.

6. C. Nakken, *The Addictive Personality: Understanding Compulsion in Our Lives* (San Francisco: Harper & Row, 1988).

7. K. S. Young, "Addictive Use of the Internet: A Case That Breaks the Stereotype," *Psychological Reports* 79 (1996): 899–902.

8. D. W. Black et al., "Characteristics of 36 Subjects Reporting Compulsive Sexual Behavior," *American Journal of Psychiatry* 154 (1997): 243–249.

9. L. Kann et al., "Youth Risk Behavior Surveillance—United States, 1997," *Journal of School Health* 68 (1998): 355–362.

10. U.S. Centers for Disease Control and Prevention, "Tobacco Use—United States, 1900–1999," *The Journal of the American Medical Association* 282 (1999): 2202–2204.

11. D. Giacopassi et al., "University Students' Perceptions of Tobacco, Cocaine, and Homicide Fatalities," *The American Journal of Drug and Alcohol Abuse* 25 (1999): 163–172.

12. D. Kandel et al., "Stages of Progression in Drug Involvement from Adolescence to Adulthood: Further Evidence for Gateway Theory," *Journal of Studies on Alcohol* 53 (1992): 447–457.

13. S. D. Winnail et al., "Relationship Between Physical Activity Level and Cigarette, Smokeless Tobacco, and Marijuana Use Among High School Adolescents," *Journal of School Health* 65 (1995): 438–442.

14. G. B. Lindsay et al., "Psychosocial and Pharmacologic Explanations of Nicotine's Gateway Drug Function," *Journal of School Health* 67 (1997): 123–127.

15. L. G. Escobedo et al., "Relationship Between Cigarette Smoking and Health Risk and Problem Behaviors Among U.S. Adolescents," *Archives of Pediatric and Adolescent Medicine* 151 (1997): 66–72.

16. V. Burke et al., "Clustering of Health-related Behaviors Among 18-year-old Australians," *Preventive Medicine* 26 (1997): 724–733.

17. A. B. Bruner et al., "Adolescents and Illicit Drug Use," *Journal of the American Medical Association* 280 (1998): 597–599.

18. J. D. Fortenberry, "Number of Sexual Partners and Health Lifestyle of Adolescents: Use of the AMA Guidelines for Adolescent Preventive Services to Address a Basic Research Question," *Archives of Pediatrics and Adolescent Medicine* 151 (1997): 1139–1141.

19. R. F. Valois et al., "Number of Sexual Intercourse Partners and Associated Risk Behaviors Among Public High School Adolescents," *Journal of Sex Education and Sex Therapy* 22 (1997): 13–22.

20. N. D. Brener et al., "Co-occurrence of Health Risk Behaviors Among Adolescents in the United States," *Journal of Adolescent Health* 22 (1998): 209–213.

21. L. Chassin et al., "Drinking During Adolescence," *Alcohol Health & Research World* 20 (1996): 175–181.

22. T. J. Johnson, J. Wendel, and S. Hamilton, "Social Anxiety, Alcohol Expectancies, and Drinking-Game Participation," *Addictive Behaviors* 23 (1998): 65–79.

23. L. Schonfeld and L. W. Dupree, "Antecedents of Drinking for Early and Late-Onset Elderly Alcohol Abusers," *Journal of Studies on Alcohol* 52 (1991): 587–592.

24. J. Wechsler, "College Binge Drinking in the 1990s: A Continuing Problem: Results of the Harvard School of Public Health 1999 College Alcohol Survey," *Journal of American College Health* 48 (2000): 199–210

25. R. C. Engs and D. J. Hanson, "Drinking Games and Problems Related to Drinking among Moderate and Heavy Drinkers," *Psychological Reports* 73 (1993): 115–120.

26. See note 23.

27. D. Kandel et al., "From Beer to Crack: Developmental Patterns of Drug Involvement," *American Journal of Public Health* 83 (1993): 851–855.

28. R. H. Durant et al., "The Relationship Between Early Age of Onset of Initial Substance Use and Engaging in Multiple Health Risk Behaviors Among Young Adolescents," *Archives of Pediatrics and Adolescent Medicine* 153 (1999): 286–300.

29. M. Durbin et al., "Factors Associated with Multiple Sex Partners Among Junior High School Students," *Adolescent Health* 14 (1993): 202–207.

30. S. R. Gambert, "Alcohol Abuse: Medical Effects of Heavy Drinking in Late Life," *Geriatrics* 52 (1997): 30–36.

31. M. A. Ichiyama, "The Social Context of Binge Drinking among Private University Freshmen," *Journal of Alcohol and Drug Education* 44 (1998): 18–33.

32. J. G. Bachman, "Explaining Recent Increases in Students Marijuana Use: Impacts of Perceived Risks and Disapproval, 1976 Through 1996," *Journal of the American Medical Association* 280 (1998): 1122–1125.

33. See note 17.

34. See note 17.

35. R. C. Engs, 1989, "Responsibility and Alcohol: Teaching Responsible Decisions about Alcohol and Its Use for Those Who Choose to Drink," *Health Education* (January/February 1989): 20–22.

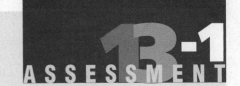

Name: _____ Date: _____ Grade: _____

Instructor: _____ Course: _____ Section: _____

The following questions were written by recovering addicts in Narcotics Anonymous.

	Yes	No
1. Do you ever use alone?		
2. Have you ever substituted one drug for another, thinking that one particular drug was the problem?		
3. Have you ever manipulated or lied to a doctor to obtain prescription drugs?		
4. Have you ever stolen drugs or stolen to obtain drugs?		
5. Do you regularly use a drug when you wake up or when you go to bed?		
6. Have you ever taken one drug to overcome the effects of another?		
7. Do you avoid people or places that do not approve of you using drugs?		
8. Have you ever used a drug without knowing what it was or what it would do to you?		
9. Has your job or school performance ever suffered from the effects of your drug use?		
10. Have you ever been arrested as a result of using drugs?		
11. Have you ever lied about what or how much you use?		
12. Do you put the purchase of drugs ahead of your financial responsibilities?		
13. Have you ever tried to stop or control your using?		
14. Have you ever been in a jail, hospital, or drug rehabilitation center because of your using?		
15. Does using interfere with your sleeping or eating?		
16. Does the thought of running out of drugs terrify you?		
17. Do you feel it is impossible for you to live without drugs?		
18. Do you ever question your own sanity?		
19. Is your drug use making life at home unhappy?		
20. Have you ever thought you couldn't fit in or have a good time without using drugs?		
21. Have you ever felt defensive, guilty, or ashamed about your using?		
22. Do you think a lot about drugs?		

23. Have you had irrational or indefinable fears?

24. Has using affected your sexual relationships?

25. Have you ever taken drugs you didn't prefer?

26. Have you ever used drugs because of emotional pain or stress?

27. Have you ever overdosed on any drugs?

28. Do you continue to use despite negative consequences?

29. Do you think you might have a drug problem?

Are you an addict? This is a question only you can answer. Members of Narcotics Anonymous found that they all answered different numbers of these questions "yes." The actual number of *yes* responses isn't as important as how you feel inside and how addiction has affected your life. If you are an addict, you must first admit that you have a problem with drugs before any progress can be made toward recovery.

NICOTINE DEPENDENCE: ARE YOU HOOKED?

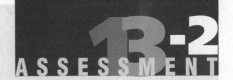

Name: _____   Date: _____   Grade: _____

Instructor: _____   Course: _____   Section: _____

Answer each question in the list below, giving yourself the appropriate points.

		0 points	1 point	2 points
☐	1. How soon after you wake up do you smoke your first cigarette?	After 30 minutes	Within 30 minutes	—
☐	2. Do you find it difficult to refrain from smoking in places where it is forbidden, such as the library, theater, doctor's office?	No	Yes	—
☐	3. Which of all the cigarettes you smoke in a day is the most satisfying?	Any other than the first one in the morning	The first one in the morning	—
☐	4. How many cigarettes a day do you smoke?	1–15	16–25	26+
☐	5. Do you smoke more during the morning than during the rest of the day?	No	Yes	—
☐	6. Do you smoke when you are so ill that you are in bed most of the day?	No	Yes	—
☐	7. Does the brand you smoke have a low, medium, or high nicotine content?	Low	Medium	High
☐	8. How often do you inhale the smoke?	Never	Sometimes	Always

☐ Total

SCORING

- More than 6 points—very dependent
- Less than 6 points—low-to-moderate dependence.

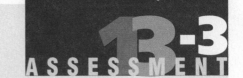

WHY DO YOU SMOKE?

Name: _____ Date: _____ Grade: _____

Instructor: _____ Course: _____ Section: _____

	Always	Fre-quently	Occa-sionally	Seldom	Never
A. I smoke cigarettes in order to keep myself from slowing down.	5	4	3	2	1
B. Handling a cigarette is part of the enjoyment of smoking it.	5	4	3	2	1
C. Smoking cigarettes is pleasant and relaxing.	5	4	3	2	1
D. I light up a cigarette when I feel angry about something.	5	4	3	2	1
E. When I have run out of cigarettes, I find it almost unbearable until I can get them.	5	4	3	2	1
F. I smoke cigarettes automatically without even being aware of it.	5	4	3	2	1
G. I smoke cigarettes to stimulate me, to perk myself up.	5	4	3	2	1
H. Part of the enjoyment of smoking a cigarette comes from the steps I take to light up.	5	4	3	2	1
I. I find cigarettes pleasurable.	5	4	3	2	1
J. When I feel uncomfortable or upset about something, I light up a cigarette.	5	4	3	2	1
K. I am very much aware of the fact when I am not smoking a cigarette.	5	4	3	2	1
L. I light up a cigarette without realizing I still have one burning in the ashtray.	5	4	3	2	1
M. I smoke cigarettes to give me a "lift."	5	4	3	2	1
N. When I smoke a cigarette, part of the enjoyment is watching the smoke as I exhale it.	5	4	3	2	1
O. I want a cigarette most when I am comfortable and relaxed.	5	4	3	2	1
P. When I feel "blue" or want to take my mind off cares and worries, I smoke cigarettes.	5	4	3	2	1
Q. I get a real gnawing hunger for a cigarette when I haven't smoked for a while.	5	4	3	2	1
R. I've found a cigarette in my mouth and didn't remember putting it there.	5	4	3	2	1

Scoring Your Test:

Enter the numbers you have circled on the test questions in the spaces provided below, putting the number you have circled to question A on line A, to question B on line B, and so on. Add the three scores on each line to get a total for each factor. For example, the sum of your scores on lines A, G, and M gives you your score on "Stimulation,"; lines B, H, and N give the score on "Handling"; and so on. Scores can vary from 3 to 15. Any score 11 and above is high; any score 7 and below is low.

A		+ G		+ M		=		Stimulation
B		+ H		+ N		=		Handling
C		+ I		+ O		=		Pleasure / Relaxation
D		+ J		+ P		=		Crutch: Tension Reduction
E		+ K		+ Q		=		Craving: Psychological Addiction
F		+ L		+ R		=		Habit

A score of 11 or above on any factor indicates that smoking is an important source of satisfaction for you. The higher you score (15 is the highest), the more important a given factor is in your smoking. See page 343 for strategies for dealing with why you smoke.

From *A Self-Test for Smokers* (U.S. Department of Health and Human Services, 1983).

DO YOU HAVE A PROBLEM WITH ALCOHOL?

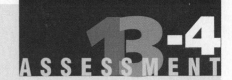

Name: _____ Date: _____ Grade: _____

Instructor: _____ Course: _____ Section: _____

Instructions

To determine if you have a problem with alcohol, answer yes (Y) or no (N) to the following questions about your drinking behavior. Refer to the scale at the end of the quiz for evaluation of your answers.

1. Do you occasionally drink heavily after a disappointment or a quarrel or when your parents or boss gives you a hard time?

2. When you have trouble or feel pressured at school or at work, do you always drink more heavily than usual?

3. Have you noticed that you are able to handle more liquor than you did when you were first drinking?

4. Did you ever wake up the "morning after" and discover that you could not remember part of the evening before, even though your friends tell you that you did not pass out?

5. When drinking with other people, do you try to have a few extra drinks that others don't notice?

6. Are there certain occasions when you feel uncomfortable if alcohol is not available?

7. Have you recently noticed that when you begin drinking, you are in more of a hurry to get the first drink than you used to be?

8. Do you sometimes feel a little guilty about your drinking?

9. Are you secretly irritated when your family or friends discuss your drinking?

10. Have you recently noticed an increase in the frequency of your memory blackouts?

11. Do you often find that you wish to continue drinking after your friends say they have had enough?

12. Do you usually have a reason for the occasions when you drink heavily?

13. When you are sober, do you often regret things you did or said while drinking?

14. Have you tried switching brands or following different plans for controlling your drinking?

15. Have you often failed to keep the promises you've made to yourself about controlling or cutting down on your drinking?

16. Have you ever tried to control your drinking by changing jobs or moving to a new location?

17. Do you try to avoid family or close friends while you are drinking?

18. Are you having an increasing number of financial and academic problems?

19. Do more people seem to treat you unfairly without good reason?

20. Do you eat very little or irregularly when you are drinking?

21. Do you sometimes have the shakes in the morning and find that it helps to have a drink?

22. Have you recently noticed that you cannot drink as much as you once did?

23. Do you sometimes stay drunk for several days at a time?

24. Do you sometimes feel very depressed and wonder whether life is worth living?

25. Sometimes after a period of drinking, do you see or hear things that aren't there?

26. Do you get terribly frightened after you have been drinking heavily?

If you answer *"yes"* to two or three of these questions, you may wish to evaluate your drinking in these areas. *Yes* answers to *several* of these questions may indicate one of the following stages of alcoholism:

- Questions 1–8 (early stage): Drinking is a regular part of your life.

- Questions 9–21 (middle stage): You are having trouble controlling when, where, and how much you drink.

- Questions 22–26 (beginning of the final stage): You no longer can control your desire to drink.

14

SEXUALLY TRANSMITTED DISEASES

OBJECTIVES

- Describe how sexually transmitted diseases are passed from one person to another.

- Discuss the reasons for the prevalence of STDs.

- List the symptoms, risks, and treatment for various STDs: chlamydia, gonorrhea, genital warts, herpes, viral hepatitis, pelvic inflammatory disease, pubic lice and scabies, syphilis, and AIDS.

- Describe guidelines for preventing and treating STDs.

JUST AS THEIR NAME IMPLIES, **sexually transmitted diseases** (STDs) are transmitted, or passed from one person to another, through sexual contact. Several STDs can also be passed in infected blood. Generally, the organisms that cause these diseases are fragile and cannot exist outside the protective environment of the human reproductive tract. Therefore, in most cases, they cannot be transmitted by toilet seats, soap dishes, towels, or doorknobs. Some sexually transmitted diseases can be cured; others can be treated but not cured. These diseases can be life-threatening and life-changing. Fortunately, most STDs can be prevented.

> More than 25 diseases are spread through sexual contact. About one in four adults in the United States has an STD.

Some STDs have been around a long time. They are mentioned in the Old Testament, and epidemics were recorded as early as the time of Columbus. Today, the more than 25 identified STDs are among the most prevalent infectious diseases in the United States. More than 15.3 million new cases are reported to the Centers for Disease Control and Prevention (CDC) every year, and more than 68 million Americans have an incurable STD.[1] Because many people who are infected show no symptoms, the CDC estimates that the number of Americans infected in any one year may be as high as 10 million. Only the common cold and flu are more prevalent. Three million cases of STDs occur each year among adolescents.[2] Figure 14.1 lists estimated new cases of common STDs.

Many STDs have reached epidemic proportions, even though some of them can be cured with proper medication. STDs are rampant for a number of reasons:

- Some STDs have no symptoms, so victims are unaware that they are infected. Others have only mild symptoms that can be easily confused with other ailments.
- When birth control pills became widely available, many people stopped using condoms as a form of birth control, and, whereas condoms offer some protection against STDs, birth control pills do not.
- As a trend, people are becoming sexually active at earlier ages and are having more than one sexual partner.
- Some STDs cannot be treated and others have developed strains that resist antibiotics.
- Fear of social stigma, disapproval, and condemnation stops some people from seeking treatment, even

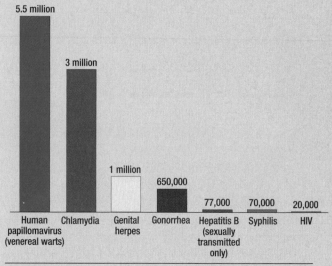

FIGURE **14.1** ESTIMATED ANNUAL U. S. CASES OF COMMON SEXUALLY TRANSMITTED DISEASES.

- 5.5 million — Human papillomavirus (venereal warts)
- 3 million — Chlamydia
- 1 million — Genital herpes
- 650,000 — Gonorrhea
- 77,000 — Hepatitis B (sexually transmitted only)
- 70,000 — Syphilis
- 20,000 — HIV

Source: Division of STD/HIV Prevention U.S. Centers for Disease Control and Prevention.

when they suspect they might be infected. Others become complacent because of the past successes of penicillin and other antibiotics.
- Many victims deny the possibility of infection, believing "it can never happen to me," or they believe STDs affect only high-risk groups.
- Some people erroneously believe that STDs are only minor irritations and are unaware of the serious complications that can result if STDs go untreated.

CAUSES

STDs are caused by pathogens, or disease-causing microorganisms. The types of pathogens that cause STDs include bacteria, viruses, parasites, and fungi. STD infections can recur with every new exposure. The body generally does not build up a resistance to the organisms that cause these diseases. Most affect the genitals, anus, mouth, and throat. Left untreated, many have serious complications that affect the entire body. Acquired immune deficiency syndrome (AIDS) is caused by the human immunodeficiency virus (HIV), which disables the immune system, leaving the body open to various opportunistic infections, and leads eventually to death.

Strictly speaking, anyone who engages in sexual activity is at risk for STDs. People who have more than one sexual partner or who have sex with someone who has or had more than one sexual partner is at greater risk. The risk also increases substantially if a person does not use condoms. Sexual behavior that tears or damages the vagina, anus, or penis increases the risk, and anal intercourse is especially dangerous. Women are at greater risk than men because they have a greater area of mucous membranes in their genital tissues. Gay and bisexual men, their sexual partners, intravenous drug users, and their partners are at highest risk. An infected mother can pass the disease to her child during gestation and birth.

SIGNS AND SYMPTOMS

Signs and symptoms are often slower to develop and more difficult to detect in women than in men, so women may not have as early an indication of infection. General signs and symptoms of STDs include

- Sores on or near the genitals, anus, or mouth
- Pain in the genitals, anus, or mouth
- A burning sensation in the genitals, anus, or mouth
- Discharge from the vagina or penis
- Itching around the genitals, in the vagina, in the rectum, around the anus, or in and around the mouth
- Abdominal pain
- Growths or warts in the genital area, anus, or mouth; these may be skin-colored or dark, flat or raised

Sores, warts, itching, rashes, and burning in areas of the body other than the genitals, vagina, rectum, and mouth usually do not indicate STDs. If you develop these symptoms and think you may have been exposed to an STD, however, you should see a physician.

COMMON STDS

Understanding the incidence, signs and symptoms, and risks for specific STDs can help you reduce your risk of becoming infected.

| Chlamydia |

Three million new cases of chlamydia occur each year.[3] An estimated 15 percent of all college students in the United States are infected. As many as half a million cases in women progress to pelvic inflammatory disease (PID), which can cause sterility and death. An estimated 4 percent of all pregnant women are infected. If left untreated, chlamydia will worsen.

Caused by *Chlamydia trachomatis* bacteria, **chlamydia** often occurs simultaneously with other STDs, most commonly gonorrhea and herpes. If unidentified for many years, the bacteria also can cause non-gonococcal urethritis (NGU) and lymphogranuloma venereum (LGV).

About 90 percent of all men who are infected have symptoms. Only about 20 percent of all women who are infected have symptoms unless the infection progresses into something more serious, such as pelvic inflammatory disease. Even when women do have symptoms, they often are mild and can disappear on their own, even though the woman is still infected. When symptoms occur, they usually appear 1 to 3 weeks after infection.

Chlamydia infects the mucous membranes that line the genitals, rectum, anus, mouth, and eyes. It is transmitted by contact with infected mucous membranes and occurs most commonly between heterosexuals. The most common complications for newborns are pneumonia and conjunctivitis (an infection of the membranes in the eyes), which are found in more than 30,000 newborn babies each year in the United States.

In men, the most common symptoms are the following:

- Whitish or pus-like discharge from the penis
- Pain during urination; a watery, clear discharge after urination
- Frequent urination
- Urethral itching
- A painful, swollen scrotum
- Abdominal discomfort

Women who experience symptoms may have any of the following:

- Whitish vaginal discharge
- Itching or burning of the genitals
- Mild pain during urination
- Abdominal discomfort
- Bleeding between periods
- Symptoms of pelvic inflammatory disease (fever, painful intercourse, pelvic pain, vaginal discharge)

Sexually transmitted disease A disease that is passed from one person to another through sexual contact.

Chlamydia An STD caused by a bacteria that infects the mucous membranes that line the genitals, rectum, anus, mouth, and eyes.

Complications of chlamydia in men include diseases of the urinary tract and sterility. In women, chlamydia is the leading cause of pelvic inflammatory disease, which also can cause sterility. Chlamydia that is untreated can damage the arteries, heart valves, and heart muscle in men and women alike. At particular risk for chlamydia are people with more than one sexual partner, people who do not use some kind of barrier (such as condoms) during intercourse, and people who have multiple sexual partners.

Treatment consists of a full course of antibiotics, usually tetracycline or erythromycin. Infected and diagnosed individuals should

1. Take all the antibiotics the doctor prescribes.
2. Have a follow-up culture 2 weeks after finishing the antibiotics to make sure the bacteria have been destroyed completely.
3. Avoid all sexual activity until the infection is gone, at least until the follow-up culture is clean.
4. Tell all sexual partners so they can get tested and treated for chlamydia; if you have sex again with an infected partner during or after your treatment, you could be reinfected.

| Gonorrhea |

Known most commonly as "the clap," 650,000 new cases of **gonorrhea** are reported each year. However, the actual number of infected people in the United States may be as many as five times that high, because only about 20 percent of all cases are believed to be reported. This STD

is most common among people aged 20 to 24, and its incidence is increasing most rapidly among non-white adolescents and young adults.

Gonorrhea is caused by a bacteria that infects the cervix, rectum, urethra, or mouth. The bacteria dies rapidly when removed from the warmth and moisture of the mucous membranes, so it cannot be transmitted by inanimate objects. It is transmitted by vaginal intercourse, anal-genital sex, and oral-genital sex. Because the environment of the vagina is so conducive to growth of the bacteria that causes gonorrhea, women who are exposed to the bacteria through intercourse have an 80 percent chance of developing gonorrhea. The most common site of infection is the cervix. If left untreated, gonorrhea is chronic and progressive. People infected with gonorrhea do not become immune to it, so they can become reinfected many times.

The symptoms of gonorrhea generally develop within 2 days to 2 weeks after infection but may not appear for as long as 30 days. As with chlamydia, it may have no symptoms at all or only mild symptoms, especially in women.

Men generally tend to have more noticeable signs and symptoms, which include the following:

- A profuse, yellowish or milky, foul-smelling discharge from the penis
- Burning, frequent urination
- Fever
- Abdominal pain
- Swollen lymph glands in the groin
- Swelling of the testicles

An estimated 80 percent of women infected with gonorrhea do not have immediate symptoms. If women develop symptoms, they are usually mild and include

- Slight burning or pain in the genital area
- Slight foul-smelling vaginal discharge that has a different color or odor than a woman's usual discharge
- Possible pain during urination
- Abnormally heavy menstrual bleeding or bleeding between periods

Gonorrhea transmitted during oral sex can cause a mild sore throat (often no more severe than the sore throat that accompanies the common cold). If gonorrhea was transmitted during anal intercourse, it can cause pain, burning, and discharge from the anus or the presence of mucous, pus, or blood in the stools.

Babies born to infected mothers may become blind. Because gonorrhea is so prevalent, the eyes of newborns are treated routinely with silver nitrate. Other complications include pneumonia and infections of the anus or rectum.

If left untreated, gonorrhea can cause permanent sterility in women and men alike. Other complications include heart damage, brain damage, liver damage, arthritis, skin lesions, and meningitis. The bacteria responsible for gonorrhea can survive in the reproductive tract for years, enabling a man or a woman without symptoms to infect multiple partners unknowingly.

Gonorrhea most often is treated with penicillin. If a chlamydia infection is present also, tetracycline is added. Gonorrhea can be stubborn to treat: As many as 40 percent of gonorrhea infections are resistant to penicillin and must be treated with newer drugs.

Anyone who is infected and diagnosed with this STD should

1. Take the full course of antibiotics prescribed by a doctor, even though the symptoms will probably ease up within 12 hours and disappear within 3 days.
2. Return for a follow-up culture a week after finishing the antibiotics.
3. Avoid sexual intercourse or other sexual contact that could spread the infection until the doctor verifies that the infection is completely gone.
4. Contact your sex partner(s) who could be infected; if they are not treated and you have sex with them during or after your treatment, you could get reinfected.

Gonorrhea is so common that some health officials recommend regular screening (usually once every 6 months) for all sexually active people.

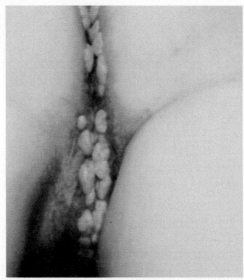

Genital warts on the male; this STD requires treatment to remove the warts.

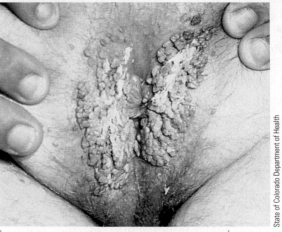

An advanced case of genital warts on the female.

| Genital Warts |

Genital warts are wart-like growths caused by the **human papilloma virus (HPV)**. The most common STD, an estimated 5.5 million Americans develop the infection each year.[4] It is epidemic on America's college campuses. More than 65 different strains of HPV cause genital warts, and a person can be infected by more than one strain at the same time.

The most common symptom—warts on the penis, scrotum, anus, cervix, vagina, or around the urethra—may develop as soon as 1 to 3 months following infection or as long as 8 months after infection. Outbreaks of warts are more common during pregnancy and in people who have weak immune systems. Genital warts can be transmitted by skin-to-skin contact during vaginal or

> Once infected with a viral STD, a person never will become uninfected.

anal intercourse or by oral-genital contact during oral sex.

Genital warts usually start with localized irritation and itching, followed by the presence of painless warts. These may be soft or hard, flat, small, yellowish, and dry. In most areas of the body, they usually are larger, shaped irregularly, and may be white, pink, or gray. Often warts are inside the vagina or rectum or on the cervix, so they may not be noticed unless a physician discovers them during an examination. Flat warts are so small that they may not be visible to the human eye.

Genital warts have been described as looking like cauliflower in their advanced stages. In women they often clump together, interfering with

Gonorrhea An STD caused by a bacteria that infects the cervix, rectum, urethra, or mouth.

Genital warts An STD caused by the human papilloma virus (HPV) and characterized by warts around the genitals or mouth.

Human papilloma virus (HPV) The virus that causes genital warts; some strains of the virus also have been linked to cervical cancer.

urination and sexual intercourse. If the infection was passed via oral sex, the warts may grow in and around the mouth.[5]

Many people have HPV and never develop obvious symptoms, however everyone with the virus is at risk for the complications. HPV presents life-threatening risks in people who have symptoms as well as those who do not have symptoms. The complications of genital warts are potentially deadly. HPV is associated with more than 90 percent of all cervical cancers, and it is associated with other genital cancers as well, including cancer of the penis.

Newborns infected by their mothers can develop warts in the mouth and bronchial passages. This can interfere with breathing.

Treatment can remove the warts, but it cannot completely kill the virus that causes the warts. Recurrence is extremely common. The typical treatment for genital warts is the drug podophyllin, which causes the wart to slough off. It normally is applied by a physician once a week for 5 or 6 weeks until the wart has disappeared completely. Podophyllin cannot be used by pregnant women or to treat warts in the cervical area.

Warts that resist treatment with podophyllin sometimes can be removed by surgery, electrocautery (burning), or cryotherapy (freezing). All these options result in scarring.

A person diagnosed and treated for genital warts should

1. Follow the physician's instructions carefully; repeated treatment usually is necessary to remove the warts.
2. Use any antibiotic ointments the physician prescribes.
3. Avoid sexual contact during an outbreak of warts; use condoms when warts are not visible.
4. For women: Have a pelvic exam, including a Pap smear, every year to monitor the risk of cervical cancer.
5. Never use over-the-counter wart removers. They are useless against genital warts and can cause tissue damage if applied to the genital area.

Because treatment does not kill the virus that causes genital warts, once infected, the person always carries the virus, even though it may be dormant for months or years at a time.

| Herpes |

Of the different strains of herpes simplex virus, the most common is herpes simplex-1, the culprit behind the common cold sore or fever blister. Other viruses in the herpes family cause chicken pox, shingles, and infectious mononucleosis. The herpes simplex-2 virus causes the herpes STD, also known as **herpes genitalis**.

Once a person gets genital herpes, it remains forever. It has no cure, but the symptoms can be treated with limited success. The virus always will reside in the body, even when the blistering sores characteristic of a herpes outbreak are not present. Some people have only one or two outbreaks a year; others may have them much more often. The virus can be spread even when no lesions are visible. Herpes is transmitted by contact with an active sore or with the virus-containing secretions from the vagina or penis, even when an outbreak is not occurring.

Approximately one million new cases of herpes are reported to the CDC each year. More than 37 million Americans have the virus. It is most common among those aged 18 to 25 years. Usually within 10 days of infection, flu-like symptoms arise that may include the following:

- Fever
- Swollen glands, especially in the groin
- Muscle aches and pains
- Fatigue
- Occasionally, shooting or stabbing pains in the abdomen and legs

During this initial period, the infected person may feel pain during intercourse or urination. The characteristic blisters that appear on the genitals or mouth follow the flu-like symptoms. These sores shed the herpes virus and are highly contagious. Herpes sores progress through four stages:

1. At the site where the virus entered the body, the skin starts to itch or tingle, turns red, and becomes extremely sensitive. This sensation, called the **prodrome**, typically precedes all outbreaks.
2. One or more small, painful blisters or sores erupt on the glans and shaft of the penis, around the anus, at the opening of the vagina, on the clitoris, on the

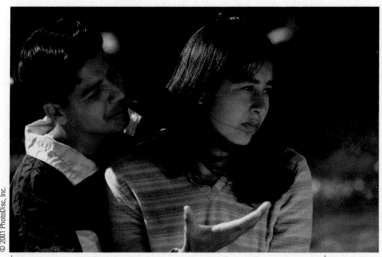

| If you care enough to hesitate, you care enough to tell your partner. |

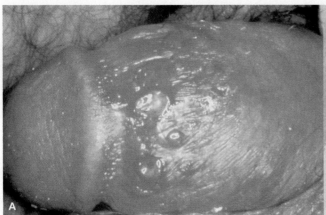
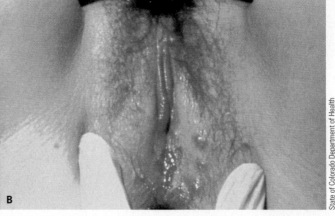

State of Colorado Department of Health

| Genital herpes appears on the penis (A) and labia (B). |

cervix, or on the labia. If oral-genital contact occurred, the sores may be in or around the mouth. The blisters rupture and the resulting painful, itching, open sores may weep a yellowish secretion or pus.

3. Without treatment, the sores diminish; scabs form and fall off within 1 to 2 weeks. Pain, fever, and other symptoms subside.

4. The virus lies dormant in the nerve endings until the next outbreak. The recurrence of blisters are usually less severe and of shorter duration. Recurrence can be caused by unrelated illness, fever, emotional stress, lack of sleep, exposure to cold or heat, sunburn, poor nutrition, and menstruation.

The most typical complication of herpes is **auto-inoculation**—in which the mouth, eyes, or other part of the body can become infected. If a person experiencing an outbreak touches a blister, then rubs their eyes, the eyes can become infected. Women are at higher risk for cervical cancer if they are infected with herpes.

Possibly the most serious complications involve babies born to mothers with herpes. If a woman with an active herpes lesion delivers a baby vaginally, the baby has a one-in-four chance of becoming infected and can suffer blindness, experience mental retardation, or damage to internal organs, and may even die. During a herpes outbreak or presence of the virus in the vagina, a pregnant woman should have a cesarean section delivery to lower the risk of infecting the baby.

Herpes is caused by a virus, and it has no known cure. Drug treatments using antiviral drugs have helped relieve symptoms. A person diagnosed with herpes should

1. Wash the hands thoroughly after touching infected areas to avoid spreading the disease to other areas of the body.

2. Keep the infected lesions clean and dry.

3. Wear loose clothing to avoid irritating the infected areas; avoid scratching, rubbing, touching, or picking at sores.

4. Avoid sexual contact of any kind during the prodrome and when lesions are active.

5. Use a latex condom to help prevent spread of the infection when blisters are not present.

6. Practice good health habits to avoid getting fatigued or stressed, which can lead to recurrences.

7. For women, have a pelvic exam including a Pap smear every 6 to 12 months to monitor the risk for cervical cancer. If pregnant, discuss the history of the infection with the doctor. Physicians usually recommend that the baby of an infected mother be delivered by Cesarean section.

| Viral Hepatitis |

Hepatitis, an infection that causes inflammation of the liver, is caused by one or more viruses. Of the four identified types of hepatitis, the most common is hepatitis A, more often called "infectious hepatitis." Hepatitis A is spread through unsanitary conditions, poor hygiene, direct exposure to the virus, or infected food and water. An estimated half of all adults in the United States have developed antibodies to hepatitis A, and it can be prevented with gamma globulin injections within 10 days of exposure.

Hepatitis B is spread through exposure to the contaminated blood or body

Herpes genitalis An infection caused by the herpes simplex-2 virus and characterized by blistering sores on the genitals.

Prodrome The stage of infection when early symptoms erupt, in the case of herpes, a sensation in which the skin starts to itch or tingle; precedes onset of the blisters and sores.

Autoinoculation Spreading an infection to other parts of one's own body.

Hepatitis B A form of hepatitis spread through exposure to the contaminated blood or body fluids of an infected person; can cause long-term liver damage.

fluids of an infected person. Besides being spread through semen and vagina secretions, it can be transmitted through breast milk, saliva, and perspiration. Hepatitis B is a resilient pathogen; it can be spread through less-direct contact.

Signs and symptoms of hepatitis B develop within 6 months of infection and include

- Mild fever
- Loss of appetite
- Nausea and vomiting
- Diarrhea
- Severe fatigue
- Pain in the muscles and joints
- Headache
- Tenderness in the upper right section of the abdomen

Within 2 weeks after symptoms first appear, signs of liver damage may become apparent, including

- **Jaundice**
- Light gray or whitish stools
- Dark urine
- Tender, enlarged liver

Because the symptoms of hepatitis B are so much like those of the flu or infectious mononucleosis, a blood test is needed for proper diagnosis. Long-term complications from hepatitis B, which can be devastating, include chronic progressive hepatitis, liver cancer, liver failure, cirrhosis of the liver, and death.

Although hepatitis B has no cure, an effective vaccine is available to make uninfected people immune and prevent infection. Anyone in the high-risk group should ask for the vaccine. High-risk individuals include

- Sexually active people and their partners
- Sexual partners of an infected person or a person living in the house with an infected person, even if not sexually involved
- Intravenous drug users and their partners
- People in health-care professions
- Natives of or travelers to Africa, Asia, Alaska, and the Pacific Islands

People diagnosed with hepatitis B should

1. Get plenty of rest. Follow the physician's guidelines for limiting activity during the acute stage of infection.
2. Avoid using drugs, including alcohol, that are metabolized by the liver, because these substances can put an excess burden on the liver.
3. Avoid sexual contact.
4. If pregnant, discuss the disease with a physician. Do not breast-feed your baby.

5. Have regular follow-up checkups to determine the risk of liver disease.

Pelvic Inflammatory Disease

Pelvic inflammatory disease (PID) can be caused by other sexually transmitted diseases, most commonly chlamydia and gonorrhea. The most dangerous of all STDs, it is a severe infection of the lining of the abdominal cavity. One of the factors that makes PID so dangerous is that it is difficult to diagnose, and, unless treated immediately, it can cause scar tissue to form in the fallopian tubes.

Signs and symptoms of PID include the following:

- Menstrual irregularities, including irregular cycles, profuse bleeding during menstruation, and vaginal bleeding between cycles
- Severe menstrual cramps
- Unusual vaginal discharge
- Pain or tenderness in the abdomen or lower back
- Fever and chills
- Nausea and vomiting
- Loss of appetite
- A burning sensation during urination

Some women who develop PID become sterile. Of those who do get pregnant, the risk of ectopic pregnancy (a fetus that attaches to the fallopian tube instead of the uterus), miscarriage, and stillbirth increases dramatically. If an ectopic pregnancy is undiagnosed, the fetus continues to grow until it ruptures the fallopian tube. This can cause severe bleeding and result in death. Therefore, PID can be life-threatening in many ways.

PID can be treated with antibiotics. Early treatment is essential. Later treatment can kill the bacteria but cannot repair the damage already done from the infection. A person who is diagnosed and treated should do the following:

1. Follow the complete course of antibiotics prescribed by a doctor, even if the symptoms disappear.
2. Stop using an IUD.
3. Avoid sexual activity until the infection has cleared.
4. Ask that any sexual partners be treated; if they are not and you have sex with them during or after treatment, you can become reinfected.
5. Do not douche, because it can spread the infection.

Pubic Lice and Scabies

Commonly called "crabs," **pubic lice** are tiny parasites that move from partner to partner during sexual activity. Pubic lice actually are one of three different kinds of lice that attach to various parts of the body. Whereas pubic lice grip the pubic hair and feed on the small blood vessels of the underlying skin, other lice attach to skin or the hair of the head.

With a life cycle of approximately 2 months, pubic lice attach to the pubic hair, where females can lay as many as 10 eggs (nits) a day. The nits adhere to the pubic hair with a thick, sticky substance. Body warmth incubates the eggs until they hatch, and the new lice start feeding on the blood vessels as the old lice drop off. As they drop off, the lice are visible to the naked eye in bedding and clothing.

The tiny mite that causes **scabies** has a similar life cycle, but the female mite burrows under the skin at night.

Common signs and symptoms of pubic lice include

- Intense itching in the pubic area
- Visible lice or whitish nits in the pubic hair
- Swollen glands in the groin

Common signs and symptoms of scabies include

- Characteristic patterns of burrowing, most commonly on the buttocks, under the breasts, between the fingers and on the wrists
- A discharge of pus from the burrowed areas
- Intense itching

Treatment options for pubic lice include shampoos and lotions available by prescription and over-the-counter. Both are applied to the pubic hair; a fine-tooth comb is then used to remove nits. Most advise against using certain products during pregnancy, so pregnant women should check with a doctor.

Individuals diagnosed with scabies should follow the doctor's directions, because scabies can also be transmitted by close nonsexual contact. If diagnosed with pubic lice or scabies, the infected person should

1. Follow treatment directions carefully.
2. Dip the comb in vinegar, then water, to dissolve the sticky substance holding nits to the pubic hair.
3. Wash all clothing, bedding, and linens contacted prior to treatment. A person who does not have sexual contact can be infected by towels or sheets.
4. Clean all upholstery and furniture contacted prior to treatment.
5. Avoid sexual contact and inform all sexual partners to seek treatment. If they are not treated, and you have sex with them during or after treatment, you could become reinfected.

| Syphilis |

Approximately 70,000 new cases of **syphilis** are reported each year. Caused by a spirochete (corkscrew-shaped type of bacteria), syphilis is transmitted through direct contact with infectious sores, skin rashes, or mucous patches caused by the disease.

Syphilis is transmitted most often through intercourse, anal-genital contact, and oral-genital contact, though it can also be transmitted by kissing a person who has a sore or mucous patches on the mouth. Syphilis also can be transmitted from a pregnant woman to her baby after the fourth month of pregnancy. (For the first four months, a special temporary membrane in the placenta protects the fetus from infectious agents in the mother's bloodstream.) After the fourth month, the bacteria that causes syphilis is passed easily across the placenta from the mother's bloodstream to the baby's circulatory system.

Syphilis has four specific stages:

1. Primary stage. Occurring 2 to 3 weeks after the bacteria enter the body, a sore (**chancre**) develops at the site where the bacteria entered, usually on the genitals. The chancre may look like a blister or pimple but is often an open sore. It may be as large as a dime but commonly is as small as a pinhead and may go unnoticed, especially if it is in the vagina, rectum, anus, or mouth. The sore looks painful but is actually painless and may be accompanied by painless swollen lymph nodes in the groin. Within 3 to 6 weeks, the chancre clears up without treatment, so many infected people assume it was something else. Even though the chancre has healed, infectious bacteria remain in the system.

2. Secondary stage. Any time from 6 weeks to a year after the chancre heals, the symptoms of secondary syphilis appear. These symptoms, which may be mild to severe and can last anywhere from a few days to a few months, include:

- Low-grade fever
- Nausea and loss of appetite
- Whitish patches on the mouth and throat (infectious patches)
- Sore throat
- Painless rash anywhere on the skin, especially on the soles of the feet and palms of the hands. Though the rash does not itch, it spreads infection.
- Headache

Jaundice Liver condition in which the skin and whites of the eyes appear yellow.

Pelvic inflammatory disease (PID) A severe infection of the lining of the abdominal cavity, usually caused by bacterial STDs.

Pubic lice Commonly called "crabs," tiny parasites that feed on the small blood vessels of the skin beneath the pubic hair.

Scabies Tiny mites that burrow under the skin at night; may be spread by nonsexual contact.

Syphilis An STD caused by a bacteria, occurring in four stages; untreated, it is fatal.

Chancre A painless, red-rimmed sore that develops at the site where syphilis bacteria enter the body.

- Swollen glands
- Hair loss, usually patchy
- Arthritic-type joint pain
- Large sores on the genitals or around the mouth

Even if untreated, these symptoms usually run their course, then disappear. This does not mean the infection is gone. The disease remains dormant, and symptoms can reappear at any time. The person remains infectious during this stage, even though symptoms have cleared up.

3. Latent stage. No outward symptoms are present during the latent stage, which usually lasts as long as 30 years. During the latent stage, the person is no longer contagious unless moist lesions erupt. One exception is a pregnant woman, who can pass syphilis to her fetus during the latent stage. Even though nothing seems to be happening on the outside during the latent stage, the spirochetes attack the body's organs, causing substantial damage to the brain, heart, and central nervous system. Maladies characteristic of the latent stage include heart disease, senility, blindness, central nervous system deterioration, and sometimes death.

4. Late (tertiary) stage. The late stage of syphilis usually begins 5 to 20 years after the initial infection. Two-thirds of people with untreated infections have no further symptoms. About one-third of people with untreated infections develop blindness, deafness, central nervous system destruction, damage to the heart, paralysis, psychosis, and, finally, death during the late stage of syphilis.

A fetus infected by the mother's blood may develop mild to severe organ damage as a result. Syphilis also can result in stillbirth.

Penicillin is the drug of choice in treating syphilis. With treatment, syphilis can be cured at any stage. Early detection and treatment is best, because treatment is effective at killing the bacteria and stopping the disease. However, it cannot repair the damage that the disease already caused. A person diagnosed and treated for syphilis should

1. Follow the complete course of antibiotics as prescribed by a doctor, even if symptoms are not apparent.
2. Discuss with the doctor the possibility of simultaneous STD infections, such as gonorrhea or chlamydia. If additional infections are present, higher doses of various antibiotics are necessary.
3. Avoid sexual activity until cured.
4. Have follow-up blood tests for a year after finishing antibiotic treatment.

HIV and AIDS

In the United States, approximately 580,000 people are infected with **HIV**, the virus that causes **AIDS**.[6] There are 20,000 new cases each year and more than 400,000 Americans have died of the consistently fatal disorder. The number of women infected with HIV is increasing faster than any other population. Currently there is no vaccine and no cure.

DIFFERENCES BETWEEN HIV AND AIDS HIV is the virus that, over time, causes AIDS. At first, people who become infected with HIV may not know they are infected. An incubation period of weeks, months, or years may go by during which no symptoms appear. The virus may live in the body 10 years or longer before symptoms develop. The person can spread HIV to others even when there are no symptoms during the early stages of infection.

As the infection progresses to the point at which certain diseases develop, the person is said to have AIDS. HIV itself does not kill people, nor do people die of AIDS. "AIDS" is the term used to define the final stage of HIV infection. Death results from a weakened immune system that is unable to fight off the opportunistic diseases that develop. To test your knowledge of AIDS, see Assessment 14-1.

Earliest symptoms of the disease include unexplained weight loss, constant fatigue, mild fever, swollen lymph glands, diarrhea, and sore throat. Advanced symptoms include loss of appetite, skin diseases, night sweats, and deterioration of mucous membranes.

Though fatal to AIDS victims, most of the illnesses AIDS patients develop are harmless and rare in the general population. The two most common fatal conditions in AIDS patients are pneumocystis carinii pneumonia (a parasitic infection of the lungs) and Kaposi's sarcoma (a type of skin cancer). The AIDS virus also may attack the nervous system, causing brain and spinal cord damage.

On the average, the individual develops the symptoms that fit the case definition of AIDS about 7 to 8 years following infection. From that point on, the person may live another 2 to 3 years. In essence, from the point of infection, the individual may endure a chronic disease for 8 to 10 years.

The only means to determine whether someone has HIV is through an HIV antibody test. Being HIV-positive does not necessarily mean the person has AIDS. Several years may go by before the person develops the diseases that fit the case definition of AIDS.

Upon HIV infection, the immune system's line of defense against the virus is to form antibodies that bind to the virus. On the average, the body takes 3 months to manufacture enough antibodies to show up positive in an HIV antibody test. Sometimes this may take 6 months or longer.

If HIV infection is suspected, a prudent waiting period of 3 to 6 months is suggested prior to testing. During this time, and from there on, individuals should refrain from further endangering themselves and others through risky behaviors such as sexual activity or IV drug use. Some people choose to be tested to be reassured that their risky behaviors are acceptable. Even if the test turns up negative for HIV, this is not a license to continue risky behaviors. Once infected with HIV, a person never will become uninfected. There is no second chance. Everyone must protect himself or herself against this chronic disease. No one should believe that it can never happen to him or her!

Although professionals disagree as to how many HIV carriers will develop AIDS, sooner or later most HIV-infected individuals will be diagnosed with AIDS. Even if a person has not developed AIDS, the virus can be passed on to others who could easily develop AIDS.

| HIV TRANSMISSION | Two basic conditions have to be present for HIV to be transmitted:

1. One person has to be infected.
2. The virus has to be transmitted to an area in the body where body fluids can be exchanged.

HIV is transmitted by the exchange of body fluids including blood, semen, vaginal secretions, and maternal milk. These fluids may be exchanged during sexual intercourse, by using hypodermic needles used previously by infected individuals, between a pregnant woman and her developing fetus, by infection of babies from the mother during childbirth, less frequently during breast-feeding, and rarely from a blood transfusion or organ transplant.

The risk of being infected with HIV from a blood transfusion today is slight. Prior to 1985, several cases of HIV infection came from blood transfusions because the blood was donated by HIV-infected individuals. Today, all donated blood is tested for HIV.

A myth regarding HIV is that it can be transmitted by donating blood. People cannot get HIV from giving blood. Health professionals use a new needle every time they withdraw blood from a person. These needles are used only once and are thrown away immediately after each person has donated blood.

People do not get HIV because of who they are but because of what they do. HIV and AIDS can threaten anyone, anywhere, regardless of gender, race, income, or education. It is considered an equal-opportunity destroyer. HIV can be transmitted between males, between females, from male to female, or from female to male. However, HIV and AIDS are preventable. Almost all of the people who get HIV do so because they choose to engage in risky behaviors.

| RISKY BEHAVIORS | You cannot tell if people are infected with HIV or have AIDS by simply looking at them or taking their word. Not you, not a nurse, not even a doctor can tell without an HIV antibody test. Although many people who have been infected with HIV look normal and healthy for years, they are capable of passing the virus to others. Therefore, every time you engage in a risky behavior, you run the risk of contracting HIV. The two most basic risky behaviors are

1. **Having unprotected vaginal, anal, or oral sex with an HIV-infected person.** Unprotected sex means having sex without the proper use of a condom. A person should select only latex (rubber or prophylactic) condoms that say "disease prevention" on the package. Although you might have unprotected sex with an infected person and not get the virus, you can also get it by having unprotected sex only once with that infected person.

   Rubbing during sexual intercourse often damages mucous membranes and causes unseen bleeding (even in the mouth). During vaginal, anal, or oral sexual contact, infected blood, semen, or vaginal fluids can penetrate the mucous membranes that line the vagina, the penis, the rectum, the mouth, or the throat. From the membrane, HIV then can travel into the previously uninfected person's blood.

   Health experts believe unprotected anal sex is the riskiest type of sex. Even though bleeding is not visible in most cases, anal sex almost always causes tiny tears and bleeding in the rectum. This happens because the rectum does not stretch easily, the mucous membrane is quite thin, and small blood vessels lie directly beneath the membrane. Condoms also are more likely to break during anal intercourse because of the greater friction produced in a smaller cavity. All of these factors greatly enhance the risk of transmitting HIV.

   Although latex condoms reduce risk if they are used correctly, they are not 100 percent foolproof. Abstaining from sex is the only way to completely protect yourself from HIV infection and other STDs.

2. **Sharing hypodermic needles or other drug paraphernalia with someone who is infected.** Following an injection, a small amount of blood remains in the needle and sometimes in the syringe itself. If the person who

Human immunodeficiency virus (HIV) The virus that weakens and destroys the immune system and gradually leads to AIDS.

Acquired immunodeficiency syndrome (AIDS) The final stage of HIV infection, characterized by opportunistic infections that are rare or harmless in people with normal immune function.

used the syringe is infected with HIV and someone else uses that same syringe, regardless of the drug used (legal or illegal), that small amount of blood is sufficient to spread the virus. All used syringes should be destroyed and disposed of immediately after they are used.

In addition, a person must be cautious when getting acupuncture, getting a tattoo, or having the ears pierced. If the needle was used previously on someone who is HIV-infected and was not disinfected properly, the person risks getting HIV as well.

Infrequent use of drugs, including alcohol, also heightens the risk of spreading HIV. Otherwise-prudent people often act irrationally and engage in risky behaviors when they are under the influence of alcohol and other drugs. Getting high can make you willing to have sex when you didn't plan to and thereby run the risk of HIV infection.

A very small risk is present in receiving donated blood. Because of the 3- to 6-month incubation period, a slight risk of receiving HIV-infected blood is present. Therefore, people who are planning to have surgery may consider storing their own blood in advance so that safe blood will be available if they need it.

HOW AIDS IS NOT TRANSMITTED There is no evidence of airborne transmission of the virus; HIV cannot be passed by coughing or sneezing. Small concentrations of the virus have been found in saliva and teardrops, but there is no record of anyone getting HIV through open-mouthed kissing or from someone else's tears. In principle, if both people have open cuts in the lips, mouth, or gums, HIV could be transmitted through openmouthed kissing, but such a case has never been documented.

The virus cannot be transmitted through perspiration (sweat), either. Sporting activities with no physical contact pose no risk to uninfected individuals, unless they have open wounds through which blood from an infected person can come in direct contact with the open wound of the uninfected person. The skin is an excellent line of defense against HIV. Blood from an infected person cannot penetrate the skin except through an opening in the skin. As an extra precaution, a person should use vinyl or latex gloves when performing work that requires direct contact with someone else's blood or open wound.

Some people fear getting HIV from health care professionals. The chances of getting infected during physical or medical procedures are extremely low. Health care workers take extra care to protect themselves and their patients from HIV.

HIV is not transmitted through normal social contact. HIV cannot be caught by spending time with, shaking hands with, or hugging an infected person; by using a public telephone, toilet seat, drinking fountain, swimming pool, dishes, or silverware used by an HIV patient; or by sharing a drink, food, a towel, or clothes with a person who has HIV.

Another myth regarding HIV transmission is that you can get it from insects or animals. The "H" in HIV stands for "human." You cannot catch HIV from insects or animals, because they do not get infected with HIV. A mosquito that picks up the virus may carry the virus in its stomach, but the virus cannot reproduce in the mosquito or travel to the mosquito's saliva.

What about dating? Dating and getting to know other people is a normal part of life. Dating, however, does not mean the same thing as having sex. Sexual intercourse as a part of dating can be risky, and one of the risks is acquiring HIV and other STDs. You can't tell if someone you are dating or would like to date has been exposed to HIV. The good news is that, as long as you avoid sexual activity and don't share drug needles, it doesn't matter whom you date.

HIV TESTING A person can be tested for HIV in several ways. Testing usually is free of charge, and the results are kept confidential. Many states also conduct anonymous testing, which means the name is never recorded. Instead, a number is assigned as a link to the test.

Two types of tests are used to detect HIV:

1. The EIA or ELISA. This simple, inexpensive screening test measures whether the person has developed antibodies to the virus. If the test is negative and the person has not been exposed to HIV within the previous 3 months, he or she can be relatively certain of not being infected. Generally, no further testing is required. If the test is positive, the person is usually asked to take a second screening test to reduce the chance of a false positive result.
2. The western blot test. If the second EIA/ELISA test is positive, this more sophisticated, expensive test is given to confirm the positive results. If the western blot is positive, HIV infection is certain. If it is negative, you can be reasonably certain of not being infected, because false negative results are rare.

Neither of these tests can tell if a person has AIDS. The tests can determine only if he or she has been infected with HIV. A diagnosis of AIDS is given only if the person is infected with HIV and

- the T-lymphocyte count is low, or
- the person has one of the opportunistic infections listed by the Centers for Disease Control and Prevention.

These infections are rare or harmless in people with normal immunity.

As with any other serious illness, people with AIDS deserve respect, understanding, and support. Rejection and discrimination are traits of immature, hateful, and ignorant people. Education, knowledge, and responsible behaviors are the best ways to minimize fear and discrimination.

HIV TREATMENT Even though several drugs are being tested to treat and slow down the disease process, AIDS has no known cure. At least 30 different approaches to an AIDS vaccine are being explored. The best advice at this point is to take a preventive approach.

Although HIV has no cure, medications are available that allow HIV-infected patients to live longer. The sooner treatment is initiated following infection, the better the chances for delaying the onset of AIDS.

Developing a vaccine to prevent HIV infection or AIDS seems highly unlikely in the next few years. People should not expect a medical breakthrough. Treatment modalities, however, should continue to improve and allow HIV-infected persons and AIDS patients to live longer and more productive lives.

Presently, several AIDS studies are being conducted in the United States. The purpose of AIDS clinical trials is to evaluate experimental drugs and various therapies for people at all stages of HIV infection. As with all HIV testing, calls are completely confidential. Eligibility to participate in an AIDS clinical trial varies, and all applicants are evaluated individually. Those who are interested will receive information on the purpose and location of the trials that are open, eligibility requirements and exclusion criteria, and names and telephone numbers of persons to contact.

PREVENTING SEXUALLY TRANSMITTED DISEASES

Knowing that STDs are life-threatening and life-changing in their consequences, you will want to avoid risk and take precautions to keep yourself from becoming a victim. The one strategy that is 100 percent effective is abstinence. More and more young people are taking this approach to secure a high quality of life. The next-best prevention technique is a mutually monogamous sexual relationship, wherein two uninfected people have a sexual relationship only with each other. A mutually monogamous relationship is effective in preventing STDs, but utilizing this strategy poses some challenges. First you need to know that you and your partner are uninfected,

and second you need to know if your partner is being monogamous or sexually faithful.

In today's society, people often have difficulty knowing when to trust a person. When it comes to sharing information about past and present sexual behavior, most people are dishonest.[7] You may be led to believe you are in a monogamous relationship when your partner actually (a) may be cheating on you and gets infected, (b) ends up having a one-night stand with someone who is infected, (c) got the virus several years before the present relationship and still doesn't know of the infection, (d) may not be honest with you and chooses not to tell you about the infection, or (e) is shooting up drugs and becomes infected. In any of these cases, an STD can be passed on to you.

In addition to the medical consequences of acquiring an STD, negative emotional outcomes result from STDs. When people develop STDs that cannot be cured, their self-esteem and self-respect plummet. They often report a loss of dignity and hope. Depression results as they experience the betrayal of a partner who cheated and lied and as they anticipate having a disease forever and having to tell a future life partner about it.

Because your future and your life are at stake, and because you cannot be completely sure if your partner is infected, you should give serious and careful consideration to postponing sex until you believe you have found a lifetime monogamous relationship. In doing so, you will not have to live with the fear of catching HIV or other STDs or deal with an unplanned pregnancy. Additionally, you won't have to deal with the stress of worrying about either of these issues. Many people postpone sexual activity until they are married. This is the best guarantee against HIV. Married life will provide plenty of time for a fulfilling and rewarding sexual relationship.

Some people would have you believe you are not a "real" man or woman if you don't have sex early in your life. Manhood and womanhood are not proven during sexual intercourse but, instead, through mature, responsible, and healthy choices. Other people may lead you to believe that love doesn't exist without sex. Sex in the early stages of a relationship is not the product of love but is simply the fulfillment of a physical, and often selfish, drive. Then there are those who enjoy bragging about their sexual conquests and mock people who choose to wait. In essence, many of these "conquests" are only fantasies or attempts to gain popularity with peers.

Sexual promiscuity never leads to a trusting, loving, and lasting relationship. Mature people respect others' choices. If someone does not respect your choice to wait, he or she certainly does not deserve your friendship or, for that matter, anything else. Sexual intercourse lasts only a few minutes. The consequences of irresponsible sex, however, may last a lifetime. In some cases, these consequences are fatal.

A loving relationship develops over a long time with mutual respect for each other. There is no greater sex relationship than that between two loving and responsible individuals who mutually trust and admire each other. Contrary to many beliefs, these relationships are possible. They are built upon unselfish attitudes and behaviors.

As you look around, you will find that many believe the same way you do. Seek them out and build your friendships and future around people who respect you for who you are and what you believe. You don't have to compromise your choices or values. In the end you will reap the greater rewards of a fulfilling and lasting relationship, free of AIDS and other STDs. Additionally, you will experience self-respect and enhanced self-esteem.

Also, be prepared for social situations and avoid being in a sexually intimate situation. Look for common interests and become involved in social settings and activities that do not involve time alone in places where sexual involvement is tempting. Communication is important; express your feelings openly: "I'm not ready for sex; I just want to have fun and kissing is fine with me."[8] If your friend does not accept your answer and is not willing to stop the advances, be prepared with a strong response. Statements like "Please stop" or "Don't!" are for the most part ineffective. Use a firm statement such as: "No, I'm not willing to do it" or "I've already thought about this and I'm not going to have sex." If this still does not work, it is effective to label the behavior rape and say: "This is rape and I'm going to call the police."

HOTLINES

Several toll-free hotlines offer more information on anonymous testing, treatment programs, support services, HIV and AIDS, and STDs in general. All information discussed during a phone call to these hotlines is kept strictly confidential.

- National AIDS Hotline: 1-800-342-AIDS (La Linea Nacional de SIDA: 1-800-344-SIDA, for Spanish-speaking people)
- STD Hotline: 1-800-227-8922.
- National Institute on Drug Abuse (NIDA) Information and Treatment Referral: 1-800-622-HELP (1-800-66-AYUDA for Spanish-speaking people) (NIDA also provides information on drug abuse and addictive behavior.)

MYTHS ABOUT AIDS

You've probably heard one or more of these statements, but they're all untrue:

- You can get AIDS by donating blood.
- You can get AIDS through casual contact, such as shaking hands with or hugging an infected person.
- You can catch AIDS if an infected person coughs or sneezes on you.
- You can get AIDS from a mosquito.
- AIDS could spread rapidly through the general population.
- If you're not gay and don't shoot drugs, you're safe.
- Infected women can't transmit AIDS.
- If you don't have symptoms, you're not contagious.
- If you're HIV-positive, you'll know it from the symptoms.
- If you test positive for HIV, you have AIDS.
- Abstinence is the only way to protect yourself against AIDS.

HIV RISK REDUCTION Observing the following precautions can reduce your risk for getting HIV and, subsequently, AIDS:

1. Postpone sex until you and your uninfected partner are prepared to enter into a lifetime monogamous relationship. Magic Johnson stated:

   [I]f I had known what I do now when I was younger, I would have postponed sex as long as I could, and I would have tried to have it the first time with somebody that I knew I wanted to spend the rest of my life with. I certainly want my children to postpone sex. Now the rest of my life may be a lot shorter than I thought it was going to be, and I may not be around to see my son, Andre, grow up and to see what happens to the baby Cookie and I are having in the summer of '92, and, of course, I may not have the long life I want with Cookie.[9]

2. Unless you are in a monogamous relationship and you know your partner is not infected (which you may never know for sure), practice safer sex every single time you have sex. This means you should use a latex condom from start to finish (before there is any sexual contact until after the penis is withdrawn) for each sexual act, including oral sex. Put the condom on as soon as the penis is erect; pinch the condom to allow a little extra space at the tip, but do not let any air get trapped in the condom. Roll it all the way to the base of the penis, and keep it all the way on until the penis is fully withdrawn. When

COMPARING SELECTED SEXUALLY TRANSMITTED DISEASES

Disease	Symptoms	Outlook	Complications	Diagnosis and Treatment
Syphilis	Spirochete infection. Curable in early stages. Transmitted by oral, genital, anal contact. After a decline, case numbers rising again in North America, mainly related to drug use or exchange of sex for drugs.	Painless sore (chancre) appears 3–6 weeks after infection on genitals, mouth, or rectal area; most obvious in men, hardly noticed if vaginal. Heals without scarring. About 4–10 weeks later, second stage: fever, rash, which disappears but may reappear.	If untreated, chronic, occasionally fatal. Third stage appears up to 30 years later with brain and spinal cord damage, blindness, insanity. Untreated, can cause miscarriage and birth defects; infants of infected mother may be born with syphilis (congenital syphilis).	Even if no symptoms, can diagnose by simple blood test; test results usually positive by time chancre (ulcer) appears. Antibiotics, taken as prescribed, a dependable cure in early stages.
Gonorrhea ("clap")	Bacterial infection, transmitted by oral, vaginal, or anal sex. Prevalent in young women, teens. Untreated, can result in pelvic inflammatory disease (PID) and infertility. Up to half of infected people have no symptoms.	Symptoms (if any) within 7 days of contact: painful urination, thick vaginal or penile discharge, bleeding between periods, sore throat (if contracted via oral sex), rectal pain or discharge (if through anal sex).	May lead to tubal scarring, PID, ectopic pregnancy (outside womb; dangerous for mother). Can cause permanent sterility in both sexes. Eye infection and possible blindness in infected newborns.	Diagnosed by smear and lab culture. Antibiotics a reliable cure, but some strains now resistant to standard antibiotics (e.g., penicillin) and require cefixime, ceftriaxone, or other new drugs.
Herpes	Viral infection due to Herpes virus types I or II. Spreads via oral, vaginal, or anal sex or kissing. Can spread silently, via asymptomatic people. Most easily transmitted by direct contact with active sores or genital secretions.	Symptoms within 10 days: slight fever, tingling, shooting pains, swollen lymph glands, then painful blisters, anywhere on genitals—mainly penis, vulva, or anal areas. Subsides without treatment, but can recur. First outbreak usually worst, but sometimes unnoticed.	Virus remains permanently in nerves, stays dormant for months or years. Newborns may get herpes during birth, resulting in central nervous system damage or death. Cesarean delivery may be advised for babies of infected mothers.	Diagnosis from blisters (scraping or culture). Medicine, not a cure, eases symptoms and reduces length of attack and its severity. Herpes support groups helpful in combating psychological problems.
Chlamydia	Bacterial infection, very common, in teens, 60–80 percent without symptoms. Spreads via anal, vaginal, or oral sex with infected partners. Often occurs together with gonorrhea.	Like gonorrhea: painful urination, vaginal or penile discharge, abdominal pain, genital itching. But often mild, unnoticed in carriers, can disappear without treatment.	In women, leading cause of PID, ectopic pregnancy, infertility. In men, can produce urinary tract diseases and prostatitis. Babies of infected mothers prone to eye infections, pneumonia.	Diagnosed by culture or other tests. Antibiotic treatment a reliable cure (if caught early).
Genital Warts	Caused by human papilloma virus (HPV). Highly contagious, spread by intimate bodily contact, especially sexual activity, often accompanies other STDs.	Warts—tiny growths on and around genitals—usually itchy, pinkish, flat, irregularly surfaced, may increase in size. Often undetectable in women in vagina or on cervix, except by physician.	Certain HPV strains linked to cervical cancer in women (and possibly penile cancer in men). Infants born to mothers with HPV may develop warts.	Removal advised—chemically, by freezing, or with lasers. Women should have regular Pap smears to detect HPV infection and early cervical cancer changes.
Hepatitis B	Virus passed on via blood, semen, vaginal secretions, saliva, needles, razors, toothbrushes. Can go from mother to infant at birth. Groups most at risk: those practicing anal sex, those with many partners, injection drug users, babies of infected mothers.	Usually subclinical with few or no symptoms. Possibly flu-like malaise, fever, fatigue typically lasting 6 weeks, perhaps jaundice/skin and eye-white yellowing. May linger in body unnoticed.	60–90 percent of infected children and 10 percent infected as adults become lifelong carriers, at risk of cirrhosis and liver cancer. Unsuspecting carriers can infect others. Fulminant is a rapidly fatal form occurring in 1 per 100 cases.	Detected by blood tests for viral markers. No cure. Effective safe vaccine recommended for all at risk—especially health care workers and those living with or close to known hepatitis B carriers.

Adapted from **Health News**. **Health News** is a bimonthly publication of the University of Toronto Faculty of Medicine. Subscriptions and back issues can be obtained by writing to Health News, 109 Vanderhoof Ave., Suite 205, Toronto, Ontario M4G 2H7 or by calling (416) 696-8818.

CONDOM DO'S AND DON'TS

- Do use condoms during every sexual encounter.
- Do use condoms for vaginal intercourse, anal intercourse, and oral sex.
- Use only latex condoms. Natural membranes have pores through which the virus can travel.
- Do use caution when opening a condom. Teeth, fingernails, or other sharp objects could tear the condom.
- Do put the condom on as soon as the penis is erect, roll it all the way to the base of the penis, and be sure it stays on until the penis is fully withdrawn. Also make sure there is no air in the tip of the condom.
- Do use plenty of water-based lubricant, not oil- or alcohol-based lubricants such as Vaseline or baby oil. These weaken latex and make condoms break more easily.
- All condoms are stamped with a date of manufacture. You should look for a date within 2½ years from this date.
- Don't use a condom more than once.
- Don't continue using a condom if it breaks during sex. Stop and put on a new condom.
- Don't expose condoms to extreme light or temperature. Don't carry condoms in wallets. These conditions may cause a condom to dry out and break.
- Don't stretch or inflate a condom before use.

HOW TO PREVENT STDS

To prevent STDs, practice the following safety measures:

- Plan before you get into a sexual situation. Determine the conditions under which you will allow sex to take place. If you decide to have sex, practice safer sex.
- Discuss STDs with the person you are contemplating having sex with before you do so. Talking about STDs might be awkward, but the short-lived embarrassment of addressing intimate questions can keep you from contracting or spreading disease. If you do not know the person well enough to address this issue, or you are uncertain about the answers, do not have sex with this individual.
- Eliminate your risk of getting an STD by not having sexual contact with anyone or by having contact only with a noninfected partner who has contact only with you. Limit the number of sexual partners you have. Having one partner lowers your chance of infection.
- Unless you're sure your partner is free of an STD, protect yourself by using a latex condom every time you have sexual intercourse. For extra protection, use a spermicide with the condom. Spermicide can kill the bacteria and viruses that cause some STDs.
- Avoid mixing alcohol or other drugs with sexual activities. They could cloud your judgment and lead you to engage in unsafe sexual practices.
- Thoroughly wash immediately after sexual activity. Washing with hot, soapy water will not guarantee safety against STDs, but it can prevent you from spreading certain germs on your fingers and may wash away bacteria and viruses that have not entered the body yet.
- If you suspect your partner is infected with an STD, ask. Also, look for signs of infection, such as sores, redness, inflammations, a rash, growths, warts, or discharge. If you are unsure, abstain.
- Consider abstaining from sexual relations if you have any kind of an illness or disease, even a common cold. Any kind of illness lowers immunity and can make you extra-vulnerable to STDs.
- See a doctor. If you think you might have an STD, go to your doctor right away. Ask your partner to get tested, too, so you won't pass STDs back and forth.

withdrawing the penis from the vagina, hold the condom tight at the base of the penis to prevent leakage. Inspect the condom for tears.

If you ask your partner to use a condom but he or she refuses to do so, say no to sex with that person.

Many experts believe greater protection can be obtained by placing a small amount of the spermicide nonoxynol–9 inside the condom at its tip and then lubricating the outside with additional spermicide. Nonoxynol–9 is used to kill the sperm for birth control purposes. In test tubes, it has been shown to kill some STD germs and HIV. This spermicide, however, should not be used in place of a condom, because it will not offer the same protection as the condom does by itself.

3. Avoid having multiple and anonymous sexual partners. Anyone you have sex with could be infected with an STD.

4. Don't have sexual contact with anyone who does not practice safer sex.

5. Avoid sexual contact with anyone who has had sex with people at risk for STDs, even if they are now practicing safer sex.

6. Be cautious when communicating on the Internet. People who seek sex using the Internet have a greater chance of having STDs.[10]

7. Don't have sex with prostitutes.

8. If you do have sex with someone who might be infected with an STD or whose history is unknown to you, avoid exchange of body fluids.

9. Don't share toothbrushes, razors, or other implements that could become contaminated with blood with anyone who is, or who might be, infected with an STD.

10. Be cautious regarding procedures such as acupuncture, tattooing, and ear piercing, in which needles or other nonsterile instruments may be reused to pierce the skin or mucous membranes. These procedures are safe only if proper sterilization methods or disposable needles are used. Before undergoing the procedure, ask about the precautions.

11. If you are planning to undergo artificial insemination, insist on frozen sperm obtained from a laboratory that tests all donors for infection with HIV. Donors should be tested twice before the lab accepts the sperm—once at the time of donation and again a few months later.

12. If you know you will be having surgery in the near future, and if you are able, consider donating blood for your own use. This will eliminate completely the already-small risk of contracting HIV through a blood transfusion. It also will eliminate the more substantial risk of contracting other blood-borne diseases, such as hepatitis, from a transfusion.

Avoiding risky behaviors that destroy quality of life and life itself are critical components of a healthy lifestyle. Learning the facts so you can make responsible choices can protect you and those around you from life-changing and life-threatening diseases. Preventing sexually transmitted diseases is a key to averting both physical and psychological damage.

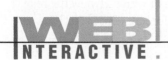
INTERACTIVE.

WEB ACTIVITIES

■ **Planned Parenthood** This excellent site features information on sexual health, including family planning, emergency contraception, and sexually transmitted diseases. It also features a clinic locator to help you find places where you can receive confidential diagnosis and treatment.
http://www.plannedparenthood.org

■ **Assess Your Risk for HIV and Other Sexually Transmitted Diseases** By completing this simple 24-question multiple choice questionnaire, you will obtain an accurate portrayal of your personal risk for acquiring HIV and other types of sexually transmitted diseases.
http://www.thebody.com/surveys/sexsurvey.html

■ **Go Ask Alice** This site offers information on sexuality from the Columbia University Health Education Department and features a series of questions and answers on sexual intercourse, abstinence, kissing, and genital wonderings.
http://www.goaskalice.columbia.edu/Cat6.html

■ **Sexually Transmitted Diseases—A quiz** Take this ten-question multiple choice quiz to test your knowledge of STDs and learn more about their symptoms, prevention, and treatment.
http://www.unspeakable.com/nph-survey.cgi?tag=std

InfoTrac

You can find additional readings related to wellness via InfoTrac College Edition, an on-line library of more than 900 journals and publications. Follow the instructions for accessing InfoTrac that came packaged with your textbook, then search for articles using a key word search.

Suggested Reading Lisa M. Lewis, Richard S. Melton, Paul A. Succop, and Susan L. Rosenthal, "Factors Influencing Condom Use and STD Acquisition Among African American College Women," *Journal of American College Health* 49, no. 1 (July 2000): 19.

1. What percent of the women studied always used condoms? Based on the study's prevalence rate of sexually transmitted diseases, why is this result significant?

2. What is the relationship among the age at first sexual intercourse, the rate of condom use, and the rate of acquiring a sexually transmitted disease? Name two reasons to explain the latter relationship.

3. What factors were most significant in predicting which women were most likely to acquire a sexually transmitted disease?

Web Activity
Sexually Transmitted Disease Risk Profiler
http://www.unspeakable.com/profiler/profiler.html

Sponsor The Naked Truth, a public health outreach project sponsored as an educational service by Pfizer Inc., a manufacturer of pharmaceuticals. Dr. Jonathan Zenilman, an associate professor in the Division of Infectious Diseases at the Johns Hopkins University School of Medicine and an expert on STDs, provides professional oversight for this very informative site. Dr. Zenilman is a former research coordinator at the U.S. Centers for Disease Control and Prevention.

Description This site has two interactive sections. The first, Risk Profiler, can help you determine where your risk of acquiring an STD lies. The second is a 10-question STD Quiz.

Available Activities The site has two interactive sections:

1. Risk Profiler takes your answers to 13 questions about your age, gender, sexual history, and behavior and shows you how these factors play a part in creating your own personal risk profile.
2. STD Quiz gives you an opportunity to test your knowledge of STDs and learn more about their symptoms, prevention, and treatment.

Web Work

1. From the home page, click on the link "Enter the Risk Profiler."
2. Read the disclaimer and then click on the "Risk Profiler" link.

3. Answer each of the 13 multiple choice questions by clicking on the appropriate radio button that corresponds to your answer.
4. When completed, click on the "Generate Report" box at the bottom of the questions.
5. You will receive your evaluation regarding your relative risk of acquiring a sexually transmitted disease and information on how to decrease your risk.
6. Upon completion of the Risk Profiler, click on the "STD Quiz" icon located at the bottom of the page.

Helpful Hints

1. The Risk Profiler provides rough estimates of the relative risks engendered by various factors: sex, age, behavior. It is not predictive. Its ratings should not be used as a model for individual behavior.
2. The most important part of your risk profile is determined by you, through the decisions you make and the actions you take. Risk to any one person depends on more factors than can be addressed within the scope of The Profiler.
3. The STD Quiz is an anonymous service provided to you solely for educational purposes. Absolutely no personal information is collected by this program. You are the only person who can view the results, which are discarded forever when your browser session ends.

For additional Web activities, links, and suggested readings, visit our Health, Fitness, and Wellness Resource Center at http://health.wadsworth.com.

NOTES

1. J. H. Tanne, "US Has Epidemic of Sexually Transmitted Disease," *British Medical Journal* 317 (1998): 1616.
2. L. Kann, "Youth Risk Behavior Surveillance—United States, 1997," *Journal of School Health* 68 (1998): 355–362.
3. Unless otherwise noted, all the statistics regarding STDs are from the Centers for Disease Control and Prevention, Atlanta.
4. Kaiser Family Foundation and American School Health Association, *Sexually Transmitted Diseases In America: How Many Cases and at What Cost?* (December, 1998).
5. G. I. Uwaifo et al., "What's Your Diagnosis?," *Consultant* 38 (1998): 2943–2945.
6. M. L. Kamb et al., "Efficacy of Risk-Reduction Counseling to Prevent Human Immunodeficiency Virus and Sexually Transmitted Diseases," *The Journal of the American Medical Association* 280 (1998): 1161–1165.
7. J. M. Ellen et al., "Individuals' Perceptions About Their Sex Partners' Risk Behavior," *The Journal of Sex Research* 35 (1998): 328–331.
8. R. Franz, "Study Examines Communication and Perceptions of Sexual Risk," *Dermatology Nursing* 10 (1998): 436.
9. J. Mason, *What You Can Do to Avoid AIDS* (New York: Random House, 1991).
10. M. McFarlane et al., "The Internet as Newly Emerging Risk Environment for Sexually Transmitted Diseases," *The Journal of the American Medical Association* 284 (2000): 443–446.

HOW MUCH DO YOU KNOW ABOUT AIDS?

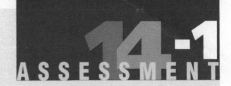

ASSESSMENT

Name: _____   Date: _____   Grade: _____

Instructor: _____   Course: _____   Section: _____

	Yes	No
1. AIDS is the end stage of infection caused by HIV.	☐	☐
2. HIV is a chronic infectious disease that spreads among individuals who engage in risky behaviors, such as unprotected sex or the sharing of hypodermic needles.	☐	☐
3. AIDS now has a cure.	☐	☐
4. Condoms are 100 percent effective in protecting you against HIV infection.	☐	☐
5. If you're sexually active, latex condoms provide the best protection against HIV infection.	☐	☐
6. Each year more and more teens are getting infected with HIV.	☐	☐
7. You can become HIV-infected by donating blood.	☐	☐
8. You can tell by looking at someone if he or she is HIV-infected.	☐	☐
9. The only means to determine whether someone has HIV is through an HIV antibody test.	☐	☐
10. HIV can completely destroy the immune system.	☐	☐
11. The HIV virus may live in the body 10 years or longer before AIDS symptoms develop.	☐	☐
12. People infected with HIV have AIDS.	☐	☐
13. Once infected with HIV, a person never becomes uninfected.	☐	☐
14. HIV infection is preventable.	☐	☐

Adapted from *Test Your Survival Smarts: Self-Quiz on Drugs and AIDS*, National Institute on Drug Abuse, U.S. Department of Health & Human Services; and Werner W. K. Hoeger and Sharon A. Hoeger, *Principles and Labs for Physical Fitness and Wellness*, 3d edition (Englewood, CO: Morton Publishing, 1994), pp. 375–376.

Answers:

1. Yes. "AIDS" is the term used to define the manifestation of opportunistic diseases and cancers that occur as a result of HIV infection (also referred to as "HIV disease").

2. Yes. People do not get HIV because of who they are but, rather, because of what they do. Almost all of the people who get HIV do so because they choose to engage in risky behaviors.

3. No. AIDS has no cure, and none seems likely soon.

4. No. Only abstaining from sex gives you 100 percent protection, but latex condoms are somewhat effective in protecting against HIV infection if they're used correctly.

5. Yes. Proper use, however, is necessary to minimize the risk of infection.

6. Yes. In the early 1990s, the number of infected teens increased by 96 percent over a short span of 2 years. Probably about 20 percent of the AIDS patients today were infected as teenagers.

7. No. A myth regarding HIV is that it can be transmitted by donating blood. People cannot get HIV from giving blood. Health professionals use a new needle every time they draw blood. These needles are used only once and are thrown away and destroyed immediately after each individual has donated blood.

8. No. The symptoms of AIDS often are not noticeable until several years after a person has been infected with HIV.

9. Yes. Nobody can tell if an HIV infection exists unless an HIV antibody test is done. Upon HIV infection, the immune system's line of defense against the virus is to form antibodies that bind to the virus. On the average the body takes 3 months to manufacture enough antibodies to show up positive in an HIV antibody test. Sometimes it may take 6 months or longer.

10. Yes. The virus multiplies, attacks, and destroys white blood cells. These cells are part of the immune system, and their function is to fight off infections and diseases in the body. As the number of white blood cells killed increases, the body's immune system gradually breaks down and may be completely destroyed.

11. Yes. Up to 10 years or more may go by before the person develops AIDS.

12. No. Being HIV-positive does not necessarily mean the person has AIDS. On the average, it takes 7 to 8 years following infection before the individual develops the symptoms that fit the case definition of AIDS. From that point on, the person may live another 2 to 3 years. In essence, from the point of infection, the individual may have the chronic disease 8 to 10 years.

13. Yes. There is no second chance.

14. Yes. The best prevention technique is to abstain from sex until the time comes for a mutually monogamous sexual relationship. In the absence of sharing needles, that one behavior, according to Dr. James Mason, director of the Centers for Disease Control in Atlanta, will almost completely remove the risk of contracting HIV or developing any other sexually transmitted disease.

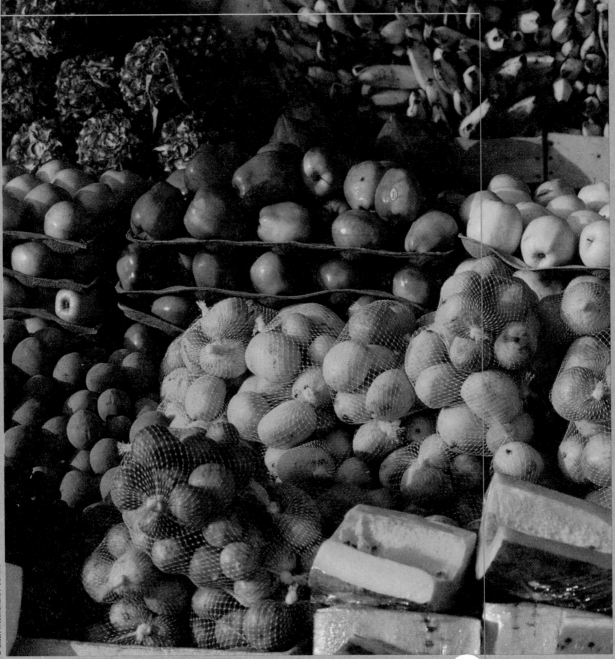

APPENDIX
NUTRITIVE VALUE OF SELECTED FOODS

Food	Amount	Weight (g)	Calories	Protein (g)	Fat (g)	Sat. Fat (g)	Cholesterol (g)	Carbohydrate (g)	Fiber (g)	Calcium (mg)	Iron (mg)	Sodium (mg)	Vit A (IU)	Thiamin (Vit B₁) (mg)	Riboflavin (Vit B₂) (mg)	Niacin (mg)	Vit C (mg)	Folate (mcg)
Apples, fresh, w/peel, lrg	1 ea	150	88	0.3	1	0.1	0	23	4.1	10	0.3	0	80	0.03	0.02	0.1	9	4.2
Applesauce, swtnd, w/o salt, cnd	1 cup	255	194	0.5	0	0.1	0	51	3.1	10	0.9	8	28	0.03	0.07	0.5	4	1.53
Apricots, pitted, fresh, whole	3 ea	114	55	1.6	0	0	0	13	2.7	16	0.6	1	2978	0.03	0.05	0.7	11	9.8
Apricots, w/skin, in heavy syrup, cnd, whole	½ cup	120	100	0.6	0	0	0	26	1.9	11	0.4	5	1476	0.02	0.03	0.5	4	2.04
Asparagus, spears, ckd w/o salt	4 ea	60	14	1.6	0	0	0	3	1	12	0.4	7	323	0.07	0.08	0.6	6	87.6
Avocado, Calif, fresh	½ ea	120	212	2.5	21	3.1	0	8	5.9	13	1.4	14	734	0.13	0.15	2.3	9	78.6
Bagel, plain, 3½" diameter	1 ea	68	187	7.1	1	0.1	0	36	1.6	50	2.4	363	113	0.37	0.21	3.1	0	59.84
Banana, fresh, med	1 ea	140	129	1.4	1	0.3	0	33	3.4	8	0.4	1	36	0.06	0.14	0.8	13	26.74
Bar, granola, hard	1 ea	24	113	2.4	5	0.6	0	15	1.3	15	0.7	71	36	0.06	0.03	0.4	0	5.52
Beans, black, mature, ckd w/o salt	1 cup	172	227	15.2	1	0.2	0	41	15	46	3.6	2	10	0.42	0.1	0.9	0	255.9
Beans, chickpea/garbanzo, mature, ckd	1 cup	164	269	14.5	4	0.4	0	45	12.5	80	4.7	11	44	0.19	0.1	0.9	2	282.0
Beans, frijoles/refried, cnd	½ cup	145	136	8	2	0.7	12	23	7.7	51	2.4	434	0	0.04	0.02	0.5	9	15.95
Beans, green, snap/string, ckd	½ cup	65	23	1.2	0	0	0	5	2.1	30	0.8	2	433	0.05	0.06	0.4	6	21.64
Beans, kidney, red, mature, cnd	1 cup	185	157	9.7	1	0.1	0	29	11.8	44	2.3	631	0	0.19	0.16	0.8	2	93.61
Beans, lima, fordhook, immature, ckd f/fzn w/o salt, drained	½ cup	85	85	5.2	0	0.1	0	16	4.9	19	1.2	45	162	0.06	0.05	0.9	11	18.02
Beans, mung, mature, sprouted, raw	½ cup	52	16	1.6	0	0	0	3	0.9	7	0.5	3	11	0.04	0.06	0.4	7	31.62
Beans, pinto, mature, ckd w/o salt	1 cup	171	234	14	1	0.2	0	44	14.7	82	4.5	3	3	0.32	0.16	0.7	4	294.1
Beef, chuck arm pot roast, brsd, choice, ¼" trim	3 oz	85	296	22.9	22	8.6	84	0	0	8	2.6	50	0	0.06	0.2	2.7	0	7.65
Beef, corned, cnd	3 oz	85	212	23	13	5.3	73	0	0	10	1.8	855	0	0.02	0.12	2.1	0	7.65
Beef, ground, hamburger patty, brld, well done, 16% fat	3 oz	85	225	24.3	13	5.3	84	0	0	8	2.4	70	0	0.06	0.27	5	0	9.35
Beef, ground, hamburger patty, brld, well done, 18% fat	3 oz	85	238	24	15	5.9	86	0	0	10	2.1	76	0	0.05	0.2	5.1	0	9.35
Beef, liver, fried	3 oz	85	184	22.7	7	2.3	410	7	0	9	5.3	90	30689	0.18	3.52	12.3	20	187
Beef, T-bone steak, brld, choice, ¼" trim	3 oz	85	263	19.7	20	7.7	57	0	0	7	2.3	54	0	0.08	0.18	3.4	0	5.95
Beef, top sirloin steak, lean, brld, choice, ¼" trim	3 oz	85	172	25.8	7	2.6	76	0	0.7	9	2.9	56	0	0.11	0.25	3.6	0	8.5
Beer	12 fl-oz	360	148	1.1	0	0	0	13	0.7	18	0.1	18	0	0.02	0.09	1.6	0	21.6
Beer, light	12 fl-oz	354	99	0.7	0	0	0	5	0	18	0.1	11	0	0.03	0.11	1.4	0	14.51
Beets, cnd, drained, diced	½ cup	80	25	0.7	0	0	0	6	1.4	12	1.5	155	9	0.01	0.03	0.1	3	24.16
Biscuits, homemade	1 ea	35	124	2.5	6	1.5	1	16	0.5	82	1	203	29	0.12	0.11	1	0	21.35
Blueberries, fresh, bilberries	½ cup	73	41	0.5	0	0	0	10	2	4	0.1	4	73	0.04	0.04	0.3	9	4.67
Brandy, 86 proof	1 oz	28	70	0	0	0	0	0	0	0	0	0	0	0	0	0	0	0
Bread, banana, prep f/recipe w/veg shortening	1 pce	50	169	2.2	6	1.5	22	28	0.7	9	0.7	99	46	0.09	0.1	0.7	1	5.5
Bread, cracked wheat	1 pce	25	65	2.2	1	0.2	0	12	1.4	11	0.7	134	0	0.09	0.06	0.9	0	15.25
Bread, French	1 pce	35	96	3.1	1	0.2	0	18	1	26	0.9	213	0	0.18	0.12	1.7	0	33.25
Bread, mixed grain	1 pce	26	65	2.6	1	0.2	0	12	1.7	24	0.9	127	0	0.11	0.09	1.1	0	20.8
Bread, pita pocket, white	1 ea	60	165	5.5	1	0.1	0	33	1.3	52	1.6	322	0	0.36	0.2	2.8	0	57
Bread, pumpernickel	1 pce	32	80	2.8	1	0.1	0	15	2.1	22	0.9	215	0	0.1	0.1	1	0	25.6
Bread, rye	1 pce	25	65	2.1	1	0.2	0	12	1.5	18	0.7	165	2	0.11	0.08	1	0	21.5
Bread, white, f/recipe w/2% milk	1 pce	25	71	2	1	0.3	1	12	0.5	14	0.7	90	20	0.1	0.1	0.9	0	22.75
Bread, whole wheat	1 pce	25	62	2.4	1	0.2	0	12	1.7	18	0.8	132	0	0.09	0.05	1	0	12.5
Broccoli, med stalk, 8" long, ckd w/o add salt	1 ea	140	39	4.2	0	0.1	0	7	4.1	64	1.2	36	1943	0.08	0.16	0.8	104	70
Broccoli, spear, raw, 5" long	1 ea	114	32	3.4	0	0.1	0	6	3.4	55	1	31	1758	0.07	0.14	0.7	106	80.94
Brownie, chocolate, w/walnuts, prep f/rec	1 ea	20	93	1.2	6	1.5	15	10	0.4	11	0.4	69	153	0.03	0.04	0.2	0	5.8
Brussels Sprouts, ckd, drained	½ cup	78	30	2	0	0.1	0	7	2	28	0.9	16	561	0.08	0.06	0.5	48	46.8
Buns, hamburger	1 ea	40	114	3.4	2	0.5	0	20	1.1	56	1.3	224	0	0.19	0.12	1.6	0	38

Food	Amount	Weight (g)	Calories	Protein (g)	Fat (g)	Sat. Fat (g)	Cholesterol (g)	Carbohydrate (g)	Fiber (g)	Calcium (mg)	Iron (mg)	Sodium (mg)	Vit A (IU)	Thiamin (Vit B_1) (mg)	Riboflavin (Vit B_2) (mg)	Niacin (mg)	Vit C (mg)	Folate (mcg)
Buns, hot dog/frankfurter	1 ea	40	114	3.4	2	0.5	0	20	1.1	56	1.3	224	0	0.19	0.12	1.6	0	38
Burger/Patty, vegetarian, Gardenburger, original	1 ea	71	130	8	3	1	11	18	5	84	0	290	50	0.11	0.15	1.1	0	10.08
Burger/Patty, vegetarian, soy	1 ea	71	142	14.9	6	1	0	6	3.3	21	1.5	390	0	0.64	0.43	7.1	0	55.38
Butter, salted	1 Tbs	5	36	0	4	2.5	11	0	0	1	0	41	153	0	0	0	0	0.15
Buttermilk, skim, cultured	1 cup	245	99	8.1	2	1.3	9	12	0	285	0.1	257	81	0.08	0.38	0.1	2	12.25
Cabbage, ckd w/o add salt, drained, shredded	½ cup	85	19	0.9	0	0	0	4	2	26	0.1	7	112	0.05	0.05	0.2	17	17
Cabbage, raw, shredded	½ cup	45	11	0.6	0	0	0	2	1	21	0.3	8	60	0.02	0.02	0.1	14	19.35
Cake, angel food, cmrcl prep	1 pce	60	155	3.5	0	0.1	0	35	0.9	84	0.3	449	0	0.06	0.29	0.5	0	21
Cake, carrot, w/cream cheese icing	1 pce	96	419	4.4	25	4.7	52	45	1.2	24	1.2	236	3310	0.13	0.15	1	1	11.52
Cake, chocolate, w/chocolate icing, 1/8th	1 pce	69	253	2.8	11	3.3	29	38	1.9	30	1.5	230	59	0.02	0.09	0.4	0	11.73
Cake, devils food, marshmallow iced	1 pce	99	408	3.5	21	5.8	52	52	1.2	47	1.3	338	0				0	
Cake, pound, w/butter	1 pce	30	116	1.7	6	3.5	66	15	0.1	10	0.4	119	182	0.04	0.07	0.4	0	12.3
Cake, white, w/chocolate icing	1 pce	71	259	1.8	8	3.7	13	46	0.8	55	0.5	219	166	0.05	0.07	0.3	0	2.11
Calamari/Squid, fried, mixed species	1 cup	150	262	26.9	11	2.8	390	12	0	58	1.5	459	52	0.08	0.69	3.9	6	21
Candy Bar, Almond Joy, fun size	1½ oz	42	196	1.8	11	7.3	2	24	2	26	0.6	61	5	0.01	0.06	0.2	0	
Candy Bar, Mars almond	1 ea	50	234	4.1	12	3.6	8	31	1	84	0.6	85	94	0.02	0.16	0.5	0	9.5
Candy Bar, Milky Way, 2.1 oz bar	1 ea	60	254	2.7	10	4.7	8	43	1	78	0.5	144	65	0.02	0.13	0.2	1	6
Candy Bar, Special Dark sweet chocolate	1 ea	41	226	2	13	8.3	0	25	2	11	1	3	14	0.01	0.03	0.2	0	0.82
Candy, caramels, plain/chocolate	1 oz	28	107	1.3	2	1.8	2	22	0.3	39	0	69	9	0	0.05	0.1	0	1.4
Candy, hard, all flvrs	1 oz	28	110	0	0	0	0	27	0	1	0.1	11	0	0	0	0	0	0
Candy, Kisses, milk chocolate	1 oz	28	144	1.9	9	5.2	6	17	1	53	0.4	23	52	0.02	0.08	0.1	0	2.24
Candy, M & M's peanut chocolate	1 oz	28	144	2.7	7	2.9	3	17	1	28	0.3	13	26	0.03	0.05	1	0	9.8
Candy, M & M's plain chocolate	1 oz	28	138	1.2	6	3.7	4	20	0.7	29	0.3	17	57	0.02	0.06	0.1	0	1.68
Candy, milk chocolate, w/almonds	1 oz	28	147	2.5	10	4.8	5	15	1.7	63	0.5	21	21	0.02	0.12	0.2	0	3.36
Carrots, ckd w/o add salt, drained, slices	½ cup	73	33	0.8	0	0	0	8	2.4	23	0.5	48	17924	0.02	0.04	0.4	2	10.15
Carrots, raw, whole, 7½" long	1 ea	81	35	0.8	0	0	0	8	2.4	22	0.4	28	22784	0.08	0.05	0.8	8	11.34
Catsup/Ketchup	1 Tbs	15	16	0.2	0	0	0	4	0.2	3	0.1	178	152	0.01	0.01	0.2	2	2.25
Cauliflower, ckd, drained	½ cup	63	14	1.2	0	0	0	3	1.7	10	0.2	9	11	0.03	0.03	0.3	28	27.72
Celery, raw, med stalk, 8" long	1 ea	40	6	0.3	0	0	0	1	0.7	16	0.2	35	54	0.02	0.02	0.1	3	11.2
Cereal, 100% Bran, rte, dry	½ cup	33	89	4.1	2	0.3	0	24	9.8	23	4.1	229	0	0.79	0.89	10.5	31	23.43
Cereal, All-Bran, rte, dry	¼ cup	21	55	2.6	1	0.1	0	16	6.8	74	3.1	43	525	0.27	0.29	3.5	10	63
Cereal, Alpha-Bits, rte, dry	1 cup	28	110	2.2	1	0.1	0	24	1.2	8	2.7	178	1235	0.36	0.42	4.9	0	98.84
Cereal, bran flakes, rte, dry	¾ cup	30	96	2.8	1	0.1	0	24	5.3	17	8.1	220	750	0.38	0.43	5	0	99.9
Cereal, Cheerios	1 cup	23	84	2.4	1	0.3	0	18	2	42	6.2	218	958	0.29	0.33	3.8	12	76.59
Cereal, Chex, corn, rte, dry	1 cup	28	105	2	0	0.1	0	24	0.5	94	8.4	270	0	0.35	0	4.7	6	93.24
Cereal, Chex, wheat, rte, dry	1 cup	46	159	4.8	1	0.2	0	37	5.1	92	13.8	412	0	0.34	0.06	4.6	6	92
Cereal, corn flakes, rte, dry	1 cup	25	91	1.6	0	0.1	0	22	0.7	1	7.8	266	625	0.32	0.35	4.2	12	88.25
Cereal, Corn Pops, rte, dry	1 cup	28	107	1	0	0.1	0	26	0.4	2	1.7	111	700	0.36	0.39	4.7	14	98.84
Cereal, Cream of Wheat, quick, ckd w/water	1 cup	244	132	3.7	0	0.1	0	27	1.2	51	10.5	142	0	0.24	0	1.5	0	109.8
Cereal, Crispy Rice, rte, dry	¾ cup	22	87	1.4	0	0	0	19	0.3	4	0.6	161	971	0.41	0.46	5.4	12	108.6
Cereal, Frosted Flakes, rte, dry	1 cup	35	135	1.4	0	0.1	0	32	0.7	1	5.1	226	847	0.42	0.49	5.6	17	105
Cereal, Frosted Mini Wheats, rte, dry	1 cup	55	186	5.2	1	0.2	0	45	5.9	20	15.4	2	0	0.38	0.44	5.4	0	110
Cereal, granola, rte, dry	½ cup	57	257	6	10	1.3	0	38	3.6	43	1.8	92	0	0.18	0.06	0.6	0	8.55
Cereal, Grape Nuts, rte, dry	½ cup	57	205	6.2	1	0.2	0	46	5	19	15.9	348	737	0.37	0.42	4.9	0	98.04
Cereal, Honey Bran, rte, dry	½ cup	30	102	2.6	1	0.2	0	25	3.3	14	4.8	173	1323	0.39	0.45	5.3	16	20.1
Cereal, Life, plain, rte, dry	1 cup	44	167	4.3	2	0.3	0	35	2.8	134	12.3	240	16	0.55	0.62	7.3	0	146.9
Cereal, Mueslix, five grain muesli, rte, dry	1 cup	82	289	6.2	5	0.7	0	63	5.6	67	8.9	107	2488	0.75	0.84	9.8	1	196.8
Cereal, Nutri-Grain, wheat, rte, dry	1 oz	28	101	2.4	0	0.1	0	24	1.8	8	0.8	190	0	0.36	0.42	4.9	15	98.84
Cereal, oatmeal, unsalted, ckd w/water	½ cup	120	74	3.1	1	0.2	0	13	2	10	0.8	1	19	0.13	0.02	0.2	0	4.8

Food	Amount	Weight (g)	Calories	Protein (g)	Fat (g)	Sat. Fat (g)	Cholesterol (g)	Carbohydrate (g)	Fiber (g)	Calcium (mg)	Iron (mg)	Sodium (mg)	Vit A (IU)	Thiamin (Vit B_1) (mg)	Riboflavin (Vit B_2) (mg)	Niacin (mg)	Vit C (mg)	Folate (mcg)
Cereal, raisin bran, rte, dry	1 cup	49	155	3.9	1	0.1	0	38	6.4	22	9	299	623	0.31	0.35	4.2	0	82.81
Cereal, Shredded Wheat, sml biscuits, rte, dry	1 cup	19	68	2.1	0	0.1	0	15	1.9	7	0.8	2	0	0.05	0.05	1	0	9.5
Cereal, Smacks, rte, dry	1 cup	37	141	2.4	1	0.4	0	32	1.3	4	2.5	70	1028	0.52	0.59	6.8	21	136.9
Cereal, Special K, rte, dry	1 cup	21	78	4.3	0	0	0	15	0.7	3	5.9	169	508	0.36	0.4	4.7	10	63
Cereal, Total, wheat, rte, dry	1 cup	33	116	3.3	1	0.2	0	26	2.9	284	19.8	218	1375	1.65	1.87	22.1	66	439.8
Cereal, Wheaties, rte, dry	1 cup	29	106	3.1	1	0.2	0	23	2	53	7.8	215	725	0.36	0.41	4.8	14	96.57
Cheese Puffs/Cheetos	1 oz	28	155	2.1	10	1.8	1	15	0.3	16	0.7	294	74	0.07	0.1	0.9	0	33.6
Cheese Spread, low fat, low sod	1 pce	34	61	8.4	2	1.5	12	1	0	233	0.1	2	92	0.01	0.13	0	0	3.06
Cheese, American, proc, shredded	1 oz	28	105	6.2	9	5.5	26	0	0	172	0.1	401	339	0.01	0.1	0	0	2.18
Cheese, blue	1 oz	28	99	6	8	5.2	21	1	0	148	0.1	391	202	0.01	0.11	0.3	0	10.19
Cheese, cheddar, diced	1 oz	28	113	7	9	5.9	29	0	0	202	0.2	174	297	0.01	0.11	0	0	5.1
Cheese, feta	1 oz	28	74	4	6	4.2	25	1	0	138	0.2	313	125	0.04	0.24	0.3	0	8.96
Cheese, monterey jack, shredded	1 oz	28	105	6.9	8	5.3	25	0	0	209	0.2	150	266	0	0.11	0	0	5.1
Cheese, mozzarella, part skm milk, low moist, shredded	1 oz	28	78	7.7	5	3	15	1	0	205	0.1	148	197	0.01	0.1	0	0	2.77
Cheese, parmesan, grated	1 Tbs	5	23	2.1	2	1	4	0	0	69	0	93	35	0	0.02	0	0	0.4
Cheese, ricotta, part skm	1 oz	28	39	3.2	2	1.4	9	1	0	76	0.1	35	121	0.01	0.05	0	0	3.67
Cheese, Swiss, shredded	1 oz	28	105	8	8	5	26	1	0	269	0	73	237	0.01	0.1	0	0	1.79
Cheesecake	1 pce	85	273	4.7	19	8.4	47	22	0.4	43	0.5	176	465	0.02	0.16	0.2	0	15.3
Cherries, sweet, fresh	10 ea	75	54	0.9	1	0.2	0	12	1.7	11	0.3	0	160	0.04	0.04	0.3	5	3.15
Chicken, broiler/fryer, breast, rstd	1 ea	98	193	29.2	8	2.1	82	0	0	14	1	70	91	0.06	0.12	12.5	0	3.92
Chicken, broiler/fryer, dark meat, w/o skin, rstd	3 oz	85	174	23.3	8	2.3	79	0	0	13	1.1	79	61	0.06	0.19	5.6	0	6.8
Chicken, broiler/fryer, drumstick, rstd	1 ea	52	112	14.1	6	1.6	47	0	0	6	0.7	47	52	0.04	0.11	3.1	0	4.16
Chicken, broiler/fryer, meat only, w/o skin, rstd	3 oz	85	162	24.6	6	1.7	76	0	0	13	1	73	45	0.06	0.15	7.8	0	5.1
Chips, corn	1 oz	28	151	1.8	9	1.3	0	16	1.4	36	0.4	176	26	0.01	0.04	0.3	0	5.6
Chips, tortilla, chili & lime	18 pce	28	110	2	2	0	0	22	1.8	60	3.6	200	1	0.02	0.05	0.4	0	2.8
Chips, tortilla, plain	1 oz	28	140	2	7	1.4	0	18	1.8	43	0.4	148	55	0.07	0.1	2.3	2	8.71
Cod, batter fried	3½ oz	100	173	17.4	8	1.6	50	7	0.2	29	0.7	91	30	0.07	0.04	2.2	3	6.6
Cod, stmd/poached	3½ oz	100	102	22.4	1	0.1	46	0	0	9	0.3	80	28	0.02	0.05	0.4	0	0.18
Coffee, brewed	¾ cup	180	4	0.2	0	0	0	1	0	4	0.1	4	0	0	0	0.5	0	
Collards, ckd w/o add salt	½ cup	95	25	2	0	0	0	5	2.7	113	0.4	9	2973	0.04	0.1	0.5	17	88.35
Cone, ice cream, wafer/cake type	1 ea	115	480	9.3	8	1.4	8	91	3.4	29	4.1	164	127	0.29	0.41	5.1	0	117.3
Cookie, chocolate chip, prep w/marg f/rec	2 ea	20	98	1.1	6	1.6	6	12	0.6	8	0.5	72	1	0.04	0.04	0.3	0	6.6
Cookie, chocolate sandwich, creme filled	4 ea	40	189	1.9	8	1.5	0	28	1.3	10	1.6	242		0.03	0.07	0.8	0	17.2
Cookie, fig bar	4 ea	56	195	2.1	4	0.6	0	40	2.6	36	1.6	196	18	0.09	0.12	1	0	15.12
Cookie, oatmeal raisin, prep f/rec	2 ea	26	113	1.7	4	0.8	9	18	0.8	26	0.7	140	167	0.06	0.04	0.3	0	7.8
Cookie, peanut butter, prep f/rec	2 ea	24	114	2.2	6	1.1	7	14	0.5	9	0.5	124	144	0.05	0.05	0.8	0	13.2
Cookie, shortbread, cmrcl, plain	4 ea	32	161	2	8	2	6	21	0.6	11	0.9	146	28	0.11	0.11	1.1	0	18.88
Cookie, vanilla, wafer type, 12–17% fat	10 ea	40	176	2	6	1.5	20	29	0.8	19	1	125	11	0.11	0.13	1.2	0	20
Coriander, raw	¼ cup	4	1	0.1	0	0.1	0	0	0.1	4	0.1	1	111	0	0		7	0.41
Corn, yellow, vac pack, cnd	½ cup	83	66	2	1	0.1	0	16	1.7	4	0.3	226	200	0.03	0.06	1	0	40.92
Cornbread, prep f/dry mix	1 ea	60	188	4.3	6	1.6	37	29	1.4	44	1.1	467	123	0.15	0.16	1.2	0	33
Cornmeal, yellow, degermed, enrich, dry	½ cup	120	439	10.2	2	0.3	0	93	8.9	6	5	4	496	0.86	0.49	6	0	224.4
Cottage Cheese, 2% fat	½ cup	113	101	15.5	2	1.4	9	4	0	77	0.2	459	79	0.03	0.21	0.2	0	14.8
Cottage Cheese, creamed, sml curd	½ cup	105	109	13.1	5	3	16	3	0	63	0.1	425	171	0.02	0.17	0.1	0	12.81
Crab, blue, cnd, drained	1 cup	135	134	27.7	2	0.3	120	0	0	136	1.1	450	7	0.11	0.11	1.8	4	57.38
Crackers, cheese	1 ea	10	50	1	3	0.9	1	6	0.2	15	0.5	100	16	0.06	0.04	0.5	0	8.4
Crackers, graham, plain/honey, 2½ square	2 ea	14	59	1	3	0.2	0	11	0.4	3	0.5	85	0	0.03	0.04	0.6	0	
Crackers, matzoh, plain, svg	1 ea	28	111	2.8	0	0.1	0	23	0.8	4	0.9	1	0	0.11	0.08	1.1	0	32.76

Food	Amount	Weight (g)	Calories	Protein (g)	Fat (g)	Sat. Fat (g)	Cholesterol (g)	Carbohydrate (g)	Fiber (g)	Calcium (mg)	Iron (mg)	Sodium (mg)	Vit A (IU)	Thiamin (Vit B_1) (mg)	Riboflavin (Vit B_2) (mg)	Niacin (mg)	Vit C (mg)	Folate (mcg)
Crackers, rye, wafers	2 ea	14	47	1.3	0	0	0	11	3.2	6	0.8	111	1	0.06	0.04	0.2	0	6.3
Crackers, saltine	1 ea	11	48	1	1	0.3	0	8	0.3	13	0.6	143	0	0.06	0.05	0.6	0	13.64
Crackers, standard, reg, snack type, round	1 ea	3	15	0.2	1	0.1	0	2	0	4	0.1	25	0	0.01	0.01	0.1	0	2.31
Crackers, triscuit	1 ea	5	24	0.5	1	0.2	0	3	0.5	1	0.2	26	0	0.01	0.01	0.1	0	0.36
Crackers, wheat	1 ea	2	9	0.2	0	0.1	0	1	0.1	1	0.1	16	0	0	0.06	0	0	3.7
Cream Cheese	1 oz	28	98	2.1	10	6.2	31	1	0	22	0.3	83	400	0.01	0.02	0	0	0.34
Cream, light	1 Tbs	15	29	0.4	3	1.8	10	1	0	14	0	6	95	0	0.02	0	0	0.56
Cream, whipping, heavy	1 Tbs	15	52	0.3	6	3.5	21	0	0	10	0	6	221	0	0.02	0	0	0.56
Croissant, butter	1 ea	57	231	4.7	12	6.6	38	26	1.5	21	1.2	424	424	0.22	0.14	1.2	0	35.34
Cucumber, w/o skin, raw, sliced	½ cup	60	7	0.3	0	0.2	0	2	0.4	8	0.1	1	44	0.01	0.01	0.1	2	8.4
Dates, fresh, whole	10 ea	83	228	1.6	0		0	61	6.2	27	1	2	42	0.07	0.08	1.8	0	10.46
Dinner, chicken, cacciatore, w/noodles, low cal, fzn	1 ea	308	311	22.5	10	2.4	59	33	3.4	29	3.2	934	732	0.28	0.4	8	26	32.22
Doughnut, cake	1 ea	47	198	2.3	11	1.7	17	23	0.7	21	0.9	257	27	0.1	0.11	0.9	0	22.09
Doughnut, raised, glazed	1 ea	60	242	3.8	14	3.5	4	27	0.7	26	1.2	205	8	0.22	0.13	1.7	0	25.8
Egg Substitute, Egg Beaters, new	¼ cup	61	30	6	0	0	0	1	0	20	1.1	125	300	0	0.85	0	0	32.0
Egg Whites, raw	1 ea	33	16	3.5	0	0	0	0	0	2	0.6	54	0	0	0.15	0	0	0.99
Egg Yolks, raw, lrg	1 ea	17	61	2.8	5	1.6	218	0	0	23	0.6	7	331	0.03	0.11	0	0	24.82
Eggs, hard ckd/bld, lrg	1 ea	50	78	6.3	5	1.6	212	0	0	25	0.6	62	280	0.03	0.26	0.1	0	22
Eggs, scrambled, plain, lrg	1 ea	64	106	7.1	8	2.4	225	1	0	45	0.8	179	436	0.03	0.28	0.1	0	19.2
Eggs, whole, fried	1 ea	46	92	6.2	7	1.9	211	1	0	25	0.7	162	394	0.03	0.24	0	0	17.48
Entree, lasagna, w/meat, prep f/rec	1 pce	220	352	20.7	14	7.2	52	36	2.5	243	2.8	351	902	0.21	0.3	3.8	13	17.82
Entree, macaroni & cheese, prep f/rec w/margarine	½ cup	100	215	8.4	11	4.4	21	20	0.6	181	0.9	543	430	0.1	0.2	0.9	0	5.15
Entree, meatloaf, beef	1 pce	111	232	20.2	14	5.6	107	5	0.2	37	2.1	185	148	0.06	0.28	3.3	1	14.28
Entree, quiche, lorraine	1 pce	242	724	20.5	56	25.9	304	34	1	318	2.6	303	1323	0.36	0.67	2.8	1	26.48
Entree, spaghetti, w/meatballs, prep f/rec	1 cup	248	332	18.6	12	3.3	74	39	7.7	124	3.7	1009	1587	0.25	0.3	4	22	9.99
Entree, spaghetti, w/tomato sauce & cheese, prep f/rec	1 cup	250	260	8.8	9	2	8	37	2.5	80	2.2	955	1075	0.25	0.17	2.2	12	8
Figs, dried, unckd	1 ea	21	54	0.6	0	0	0	14	2.5	30	0.5	2	28	0.01	0.02	0.1	0	1.57
Fish Sticks/Portions, heated f/fzn, 4x1x.5	2 ea	56	152	8.8	7	1.8	63	13	0	11	0.4	326	59	0.07	0.1	1.2	0	10.19
Flour, all purpose, white, bleached, enrich	1 cup	125	455	12.9	1	0.2	0	95	3.4	19	5.8	2	0	0.98	0.62	7.4	0	192.5
Flour, whole wheat	1 cup	120	407	16.4	2	0.4	0	87	14.6	41	4.7	6	0	0.54	0.26	7.6	0	52.8
Frankfurter/Hot Dog, beef & pork, 10 pack	1 ea	57	182	6.4	17	6.1	28	1	0	6	0.7	638	0	0.11	0.07	1.5	0	2.28
Frankfurter/Hot Dog, beef, 8 pack	1 ea	57	180	6.8	16	6.9	35	1	0	11	0.8	585	0	0.03	0.06	1.4	0	2.28
Frankfurter/Hot Dog, turkey	1 ea	45	102	6.4	8	2.7	48	1	0	48	0.8	642	0	0.02	0.08	1.9	0	3.6
Frozen Yogurt, vanilla/strawberry, nonfat, sml scoop	4 oz	113	112	5.6	0	0.1	2	22	1.7	196	0.1	75	7	0.05	0.23	0.1	1	11.99
Fruit Cocktail, in heavy syrup, cnd	1 cup	245	179	1	0	0	0	46	2.5	15	0.7	15	502	0.04	0.05	0.9	5	6.37
Fruit Cocktail, in juice	1 cup	248	114	1.1	0	0	0	29	2.5	20	0.5	10	756	0.03	0.04	1	7	6.2
Fruit Punch, prep f/pwd	1 cup	240	89	0	0	0	0	23	0	38	0.1	34	51	0	0	0	28	0.24
Fudge, chocolate, prep f/rec	1 oz	28	107	0.5	2	1.4	4	22	0.2	12	0.1	17	53	0	0.02	0	0	0.56
Grapefruit, pink, fresh, 3¾" diameter	½ ea	123	37	0.7	0	0.1	0	9	1.7	14	0.1	0	319	0.04	0.02	0.2	47	15.01
Grapes, tokay/empress/red flame, fresh	10 ea	50	36	0.3	0	0.1	0	9	0.5	6	0.1	1	36	0.05	0.03	0.2	5	1.95
Haddock, fillet, brd, fried	3 oz	85	184	17.1	9	1.9	65	7	0	53	1.5	145	69	0.08	0.09	3.7	0	11.6
Halibut, Greenland, fillet, bkd/brld	3 oz	85	203	15.7	15	2.6	50	0	0	3	0.7	88	51	0.06	0.09	1.6	0	0.85
Honey, strained, extracted	1 Tbs	21	64	0.1	0	0	0	17	0	1	0.1	1	0	0	0.01	0	0	0.42
Hot Cocoa/Choc, prep f/rec w/whole milk	1 cup	250	192	9.8	6	3.6	20	29	2	315	1.1	128	515	0.1	0.44	0.4	2	15
Hummus/Hummos, raw	1 cup	246	421	12.1	21	3.1	0	50	12.5	123	3.9	600	62	0.23	0.13	1	19	146.1
Instant Breakfast, prep f/dry mix w/nonfat milk	1 cup	282	216	15.7	1	0.7	9	36	0.2	407	4.8	268	2343	0.4	0.42	5.5	31	118.2

Food	Amount	Weight (g)	Calories	Protein (g)	Fat (g)	Sat. Fat (g)	Cholesterol (g)	Carbohydrate (g)	Fiber (g)	Calcium (mg)	Iron (mg)	Sodium (mg)	Vit A (IU)	Thiamin (Vit B₁) (mg)	Riboflavin (Vit B₂) (mg)	Niacin (mg)	Vit C (mg)	Folate (mcg)
Instant Breakfast, prep f/dry mix w/whole milk	1 cup	281	280	15.4	9	5.4	38	36	0.2	396	4.9	262	2151	0.41	0.47	5.5	31	117.7
Jam/Preserves, pkt	1 ea	14	39	0.1	0	0	0	10	0.2	3	0.1	4	2	0	0	0	1	4.62
Jelly	1 Tbs	18	51	0	0	0	0	13	0.2	1	0	5	3	0	0	0	0	0.18
Juice, apple, unswtnd, cnd/btld	½ cup	124	58	0.1	0	0	0	14	0.1	9	0.5	4	1	0.03	0.02	0.1	1	0.12
Juice, cranberry cocktail	1 cup	253	144	0	0	0	0	36	0.3	8	0.4	5	10	0.02	0.02	0.1	90	0.51
Juice, grape, unswtnd, btld/cnd	½ cup	127	77	0.7	0	0	0	19	0.1	11	0.3	4	10	0.03	0.05	0.3	0	3.3
Juice, grapefruit, unswtnd, cnd	½ cup	124	47	0.6	0	0	0	11	0.1	9	0.2	1	9	0.05	0.02	0.3	36	12.9
Juice, grapefruit, unswtnd, prep f/fzn conc	1 cup	247	101	1.4	0	0	0	24	0.2	20	0.3	2	22	0.1	0.05	0.5	83	8.89
Juice, lemon, fresh	1 Tbs	15	4	0.1	0	0	0	1	0.1	1	0	0	3	0	0	0	7	1.94
Juice, orange, prep f/fzn	½ cup	125	56	0.9	0	0	0	13	0.2	11	0.1	1	98	0.1	0.02	0.3	49	54.75
Juice, prune, w/o pulp	½ cup	88	60	0.7	0	0	0	14	0.5	2	0.9	4	54	0.1			3	
Juice, tomato, w/salt, cnd	1 cup	244	41	1.9	0	0	0	10	1	22	1.4	881	1357	0.11	0.08	1.6	45	48.56
Kale, ckd w/o add salt, drained	½ cup	55	15	1	0	0	0	3	1.1	40	0.5	13	4070	0.03	0.04	0.3	23	7.32
Kiwifruit/Chinese Gooseberries, fresh, med	1 ea	76	46	0.8	0	0	0	11	2.6	20	0.3	4	133	0.02	0.04	0.4	74	28.88
Lamb, leg, whole, lean, rstd, choice, ¼" trim	3 oz	85	162	24.1	7	2.3	76	0	0	7	1.8	58	0	0.09	0.25	5.4	0	19.55
Lamb, loin chop, lean, brld, choice, ¼" trim	3 oz	84	181	25.2	8	2.9	80	0	0	16	1.7	71	0	0.09	0.24	5.8	0	20.16
Lemonade, white, fzn conc	12 oz	340	615	1	1	0.1	0	160	1.4	24	2.4	14	323	0.09	0.33	0.3	60	34
Lentils, sprouts, stir fried	1 cup	124	125	10.9	1	0.1	0	26	4.8	17	3.8	12	51	0.27	0.11	1.5	16	83.08
Lentils, unsalted, ckd	1 cup	200	232	18	1	0.1	0	40	15.8	38	6.7	4	16	0.34	0.15	2.1	3	361.6
Lettuce, butterhead, Boston/bibb, leaf, raw	2 pce	15	2	0.2	0	0	0	1	0.2	5	0.6	1	146	0.01	0.01	0.3	13	11
Lettuce, romaine, raw, chpd	1 cup	55	8	0.9	0	0	0	1	0.9	20	0.6	4	1430	0.06	0.06	0.3	13	74.64
Lobster, northern, stmd	1 cup	145	142	29.7	1	0.2	104	2	0	88	0.6	551	126	0.01	0.1	1.6	0	16.1
Lunchmeat Spread, liverwurst, cnd	1 oz	28	87	3.6	7	2.5	33	2	0.5	0	2.3	193	3818				1	
Lunchmeat, bologna, beef & pork	1 pce	28	88	3.3	8	3	15	1	0	3	0.4	285	0	0.05	0.04	0.7	0	1.4
Lunchmeat, bologna, turkey	2 pce	57	113	7.8	9	2.9	56	1	0	48	0.9	500	0	0.03	0.09	2	0	3.99
Lunchmeat, roast beef, deli style, pouch	3 oz	85	96	17.2	3	1.1	41	1	0	5	1.6	860	0				0	
Lunchmeat, turkey breast, rstd, fat free	1 pce	28	24	4.2	0	0.1	9	1	0	3	0.3	334	0				0	
Mayonnaise, imit, low cal	1 Tbs	15	35	0.1	3	0.5	4	2	0	0	0	75	0				0	
Mayonnaise, soybean oil, w/salt	1 tsp	5	36	0.1	4	0.6	3	0	0	1	0	28	14				0	0.38
Melon, cantaloupe/musk, med 5" diameter	¼ ea	239	84	2.1	1	0.2	0	20	1.9	26	0.5	22	7705	0.09	0.05	1.4	101	40.63
Melon, honeydew, fresh, wedge, 1/8 melon	1 pce	129	45	0.6	0	0	0	12	0.8	8	0.1	13	52	0.1	0.02	0.8	32	7.74
Milk Shake, chocolate, fast food	10 fl-oz	340	432	11.6	13	7.9	44	70	2.7	384	1.1	330	316	0.2	0.83	0.5	2	11.9
Milk, evaporated, whole, w/add vit A, cnd	½ cup	126	169	8.6	10	5.8	37	13	0	329	0.2	133	500	0.06	0.4	0.2	2	9.95
Milk, low fat, 1%, w/add vit A	1 cup	244	102	8	3	1.6	10	12	0	300	0.1	123	500	0.1	0.41	0.2	2	12.44
Milk, low fat, 2%, chocolate	1 cup	250	179	8	5	3.1	17	26	1.2	284	0.6	150	500	0.09	0.41	0.3	2	12
Milk, low fat, 2%, w/add vit A	1 cup	244	121	8.1	5	2.9	18	12	0	297	0.1	122	500	0.1	0.4	0.2	2	12.44
Milk, nonfat/skim, w/add vit A	1 cup	245	86	8.4	0	0.3	4	12	0	302	0.1	126	500	0.09	0.34	0.2	2	12.74
Milk, whole, 3.3%	1 cup	244	150	8	8	5.1	33	11	0	291	0.1	120	307	0.09	0.4	0.2	2	12.2
Milkshake, strawberry, fast food	10 fl-oz	340	384	11.6	10	5.9	37	64	1.4	384	0.4	282	408	0.15	0.66	0.6	3	10.2
Mixed Vegetables, cnd, drained	1 cup	182	86	4.7	1	0.1	0	17	5.5	49	1.9	271	21198	0.08	0.09	1.1	9	42.95
Muffin, English, plain	1 ea	57	134	4.4	1	0.1	0	26	1.5	99	1.4	264	0	0.25	0.16	2.2	0	46.17
Muffin, English, plain, tstd	1 ea	52	133	4.4	1	0.1	0	26	1.5	98	1.4	262	0	0.2	0.14	2	0	38.48
Muffin, wheat bran, prep f/rec w/whole milk	1 ea	45	130	3.2	6	1.2	16	19	3.2	84	1.9	265	363	0.15	0.2	1.8	4	23.4
Mushrooms, raw, pces/slices	1 cup	35	9	1	0	0	0	1	0.4	2	0.4	1	0	0.03	0.15	1.4	1	4.2
Mustard Greens, ckd w/o add salt, drained	½ cup	70	10	1.6	0	0	0	1	1.4	52	0.5	11	2122	0.03	0.04	0.3	18	51.38
Nuts, almonds, dried, unblanched, whole	¼ cup	36	208	7.7	18	1.4	0	7	4.2	89	1.5	0	4	0.09	0.29	1.4	0	10.44
Nuts, Brazil, dried, shelled, 32 kernels	1 oz	28	184	4	19	4.5	0	4	1.5	49	1	1	0	0.28	0.03	0.5	0	1.12
Nuts, cashews, dry rstd, salted	1 cup	137	786	21	63	12.5	0	45	4.1	62	8.2	877	0	0.27	0.27	1.9	0	94.8
Nuts, coconut, unswtnd, dried	½ cup	65	429	4.5	42	37.2	0	16	10.6	17	2.2	24	0	0.04	0.06	0.4	1	5.85

Food	Amount	Weight (g)	Calories	Protein (g)	Fat (g)	Sat. Fat (g)	Cholesterol (g)	Carbohydrate (g)	Fiber (g)	Calcium (mg)	Iron (mg)	Sodium (mg)	Vit A (IU)	Thiamin (Vit B₁) (mg)	Riboflavin (Vit B₂) (mg)	Niacin (mg)	Vit C (mg)	Folate (mcg)
Nuts, peanuts, oil rstd, unsalted, chpd	1 oz	28	163	7.4	14	1.9	0	5	1.9	25	0.5	2		0.07	0.03	4	0	35.2
Nuts, pecans, dried, halves	1 oz	28	193	2.6	20	1.7	0	4	2.7	20	0.7	0	22	0.18	0.04	0.3	0	6.16
Nuts, walnuts, black, dried, chpd	1 oz	28	170	6.8	16	1	0	3	1.4	16	0.9	0	83	0.06	0.03	0.2	1	18.34
Oil, canola	1 cup	218	1927	0	218	15.5	0	0	0	0	0	0	0	0	0	0	0	0
Oil, corn	1 Tbs	15	133	0	15	1.9	0	0	0	0	0	0	0	0	0	0	0	0
Oil, olive	1 Tbs	15	133	0	15	2	0	0	0	0	0	0	0	0	0	0	0	0
Oil, peanut	1 cup	216	1909	0	216	36.5	0	0	0	0	0.1	0	0	0	0	0	0	0
Oil, safflower, greater than 70% linoleic	1 Tbs	15	133	0	15	0.9	0	0	0	0	0.1	0	0	0	0	0	0	0
Oil, soybean	1 tsp	5	44	0	5	0.7	0	0	0	0	0	0	0	0	0	0	0	0
Okra, bindi, ckd w/o add salt f/raw, drained, pods	8 ea	85	27	1.6	0	0	0	6	2.1	54	0.4	4	489	0.11	0.05	0.7	14	38.85
Olives, w/o pits, ripe, lrg, cnd	10 ea	44	51	0.4	5	0.6	0	3	1.4	39	1.5	384	177	0	0	0	0	0
Olives, w/o pits, ripe, sml, cnd	10 ea	32	37	0.3	3	0.5	0	2	1	28	1.1	279	129	0	0	0	0	0
Onions, yellow, ckd w/o add salt, drained, chpd	½ cup	105	46	1.4	0	0	0	11	1.5	23	0.3	3	0	0.04	0.02	0.2	5	15.75
Oranges, fresh, med	1 ea	180	85	1.7	0	0	0	21	4.3	72	0.2	0	369	0.16	0.07	0.5	96	54.54
Oysters, eastern, brd, fried, med	1 ea	45	89	3.9	6	1.4	36	5	0.1	28	3.1	188	136	0.07	0.09	0.7	4	13.95
Oysters, eastern, raw, wild	½ cup	120	82	8.5	3	0.9	64	5	0	54	8	253	120	0.12	0.11	1.7	4	12
Pancake, buckwheat, prep f/incomplete dry mix, 4"	1 ea	27	56	2.1	2	0.5	18	8	0.6	69	0.5	144	63	0.05	0.07	0.4	0	4.59
Pancake, plain, homemade, 4"	1 ea	73	166	4.7	7	1.5	43	21	1.1	160	1.3	320	143	0.15	0.21	1.1	0	27.74
Papaya, fresh, med	½ ea	227	89	1.4	0	0.1	0	22	4.1	54	0.2	7	645	0.06	0.07	0.8	140	86.26
Pasta, egg noodles, enrich, ckd	½ cup	80	106	3.8	1	0.2	26	20	0.9	10	1.3	6	16	0.15	0.07	1.2	0	51.2
Pasta, macaroni noodles, enrich, ckd	½ cup	70	99	3.3	0	0.1	0	20	0.9	5	1	1	0	0.14	0.07	1.2	0	49
Pasta, spaghetti noodles, enrich, salted, ckd	1 cup	140	197	6.7	1	0.1	0	40	2.4	10	2	140	0	0.29	0.14	2.3	0	98
Pasta, spaghetti noodles, whole wheat, ckd	1 cup	125	155	6.7	1	0.1	0	33	5.6	19	1.3	4	0	0.14	0.06	0.9	0	6.25
Pastry, cinnamon danish	1 ea	110	443	7.7	25	6.2	23	49	1.4	78	2.2	408	13	0.33	0.29	3.2	0	68.2
Peaches, fresh, sliced	½ cup	85	37	0.6	0	0	0	9	1.7	4	0.1	0	455	0.01	0.03	0.8	6	2.89
Peaches, in heavy syrup, cnd	½ cup	96	71	0.4	0	0	0	19	1.7	3	0.3	6	319	0.01	0.02	0.6	3	3.07
Peaches, in juice, cnd, whole	½ tsp	77	34	0.5	0	0	0	9	1	5	0.2	3	293	0.01	0.01	0.4	3	2.62
Peanut Butter, smooth, salted	1 Tbs	32	190	8.1	16	3.3	0	6	1.9	12	0.6	149	0	0.03	0.03	4.3	0	23.68
Pears, bartlett, fresh, med	1 ea	180	106	0.7	1	0	0	27	4.3	20	0.4	0	36	0.04	0.07	0.2	7	13.14
Pears, in heavy syrup, cnd, halves	½ ea	103	76	0.2	0	0	0	20	1.6	5	0.2	5	0	0.01	0.02	0.2	0	1.24
Pears, in juice, cnd, halves	½ ea	77	38	0.3	0	0	0	10	1.2	9	0.2	3	5	0.01	0.01	0.2	1	0.92
Peas, cnd, drained	½ cup	85	59	3.8	0	0.1	0	11	3.5	17	0.8	214	653	0.1	0.07	0.6	8	37.65
Peas, green, ckd f/fzn w/o add salt, drained	½ cup	80	62	4.1	0	0.1	0	11	4.4	19	1.3	70	534	0.23	0.08	1.2	8	46.88
Peppers, bell, green, sweet, raw, med	1 ea	200	54	1.8	0	0.1	0	13	3.6	18	0.9	4	1264	0.13	0.06	1	179	44
Peppers, bell, red, sweet, raw, sml	1 ea	74	20	0.7	0	0	0	5	1.5	7	0.3	2	4218	0.05	0.02	0.4	141	16.28
Peppers, bell, yellow, sweet, raw, lrg	1 ea	186	50	1.9	0	0.1	0	12	1.7	12	0.9	4	443	0.05	0.05	1.7	341	48.36
Pickles, dill	1 ea	135	24	0.8	0	0.1	0	6	1.6	12	0.7	1731	444	0.02	0.04	0.1	3	1.35
Pickles, sweet, med	1 ea	35	41	0.1	0	0	0	11	0.4	1	0.2	329	44	0	0.01	0.1	0	0.35
Pie, apple, bkd f/fzn, 1/6th of 8"	1 pce	118	280	2.2	13	4.5	0	40	1.9	13	0.5	314	146	0.03	0.03	0.3	4	25.96
Pie, bluberry, prep f/rec, 1/8th of 9"	1 pce	158	387	4.3	19	4.6	0	53	2.2	11	1.9	292	66	0.24	0.21	1.9	1	36.34
Pie, cherry, prep f/rec, 1/8th of 9"	1 pce	118	319	3.3	14	3.5	0	45	1.8	12	2.2	225	483	0.17	0.15	1.5	1	31.86
Pie, chocolate cream, rts, 1/6th of 8"	1 pce	175	532	4.5	34	8.7	9	59	3.5	63	1.9	238	0	0.06	0.19	1.2	0	22.75
Pie, lemon meringue, rts, 1/6th of 8"	1 pce	140	375	2.1	12	2.5	63	66	1.7	78	0.9	204	245	0.09	0.29	0.9	4	18.2
Pie, pecan, rts, 1/6th of 8"	1 pce	138	552	5.5	26	4.9	44	79	4.8	23	1.4	585	242	0.13	0.17	0.3	2	37.26
Pie, pumpkin, rts, 1/6th of 8"	1 pce	114	239	4.4	11	2	23	31	3.1	68	0.9	321	3915	0.06	0.17	0.2	1	22.8
Pineapple, chunks, fresh	½ cup	78	38	0.3	0	0	0	10	0.9	5	0.3	1	18	0.07	0.03	0.3	12	8.27
Pineapple, in heavy syrup, cnd, tidbits	½ cup	128	100	0.4	0	0	0	26	1	18	0.5	1	18	0.12	0.03	0.4	9	5.89
Pineapple, in juice, cnd	½ cup	125	75	0.5	0	0	0	20	1	18	0.3	1	48	0.12	0.02	0.4	12	6
Popcorn, air popped, plain	1 cup	6	23	0.7	0	0	0	5	0.9	1	0.2	0	12	0.01	0.02	0.1	0	1.38

Food	Amount	Weight (g)	Calories	Protein (g)	Fat (g)	Sat. Fat (g)	Cholesterol (g)	Carbohydrate (g)	Fiber (g)	Calcium (mg)	Iron (mg)	Sodium (mg)	Vit A (IU)	Thiamin (Vit B_1) (mg)	Riboflavin (Vit B_2) (mg)	Niacin (mg)	Vit C (mg)	Folate (mcg)
Popcorn, ckd in oil, salted	1 cup	11	55	1	3	0.5	0	6	1.1	1	0.3	97	17	0.01	0.01	0.2	0	1.87
Pork, bacon/cracklings, brld/pan fried/rstd	2 pce	15	86	4.6	7	2.6	13	0	0	2	0.2	239	0	0.1	0.04	1.1	0	0.75
Pork, cured, ham, reg, 11% fat, rstd	3 oz	85	151	19.2	8	2.7	50	0	0	7	1.1	1275	0	0.62	0.28	5.2	0	2.55
Pork, ham, whole, rstd	3 oz	85	232	22.8	15	5.5	80	0	0	12	0.9	51	8	0.54	0.27	3.9	0	8.5
Pork, ribs, spareribs, brsd	3 oz	85	337	24.7	26	9.5	103	0	0	40	1.6	79	8	0.35	0.32	4.7	0	3.4
Potato Chips, plain, salted	10 pce	20	107	1.4	7	2.2	0	11	0.9	5	0.3	119	0	0.03	0.04	0.8	6	9
Potatoes, au gratin, prep w/milk & butter f/dry mix	1 cup	245	228	5.6	10	6.3	37	31	2.2	203	0.8	1076	522	0.05	0.2	2.3	8	16.17
Potatoes, baked, w/flesh & skin, long	1 ea	202	220	4.6	0	0.1	0	51	4.8	20	2.7	16	0	0.22	0.07	3.3	26	22.22
Potatoes, hash browns, prep f/fzn	½ cup	78	170	2.5	9	3.5	0	22	1.6	12	1.2	27	0	0.09	0.02	1.9	5	5.07
Potatoes, mashed, w/whole milk	½ cup	105	81	2	1	0.3	2	18	2.1	27	0.3	318	20	0.09	0.04	1.2	7	8.61
Potatoes, sweet, flesh, bkd in skin, med, peeled	1 ea	146	150	2.5	0	0	0	35	4.4	41	0.7	15	31860	0.11	0.19	0.9	36	33
Pretzels, hard, salted, twisted	1 oz	28	107	2.5	1	0.2	0	22	0.9	10	1.2	480	0	0.13	0.17	1.5	0	47.88
Prunes, dried	5 ea	61	146	1.6	0	0	0	38	4.3	31	1.5	2	1212	0.05	0.1	1.2	2	2.26
Pudding, choc, rte, 5oz can	5 oz	142	189	3.8	6	1	4	32	1.4	128	0.7	183	51	0.04	0.22	0.5	2	4.26
Pudding, tapioca, 5oz can	5 oz	142	169	2.8	5	0.9	1	28	0.1	119	0.3	226	30	0.03	0.14	0.4	3	4.26
Pudding, vanilla, 5oz can	5 oz	142	185	3.3	5	0.8	10	31	0.1	125	0.2	192	2	0.03	0.2	0.4	1	0
Raisins, seedless, unpacked	1 oz	28	84	0.9	0	0	0	22	1.1	14	0.6	3	2	0.04	0.02	0.2	1	0.92
Raspberries, fresh	1 cup	123	60	1.1	1	0	0	14	8.3	27	0.7	3	160	0.04	0.11	1.1	31	31.98
Raspberries, swtnd, fzn	1 cup	250	258	1.8	0	0	0	62	5.5	38	1.6	3	160	0.05	0.11	0.8	1	27.5
Rice, brown, ckd	½ cup	96	107	2.5	1	0.2	0	22	1.7	10	0.4	5	0	0.09	0.02	1.5	0	3.84
Rice, white, reg, ckd	½ cup	103	134	2.8	0	0.1	0	29	0.4	10	1.2	1	0	0.17	0.01	1.5	0	59.74
Rice, wild, ckd	½ cup	100	101	4	0	0	0	21	1.8	3	0.6	3	0	0.05	0.09	1.3	0	26
Rolls, hard, white	1 ea	50	146	4.9	2	0.3	0	26	1.1	48	1.6	272	0	0.24	0.17	2.1	0	47.5
Salad Dressing, blue cheese/roquefort	1 Tbs	15	76	0.7	8	1.5	3	1	0	12	0	164	32	0	0.02	0	0	1.21
Salad Dressing, french	1 Tbs	16	69	0.1	7	1.5	0	3	0	2	0.1	219	208	0	0	0	0	0.67
Salad Dressing, French, low cal	1 Tbs	15	20	0.1	1	0.1	0	3	0	2	0.1	118	195	0	0	0	0	0
Salad Dressing, Italian	1 Tbs	15	70	0.1	7	1.1	0	2	0	2	0	118	12	0	0	0	0	0.73
Salad Dressing, Italian, diet, 2cal/tsp, cmrcl	1 Tbs	15	16	0	1	0.2	1	1	0	0	0	118	0	0	0	0	0	0
Salad Dressing, ranch	1 Tbs	15	80	0	8	1.2	5	2	0	0	0.1	105	0	0	0	0	0	0
Salad Dressing, thousand island	1 Tbs	15	57	0.1	5	0.9	4	2	0	2	0.1	105	48	0	0	0	0	0.94
Salad Dressing, thousand island, low cal	1 Tbs	15	24	0.1	2	0.2	2	2	0.2	2	0.1	150	48	0	0	0	0	0.84
Salad, chicken, w/celery	½ cup	78	268	10.6	25	3.1	48	1	0.2	16	0.6	201	155	0.03	0.07	3.3	1	8.46
Salad, pasta, garden primavera, prep f/dry	¾ cup	142	280	8	12	2.5	2	34	2	80	1.8	730	200	0.15	0.17	2	1	
Salad, potato	½ cup	125	179	3.4	10	1.8	85	14	1.6	24	0.8	661	261	0.1	0.07	1.1	12	8.38
Salad, tuna	1 cup	205	383	32.9	19	3.2	27	19	0	35	2	824	199	0.06	0.14	13.7	5	16.4
Salami, beef & pork, dry	1 oz	28	117	6.4	10	3.4	22	1	0	4	0.4	521	0	0.17	0.08	1.4	0	0.56
Salmon, pink, w/bone, cnd, not drained	3 oz	85	118	16.8	5	1.3	47	0	0	181	0.7	471	47	0.02	0.16	5.6	0	13.09
Salmon, sockeye, fillet, bkd/brld	3 oz	85	184	23.2	9	1.6	74	0	0	6	0.5	56	178	0.18	0.15	5.7	0	4.25
Salsa, homemade, Mexican sauce	1 Tbs	15	3	0.1	0	0	0	1	0.2	1	0.1	1	57	0.01	0	0.1	2	1.74
Sandwich, bacon, lettuce & tomato, on soft white	1 ea	130	323	10.8	18	4.7	22	30	1.7	54	2.1	619	271	0.36	0.2	3.4	12	35.5
Sandwich, egg salad, on soft white	1 ea	111	361	9.1	24	4.2	149	29	1.2	67	2.1	499	239	0.25	0.3	1.9	0	35.39
Sandwich, peanut butter & jam, on soft white, unsalted	1 ea	100	348	11.5	15	3.1	2	46	3	60	2.2	290	2	0.27	0.17	5.3	0	40.04
Sandwich, reuben, grilled	1 ea	237	458	27.6	29	9.8	80	25	2.2	286	4.2	1933	453	0.21	0.34	2.8	13	37.79
Sardines, Atlantic, w/bones, cnd in oil, drained	1 oz	28	58	6.9	3	0.4	40	0	0	107	0.8	141	63	0.02	0.06	1.5	0	3.3
Sauce, soy, made f/soy & wheat	1 Tbs	16	9	1.3	0	0	0	1	0.1	3	0.3	871	0	0.01	0.03	0.4	0	2.56
Sauce, teriyaki, rts	1 Tbs	18	15	1.1	0	0	0	3	0	4	0.3	690	0	0.01	0.01	0.2	0	3.6
Sauerkraut, w/liquid, cnd	½ cup	118	22	1.1	0	0	0	5	2.9	35	1.7	780	21	0.02	0.03	0.2	17	27.97

Food	Amount	Weight (g)	Calories	Protein (g)	Fat (g)	Sat. Fat (g)	Cholesterol (g)	Carbohydrate (g)	Fiber (g)	Calcium (mg)	Iron (mg)	Sodium (mg)	Vit A (IU)	Thiamin (Vit B_1) (mg)	Riboflavin (Vit B_2) (mg)	Niacin (mg)	Vit C (mg)	Folate (mcg)
Sausage, pork, smkd, link	1 ea	68	265	15.1	22	7.7	46	1	0	20	0.8	1020	0	0.48	0.17	3.1	1	3.4
Scallops, brd, fried, mixed species, lrg	2 ea	31	67	5.6	3	0.8	19	3	0	13	0.3	144	23	0.01	0.03	0.5	1	11.47
Seaweed, spirulina, dried	1 cup	119	345	68.4	9	3.2	0	28	4.3	143	33.9	1247	678	2.83	4.37	15.3	12	111.8
Shrimp/Prawns, brd, fried, lrg	7 ea	85	206	18.2	10	1.8	150	10	0.3	57	1.1	292	161	0.11	0.12	2.6	1	6.89
Shrimp/Prawns, ckd, lrg	3 oz	85	84	17.8	1	0.2	166	0	0	33	2.6	190	186	0.03	0.03	2.2	2	2.98
Soda, cola	12 fl-oz	369	151	0	0	0	0	38	0	11	0.1	15	0	0	0	0	0	0
Soda, cola/Coke, diet, w/sacc, low sod	12 fl-oz	340	0	0	0	0	0	0	0	14	0.1	54	0	0	0	0	0	0
Soda, ginger ale	12 fl-oz	366	124	0	0	0	0	32	0	11	0.7	26	0	0	0	0.1	0	0
Soda, lemon lime	12 fl-oz	340	136	0	0	0	0	35	0	7	0.2	37	0	0	0	0	0	0
Soda, root beer	12 fl-oz	340	139	0	0	0	0	36	0	17	0.2	44	0	0	0	0.1	0	0
Sole/Flounder, fillet, bkd/brld	3 oz	85	99	20.5	1	0.3	58	0	0	15	0.3	89	32	0.07	0.1	1.9	0	7.82
Soup, beef bouillon/broth, cnd, prep w/water	1 cup	240	17	2.7	1	0.3	0	0	0	14	0.4	782	0	0	0.05	1.9	0	4.8
Soup, chicken noodle, prep w/water	1 cup	241	75	4	2	0.7	7	9	0.7	17	0.8	1106	711	0.05	0.06	1.4	0	21.69
Soup, clam chowder, Manhattan, prep f/cnd	1 cup	244	112	12.3	2	0	10	11	3.1	41	1.8	725	2297				4	
Soup, clam chowder, New England, prep w/milk	1 cup	248	164	9.5	7	3	22	17	1.5	186	1.5	992	164	0.07	0.24	1	3	9.67
Soup, cream of chicken, prep w/milk	1 cup	248	191	7.5	11	4.6	27	15	0.2	181	0.7	1047	714	0.07	0.26	0.9	1	7.69
Soup, cream of mushroom, prep w/milk	1 cup	245	201	6	13	5.1	20	15	0.5	176	0.6	906	152	0.08	0.28	0.9	2	9.8
Soup, minestrone, prep w/water	1 cup	241	82	4.3	3	0.6	2	11	1	34	0.9	911	2338	0.05	0.04	0.9	1	36.15
Soup, pea, split, w/ham, prep w/water	1 cup	245	184	10	4	1.7	7	27	2.2	22	2.2	975	431	0.14	0.07	1.4	1	2.45
Soup, tomato, prep w/milk	1 cup	248	161	6.1	6	2.9	17	22	2.7	159	1.8	744	848	0.13	0.25	1.5	68	20.83
Soup, tomato, prep w/water	1 cup	245	86	2.1	2	0.4	0	17	0.5	12	1.8	698	691	0.09	0.05	1.4	67	14.7
Soup, vegetable beef, prep w/water	1 cup	245	78	5.6	2	0.9	5	10	0.5	17	1.1	794	1899	0.04	0.05	1	2	10.54
Soup, vegetable, vegetarian, prep w/water	1 cup	250	75	2.2	2	0.3	0	12	0.5	22	1.1	852	3118	0.05	0.05	0.9	2	11
Sour Cream, cultured	1 Tbs	14	30	0.4	3	1.8	6	1	0	16	0	7	111	0	0.02	0	1	1.51
Spinach, ckd w/o add salt, drained	1/2 cup	103	24	3.1	0	0	0	4	2.5	140	3.7	72	8436	0.1	0.24	0.5	10	150.1
Spinach, raw, chpd	1/2 cup	55	12	1.6	0	0	0	2	1.5	54	1.5	43	3693	0.04	0.1	0.4	15	106.9
Spinach, w/o add salt, cnd, drained	1/2 cup	103	24	2.9	1	0.1	0	4	2.5	131	2.4	28	9039	0.02	0.14	0.4	15	100.7
Squash, acorn, ckd	1 cup	245	83	1.6	0	0	0	22	6.4	64	1.4	7	632	0.25	0.02	1.3	16	27.69
Squash, summer, ckd w/o add salt, drained	1/2 cup	90	18	0.8	0	0.1	0	4	1.3	24	0.3	1	258	0.04	0.04	0.5	5	18.09
Squash, winter, avg, bkd, mashed	1/2 cup	103	40	0.9	1	0.1	0	9	2.9	14	0.3	1	3664	0.09	0.02	0.7	10	28.84
Strawberries, fresh, whole	1 cup	149	45	0.9	1	0	0	10	3.4	21	0.6	1	40	0.03	0.1	0.3	84	26.37
Strawberries, slices, swtnd, fzn	1 cup	250	240	1.3	6	1.2	0	65	4.8	28	1.5	8	60	0.04	0.13	1	104	37.25
Stuffing, bread, prep f/dry mix	1/2 cup	70	125	2.2	6	1.2	0	15	2	22	0.8	380	219	0.1	0.07	1	0	70.7
Sugar, beet/cane, brown, packed	1 tsp	5	19	0	0	0	0	5	0	4	0.1	2	0	0	0	0	0	0.05
Sugar, white, granulated	1 tsp	4	15	0	0	0	0	5	0			0	0	0	0	0	0	0
Syrup, maple	1 Tbs	20	52	0	0	0	0	13	0	13	0.2	2	0	0	0	0	0	0
Taco Shells	1 ea	10	47	0.7	2	0.3	0	7	0.7	20	0.2	67	33	0.05	0.03	0.2	0	23.66
Tangerines/Mandarin oranges, fresh, med	1 ea	116	51	0.7	0	0	0	13	2.7	16	0.1	1	1067	0.12	0.03	0.2	36	9.36
Tea, brewed	1/4 cup	180	2	0	0	0	0	1	0	5		5	5				0	
Tempeh	1 cup	166	320	30.8	18	3.7	0	16	9	184	4.5	15	0	0.13	0.59	4.4	0	39.67
Tofu, firm, silken	1/2 cup	126	78	8.7	3	0.5	15	3	0.1	40	1.3	45	0	0.13	0.05	0.3	0	
Tomatoes, red, ripe, raw, med, whole	1 ea	100	21	0.9	0	0	0	5	1.1	5	0.4	9	623	0.06	0.05	0.6	19	15
Tomatoes, red, ripe, cnd w/o add salt, cnd, in liquid	1/2 cup	121	23	1.1	0	0	0	5	1.2	36	0.7	179	720	0.05	0.04	0.9	17	9.44
Tortilla/Taco/Tostada Shell, corn	1 ea	148	693	10.7	33	5	0	92	11.1	237	3.7	543	518	0.34	0.08		0	8.88
Trout, rainbow, fillet, bkd/brld, wild	3 oz	85	128	19.5	5	1.4	59	0	0	73	0.3	48	42	0.13	0.08	4.9	2	16.15
Tuna, light, cnd in oil, drained	3 oz	85	168	24.8	7	1.3	15	0	0	11	1.2	301	66	0.03	0.1	10.5	0	4.51
Tuna, light, cnd in water, drained	3½ oz	99	115	25.3	1	0.2	30	0	0	11	1.5	335	55	0.03	0.07	13.1	0	3.96
Turkey, average, w/o skin, rstd	3 oz	85	144	24.9	4	1.4	65	0	0	21	1.5	60	0	0.05	0.15	4.6	0	5.95

Food	Amount	Weight (g)	Calories	Protein (g)	Fat (g)	Sat. Fat (g)	Cholesterol (g)	Carbohydrate (g)	Fiber (g)	Calcium (mg)	Iron (mg)	Sodium (mg)	Vit A (IU)	Thiamin (Vit B₁) (mg)	Riboflavin (Vit B₂) (mg)	Niacin (mg)	Vit C (mg)	Folate (mcg)
Turnip Greens, ckd f/fzn, drained	½ cup	73	22	2.4	0	0.1	0	4	2.5	111	1.4	11	5822	0.04	0.05	0.3	16	28.76
Turnips, ckd w/add salt, raw, cubes	½ cup	78	16	0.6	0	0	0	4	1.6	17	0.2	39	0	0.02	0.02	0.2	9	7.18
Veal, loin, brsd	3 oz	85	241	25.7	15	5.7	100	0	0	24	0.9	68	0	0.03	0.26	7.7	0	11.9
Veal, loin, lean, brsd	3 oz	85	192	28.5	8	2.2	106	0	0	27	0.9	71	0	0.04	0.29	8.5	0	12.75
Vinegar, balsamic, 60 grain	1 Tbs	15	21	1	1	0.1	0	5	0	2	0.1	3	0	0.08	0.08	0.1	0	
Watermelon, fresh, diced	1 cup	160	51	1	1	0.1	0	11	0.8	13	0.3	3	586	0.13	0.03	0.3	15	3.52
Wheat, bulgur, ckd	1 cup	135	112	4.2	0	0.1	0	25	6.1	14	1.3	7	0	0.08	0.04	1.4	0	24.3
Wheat, flakes, rolled, dry	1 cup	30	97	3.5	0	0	0	21	4.4	18	1	0	0	0.13	0.03	1.4	0	
Wheat, germ, tstd	1 Tbs	6	23	1.7	1	0.1	0	3	0.8	3	0.5	0	0	0.1	0.05	0.3	0	21.12
Whiskey, 90 proof	2 fl-oz	42	110	0	0	0	0	0	0	0	0.3	0	0	0	0	0	0	
Wine, cooler	4 oz	113	56	0.1	0	0	0	7	0	6	0.3	9	1	0.01	0.01	0.1	2	1.34
Wine, red	⅛ cup	30	22	0.1	0	0	0	1	0	2	0.1	2	0	0	0.01	0.1	0	0.6
Wine, Rose	2 fl-oz	59	42	0.1	0	0	0	1	0	5	0.2	3	0	0	0.01	0	0	0.65
Wine, white, med	2 fl-oz	59	40	0.1	0	0	0	0	0	5	0.2	3	0	0	0	0	0	0.12
Yogurt, fruit, low fat, 10g prot/8 oz	1 cup	227	231	9.9	2	1.6	10	43	0	345	0.2	133	104	0.08	0.4	0.2	1	21.11
Yogurt, plain, low fat, 12g prot/8 oz	8 oz	226	143	11.9	4	2.3	14	16	0	413	0.2	159	149	0.1	0.48	0.3	2	25.31
FAST FOOD RESTAURANTS																		
General																		
Burrito, bean	1 ea	166	342	10.8	10	5.3	3	55	6.3	86	3.5	754	254	0.48	0.46	3.1	1	66.4
Chili, con carne	1 cup	255	258	24.8	8	3.5	135	22	4	69	5.2	1015	1675	0.13	1.15	2.5	2	45.9
Cole Slaw, fast food	1 cup	120	178	1.8	13	1.9	6	15	2	41	0.9	324	409	0.05	0.04	0.1	10	46.8
English Muffin, w/butter	1 ea	63	189	4.9	6	2.4	13	30	1.9	103	1.6	386	136	0.25	0.31	2.6	1	56.7
Entree, enchilada, cheese	1 ea	230	451	13.6	27	14.9	62	40		458	1.9	1106	1638	0.12	0.6	2.7	1	92
Hot Dog, plain	1 ea	98	242	10.4	15	5.1	44	18		24	2.3	670	0	0.24	0.27	3.6	0	48.02
Pancake, w/butter & syrup	2 ea	232	520	8.3	14	5.9	58	91	1.2	128	2.6	1104	281	0.39	0.56	3.4	3	51.04
Sandwich, chicken, fillet, plain	1 ea	157	444	20.8	25	7.4	52	33	1.1	52	4	826	86	0.28	0.2	5.9	8	86.35
Sundae, hot fudge, fast food	1 ea	164	295	5.9	9	5.2	21	49	0	215	0.6	189	230	0.07	0.31	1.1	2	9.84
Arby's																		
Salad, chef	1 ea	273	136	12.3	6	2.6	84	9		113	3.3	529	3321	0.26	0.25	4.6	35	
Sandwich, beef, Arby Q	1 ea	190	389	17.6	15	5.4	29	48		70	9.2	1268		0.27	0.39	9.2		
Sandwich, beef, French dip & swiss cheese	1 ea	154	369	24.7	16	7.5	58	31	0.9	232	3.6	1237	0	0.18	0.47	7.4	0	16.35
Sandwich, beef 'n cheddar	1 ea	194	508	24.6	26	7.7	52	43		150	6.1	1166	250	0.42	0.63	9.8	2	
Sandwich, chicken, grilled, deluxe	1 ea	195	365	20	17	3	37	35		59	2.1	764	339	0.27	0.25	11.5	7	
Sandwich, roast beef, regular	1 ea	155	383	22	18	6.9	43	35	1.1	60	4.9	936	0	0.28	0.48	11	1	14
Sauce, Arby's	½ oz	14	15	0.1	0		0	3			0.4	113	203					
Sauce, horsey	½ oz	14	110	0.1	5	1.2	0	3		20		105	100					
Burger King Corporation																		
Cheeseburger, Whopper	1 ea	294	730	33	46	16	115	46	3	250	4.5	1350	750	0.34	0.48	7	9	
Croissant, w/egg, sausage & cheese	1 ea	110	375	13.8	29	10	162	16	0.6	94	2.2	712	250				0	
Hamburger, Whopper	1 ea	270	640	27	39	11	90	45	3	80	4.5	870	500	0.33	0.41	7	9	
Onion Rings, reg svg	3 ea	30	75	1	3	0.5	0	10	1.5	24	0.3	196	0				0	
Potatoes, french fries, salted, med svg	1 ea	116	370	5	20	5	0	43	3	24	1.1	240	0				4	
Sandwich, chicken, broiler	1 ea	168	373	20.3	20	4.1	54	28	1.4	41	3.7	325	203				4	
Sandwich, fish, big	1 ea	255	700	26	41	6	90	56	3	60	2.7	980	100				1	
Dunkin Donuts, Inc.																		
Croissant, plain	1 ea	18	81	1.2	5	1.2	2	8	0	6	0.5	78	0					
Hidden Valley																		
Salad Dressing, ranch, reduced fat & cal	2 Tbs	28	58	0.5	5	0.9	10	2	0	11	0.1	237	15				0	
International Dairy Queen Inc.																		
Frozen Yogurt Cone, med	4 oz	113	148	5.1	1	0.3	3	32	0	143	1	91	0	0.05	0.2		1	
Frozen Yogurt, nonfat	4 oz	113	133	4	0	0		28	0	133	1	93	0				0	

Food	Amount	Weight (g)	Calories	Protein (g)	Fat (g)	Sat. Fat (g)	Cholesterol (g)	Carbohydrate (g)	Fiber (g)	Calcium (mg)	Iron (mg)	Sodium (mg)	Vit A (IU)	Thiamin (Vit B₁) (mg)	Riboflavin (Vit B₂) (mg)	Niacin (mg)	Vit C (mg)	Folate (mcg)
Hamburger, homestyle	1 ea	138	290	17	12	5	45	29	2	60	2.7	630	200	0.29	0.25	3.9	4	
Ice Cream Cone, vanilla, med	1 ea	142	237	5.7	6	4.3	22	38	0	179	1.3	115	538	0.06	0.26	0.1	2	
Milk Shake, vanilla, med	1 ea	397	520	12	14	8	45	88	0.3	400	1.4	230	400	0.12	0.6	0.8	0	
Onion Rings, svg	3 oz	85	241	3.8	12	3	0	29	2.3	15	1.1	135	0	0.09	0.05	0.4	0	
Sandwich, fish, fillet	1 ea	182	396	17.1	17	3.7	48	42	2.1	43	1.9	674	0	0.32	0.24	3.2	0	
Sundae, chocolate, med	1 ea	184	315	6.3	8	4.7	24	56	0	197	1.1	165	590	0.06	0.27	0.3	0	
Jack In the Box																		
Bowl, chicken, teriyaki	1 ea	502	670	26	4	1	15	128	3	100	4.5	1730	6500				24	
Cheeseburger, Jumbo Jack	1 ea	296	640	31	38	15	105	44	2	250	4.5	1340	750	0.44	0.54	2	9	
Hamburger	1 ea	104	250	12	9	3.5	30	30	2	100	3.6	610	0	0.16	0.28	2.1	9	
Hamburger, sourdough, jack	1 ea	233	690	34	45	15	105	37	2	200	4.5	1180	750	0.68	0.5	8.4	9	
Sandwich, chicken, supreme	1 ea	305	830	33	49	7	65	66	3	200	3.6	2140	500	0.49	0.4	13.7	9	
Kentucky Fried Chicken Corporation																		
Chicken, leg, original recipe	1 ea	54	124	11.5	8	1.8	66	4	0	18	0.6	374	89				1	
Chicken, wing, hot & spicy	1 ea	55	210	10	15	4	55	9	1	20	0.7	350	100				1	
Chicken, wing, original recipe	1 ea	45	134	8.6	10	2.4	53	5	0	19	0.3	396	96				1	
Long John Silver's																		
Dinner, fish & fries, batter fried, 2pce	1 ea	261	610	27	37	7.9	60	52		40	1.8	1480		0.38	0.34	8	9	
McDonald's Nutrition Information Center																		
Biscuit, sausage & egg	1 ea	175	541	17.7	36	9.8	241	34	1	98	2.7	1140	295	0.53	0.57	4.1	0	27.73
Cheeseburger	1 ea	115	304	14.3	12	5.7	38	33	1.9	190	2.6	779	285	0.31	0.29	3.6	2	22.37
Cheeseburger, Quarter Pounder	1 ea	186	493	26	28	12.1	88	35	1.9	279	4.2	1200	465	0.37	0.4	6.3	0	31.06
Chicken, nuggets, McNuggets, 4 pce, svg	1 ea	71	190	12	11	2.5	40	10	0	9	0.7	340	0	0.08	0.11	5	1	
Danish, apple	1 ea	115	394	5.5	18	5.5	44	56	1.1	88	1.2	318	548	0.33	0.19	2.2	1	
Frozen Yogurt Cone, vanilla, low fat	3 oz	85	142	3.8	4	2.8	19	22	0	94	0.3	71	283				1	46.53
Hamburger, Big Mac	1 ea	204	529	24.6	29	9.4	80	42	2.8	236	4.2	1011	283	0.46	0.42	5.7	3	25.63
Hamburger, Quarter Pounder	1 ea	160	391	21.4	20	7.4	65	34	1.9	140	4.2	763	93	0.37	0.3	6.3	1	33.47
McMuffin, egg	1 ea	138	294	17.2	12	4.6	238	27	1	203	2.7	802	507	0.5	0.45	3.3	1	18.95
McMuffin, sausage	1 ea	135	434	15.7	28	9.6	54	31	1.2	241	2.2	892	241	0.68	0.33	4.5	0	5.03
Milk Shake, vanilla, sml	1 ea	289	355	10.8	9	5.9	39	58	0	345	0.4	246	296	0.12	0.5	0.3	1	33.16
Muffin, apple bran, fat free	1 ea	75	197	3.9	2	0.3	0	40	2	66	0.9	250	0	0.14	0.14	1.3	1	25.57
Pie, apple	1 ea	307	1037	12	52	14	0	136	4	80	4.3	797	0	0.71	0.43	5.6	96	8.64
Potatoes, french fries, sml svg	1 ea	68	210	3	10	1.5	0	26	2	7	0.4	135	0	0.05	0.02	1.9	2	
Potatoes, hash browns	1 ea	55	135	1	8	1.6	0	15	1	7	0.4	342	0	0.08		0.9		
Salad, garden, shaker	1 ea	149	100	7	6	3	75	4	2	150	1.1	120	1500				15	
Sandwich, Filet O Fish	1 ea	131	378	13.4	21	3.8	42	35	1.7	126	1.5	731	168	0.29	0.21	2.3	0	26.73
Sauce, sweet & sour, pkt 1	1½ oz	32	57	0	0	0	0	13	0	2	0.2	160	343		0.01	0.1	0	
Pizza Hut, Inc.																		
Pizza, cheese, pan, med, 12"	2 pce	205	495	22.8	21	9.5	47	53	3.8	273	2.8	951	1000	0.57	0.61	5.2	7	
Pizza, cheese, thin n' crispy, med, 12"	2 pce	148	350	18.8	14	6.8	43	36	3.4	247	1.8	911	922	0.39	0.39	4.8	5	
Pizza, pepperoni, pan, med, 12"	2 pce	211	539	22.4	24	8.1	49	57	4.1	209	3.3	1157	966	0.63	0.49	5.4	8	0
Pizza, pepperoni, personal pan	1 ea	255	637	27	28	10	55	69	5	250	4	1339	1164	0.56	0.66	8.2	10	
Pizza, supreme, pan, med, 12"	2 pce	255	581	28	28	11.2	56	52	5.6	219	4.3	1428	912	0.8	0.79	6	10	
Subway International																		
Sandwich, chicken breast, rstd, on white, 6"	1 ea	246	332	26	6	1	48	41	3	35	3	967	617				15	
Sandwich, Italian bmt, on white, 6"	1 ea	246	445	21	21	8	56	39	3	44	4	1652	753				15	
Sandwich, meatball, on white, 6"	1 ea	260	404	18	16	6	33	44	3	32	4	1035	712				16	
Sandwich, roast beef, deli style	1 ea	180	245	13	4	1	13	38	2	23	3	638	565				14	
Sandwich, tuna, w/lt mayonnaise, on wheat, 6"	1 ea	253	391	19	15	2	32	46	3	38	3	940	729				15	
Sandwich, turkey, on white, 6"	1 ea	232	273	17	4	1	19	40	3	30	4	1391	601				15	

Food	Amount	Weight (g)	Calories	Protein (g)	Fat (g)	Sat. Fat (g)	Cholesterol (g)	Carbohydrate (g)	Fiber (g)	Calcium (mg)	Iron (mg)	Sodium (mg)	Vit A (IU)	Thiamin (Vit B₁) (mg)	Riboflavin (Vit B₂) (mg)	Niacin (mg)	Vit C (mg)	Folate (mcg)
Taco Bell Inc.																		
Burrito, beef, big supreme	1 ea	298	520	24	23	10	55	54	11	150	2.7	1520	3000				5	
Burrito, seven layer	1 ea	234	438	13.2	19	5.8	21	55	10.7	165	3	1058	1240				5	
Burrito, supreme	1 ea	255	440	17	19	8	35	51	10	150	9	1230	2500	0.4	2.1	2.9	5	
Taco	1 ea	83	192	9.6	11	4.3	27	13	3.2	85	1.1	351	532	0.05	0.15	1.3	0	
Taco, soft	1 ea	92	225	9.2	10	4.1	26	12	3.1	82	1.1	337	511	0.39	0.22	2.7	0	
Wendy's Foods International																		
Cheeseburger, w/bacon, jr	1 ea	170	393	20.5	19	7.5	58	35	1.9	171	3.6	895	390	0.31	0.32	6.6	9	28.85
Chicken, nuggets	6 pce	94	292	13.9	20	3.6	37	14	0	24	0.5	589	0	0.15	0.14	9	1	
Frosty, dairy dessert, med	1 ea	298	440	11	11	7	50	73	0	410	1.4	260	1000	0.14	0.62	0.4	0	22.9
Hamburger, bacon classic, big	1 ea	251	517	30.1	26	10.7	88	41	2.4	206	4.5	1298	622	0.4	1.36	5.3	13	
Salad, caesar, w/o dressing, side	1 ea	130	151	12.4	8	3.4	25	9	2	190	1.6	538	2501				22	
Salad, chicken, grilled, w/o dressing	1 ea	338	195	22.1	8	1.7	46	10	4	188	2.1	676	5872				35	
Salad, garden, deluxe, w/o dressing	1 ea	271	110	6.7	6	1	1	10	3.9	189	1.5	319	5883				35	
Salad, taco, w/o chips	1 ea	510	411	28.7	20	10.5	69	31	8.7	403	4.5	1132	2582	0.29	0.5	3.2	28	88.27
Sandwich, chicken, brd	1 ea	208	433	27.4	16	3.1	54	47	1.8	93	2.7	754	217	0.43	0.32	13.3	13	
Sandwich, chicken, club	1 ea	220	483	30.6	20	4.4	64	48	1.9	95	2.9	957	222				14	
Sandwich, chicken, grilled	1 ea	177	283	22.6	7	1.5	61	34	1.8	84	2.7	698	201				9	
CONVENIENCE FOODS & MEALS																		
El Charrito																		
Entree, enchilada, beef, family size, 6 pack	1 ea	200	353	11.8	17	6.5	33	39	5.2	196	2.4	837	1961				3	
Healthy Choice																		
Dinner, fish, herb baked, fzn	1 ea	273	300	14.1	6	1.3	31	48	4.4	35	0.6	424	2650				0	
Dinner, meatloaf, traditional, fzn	1 ea	340	316	15.3	5	2.5	37	52	6.1	48	2.2	459	745				55	
Entree, burrito, chicken, con queso, fzn	1 ea	216	253	10.1	4	1.8	25	43	4.3	29	1.3	426	1084				4	
Entree, lasagna, roma, fzn	1 ea	284	311	19.3	7	2.2	26	44	4.4	111	2.7	430	371	0.22	0.19	1.5	4	
Entree, spaghetti, bolognese, fzn	1 ea	284	280	14	6	2	30	43	5	40	3.6	470	500				15	
Lean Cuisine																		
Entree, chow mein, chicken, w/rice	1 ea	241	198	12.3	5	0.9	33	26	1.9	19	0.3	482	95	0.14	0.16	4.7	6	
Entree, lasagna, w/meat sauce	1 ea	291	270	19	8	2.5	25	34	5	150	1.8	560	500	0.15	0.25	3	12	
Entree, ravioli, cheese	1 ea	241	250	12	8	3	55	32	4	200	1.1	500	750	0.06	0.25	1.2	6	48
Entree, spaghetti, w/meatballs, fzn	1 ea	290	322	19.4	8	2.2	6	43	4.9	102	2.6	502	0					
The Budget Gourmet																		
Dinner, chicken, teriyaki, 3 dish	1 ea	340	360	20	12		55	44		80	1.4	610	1500	0.15	0.34	6	12	
Dinner, veal, parmigiana, 3 dish	1 ea	340	440	26	20		165	39		30	4.5	1160	5000	0.45	0.6	6	6	
Entree, beef, sirloin tips, w/country gravy	1 ea	334	365	18.8	21		47	25		71	0.4	670	882	0.18	0.2	4.7	3	
Entree, linguini, w/shrimp	1 ea	284	330	15	15		75	33		10	3.6	1250	5000	0.3	0.17	3	2	
The Budget Gourmet-Slim Select																		
Entree, stroganoff, beef	1 ea	238	269	17.3	10		58	28		58	2.6	537	288	0.25	0.33	3.8	9	
Weight Watchers																		
Entree, chow mein, chicken	1 ea	255	200	12	2	0.5	25	34	3	40	0.7	430	1499				36	

This food composition table has been prepared for West-Wadsworth Publishing Company and is copyrighted by ESHA Research in Salem, Oregon—the developer and publisher of the Food Processor®, Genesis® R&D, and the Computer Chef® nutrition software systems. The major sources for the data are from the USDA, supplemented by more than 1200 additional sources of information. Because the list of references is so extensive, it is not provided here, but is available from the publisher.

A

Acquired immunodeficiency syndrome (AIDS) The final stage of HIV infection, characterized by opportunistic infections that are rare or harmless in people with normal immune function.

Action stage Stage of change in which people are actively changing a negative behavior or adopting a new, healthy behavior.

Adaptation energy stores Reserves of physical, mental, and emotional energy that give us the ability to cope with stress.

Addiction An abnormal or disordered relationship with an object, event, or behavior.

Adequate Intakes (AI) The average amount of a nutrient that appears sufficient to maintain a specific criteria; a value used as a guide for nutrient intake when a RDA cannot be determined.

Aerobic capacity The maximal amount of oxygen the human body is able to utilize per minute of physical activity (also see maximal oxygen uptake).

Aerobic exercise Exercise that requires oxygen to produce the necessary energy (ATP) to carry out the activity.

Affirmations Positive statements that help reinforce the positive aspects of personality and experience.

Air displacement Technique to assess body composition by calculating the body volume from the air displaced by an individual sitting inside a small chamber.

Alarm The first stage of the general adaptation syndrome, characterized by the release of stress hormones.

Altruism The act of giving of oneself out of a genuine concern for other people; unselfish devotion to the interests and welfare of others.

Amino acids Building blocks of protein; "amino" means "containing nitrogen."

Anaerobic activity Activity that does not require oxygen to produce the necessary energy (ATP) to carry out the activity.

Anger A feeling of extreme hostility, indignation, or exasperation; rage.

Anorexia nervosa An eating disorder characterized by self-imposed starvation to lose and maintain very low body weight.

Anthropometric measurement techniques Measurement of body girths at different sites.

Antibodies Substances produced by the white blood cells in response to an invading agent.

Antioxidants A compound that protects other compounds from oxidation by being oxidized itself. This process protects valuable cellular substances from being altered or destroyed; in the body it helps prevent damage to cells and body fluids.

Anxiety A state of intense worry that is not grounded in reality.

Aquaphobic Having a fear of water.

Atrophy Decrease in size of a cell.

Autogenics A relaxation technique in which the person is trained, with the aid of specialized equipment, to relax all major muscle groups through a form of self-hypnosis, followed by imagery.

Autoimmune disorder A condition in which the immune system attacks the body.

Autoinoculation Spreading an infection to other parts of one's own body.

B

Ballistic stretching Exercises performed using jerky, rapid, and bouncy movements.

Basal metabolic rate (BMR) The lowest level of oxygen consumption necessary to sustain life.

Behavior modification A process to permanently change destructive or negative behaviors and replace them with positive behaviors.

Behavioral health The role of lifestyle in health.

Benign Noncancerous.

Bereavement The process of "disbonding" from someone who played an important role in one's life and is now gone.

Beta-carotene An orange pigment with antioxidant activity; a vitamin A precursor made by plants.

Binge drinking Imbibing at least five alcoholic beverages in one sitting for men, and four for women.

Bioelectrical impedance Technique to assess body composition by running a weak electrical current through the body.

Biofeedback A relaxation technique that involves measuring and controlling physiological functions.

Blood pressure A measure of the force exerted against the walls of blood vessels by the blood flowing through them.

Bod Pod Commercial name of the equipment used for the air displacement technique.

Body composition The fat and nonfat components of the human body; important in assessing recommended body weight.

Body mass index (BMI) Ratio of weight to height, used to determine thinness and fatness.

Bulimia nervosa An eating disorder characterized by a pattern of binge eating and purging in an attempt to lose and maintain low body weight.

Burnout A state of physical and mental exhaustion in which few resources remain.

C

Calisthenics The exercise of muscles for the purpose of gaining health, strength, and grace of form and movement.

Calories Units used to measure energy; determined from the heat food releases when burned. Calories reflect the extent to which a food's energy can be stored in body fat.

Cancer A group of more than a hundred diseases in which cells grow at an uncontrolled rate, mature in an abnormal way, and invade nearby tissues.

Cancer-prone personality An emotionally nonexpressive person who demonstrates ambivalence and is at increased risk for cancer; sometimes called Type C personality.

Carbohydrates Compounds composed of carbon, oxygen, and hydrogen atoms. Carbohydrates provide about half of all energy needed by muscles and other tissues and is the preferred fuel for the brain and nervous system.

Carcinogens Cancer-causing substances.

Cardiac arrhythmias Irregular heart rhythms.

Cardiac output Amount of blood ejected by the heart in 1 minute.

Cardiorespiratory endurance The ability of the lungs, heart, and blood vessels to deliver adequate amounts of oxygen to the cells to meet the demands of prolonged physical activity.

Cardiovascular diseases The array of conditions that affect the heart and the blood vessels.

Cellulite Term frequently used in reference to fat deposits that "bulge out"; these deposits are enlarged fat cells from excessive accumulation of body fat.

Chancre A painless, redrimmed sore that develops at the site where syphilis bacteria enter the body.

Chlamydia An STD caused by a bacteria that infects the mucous membranes that line the genitals, rectum, anus, mouth, and eyes; the most common STD in the United States.

Cholesterol A waxy substance, technically a steroid alcohol, found only in animal fats and oil; used in making cell membranes, as a building block for some hormones, in the fatty sheath around nerve fibers, and in other necessary substances; necessary for synthesis of sex hormones, adrenal hormones, and vitamin D; cholesterol is obtained from the diet and made in the body.

Chronic diseases Illnesses that linger over time and may get progressively worse.

Chylomicrons Triglyceride-transporting molecules in the blood.

Complete protein A dietary protein containing all nine essential amino acids in the same relative amounts that human beings require.

Complex carbohydrates Polysaccharides composed of straight or branched chains of monosaccharides.

Conflict The stress that results from two opposing and incompatible goals, demands, or needs.

Contemplation stage Stage of change in which people are considering changing behavior in the next 6 months.

Coronary heart disease (CHD) Condition in which the arteries that supply the heart muscle with oxygen and nutrients are narrowed by fatty deposits, such as cholesterol and triglycerides.

Coronary-prone personality A hard-driving, competitive person who is also hostile, angry, suspicious, and at increased risk for heart attack; sometimes referred to as Type A personality.

Crack A particularly dangerous and addictive form of cocaine.

D

Daily Values Reference Values of daily requirements developed by the Food and Drug Administration (FDA) specifically for use on food labels.

Diabetes mellitus A disease in which the body doesn't produce or utilize insulin properly.

Diastolic pressure Pressure exerted by the blood against the walls of the arteries during the relaxation phase (diastole) of the heart.

Dietary fiber The part of the plant that is not digested in the small intestine and that provides the bulk needed to keep the digestive system running smoothly; found in vegetables, fruits, grains, and legumes.

Dietary Reference Intakes (DRI) A set of nutrient values for the dietary nutrient intakes of healthy people; these values are used for planning and assessing diets and include Estimated Average Requirements, Recommended Dietary Allowances, Adequate Intakes, and Tolerable Upper Intake Levels.

Distress Negative stress, usually consisting of too much stress in a short time, chronic stress over a prolonged time, or a combination of stressors.

Duration of exercise How long a person exercises.

Dynamic Strength-training method that uses muscle contractions with movement.

E

Emotional wellness The ability to understand your own feelings, accept your limitations, and achieve emotional stability.

Energy The capacity to do work or produce heat.

Energy-balancing equation A principle holding that as long as caloric input equals caloric output, the person will not gain or lose weight. If caloric intake exceeds output, the person gains weight; when output exceeds input, the person loses weight.

Environmental wellness The capability to live in a clean and safe environment that is not detrimental to health.

Essential amino acids Amino acids that cannot be produced by the body at all or are produced in the body in insufficient amounts to meet its needs; they must be provided by the diet.

Essential fat Minimal amount of body fat needed for normal physiological functions; constitutes about 3 percent of total weight in men and 12 percent in women.

Essential hypertension Persistent high blood pressure, having no known cause.

Estimated Average Requirement (EAR) The amount of a nutrient that will maintain a specific biochemical or physiological function in half of the population.

Eustress Positive, desirable stress.

Exercise Physical activity that requires planned, structured, and repetitive bodily movement done to improve or maintain one or more components of physical fitness.

Exercise ECG An exercise test during which workload is increased gradually (until the subject reaches maximal fatigue) with blood pressure and 12-lead electrocardiographic monitoring throughout the test.

Exhaustion The final stage of the general adaptation syndrome, characterized by depletion of the body's resources and loss of adaptive abilities.

Explanatory style The way people perceive the events in their lives, from an optimistic or a pessimistic perspective.

External locus of control One's prevailing belief that the things that happen are unrelated to one's own behavior.

F

Faith Belief and trust in God, God's promises, or religion.

Fat Lipids in food or in the body that provide the body with a continuous fuel supply, protect it from mechanical shock, and carry fat-soluble vitamins.

Fear A state of escalated worry and apprehension that causes distinct physical and emotional reactions.

Fetal alcohol syndrome A set of mental and physical characteristics in a newborn caused by moderate-to-heavy alcohol drinking during pregnancy.

Fight-or-flight response A series of rapid-fire physical reactions to stress that provides maximum physical readiness to face threats in the environment.

Fighting spirit Determination; the open expression of emotions, whether negative or positive.

Flexibility Ability of a joint to move freely through its full range of motion.

Food Guide Pyramid A food group plan that assigns foods to five major food groups; developed by the U.S. Department of Agriculture.

Forgiveness The ability to release from the mind all past hurts and failures, all sense of guilt and loss.

Free fatty acids (FFA) Fats formed by glycerol and three fatty acids. Also known as "triglycerides."

Freebasing Smoking cocaine that has been separated from its hydrochloric salt by mixing it with a volatile chemical.

Frequency of exercise How often a person engages in an exercise session.

G

General adaptation syndrome A three-stage attempt of the body to react and adapt to stressors that disrupt its normal balance.

Genital warts An STD caused by the human papilloma virus (HPV) and characterized by warts around the genitals or mouth.

Girth measurements Technique to assess body composition by measuring circumferences at specific body sites.

Glucose intolerance A condition characterized by slightly elevated blood glucose levels.

Glycemic index A scale of 1 to 100 that rates the body's speed of absorption of various carbohydrates; 100 is the fastest. Formulated by rating the plasma glucose response of carbohydrate-containing foods with the response produced by the same amount of carbohydrate from a standard source, usually glucose or white bread.

Glycogen A storage form of carbohydrate in the liver and muscle.

Gonorrhea An STD caused by a bacteria that infects the cervix, rectum, urethra, or mouth.

Grief The overwhelming sorrow that follows a loss.

H

Hardiness A set of personality traits marked by commitment, control, and challenge.

Hassles Seemingly minor, irritating, everyday annoyances that increase the level of stress.

HDL cholesterol Cholesterol-transporting molecules in the blood ("good cholesterol").

Health A state of complete well-being and not just the absence of disease or infirmity.

Health locus of control The extent to which a person believes his or her behavior affects their health status.

Healthy life expectancy (HLE) Number of years a person is expected to live in good health. This number is obtained by subtracting ill-health years from the overall life expectancy.

Hepatitis B A form of hepatitis spread through exposure to the contaminated blood or body fluids of an infected person; can cause long-term liver damage.

Herpes genitalis An infection caused by the herpes simplex-2 virus and characterized by blistering sores on the genitals.

Homeostasis A stable sense of physiological balance wherein all of the body's systems are functioning normally.

Homocysteine An amino acid that, when allowed to accumulate in the blood, may lead to plaque formation and blockage of arteries.

Hope To desire and expect optimism; positive anticipation and expectation.

Hopelessness A mental state marked by negative expectations about the future; despairing.

Hostility An ongoing accumulation of anger and irritation; a permanent, deep-seated type of anger that hovers quietly until some trivial incident causes it to erupt.

Human immunodeficiency virus (HIV) The virus that weakens and destroys the immune system and gradually leads to AIDS.

Human papilloma virus (HPV) The virus that causes genital warts; some strains of the virus also have been linked to cervical cancer.

Hydrogenation A chemical process by which hydrogens are added to monounsaturated or polyunsaturated fats to reduce the number of double bonds and make the product more saturated (solid) and more resistant to spoilage.

Hydrostatic weighing Underwater weighing technique to assess body composition; considered one of the most accurate techniques for body composition assessment.

Hypertension Chronically elevated blood pressure.

Hypertrophy An increase in the size of the cell (for example, muscle hypertrophy).

Hypokinetic disease Condition associated with a lack of physical activity (for example, hypertension, coronary heart disease, obesity, and diabetes).

I

Immunity The function that guards the body from invaders, both internal and external.

Incomplete proteins Dietary proteins that do not contain all the essential amino acids in sufficient quantities for human protein synthesis.

Insulin Hormone secreted by the pancreas; essential for proper metabolism of blood glucose (sugar) and maintenance of blood glucose level.

Insulin resistance The inability of the cells to respond appropriately to insulin.

Intensity of exercise In cardiorespiratory exercise, how hard a person has to exercise to improve or maintain fitness.

Internal locus of control One's prevailing belief that events are a consequence of one's own actions and, thus, potentially can be controlled.

Irradiation Sterilizing a food by exposure to energy waves; this process kills microorganisms and insects.

Isokinetic Strength-training method in which the speed of the muscle contraction is kept constant because the equipment (machine) provides an accommodating resistance to match the user's force through the range of motion.

Isometric Strength-training method that uses muscle contractions producing little or no movement, such as pushing or pulling against immovable objects.

J

Jaundice Liver condition in which the skin and whites of the eyes appear yellow.

L

LDL cholesterol Cholesterol-transporting molecules in the blood ("bad cholesterol").

Lean body mass Body weight without body fat.

Life expectancy Number of years a person is expected to live based on the person's birth year.

Lifetime sports Sports that a person can do throughout the lifespan.

Loneliness A condition that occurs when a person's network of social relationships is significantly deficient in either quality or quantity.

Lymphocytes Specialized immune system cells.

M

Maintenance stage Stage of change in which people maintain behavioral change for up to 5 years.

Major minerals Essential mineral nutrients found in the human body in amounts larger than 5 grams; sometimes called "macrominerals."

Malignant Cancerous.

Maximal exercise test Any test that requires the participant's all-out or nearly all-out effort.

Maximal heart rate (MHR) Highest heart rate for a person, primarily related to age.

Maximal oxygen uptake (VO$_{2max}$) The maximum amount of oxygen the body is able to utilize per minute of physical activity, commonly expressed in ml/kg/min. The best indicator of cardiorespiratory or aerobic fitness.

Meditation A mental exercise to help gain control over thoughts.

Mental wellness A state in which your mind is engaged in lively interaction with the world around you.

Metabolism All of the chemical reactions that occur within living cells; energy metabolism includes the reactions by which the body obtains and spends the energy from food.

Metastasis The process that occurs when cancer cells from one growth break off, enter the bloodstream or lymph system, and are carried to a distant part of the body, where they cause another cancerous growth to begin.

Minerals Inorganic elements; some minerals are required in small amounts and are therefore essential.

Mode of exercise Form of exercise.

Moderate-intensity physical activity Physical activity that uses 150 calories of energy per day or 1,000 calories per week.

Monounsaturated fats Fatty acids that lack two hydrogen atoms and have one double bond between carbons; found in olive oil, canola oil, and peanut oil.

Motivation The desire and will to do something.

Muscular endurance The ability of a muscle to exert submaximal force repeatedly over a period of time.

Muscular strength The ability to exert maximum force against resistance.

N

Nicotine A poisonous, addictive component of tobacco, inhaled by smokers or absorbed through the lining of the mouth by people who chew it.

Nutrients Substances obtained from food and used in the body to promote growth, maintenance, and repair. The essential nutrients are those the body cannot make for itself in sufficient quantity to meet physiological need and which, therefore, must be obtained from food.

Nutrition The science of foods, of the nutrients and other substances they contain, and of their actions within the body.

O

Obesity An excessive accumulation of body fat, usually at least 30 percent above recommended body weight.

Occupational wellness The ability to perform one's job skillfully and effectively under conditions that provide personal and team satisfaction and adequately reward each individual.

Oncogenes Pieces of genetic material that serve as markers to predict later mutation and development of certain cancers, probably by encouraging mutation of related cells.

One repetition maximum (1 RM) The maximal amount of resistance (weight) that an individual is able to lift in a single effort.

Open circuit indirect calorimetry (direct gas analysis) The most precise way to determine VO$_{2max}$ using a metabolic cart to measure the amount of oxygen consumed by the body.

Overweight Excess weight according to a given standard, such as height or recommended percent body fat; less than obese.

Oxygen free radicals Substances, formed during metabolism, that attack and damage proteins and lipids, in particular the cell membrane and DNA, leading to the development of diseases such as heart disease, cancer, and emphysema.

P

Pelvic inflammatory disease (PID) A severe infection of the lining of the abdominal cavity, usually caused by bacterial STDs.

Percent body fat Proportional amount of fat in the body based on the person's total weight; includes both essential and storage fat.

Personality The whole of a person's behavioral characteristics.

Physical activity Bodily movement produced by skeletal muscles that requires energy expenditure and produces progressive health benefits.

Physical fitness The general capacity to adapt and respond favorably to physical effort.

Physical wellness Flexibility, endurance, strength, and optimism about your ability to take care of health problems.

Polyunsaturated fats Fatty acids that lack four hydrogen atoms and have two or more double bonds between carbons; found in safflower, sunflower, corn, soybean, and cottonseed oils.

Precancerous A condition in which a benign (noncancerous) condition has the potential to become cancerous.

Precontemplation stage Stage of change in which people are considering changing behavior in the next 6 months.

Preparation stage Stage of change in which people are getting ready to make a change within the next month.

Prodrome The stage of infection when early symptoms erupt, in the case of herpes, a sensation in which the skin starts to itch or tingle; precedes onset of the blisters and sores.

Progressive overload principle Training concept stating that the demands placed on a system (for example, cardiorespiratory or muscular) must be increased systematically and progressively over time to cause physiological adaptation (development or improvement).

Progressive relaxation A method of reducing stress that consists of tensing, then relaxing, small muscle groups.

Proprioceptive neuromuscular facilitation (PNF) Stretching technique in which muscles are stretched out progressively with intermittent isometric contractions.

Protein Compounds composed of amino acids necessary for growth or tissue repair; protein also functions as enzymes, hormones, regulators of fluid and electrolyte balance, acid-base regulators, transporters, and antibodies.

Psychoneuroimmunology (PNI) The scientific investigation of how the brain affects the body's immune cells and how the immune system can be affected by behavior.

Pubic lice Commonly called "crabs," tiny parasites that feed on the small blood vessels of the skin beneath the pubic hair.

R

Rate of perceived exertion (RPE) A perception scale to monitor or interpret the intensity of aerobic exercise.

Recommended body weight Body weight at which there seems to be no harm to human health; healthy weight.

Recommended Dietary Allowances (RDA) The average daily amount of a nutrient considered adequate to meet the known nutrient needs of most healthy people; a goal for dietary intakes by individuals.

Recovery The return to homeostasis after a stressful event.

Reframing Changing the way you look at things.

Relapse To slip or fall back into unhealthy behavior(s) or fail to maintain healthy behaviors.

Relaxation response The body's ability to enter a scientifically defined state of relaxation.

Religion The system of how to know God; system of belief and worship.

Resistance The second stage of the general adaptation syndrome, characterized by meeting the perceived challenge; amount of weight lifted in strength training.

Resting heart rate Heart rate after a person has been sitting quietly for 15–20 minutes.

Resting metabolism The amount of energy (expressed in milliliters of oxygen per minute or in total calories per day) an individual requires during resting conditions to sustain proper body function.

Retroviruses Viruses that invade a cell's genetic structure and are passed on to each succeeding generation of cells as the cells divide.

Reverse cholesterol transport A process in which HDL molecules attract cholesterol and carry it to the liver, where it is changed to bile and eventually excreted in the stool.

S

Saturated fats Fats carrying the maximum possible numbers of hydrogen atoms; usually found in animal products such as butter and lard.

Scabies Tiny mites that burrow under the skin at night; may be spread by nonsexual contact.

Secondhand smoke A mixture of smoke exhaled by smokers and smoke from the burning portion of a cigarette, pipe, or cigar.

Self-esteem A sense of positive self-regard and self-respect.

Set Number of repetitions in strength training (e.g., 1 set of 12 repetitions).

Setpoint Weight control theory proposing that the body has an established weight and strongly attempts to maintain that weight.

Sexually transmitted disease A disease that is passed from one person to another through sexual contact.

Simple carbohydrates Sugars in the form of fruits and milk or honey, sucrose, corn syrup, and fructose.

Skinfold thickness Technique to assess body composition by measuring a double thickness of skin at specific body sites.

Slow-sustained stretching Technique whereby the muscles are lengthened gradually through a joint's complete range of motion and the final position is held for a few seconds.

Social support The network of support that people provide to each other, including instrumental, emotional, informational, and appraisal support.

Social wellness The ability to relate well to others, both within and outside the family unit.

Specificity of training Targeting the specific body system or area the person is attempting to improve (aerobic endurance, anaerobic capacity, strength, flexibility).

Sphygmomanometer An inflatable bladder contained within a cuff and a mercury gravity manometer (or an aneroid manometer) from which the blood pressure is read.

Spiritual health Dimension of health related to a person's moral or religious nature; a relationship with a higher being.

Spiritual wellness The sense that life is meaningful, that life has purpose, and that some power brings all humanity together; the ethics, values, and morals that guide us and give meaning and direction to life.

Spontaneous remission Inexplicable recovery from incurable illness.

Spot reducing Fallacious theory claiming that exercising a specific body part will result in significant fat reduction in that area.

Storage fat Body fat in excess of essential fat; stored in adipose tissue.

Stress An automatic biological response to stressors, or demands made on an individual; the result of any event or condition that requires adaptation.

Stressor Any situation or event that makes us adapt or adjust.

Subluxation Partial dislocation of a joint.

Suppressor genes Pieces of genetic material that are part of a cell's normal protective mechanism against development of cancer.

Synergistic effect A phenomenon in which the effects of using more than one drug simultaneously are different and greater than using any of the drugs alone.

Syphilis An STD caused by a bacteria, occurring in four stages; untreated, it is fatal.

Systolic pressure Pressure exerted by the blood against the walls of the arteries during the forceful contraction (systole) of the heart.

T

Termination/adoption stage Stage of change in which people have eliminated an undesirable behavior or maintained a positive behavior for over 5 years.

THC (tetrahydrocannabinol) The psychoactive ingredient in marijuana.

Tolerable Upper Intake Level (TUIL) The maximum amount of a nutrient that appears safe for most healthy people and beyond which there is an increased risk of adverse effects.

Toxic core Type A personality traits most detrimental to health: anger, cynicism, suspiciousness, and excessive self-involvement.

Trace minerals Essential mineral nutrients found in the human body in amounts less than 5 grams; sometimes called "microminerals."

Triglycerides Fats formed by glycerol and three fatty acids. Also known as "free fatty acids."

Type A personality Sometimes referred to as "hurry sickness," a person who is hard-driving and competitive and also is hostile, angry, and suspicious; sometimes referred to as coronary-prone behavior.

Type B personality A person who is easy-going and generally free of hostility, anger, and suspicion.

Type C personality An emotionally nonexpressive person who demonstrates ambivalence and is at increased risk for cancer; sometimes referred to as cancer-prone personality.

Type D personality A distressed personality characterized by negative emotions, social inhibition, and isolation.

Type I diabetes Insulin-dependent diabetes mellitus (IDDM), a condition in which the pancreas produces little or no insulin. Also known as juvenile diabetes because it is seen primarily in young people.

Type II diabetes Non-insulin-dependent diabetes mellitus (NIDDM), a condition in which insulin is not processed properly. Also known as adult-onset diabetes.

U

Underweight Extremely low body weight.

V

Vegetarians People who omit meat, fish, and poultry from their diets. Lacto-ovo-vegetarians use milk and milk products and eggs as well as plant foods; strict vegetarians eat only plant foods.

Vigorous activity Any activity that requires a MET level equal to or greater than 6 METs (21 ml/kg/min).

Vitamins Organic, essential nutrients required in small amounts to perform specific functions that promote growth, maintenance, or repair; vitamins do not provide energy, but are necessary in energy-yielding reactions.

W

Waist-to-hip ratio A measurement to assess potential risk for disease based on distribution of body fat.

Warm-up Starting a workout slowly.

Weight-regulating mechanism (WRM) A feature of the hypothalamus (an area of the brain) that controls how much the body should weigh.

Wellness Full integration of physical, mental, emotional, social, environmental, occupational, and spiritual well-being into a quality life.

Worry A state in which we dwell on something so much that we become apprehensive.

Y

Yoga An exercise technique involving stretching, used to relieve stress and induce calm.

Yo-yo dieting Constantly losing and gaining weight